Improve International

MANUAL OF SMALL ANIMAL ONCOLOGY

Improve
Veterinary Education

First published 2024

Published by
Improve International Ltd.
Alexandra House, Whittingham Drive
Wroughton, Swindon,
Wiltshire SN4 0QJ
United Kingdom

Tel: +44 (0) 1 793 759 159
https://improveinternational.com/uk/

Important note
Veterinary medicine is an ever-changing science, so the contents of this publication, especially recommendations concerning diagnostic and therapeutic procedures, can only give an account of the knowledge at the time of publication. While utmost care has been taken to ensure that all specifications regarding drug selection and dosage and treatment options are accurate, readers are urged to review the product information sheet and any relevant material supplied by the manufacturer, and, in case of doubt, to consult a specialist. From both an editorial and public interest perspective, the publisher welcomes notification of possible inconsistencies. The ultimate responsibility for any diagnostic or therapeutic application lies with the reader.

A catalogue record for this book is available from the British Library.

ISBN: 978-1-913352-20-2

Illustrator: Elaine Leggett
Photos by the authors unless otherwise indicated.

Any comments regarding this publication will be considered to improve future editions.

Please contact us via email:

info.es@improveinternational.com

Or via our website:

https://www.improveinternational.com

The erratum and other updates will be published on the following website:

https://publication.improveinternational.com

Authors

Judith Bertrán Trepat

DVM, MS, Dipl. ACVS-SA, ACVS Fellow Oncology Surgery
Judith obtained her degree in veterinary medicine from the Autonomous University of Barcelona (UAB). After graduating, she completed an internship in internal medicine and small animal surgery at Washington State University (WSU, United States). After her time at WSU she completed an internship in small animal surgery at Fitzpatrick Referrals (United Kingdom) and received a research fellowship in the same speciality area at Ohio State University (OSU, USA) and returned to the United States. Upon completion of the fellowship, she joined the Small Animal Surgery Residency Program at Ohio State University and completed a Master's project on the biomechanics and kinematics of knee prosthesis in dogs using robotic technology. Her interest in oncology led her to specialise in surgical oncology (ACVs Fellow Surgical Oncology). Her main interests are conservative limb surgery and osteosarcoma, lymph node mapping and metastatic processes, immunotherapy, maxillofacial surgery, wound therapy, minimally invasive surgery and skin reconstruction.

Juan Francisco Borrego

DVM, PhD, Dipl. ACVIM (Oncology)
Juan graduated in veterinary medicine from the Cardenal Herrera-CEU University (Valencia) in 2003. In 2008 he completed an internship in medical oncology and radiotherapy at the Angell Animal Medical Center (Boston, USA). Between 2009 and 2012 Juan completed a residency in medical oncology at the University of Wisconsin-Madison. He became a diplomate of the American College of Internal Medicine specializing in oncology (ACVIM Oncology) in 2012. Juan then became an associate lecturer at the Cardenal Herrera CEU University for a year and spent the following 6 years as associate lecturer at the Catholic University of Valencia San Vicente Mártir. He completed his PhD in veterinary medicine at the Cardenal Herrera CEU University with his thesis titled "New therapies in canine and feline mammary tumours" in collaboration with the laboratory of molecular biology of human cancer medicine. He is co-founder and has been a partner of Auna Especailidades Veterinarias Hospital and head of the oncology service since 2015, and since 2021 has been co-director of Aúna Veterinary Specialists - IVC Evidensia. He has published in both national and international scientific journals and has given talks both nationally and internationally. He has presented more than 70 communications at international conferences related to oncology, as well as being a reviewer for indexed journals. Juan has also contributed to several chapters of the eighth and ninth editions of the Ettinger textbook of internal medicine. He is accredited by the Spanish Association of Small Animal Veterinarians (AVEPA) in oncology and is the coordinator of the practitioner certificate program in oncology (Master Improve). He is a member of several scientific boards including Zoetis, Boehringer, Qbiotics and is conducting clinical studies with various companies such as Royal Canin. Juan is also currently a member of the executive committee of the European Society of Oncology (ESVONC) as its scientific co-director. His main areas of interest are the development and application of new therapies in dogs and cats through clinical studies.

Sofia Carvalho

DVM MVetMed MRCVS Dipl. ACVIM (Oncology), American Specialist in Veterinary Oncology, RCVS recognised Specialist in Veterinary Oncology
Sofia is a board certified oncology specialist by the American College of Veterinary Internal Medicine (ACVIM) and the Royal College of Veterinary Surgeons (Oncology). She completed her residency training in medical oncology at the Royal Veterinary College (RVC) in London in 2016 and obtained her ACVIM (Oncology) diploma in the same year. During her time at the RVC Sofia completed a Master's degree in veterinary medicine and was involved in various research projects, including clinical trials in small animal oncology. Sofia recently completed an integrative oncology and a food therapy course at the Chi University. Sofia has worked at several referral hospitals in the United Kingdom and she currently combines clinical referral work and specialist medical oncology telemedicine.

Mónica Clemente

DVM, PhD, Dipl. ACVIM, Board-Certified Veterinary Oncologist
Mónica obtained her degree in veterinary medicine from the Complutense University of Madrid in 2004 with a distinction. Between 2004 and 2009 she completed her doctoral studies at the same university, where she participated in multiple research projects, as well as teaching in subjects related to veterinary internal medicine, in addition to multiple stays at the Oncology and Clinical Pathology departments at Ohio State University and the University of Florida. After completing her PhD in 2009, she moved to the United States to continue her studies. Between 2009 and 2011 she completed her postdoctoral studies and residency in oncology (ACVIM-Oncology) at the University of Florida Veterinary Hospital, also becoming a diplomate of the American College of Veterinary Internal Medicine, specialising in Oncology (DACVIM Oncology). She has published research in national and international journals and actively collaborates as a speaker at numerous veterinary oncology congresses and Master degree courses in Europe, Asia and Latin America, in addition to being a reviewer and editor

of various indexed scientific journals. She is currently an active member of ACVIM, ESVONC and is part of the scientific committee of AVEPA/GEVONC. In 2012 she set up the first Middle East Oncology Service, and she is currently Director of the Oncology Service at the British Veterinary Centre Veterinary Hospital in Abu Dhabi (United Arab Emirates) and is the only recognised veterinary oncology specialist in the Middle East.

Pachi Clemente

DVM, MS, Dipl. ACVIM Oncology
Francisco graduated in Veterinary Medicine from the University of Extremadura in 1993 and he has since dedicated his career to small animal medicine, with a special interest in oncology. From 2003 to 2012 he combined clinical work with teaching as an associate professor at the Cardenal Herrera CEU University of Valencia, where he was responsible for the Oncology service at the University Hospital. Between 2012 and 2015 he completed a residency in Medical Oncology at the American College of Veterinary Internal Medicine, Ohio State University, where he also completed a master's degree in Comparative and Veterinary Medicine. Since August 2015 he has worked at La Merced OncoVet, a clinic specialised in veterinary oncology in Calpe (Alicante), in addition to collaborating with other veterinary centres.

Keita Kitagawa

DVM, MSc
Keita obtained his Bachelor of Veterinary Science from Rakuno Gakuen University, Hokkaido, Japan in 2013. After 5 years in private practice and at the veterinary oncology service at Gifu University, Japan, he moved to Michigan State University (MSU) to complete the international medical oncology fellowship (2018-2020). Subsequently, he completed a Master's degree in comparative medicine and integrated biology at MSU between 2020 and 2022. When he was given the opportunity to follow his passion for research in veterinary clinical oncology, he happily accepted the position of PhD student at the University of Florida, College of Veterinary Medicine where he is currently based. His research interests include chemotherapeutic toxicity against the gut microbiota, tyrosine kinase inhibitor resistance, the molecular biology of cancer, cancer genetics, and precision medicine in veterinary oncology.

Ana Lara García

DVM, MSc, PhD, PGcert Med Ed, Dipl. ACVIM and ECVIM-CA (Oncology), RCVS and European Recognised Specialist in Veterinary Oncology
Ana graduated in Veterinary Medicine from the University of Las Palmas, Canary Islands (ULPGC), Spain in 1998 and obtained accreditation of her academic degree (DVM) by the American Veterinary Medical Association (AVMA, ECFVG) in 2007. Ana then completed a PhD looking at platelet function in dogs with cancer at ULPGC between 1999-2003. She continued her studies completing a Master's degree in small animal medicine, internship in oncology and residency in haematology and oncology between 2003 and 2007 at The Ohio State University (OSU), Columbus, OH, USA. In 2008 Ana became the first Spanish veterinarian to hold a diploma in oncology from both the American and European Colleges of Veterinary Internal Medicine (ACVIM and ECVIM-CA).After working for a year as a clinical instructor at the University Teaching Hospital she moved to London, UK where she became senior lecturer at the Royal Veterinary College (RVC) in London. She combined teaching with the development of the RVC Oncology Service at the Queen Mother Hospital for Animals, for which she was responsible between 2009 and 2014. She also founded and directed the ACVIM Oncology residency program from 2009 to 2017. Since 2018 she has worked as an oncology consultant at IDEXX UK and in 2021 this work has expanded to IDEXX Spain. She combines consultancy with part time clinical work at AUNA Veterinary Specialists (Valencia, Spain). Ana was a member of the executive committee of the European Society of Veterinary Oncology (ESVONC) for 10 years, holding different roles, including president from 2017 to 2021. She has been a member of the examining committee for the ECVIM-CA Diploma in Oncology and currently is the director of the ECVIM-CA Oncology Residency Program at AUNA Veterinary Specialists (Valencia, Spain). Her main research interests are new anticancer therapies in pets, diagnosis and treatment of lymphoproliferative diseases, quality of life and clinical reasoning in veterinary oncology. She has numerous publications in international scientific journals https://orcid.org/0000-0003-3672-5460 and has presented her research at international scientific meetings. Ana has been an invited speaker at numerous Spanish and European veterinary meetings and enjoys transmitting her passion for oncology through teaching postgraduate courses and continuing education.

Antonio Meléndez

DVM, MSc, PhD, Dipl. ECVCP
Antonio gained his degree and PhD in Veterinary Medicine from the Complutense University of Madrid and the Autonomous University of Barcelona (UAB) respectively. He then completed a rotating internship at the veterinary teaching hospital of the UAB (HCV-UAB) from 2010 to 2011. He completed a master's degree in clinical research from the Faculty of Medicine at the UAB and undertook a residency with the European College of Veterinary Clinical Pathology (ECVCP) at the HCV-UAB, becoming a specialist Diplomate (Dipl. ECVCP)

in 2015. He is accredited by and founded a specialist group in Clinical Pathology with AVEPA and has also spent time visiting departments in the United Kingdom and United States and has authored and participated in various publications and communications both nationally and internationally. After working as Director of the Clinical Pathology Service at Puchol Veterinary Hospital and as Laboratory Director at LABOKLIN Spain in Madrid for several years he founded T-CITO in January 2021, a service specialising in veterinary cytological and haematological diagnosis where he currently works at its headquarters in Barcelona.

Carolina Naranjo

LV, Dipl. ACVP, Dipl. ECVP, PhD
Carolina Naranjo graduated from veterinary school at the Universitat Autònoma de Barcelona (UAB), where she also obtained a PhD in veterinary medicine. She then completed a 1-year fellowship on ocular pathology at the Comparative Ocular Pathology Laboratory of Wisconsin (COPLOW) under the supervision of Dr. Richard Dubielzig. Following this she transitioned into a 3-year residency program in anatomic pathology at the University of Wisconsin. She is a diplomate of both the American and European Colleges of Veterinary Pathology (ACVP and ECVP, respectively). She has been assistant professor at the UAB and Universidad Complutense de Madrid (UCM) and managed a pathology service with a main interest in ocular pathology as a freelance. She joined IDEXX Laboratories in Barcelona in July 2015, with a special interest in ocular and periocular samples. She is co-author of several national and international papers and frequently lectures for clinicians at international venues, including the William Magrane Basic Science Course in Veterinary and Comparative Ophthalmology.

Audrey Petite

DMV, DVDI, Dipl. ECVDI MRCVS, EBVS® European Specialist in Veterinary Diagnostic Imaging, RCVS Recognised Specialist in Veterinary Diagnostic Imaging
Audrey graduated as a veterinarian from the Liège Veterinary School (Belgium) in 1999. After a couple of years in first opinion practice at a small animal clinic she completed a radiology internship. Following this she completed a three-year residency program at the Animal Health Trust (Newmarket, UK). During this period, she obtained the RCVS certificate in Veterinary Radiology in 2003 and the RCVS Diploma in Diagnostic Imaging in 2004. She became an EBVS graduate recognised by the European College of Veterinary Diagnostic Imaging in 2005 and a RCVS Specialist in veterinary diagnostic imaging in 2007. After her residency, she spent three years at a large multidisciplinary referral centre in the UK and then two years at a referral centre with a large oncology caseload. During this time, she developed an interest in CT and MRI, particularly in the fields of neurology and oncology. She especially enjoys all aspects of image-guided biopsy techniques. Audrey is the author and co-author of several scientific manuscripts and book chapters. She is a regular speaker at courses and conferences both in the UK and abroad. Audrey has also developed her own mobile ultrasound service for first opinion practitioners in South East England in 2011 and has been a consultant at Fitzpatrick Referrals since 2014.

Paulo Vilar Saavedra

DVM, MS, Dipl. ACVIM Oncology
Paulo obtained his degree in veterinary medicine from the University of Santiago de Compostela (USC) in 2004. Following this he obtained a Master's degree in clinical science from The Ohio State University in 2008 and completed his postgraduate academic studies with a PhD at the USC. During his specialist clinical training he completed an international oncology fellowship-internship at Michigan State University (MSU) in 2011, followed by a residency in clinical oncology with the American College of Veterinary Internal Medicine (ACVIM) at MSU and Virginia Tech between 2011 and 2014. Paulo's research is focused on thromboelastographic analysis of paraneoplastic haemostatic disorders, molecular biology of cancer, intestinal flora and personalised cancer therapies. From 2014 to 2021 he was associate lecturer and head of the small animal oncology service at the department of clinical science at the faculty of veterinary medicine at Michigan State University and since 2021 has been based at the University of Florida.

Jarno Schmidt

DVM, Dipl. ECVIM-CA (Oncology) MRCVS, EBVS European Specialist in Veterinary Oncology, Fachtierarzt fuer Innere Medizin der Klein-und Heimtiere M.A. (mediation and conflict management)
After graduating from the Faculty of Veterinary Medicine in Hannover (Germany), Jarno completed his PhD looking at tumoural angiogenesis whilst also completing an oncology residency with the ECVIM-CA in the United Kingdom at the VRCC veterinary referral practice. He is currently Director of the Medical Oncology Service at the Hofheim Veterinary Practice (Germany). In addition, he also works part time as a coach, and as a corporate mediator and educator in business and health. Similarly, he teaches conflict management and communication skills in highly emotionally charged professional situations to both veterinarians and non-veterinarians.

Contents

Introduction to Veterinary Oncology
Ana Lara García and Sofía Carvalho
The Aetiology of Cancer . . . 2
Principles of Tumour Biology and General Pathology of Neoplasms . . . 7
Diagnosis in the Cancer Patient . . . 12
Palliative Care in the Pet with Cancer . . . 16
Nutritional Approach to Cancer Patients . . . 22
Bibliography . . . 29
Self-assessment . . . 32

Paraneoplastic Syndromes
Sofia Carvalho
Haematological Paraneoplastic Syndromes . . . 36
Gastrointestinal Paraneoplastic Syndromes . . . 39
Endocine Paraneoplastic Syndromes . . . 40
Neurological Paraneoplastic Syndromes . . . 42
Dermatological Paraneoplastic Syndromes . . . 43
Other Paraneoplastic Syndromes . . . 44
Bibliography . . . 46
Self-assessment . . . 48

Diagnostic Imaging of the Cancer Patient
Audrey Petite
Advantages and Disadvantages of the Different Methods of Diagnostic Imaging . . . 52
Conventional Radiography: Principles and Interpretation of Clinical Cases . . . 53
Ultrasound: Principles and Interpretation of Clinical Cases . . . 60
Computed Tomography: Principles and Interpretation of Clinical Cases . . . 70
Other Advanced Imaging Techniques: Scintigraphy, PET-CT, MRI, and DCE-MRI . . . 79
Bibliography . . . 81
Self-assessment . . . 83

Practical Chemotherapy for Dogs and Cats
Ana Lara García
Tumour Biology and Mechanism of Action of Chemotherapeutic Agents . . . 88
Considerations Regarding the Choice and Dose of Cytotoxic Drugs . . . 90
Chemotherapy Strategies in Veterinary Medicine . . . 91
Guidelines for Chemotherapy . . . 92
Metronomic Therapy in Veterinary Oncology . . . 102
Tyrosine Kinase Inhibitors in Veterinary Oncology . . . 108
Annex: Chemotherapy Protocols . . . 116
Bibliography . . . 118
Self-assessment . . . 120

Diagnosis and Treatment of Lymphoma and Leukaemia in Dogs and Cats
Ana Lara García
Diagnosis of Lymphoma in Dogs and Cats . . . 126
Practical Considerations of Multicentric and Non-multicentric Canine Lymphoma . . . 130
Canine Lymphoid Leukaemia . . . 134
Plasma Cell Tumours and Multiple Myeloma . . . 137
Solitary or Extramedullary Plasma Cell Tumours . . . 140
Canine Cutaneous Plasmacytosis . . . 140
Bibliography . . . 141
Self-assessment . . . 143

Mast Cell Tumours, Skin Neoplasms, Soft-tissue Sarcomas, and Feline Injection Site Sarcoma
Mónica Clemente
Canine Mast Cell Tumours . . . 148
Feline Mast Cell Tumours . . . 161
Skin Neoplasms in Dogs and Cats . . . 164
Soft-tissue Sarcomas . . . 179
Feline Injection Site Sarcoma . . . 184
Bibliography . . . 189
Self-assessment . . . 196

Neoplasms of the Nervous System: Diagnosis, Treatment, and Prognosis
Mónica Clemente
Brain Tumours . . . 205
Spinal Tumours . . . 211
Tumours of Cranial, Paraspinal and Peripheral Nerves . . . 214
Bibliography . . . 215
Self-assessment . . . 217

Fundamentals of Radiation Oncology: Principles and Practices
Mónica Clemente
The History of Radiation . . . 222
Biological Basis . . . 223
Bibliography . . . 235
Self-assessment . . . 237

Ocular Neoplasms
Carolina Naranjo Freixa
Neoplasms of the Eyelid . . . 242
Neoplasms of the Eyelid Margins . . . 244
Conjunctival and Nictitating Membrane Neoplasms . . . 246
Corneal Neoplasms . . . 250
Uveal Neoplasms . . . 251
Retina and Optic Nerve Tumours . . . 261
Orbital Tumours . . . 262
Bibliography . . . 266
Self-assessment . . . 268

Gastrointestinal Neoplasms in Cats and Dogs
Pachi Clemente Vicario
Tumours of the Oral Cavity 274
Gastrointestinal Lymphoma 278
Gastric Carcinoma 279
Hepatic Tumours 280
Intestinal Carcinoma 281
Gastrointestinal Stromal Tumours 282
Perianal Tumours: Anal Sac Adenocarcinoma 282
Bibliography 284
Self-assessment 288

Tumours of the Musculoskeletal System
Pachi Clemente Vicario
Osteosarcoma 292
Other Tumours of the Bone and Musculoskeletal System 295
Joint Tumours 298
Bibliography 300
Self-assessment 302

Tumours of the Nasal Cavity and Pulmonary Tumours
Pachi Clemente Vicario
Nasal Tumours 306
Pulmonary Tumours 310
Bibliography 314
Self-assessment 316

Practical Principles of Oncology Surgery
Judith Bertrán
Principles of Surgical Oncology of the Respiratory System 320
Principles of Oncological Surgery of the Digestive System 329
Principles of Oncological Skin Surgery 340
Bibliography 346
Self-assessment 347

Urogenital System and Mammary Tumours
Juan Francisco Borrego
Kidneys 352
Bladder and Urethra 353
Prostate 357
Penile, Scrotum, and Prepuce Tumours 359
Testicles 359
Vagina and Vulva 360
Uterus 361
Ovaries 362
Mammary Gland 364
Bibliography 369
Self-assessment 374

Tumours of the Endocrine System
Jarno Schmidt
Thyroid Tumours 378
Parathyroid Tumours 380
Insulinoma 383
Hypersomatotropism or Acromegaly 385
Hyperadrenocorticism 387
Pheochromocytoma 389
Feline Primary Hyperaldosteronism (Conn Syndrome) 389
Bibliography 391
Self-assessment 392

Cytological Diagnosis of Neoplastic Processes
Antonio Meléndez Lazo
Sample Handling: Cytological Preparation Quality 396
Sampling and Types of Preparations 397
Malignancy Criteria: Neoplasm vs Non-neoplasm 398
Classification of Neoplastic Lesions 400
Cutaneous and Subcutaneous Neoplasms 403
Neoplasms of Lymphoid Organs 410
Neoplasms of the Endocrine System 412
Neoplasms of Internal Organs 415
Bibliography 418
Self-assessment 419

Annex 1. New Developments in Immunotherapy in Veterinary Oncology
Keita Kitagawa and Paulo Vilar Saavedra
The Innate and the Acquired Immune Response 424
Mechanism of Immune Evasion 424
Non-specific Immunotherapy 425
Specific Immunotherapy 428
Antibody Therapy 429
Adoptive Transfer T-cell Therapy (ACT) 429
Other Treatments 429
Bibliography 430

Annex 2. Histiocytic Diseases
Keita Kitagawa and Paulo Vilar Saavedra
Canine Histiocytic Disease 432
Feline Histiocytic Disease 435
Bibliography 438

Annex 3. Biopsy
Sofia Carvalho
Types of Biopsy 440
Methods for Performing Biopsies 441
Recommendations for Sample Collection, Presentation, Cutting and Histopathological Margin Evaluation 443
Interpretation of Histopathology Results and Some Examples 444
Bibliography 445

Introduction to Veterinary Oncology

Ana Lara García and Sofia Carvalho

The Aetiology of Cancer

The Genetic Basis of Cancer

The word cancer describes a large number of diseases that share the common characteristic of **uncontrolled cell growth and proliferation**. Cancer is a genetic disease, although it is not necessarily always heritable.

Initiation, Promotion, Tumoural Progression

- **Onset**: a genetic mutation endows a somatic cell with unlimited replication potential or other growth or survival advantage over cells in its environment.
- **Promotion**: a second mutation or series of mutations provides cells with the ability to outcompete neighbouring cells, leading to potential expansion into a recognisable tumour.
- **Progression**: third series of mutations that reinforces the potential for malignancy leading to invasion and destruction of surrounding tissue and metastasis. There is no one single gene responsible for carcinogenesis. At least 5–6 mutations must be present.

The Key Characteristics of Cancer

In 2011 Hanahan and Weimberg published the 10 key characteristics of cancer, continuing their work which was published in 2000. As knowledge of cancer development increases it is now recognised that the following are necessary for cellular transformation into neoplastic cells.

1. Self-sufficiency in Growth Signals

The **cellular capacity to undergo proliferation in a chronic, persistent way**. Under normal circumstances, cells respond to signals from the environment and adapt their behaviour to the message which they receive from outside that regulates their growth, depending on the needs of the organism. The tumour cell does not respond to these external stimuli, since the mutations it possesses make it insensitive to regulatory mechanisms and it continues to grow independently.

2. Insensitivity to Antigrowth Signals

In addition to having the ability to induce and maintain sustained growth, neoplastic cells also develop a **way around the powerful systems that negatively regulate uncontrolled proliferation**. At a cellular level many of these systems depend on so-called tumour suppressor genes (e.g. P53, RB1, PTEN, and CDKN2A). There are signals that stop growth that are usually dispatched and integrated by the products of tumour suppressor genes. When the function of these genes is lost due to mutations or gene silencing, the balance between their function and that of the proto-oncogenes that promote cell growth is lost.

Another important concept is **autophagy**. Tumour cells possess intracellular vesicles called autophagosomes. These can fuse with lysosomes and intracytoplasmic organelles to form new molecules that provide the cellular energy-producing machinery, allowing the tumour cell to survive in a nutrient-deficient environment that would normally cause cellular stress.

3. Ability to Avoid Apoptosis

Programmed cell death is the last phase for every cell. Survival depends on survival factors and nutrients present in the environment. Tumour cells usually avoid apoptosis after the **loss of pro-apoptotic tumour suppressor genes** (P53, PTEN) or by **gaining genes with an anti-apoptotic function** such as BCL2. Apoptosis avoidance appears to be an important mechanism in the pathogenesis of indolent tumours (e.g. low-grade T-zone lymphoma, follicular lymphoma, or chronic lymphocytic leukaemia).

4. Unlimited Replication Capacity

Immortality is essential in neoplastic cells. Normally, the genetic program of a normal cell limits the number of times it can replicate. Cells that are capable of replicating must maintain the integrity of telomeres, which are the protective terminals of chromosomes and are made up of repetitive DNA sequences that protect them from destruction. Solid tumours acquire immortality by activating the telomerase enzyme system that helps maintain telomere integrity.

5. Sustained Angiogenesis

Development of the **tumour vasculature** provides a constant supply of oxygen and nutrients. Factors such as vascular endothelial growth factor (VEGF) and its receptors and platelet-derived growth factor (PDGF) and its receptors, among others, are necessary. Tumour cells can produce these factors in order to maintain and increase the blood supply to the tumour.

6. Ability to Invade Tissues and Metastasise

Ultimately, this is the acquisition of characteristics that allow tumour cells to **travel from the site of the primary tumour** through blood or lymph, invade the stroma in favourable locations, and establish themselves in distant locations. The most important step in this process is achieving the ability to survive in the capillary beds.

7. Genomic Instability and Mutation

In tumour genomes, **aneuploidy** (an abnormal number of DNA copies) is present, as well as **chaotic changes indicative of multiple numerical and structural abnormalities in the DNA**. It is possible that the initiation events in many tumours occur early during highly proliferative phases of growth and tissue restructuring.

This may explain why aneuploidy in tissue such as epithelial tissue promotes changes that lead from hyperplasia to atypical hyperplasia (dysplasia) and hence to the development of adenoma and, over time, to the formation of a localised carcinoma that can evolve into invasive carcinoma and metastatic carcinoma.

Boveri's "**cancer aneuploidy theory**" is based on the idea that this aneuploidy is necessary for carcinogenesis. The "**mutant phenotype**" proposed by Loeb shows that there are cells predisposed to undergoing multiple mutations, especially when they divide rapidly, which increases the number of errors in DNA replication and chromosomal segregation and triggers the appearance of cancer.

On the other hand, the **rate of mutations may be different depending on the type of neoplasia**, it is much higher in solid tumours (carcinomas, sarcomas, melanomas) than in leukaemia. For example, haematopoietic tumours do not appear to have the chaotic chromosomal instability associated with solid tumours.

8. Tumour Maintenance Caused by Inflammation

Cancer is like a **wound that never heals**. Although there are inflammatory populations that retard tumour growth and even kill tumour cells, **there are a group of inflammatory cells that contribute to tumour growth** and survival by providing proliferation-promoting factors, factors that limit cell death, proangiogenic factors, enzymes that modify the extracellular matrix facilitating angiogenesis, invasion and metastasis, among other protumoural actions.

9. Cell Energy Dysregulation

Many tumour cells preferentially use the **lactate-generating anaerobic glycolytic pathway** to generate energy even when oxygenation conditions are appropriate. This is called the "**Warburg effect**", which appears to be mediated by various activated oncogenes and the loss of tumour suppressor genes. This metabolic pathway provides tumour cells with selective growth and survival advantages, increasing cell proliferation, avoiding cytostatic controls and decreasing the capacity for apoptosis. **While some cancer cells secrete lactate, others consume it for energy**. This is a homeostatically unbalanced energetic environment characteristic of tumour growth. All of this occurs in conditions where oxygenation is not static, but instead fluctuates temporarily as a result of the chaotic tumoural neovasculature. This unique energy dysregulation that is effective for tumoural cells is considered one of the main characteristics of cancer.

Clonal Evolution Theory

The interaction of the tumour with its microenvironment relies on mutual support that **promotes tumour growth and prevents inflammatory attack by the host immune system**. It is based on the ability of tumours to modulate stromal cells to support their own growth by supplying an appropriate matrix and an abundance of nutrients, while curbing antitumour responses.

The normal stroma prevents tumour growth, but the tumour synthesises factors that influence the generation of a supportive stromal environment and thus prevents the host from initiating an effective antitumoural response, for example by transforming growth factor B and cytokines that activate the Stat-3 protein. Descendant tumoural cells can evolve to form stromal or vascular structures that support tumour growth.

Paget's Seed and Soil Hypothesis

This hypothesis consists of the gradual acquisition of advantages that allow the "seeds" (tumour cells) to leave the site of the primary tumour, travel through the blood or lymph, invade the stroma in specific favourable areas, the "soil", based on an affinity for the microenvironment of specific organs depending on the tumour type and thus re-establish in distant organs following a specific pattern of metastasis. Organs with extensive capillary networks such as the lungs and liver are often the targets for haematogenous metastasis.

Genetic Instability in Carcinogenesis

Epigenetic Events and Cancer

Epigenetic changes are those that **alter the phenotype without modifying the genotype**. **Gene silencing occurs through methylation** of cytosine-containing dinucleotide residues followed by guanine (CpG) in promoter regions and by deacetylation of histones. Both events **interfere with the transcription mechanism and repress gene expression**.

The silencing of specific genes through methylation is implicated in numerous types of cancer in humans and animals. Silencing by methylation in a particular gene, for example, the Ink4a gene, can lead to T-cell leukaemia, while mutations of this gene or deletion can lead to the development of melanoma.

Some epigenetic changes can be inherited, in such a way that, for a given gene, instead of expressing one allele from the father and another from the mother, a single allele is expressed and the other (from a parent gene where there is silencing) is permanently repressed (sealed allele). This is called **genetic stamping**. Epigenetic changes in Wilms tumour and hereditary colon cancer alter allele expression leading to overexpression of the insulin growth factor (IGF2) gene.

Hereditary Tumour Syndromes: Gene-environment Interactions in Cancer

Hereditary cancer syndromes represent 5–10% of human cancers. They tend to be **dominant inheritance patterns** and have high penetrance or inheritance from one mutant allele followed by inactivation of the second allele through loss of heterozygosity. All but two of the known inherited neoplastic syndromes originate from mutations that inactivate some type of "tumour suppressor" gene.

In dogs, at least one hereditary tumour syndrome is known of: **renal carcinoma and nodular dermatofibrosis syndrome in German Shepherds**. The heritable factor (RCND gene) that causes this syndrome is found on chromosome 5 (CFA5), specifically in the folliculin gene, which has been described as responsible for the equivalent disease in humans (Birt-Hogg-Dube syndrome).

Tumoural Stem Cells

Also called **tumour initiation cells**. It is believed that these cells retain or acquire the capacity for self-renewal and that they are capable and responsible for initiating the process of tumour genesis, as well as for keeping the neoplasm alive.

It is postulated that there is a subpopulation derived from these cells that undergoes differentiation towards the tumour phenotype and loses the ability to self-renew and, thus, supports the neoplasm indefinitely. It is believed these cells exist and are characterised by a peculiar phenotype and a defined number of mutations of a small number of genes.

The parallel hypothesis is that of the stochastic model, where all tumour cells have an equal capacity for self-renewal. It is possible that both models of growth and perpetuation of cancer actually coexist.

Pharmacoresistance Models in Tumours

Tumour cells **acquire resistance mechanisms to cytotoxic drugs**, and this explains that after an initial and sustained response to chemotherapy there may be tumour progression.

Sometimes, although some lesions can be seen to maintain their response to treatment, others progress, due to the mechanisms explained below.

1. The Conventional Model

The cell acquires a drug-resistant phenotype by random mutation that promotes the expression of intracellular pumps for the expulsion of substances toxic to the cell (one of the most common is the P-glycoprotein, which is encoded by the multidrug resistance gene, MDR), and this becomes the dominant phenotype through selective pressure caused by exposure to chemotherapy and non-mutated cells die.

2. Tumoural Stem Cell Model

The tumour contains a small number of stem cells that express drug transporters as part of their normal phenotype, which undergo selection through chemotherapy; non-precursor cells die.

3. Acquired Resistance

Stem cells become drug resistant after chemotherapy and the compromised cells die; mutations in tumour stem cells and their descendants proliferate, conferring a drug-resistant phenotype; non-precursor and mutated cells die.

4. Intrinsic Resistance

Stem cells and cells of variable differentiation have inherent drug resistance, so treatments are ineffective, leading to tumour growth. There is no clinical response.

An example would be high-grade T-cell lymphomas that are initially inherently resistant to doxorubicin and therefore do not go into remission with protocols that are based on this drug.

Carcinogenesis: Chemical, Physical and Hormonal Factors

In humans there are lists of carcinogenic and potentially carcinogenic substances created by official institutions in each country. There is no similar list for companion animals, but **it can be assumed that substances that have been shown to be carcinogenic to humans will most likely be carcinogenic to pets as well**. Different chemical, physical, hormonal and viral factors that have been shown to be carcinogenic in animals are described below.

Chemical Products

Cigarette Smoke

There is an increased risk of cancer in people who smoke (lung, oesophagus, urinary bladder, pancreas, and others). Pets are not primary smokers, but they share our environment and are **regularly exposed to smoke from people who smoke**. There are studies that associate this with an increased risk of developing nasal cancer in dolichocephalic breeds, as well as an increased risk of developing lymphoma, but not lung cancer. An increased risk of lymphoma has also been found in cats living in smokers' households and an increase in P53 mutations in cats with oral squamous cell carcinoma exposed to tobacco smoke, although a direct relationship with the development of this neoplasm has not been demonstrated.

Pesticides/Herbicides/Petrochemicals

Dichlorophenoxyacetic acid (2–4D) garden herbicides have been associated with increased risk of developing canine lymphoma, but there are some studies that have not found this association. On the other hand, an increased risk of lymphoma has been detected in dogs located in industrial areas whose owners used paints, solvents or pesticides. An increase in the urinary excretion of various herbicides including 2–4D has been detected in dogs that live in houses with gardens treated with these products.

Scottish terrier-type dogs that are predisposed to transitional cell carcinoma of the bladder **are at increased risk if exposed to phenoxy-type herbicides such as 2–4D**.

Also, topical insecticides have been associated with the risk of transitional cell carcinoma of the bladder, especially in obese dogs. It thus seems reasonable to try to **avoid exposing dogs to phenoxy-type herbicides**.

Higher rates of oral squamous cell carcinoma have been observed in cats that have worn flea collars. **No association of flea or tick products with canine lymphoma** or of these products in spot-on format has been found in Scottish terriers with transitional cell carcinoma of the urinary bladder.

Food Preservatives and Cooking Methods

Nitrites, nitrates, and polyvinyls are carcinogenic in laboratory animal studies. Cooking at high temperatures and on the grill can form **acrylamides and tricyclic amines** which are carcinogenic.

Cyclophosphamide

The chronic use of cyclophosphamide is associated in people and dogs with the development of **sterile haemorrhagic cystitis**, and in the case of humans also with the development of urinary bladder tumours, and in dogs, although rare, it has also been described.

The metabolite of this cytotoxic drug, acrolein, causes a pyroptotic reaction that leads to ulceration of the urothelium and increases nitric oxide production. Chronic damage to the urothelium leads to the development of cystitis and in some cases can end up triggering the development of neoplasia.

Physical Factors

Exposure to Sunlight/Ultraviolet (UV) Radiation

Chronic prolonged exposure to sunlight and/or lack of pigmentation are proven risk factors for the development of squamous cell carcinoma in humans. They are also important in the development of feline **squamous cell carcinoma** on the nasal plane, pinna or face, as well as in cutaneous locations in dogs.

The fraction of the ultraviolet spectrum most likely responsible for non-melanocytic skin lesions in humans and animals is **UV-B which is in the 280 nm range**. Pets are exposed to UV-B around midday and early afternoon and should be protected especially if they have a light coat or a predominance of depigmented skin areas.

Ionising Radiation (X and γ-rays)

Exposure to ionising radiation in the environment or at work increases the risk of various neoplastic processes such as leukaemia and thyroid cancer. **Carcinogenesis associated with radiotherapy** is defined as the development of neoplasms in anatomical areas that have previously received radiation treatment for another type of cancer.

This has been described in veterinary literature mainly after radiotherapy with Cobalt 205 units with an estimated incidence of 3.5% and appearance after prolonged periods (several years), where it could be a concern in very young dogs receiving radiotherapy, since that their life expectancy is longer.

Chronic Trauma/Inflammation

In some situations where there is chronic, continuous inflammation, it is possible that, neoplastic development is promoted in a non-specific way, since the **development of**

mutations in inflammatory cells such as fibroblasts can be triggered when they are subjected to high proliferation conditions as part of the inflammatory process. The rest of the participants in the process, such as growth factors, cytokines and other inflammatory cells, can contribute in a non-specific way to the continued proliferation of these abnormal cells, leading to the development of a neoplasm.

Examples in veterinary oncology are **feline injection site sarcomas or feline ocular sarcomas secondary to ocular trauma** that induces secondary uveitis and lens rupture. Cases with **chronic pigmentary keratitis** where squamous cell carcinoma has developed have been described in dogs.

Surgery and Surgical Implants

The development of **sarcomas in anatomical locations with metallic orthopaedic implants** has been described in human patients, dogs and laboratory animals. The studies that exist have not concluded whether the development of neoplasia is due to the implant itself or to other factors such as complications in healing or chronic osteomyelitis.

Although there are several studies in dogs with orthopaedic implants for fixation of fractures or repair of the anterior cruciate ligament that describe a prevalence of osteosarcomas, they have also concluded that statistically a cause-effect relationship cannot be established: the small number of cases that develop neoplasia and the design of these studies may have been responsible for these results.

There are reported cases of dogs that have developed sarcomas associated with a pacemaker or forgotten surgical gauze in the abdomen after a surgical procedure. These data mean that neoplasia in animals with pain or lameness in anatomical locations where there are surgical implants should be considered as a differential diagnosis, especially years after the procedure.

Asbestos

Humans and dogs exposed to asbestos are at **increased risk of developing pleural mesothelioma**. Pleural mesothelioma has been found in dogs whose owners had an asbestos-related profession, but there are also other factors that are related to the aetiology of mesothelioma, such as chronic inflammation.

Parasitic Infestations

Spirocerca lupi is associated with fibrosarcoma and oesophageal osteosarcoma.

Hormonal Factors

The debate around neutering in pets has increased since although it can help prevent certain types of cancer, in certain breeds it may have an association with the development of cancer.

Now, when looking at the entire population of pets, the **risk of association with cancer is low** compared to the benefits of population control and the reduction of deadly diseases.

Canine Mammary Tumours

Mammary tumours are the most common neoplasm in unsterilised bitches and primarily affect middle-aged intact females (9–11 years), with an incidence that increases from 6 years of age, and 50% are malignant. **Spaying before the first season or oestrous cycle greatly reduces the dog's risk of developing mammary tumours**. The risk increases from 0% in females spayed before the first season to 26% if they are spayed after their second season.

The use of products containing **medroxyprogesterone acetate** for the prevention of heat or to treat pseudo-pregnancy increases the risk of mammary tumours developing in bitches.

Bitches that are spayed while having a malignant mammary tumour removed have a lower risk of developing non-malignant mammary tumours in the future. There is a small group of bitches with oestrogen receptor-positive and intermediate-grade malignant mammary tumours (although this information is not a routine part of histopathological analysis) who also benefit from spaying.

Steroid sex hormones are believed to have a primary effect on target cells during the early stages of mammary carcinogenesis in dogs, as supported by the absence of a protective effect of spaying after two seasons and the presence of receptors for oestrogen and progesterone in higher concentrations in normal mammary tissue and benign lesions, compared to mammary cancer tissue and metastatic lesions.

Progesterone-induced growth hormone is believed to have an autocrine/paracrine action causing cyclic epithelial changes and possibly carcinogenesis.

Feline Mammary Tumours

Oestrogens and progestogens play an important role in the development of feline mammary carcinogenesis. Intact female cats and cats regularly exposed to progesterone are at increased risk of developing mammary tumours and 80–90% of these are malignant. Compared to unspayed cats, there is a statistically significant reduction of risk in the development of mammary tumours when female cats are **spayed before the first year of age, with a reduction in occurrence by 91%** if they are spayed before 6 months of age, compared with an 86% reduction in those spayed before one year old.

Lymphoma

Non-Hodgkins LSA (NHL) is 50% more common in men than women. **Male dogs show a predisposition to suffering from LSA**. Intact females were significantly less susceptible to developing LSA than other sexes. An increased risk has also been described in Labrador Retrievers and the Hungarian Vizsla. Another study concluded that both intact males and females had a lower risk of developing lymphoma than neutered males and spayed females respectively.

Osteosarcoma (OSA)

The risk ratio for developing osteosarcoma between males and females is the same, although **studies that have described the risk as being twice as much for the development of this neoplasia in sterilised animals exist**.

A study in the United States showed that in the Rottweiler, a breed already predisposed to OSA, spaying before 12 months of age increased the risk.

Mast Cell Tumours

Spayed females appear to be at higher risk than other gonadal states for developing this type of tumour, but the hormonal influence remains unclear.

Perianal Adenomas

Perianal adenomas are androgen-dependent and **occur primarily in non-neutered males and in dogs with hyperadrenocorticism that produce excess testosterone**. In bitches they occur secondary to testosterone secretion from the adrenal glands. Most of these adenomas in intact males **resolve after castration**.

Prostate Cancer

Prostatic adenocarcinomas do not appear in higher proportions in uncastrated dogs, in fact **castrated dogs seem to have a higher risk than intact dogs for this disease**. Castration does not appear to be related to carcinogenesis, but it may be that it favours its progression.

Principles of Tumour Biology and General Pathology of Neoplasms

A tumour is a mass or inflammation and may or may not be neoplastic.

A neoplasm is the abnormal growth of a tissue causing a mass, which can be benign or malignant, and which does not respond to the usual control mechanisms. The growth of this mass does not stop even when the initial stimulus that caused it is eliminated.

A cancer is a malignant neoplasm and, since it originates from normal tissue, it is composed of parenchymal and stromal cells along with inflammatory cells and others that make up the tumour microenvironment.

- Differentiation is controlled by gene expression and is defined as the appearance and organisation of cells and their association with the supporting stroma.
- It can be difficult to distinguish between a well-differentiated cancer and a normal reversible process such as hyperplasia or atrophy. In many cases, this differentiation is only possible if the inciting stimulus is removed.
- A cancer is a clonal population of cells that no longer responds to homeostatic tissue mechanisms.
- Molecular techniques that determine the clonal expansion of cells by their similar DNA sequence can help differentiate these processes even before any microscopic change in cell morphology and tissue structure occurs.

Metaplasia is not a neoplastic process but is the dedifferentiation of one type of tissue and its transformation into another type of differentiated tissue. Metaplasia should stabilise or regress when the inciting stimulus ceases. For example, squamous metaplasia in the prostate occurs when epithelial cells are converted into squamous cells under the influence of oestrogens. **Metaplastic cells** can be carcinogenic if the stimulus remains long-term. For example, in the lungs of a smoker, squamous metaplasia may undergo dysplastic changes and may eventually develop into squamous cell carcinoma of the bronchi.

Dysplasia is abnormal development of tissue, not necessarily a neoplastic condition.

Anaplasia is a loss of differentiation or atypical differentiation. This is a feature of many malignant tumours, but it does not necessarily happen in all of them. Including **cellular pleomorphism, anisocytosis and anisokaryosis**.

A **desmoplastic, scirrhous response** is an abundant fibroblastic proliferation with collagen formation that can be seen in some invasive cancers.

Terminology for Definition of Benign and Malignant

In general, with a few exceptions, the first part of the lesion name refers to the **tissue of origin** and the end of the word will vary depending on the **benign or malignant nature of the lesion** (Table 1).

- **Benign lesions**:
  - epithelial: adenoma/papilloma/epithelioma
  - mesenchymal: tissue + -oma
- **Malignant lesions**:
  - epithelial: carcinoma
  - mesenchymal: sarcoma

Table 1. Nomenclature of the main types of tumour in veterinary medicine.

Tissue or cell of origin	Benign	Malignant
	EPITHELIAL	
Squamous	Squamous papilloma	Squamous cell carcinoma
Transitional	Transitional cell papilloma	Transitional cell carcinoma
Glandular	Adenoma, cystadenoma	Adenocarcinoma
Non-glandular	Adenoma	Carcinoma
	MESENCHYMAL	
Fibrous tissue	Fibroma	Fibrosarcoma
Fat	Lipoma, infiltrative lipoma	Liposarcoma
Cartilage	Chondroma	Chondrosarcoma
Bone	Osteoma	Osteosarcoma, multilobed osteochondrosarcoma
Muscle (smooth)	Leiomyoma	Leiomyosarcoma
Muscle (skeletal)	Rhabdomyoma	Rhabdomyosarcoma
Endothelial cells	Haemangioma	Haemangiosarcoma
Synovial	-	Synovial sarcoma
Mesothelium	-	Mesothelioma
Melanocytes	Benign melanoma, melanocytoma	Malignant melanoma, melanosarcoma
Peripheral nerve	-	Malignant Schwannoma, neurofibrosarcoma, peripheral nerve sheath tumour
Of unknown origin*	-	Malignant fibrous histiocytoma, haemangiopericytoma
	HAEMATOPOIETIC AND LYMPHORETICULAR	
Lymphocytes	-	
Plasmatic cells	Cutaneous plasmacytoma	Multiple myeloma, plasmacytoid lymphoma
Granulocytes	-	Myeloid leukaemia
Red blood cells	-	Erythroid leukaemia
Macrophages	Histiocytoma	Histiocytic sarcoma (malignant histiocytosis)
Mastocytes	-	Mast cell tumour**
Thymus	Encapsulated thymoma	Invasive thymoma
	CEREBRAL	
Glial cells	Astrocytoma, oligodendroglioma	Astrocytoma, glioblastoma multiforme, oligodendroglioma
Meninges	Meningioma	Malignant meningioma
	GONADAL	
Germinal cells***	Seminoma, dysgerminoma	Seminoma, dysgerminoma
Support cells***	Sertoli cell tumour, granulosa cell tumour	Sertoli cell tumour, granulosa cell tumour
Interstitial cells***	Interstitial cell tumour (Leydig), thecoma, luteoma	Interstitial cell tumour (Leydig)

*Pathologists disagree regarding the origin of these tumours; some consider them to be a type of tumour of the peripheral nerve sheath or perivascular wall tumours.
**In theory all mast cell tumours are potentially malignant, but grade 1 mast cell tumours are clinically benign.
***Unfortunately, the terminology used to describe these tumours does not distinguish between benign and malignant forms.

Histologic Characteristics of Neoplasms

Together with information on the histological characteristics of a tumour (Table 2), the clinical information on the involvement of the lymph nodes or the presence of metastases makes it possible to differentiate a benign tumour from a malignant one.

Table 2. Histological characteristics of hyperplasia and benign and malignant neoplasms.

Characteristics	Hyperplasia	Benign neoplasia	Malignant neoplasia
General differentiation	Normal	Disorganised, but well differentiated	Disorganised, from well to poorly differentiated
Nuclear and cellular pleomorphism	None	Minimum	Moderate to notable
Mitotic index	Variable, generally low	Generally low	Often high
Nucleoli	Normal	Normal	Large and/or multiple
Presence of necrosis	None	Minimal in genera	Minimum to abundant
Tissue delimitation	Mixed with normal tissue	Expansive and/or compressive	Invasive

Metastasis

Vascular or lymphatic invasion by a malignant tumour is an indication of early metastasis. Malignant tumours can metastasise via both routes.

Normally, **carcinomas and melanomas prefer the lymphatic route**, and invade the regional and distant lymph nodes first, and then spread to distant organs such as the lungs, spleen and liver.

Sarcomas usually metastasise directly via the haematogenic route and first spread to distant organs such as the lungs, spleen and liver. However, they sometimes also invade regional and distant lymph nodes.

Grading or Classification of Neoplasms

Histological classification or grading systems for specific types of neoplasms in domestic animals are of prognostic significance (Table 3), as they predict the biological behaviour of the tumour. However, as important as the histological degree is the TNM (tumour, lymph node, metastasis) clinical stage when establishing a prognosis.

There are **several systems for grading neoplasms** in domestic animals, such as the Patnaik or Kiupel classification for canine skin mast cell tumours or grading of soft-tissue sarcomas. There are also classifications that provide different categories and grades for a particular type of neoplasm, such as canine mammary carcinomas and feline lymphomas. However, there are no classification or grading systems for all types of tumours and, in many cases and due to the heterogeneity of tumour tissue, grading of small pieces of tissue is not possible.

The grading or classification of a tumour is directly correlated with **survival, metastasis rate, disease-free interval**, and **local recurrence frequency and/or rate**.

Malignancy characteristics are used to establish the degree of malignancy.

1. Degree of differentiation.
2. Mitotic index (number of mitotic figures in 10 fields of high magnification 400x).
3. Degree of cellular or nuclear polymorphism.
4. Amount of necrosis.
5. Invasiveness.
6. Stromal reaction.
7. Number and size of the nucleolus.
8. Global cellularity.
9. Lymphatic response.

In cases where there is no validated system for tumour grading, **evaluation of the histopathology report** is useful. For example, in the case of solid neoplasms (carcinomas, sarcomas, melanomas). In this report, it is appropriate to look at the histological characteristics commonly used to perform grading and attempt to estimate the clinical behaviour of the tumour according to the differentiation of the neoplasm (well, moderate or poorly differentiated) and its proliferative capacity (according to the mitotic index values). Thus, in some tumours such as oral and skin melanomas in the dog and cat, in which there is no grading system, the literature has found that some histological prognostic factors, such as the mitotic index, can be identified.

Analysis and Evaluation of Tissue Samples

It is **very important for clinicians and pathologists to work together**, since the more information the clinician provides the pathologist with, the greater the precision of the histopathological diagnosis and the assessment of the integrity of the tumour margins.

In some cases, the use of immunohistochemistry in order to accurately define the type of tumour is necessary. This occurs, for example, in the case of undifferentiated neoplasms or round cell tumours in which the morphological characteristics are not sufficient to reach a definitive diagnosis.

Table 3. Grades and histological characteristics of prognostic importance in neoplasms.

Type of tumour	Grade	Important characteristics
Cutaneous mastocytoma (dog)	I, II, II	Cellularity, nucleus: cytoplasm ratio, cellular morphology, mitotic index, depth, necrosis, granularity
	2 levels: high, low	Mitotic index, karyomegaly, multinucleation anomalous nuclei
	SC: high, low	Mitotic index ≤4, >4, invasiveness, multinucleation
Cutaneous mastocytoma (cat)	Well and poorly differentiated, histiocytic	Nuclear and cellular pleomorphism, mitotic index
Lymphoma	Low, intermediate, high	Architecture, mitotic index, nucleus size, morphology, T and B-cell immunophenotypes
Cutaneous melanoma	Well and poorly differentiated	Mitotic index: ≥3/10 HPF*
Oral melanoma and labial melanoma	Well and poorly differentiated	Mitotic index: ≥3/10 HPF
Uveal melanoma of the anterior chamber (cat, dog)	I–VI (or early, moderate, advanced); benign, malignant (dog)	Mitotic index, invasiveness
Soft-tissue sarcoma (dog)	1, 2, 3 or mitotic index >9**, mitotic index <9**	General differentiation, mitotic index, necrosis
Pulmonary carcinoma (dog)	1, 2, 3	General differentiation, nuclear pleomorphism, mitotic index, necrosis, nucleolus size, fibrosis, invasion
Pulmonary carcinoma (cat)	Moderate and poorly differentiated	Organisation, pleomorphism, vascular and pulmonary invasion
Mammary gland carcinoma (dog)	System 1: well, moderately and poor differentiated	Invasiveness, nuclear differentiation, lymphoid response
	System 2: grades I, II, III	Tubule formation, nuclear pleomorphism, mitotic index, simple carcinoma as opposed to others, lymph node metastasis
Mammary gland carcinoma (cat)	System 1: well, moderately and poor differentiated	Differentiation, cellular pleomorphism, mitotic index
	System 2: grades I, II, III	Same as system 2 in the dog
Synovial cell sarcoma	1, 2, 3	Nuclear pleomorphism, mitotic index, necrosis
	Histiocytic or non-histiocytic	CD18 ±
	Myxoma or non-myxoma	Abundant myxomatous matrix
Primary and metastatic osteosarcoma (dog)	I–III	Tumoural pleomorphism, mitosis, tumoural matrix, cellular density, necrosis, vascular invasion
Multilobed osteosarcoma	1, 2, 3	Borders, lobar size, organisation, mitotic index, nuclear pleomorphism, necrosis
Mandibular osteosarcoma	1, 2, 3	Nuclear pleomorphism, mitotic index, necrosis
Appendicular chondrosarcoma	1, 2, 3	Tumoural pleomorphism, mitosis, tumoural matrix, cellularity, necrosis, architecture
Haemangiosarcoma	1, 2, 3	General differentiation, nuclear pleomorphism, mitotic index, necrosis
Non-lymphoid splenic sarcoma, non-angiomatous	Mitotic index 0–9, mitotic index >9	Mitotic index
Splenic fibrohistiocytic nodules	1, 2, 3	Proportion of lymphocytes and multinucleated cells, mitotic index
Transitional cell carcinoma	1, 2, 3	Cytoplasmatic and nuclear variation, nucleus location, number and size of nucleoli, mitosis
Squamous cell carcinoma	1, 2, 3	General differentiation, mitotic index, nuclear pleomorphism, invasion, stromal reaction

* Mitotic index: ≥3/10 HPF (high power fields): mitosis ≥3 per 10 high power fields.
**Total amount of mitosis in 10 fields at 400× magnification.
SC: subcutaneous.

Surgical margins and histoprognostic grading systems are key parts of making the most accurate prognostic prediction possible and establishing an adequate treatment plan.

Evaluation of Tumoural Margins

Available when surgery is performed with curative intentions.

- **Macroscopically**: the surgical margin is the margin below which the tissue remains in the surgical wound bed.
- **Microscopically**: the surgical margin is the region between the neoplastic process and the surgical border of the biopsy sample. Observation of the margins depends on the sample, the dissection method and the observer.

It is recommended that the clinician marks and draws the margins with different coloured surgical ink to facilitate the pathologist's work in accurately delineating the tumour margins.

Histological margins should be measured and should also be interpreted according to the type of tumour. The retraction which the tissues suffer after processing (fixation with formalin and dehydration) must be taken into account, and in the case of skin biopsies, can be up to 30%.

Depending on the type of tumour and its grade, the existence of clean margins does not always imply that the surgery has been curative and, conversely, infiltrated margins do not always cause recurrence. For example, in grade II canine cutaneous mast cell tumours, only 30% of those that have been incompletely removed will experience a recurrence. To the contrary, for feline injection site sarcomas, which have a highly infiltrative behaviour, the recurrence rate is 80% even when the margins are clean (this rate drops to 14% if the surgical margins are 5 cm).

Immunohistochemistry (IHC)

Immunohistochemistry is a staining procedure that uses **antibodies to identify specific intra- or extracellular molecules** (these can be cytoplasmic filaments, secretory substances, extracellular markers, membrane receptors). It can be carried out on frozen sections of tissue or on paraffinised tissue blocks. Immunohistochemistry should always be interpreted in conjunction with findings from routine light microscopy.

IHC is of **great help for identification of tumour type** when the morphological characteristics are not clear or are not sufficient for the pathologist to establish a final diagnosis. In addition, it provides **additional information that can help establish a prognosis** for certain types of neoplasia. For example, it can help distinguish between B-cell and T-cell lymphoma and, in the case of canine cutaneous mast cell tumours, can be useful in determining the KI67 cell proliferation index.

The **main marker antibodies** used in IHC are:

- epithelial neoplasia: cytokeratin
- mesenchymal neoplasia: vimentin
- lymphatic cells: CD3 (T cells), CD79 or PAX5 (B cells)
- melanomas: melan-A, PNL2, S-100, vimentin, tyrosinase, TRP1, TRP2.

Guidelines for Handling of Samples

Specimens should be **greater than 1 mm thick** (or multiple 1 × 5 mm in the case of core needle biopsies). Small samples should be identified (placed in a biopsy container or on filter paper). It is advisable to mark the margins of excisional biopsies and surgical specimens with surgical ink. Also, when these specimens are large, at least 4–5 representative samples should be taken.

To fix the sample, **10% buffered neutral formalin** is used (20% ethylene glycol can be added in cold conditions) with a **1:10 tissue/fixative ratio**. Sample processing takes 24 hours or even longer if there is fat, haemorrhagic tissue, or bone in the sample.

Molecular techniques such as IHC are often used with wax embedded specimens on slides. In the case of the PCR technique, thicker samples are needed.

It is **advisable to request several tests at the same time** at the time the samples are shipped as they will be of better quality. For example, IHC for B cells or T cells can be requested and at the same time a lymph node from a dog with a high suspicion of lymphoma can be submitted.

It is **essential samples are accompanied by**:

- complete clinical history
- illustrations on the location of the lesion on the animal
- the margins of the lesion should be marked and labelled
- photographs can also be sent if deemed necessary.

Clinicopathological Correlation and Second Opinions

On some occasions, histology alone is not enough to establish a definitive diagnosis and therefore it is necessary to relate it to the clinical findings.

In case of discrepancy between histology and the symptoms, a second opinion should be sought.

- After a second opinion, there is a greater probability of diagnosis in 1.4–5.8% of samples.
- During the processing of the samples, there may be errors such as, for example, mistakes in the labelling of the samples, failures when processing them or omitting the processing of critical tissues sent by the clinician.

Diagnosis in the Cancer Patient

It is important to adopt a comprehensive diagnostic approach to the cancer patient and to remember that there is **always a patient attached to any tumour**. Considering the approach globally and not just the tumour itself significantly increases the probability of not missing any underlying cause, comorbidity, or paraneoplastic conditions, which in turn may also require specific treatment. An important part of this approach is tumour staging.

Clinical History

Taking a **complete and detailed clinical history** from the owner is very important, as it helps with diagnosis, prognosis, and biological behaviour.

Data such as the duration of clinical signs and the growth rate of the tumour provide information about how aggressive it is. The previous existence of another tumour may indicate that recurrence and/or metastasis has occurred and help formulate a diagnostic plan. Likewise, a history of other serious medical conditions can influence the diagnostic plan, prognosis, and treatment options.

Physical Examination

A complete physical examination (Box 1) is essential to correctly characterise the primary lesion, multifocal lesions and in order not to miss possible metastases or other underlying or concurrent diseases that may be detected. It is important that the tumour(s) are **correctly documented in the clinical history**, preferably with photographs that allow monitoring of the response to treatment, which can be decisive for the planning of any type of adjuvant therapy, such as radiotherapy.

In some circumstances, the clinical evolution of a tumour can provide useful information about its biological behaviour (benign or malignant). Rapid growth, ulcer generation, adherence to underlying tissues, and enlargement of regional lymph nodes are factors commonly associated with malignant behaviour. An example would be canine mastocytoma, in which rapid growth, intense oedema, ulceration and possibly their anatomical location (for example oral, mucous or nail) can be associated with a more aggressive phenotype.

Box 1. Details which should be taken into account when performing a physical examination on a patient

- The patient's temperament and level of response to stimuli, temperature, capillary refill time and hydration state.
- In the case of cutaneous masses, establishing whether their origin is dermal or whether they originate from internal structures and whether they are connected to adjacent structures.
  - Tumours which invade adjacent structures are harder to remove and this worsens the prognosis.
  - Obtaining exact measurements, or, at least, an approximation of the three-dimensional size of the tumour helps to determine the response to treatment and should be noted in the clinical file.
- Careful palpation of regional lymph nodes to establish whether these are affected or not.
  - Cytology of lymph node aspirations should be performed whether they are enlarged or not.
  - The size of the lymph nodes should be noted in the clinical file.
- Rectal palpation is an essential part of examination of the prostate, urethra, anal glands and lymph nodes of the pelvic canal.
- Thoracic auscultation allows cardiac and pulmonary function to be assessed.
  - In cats, gentle compression of the cranioventral portion of the chest can help to identify whether there is a cranial mediastinal mass.
  - Auscultation helps to detect pleural effusions.
- Detailed oral examination and of nasal structures.
- Evaluation and documentation of the musculoskeletal and integumentary systems.
  - Note if there is lameness.
  - Observe the body condition.
  - Presence of dermatological abnormalities.
- Abdominal palpation to detect masses and/or organomegaly, as well as the size and structure of abdominal organs.
- Full ophthalmologic examination, which includes a fundus examination, as neoplasms can cause anterior uveitis and other ophthalmological anomalies such as retinopathies.
- Basic neurological examination which includes evaluation of cranial nerves, level of conscience, and proprioceptive deficits.
- Full neurological examination when the initial history, clinical signs and physical examination suggest neurological dysfunction.

Routine Complete Blood Count

A complete blood count is always recommended. While it rarely provides information directly applicable to tumour treatment (other than haematopoietic tumours), it can be used to identify some important features, such as neutrophilia (infection, inflammation, paraneoplasia), neutropaenia, polycythaemia (renal tumours, other neoplastic causes), anaemia (immune-mediated secondary haemolytic anaemia, IMHA), bone marrow involvement, (gastrointestinal bleeding due to mast cell involvement) and thrombocytopaenia (immune-mediated secondary thrombocytopaenia, IMTP), disseminated intravascular coagulation (DIC), haemorrhage. It can also be used to identify paraneoplastic disorders, such as eosinophilia, or even concomitant disorders, such as leukaemia.

Routine biochemistry can be used to detect elevated liver enzymes caused by tumour infiltration or liver disease, electrolyte imbalances, and reduced liver or kidney function. It is important to have a good knowledge of the patient's liver and kidney status because this could also alter the metabolism of the drug and affect the dosage of chemotherapy. Baseline values before treatment are also helpful, considering the potentially nephrotoxic or hepatotoxic nature of some chemotherapeutics. Sometimes with some types of neoplasms (e.g. myeloma or lymphoid tumours) abnormal protein levels (hyperglobulinaemias, dysproteinaemias) are seen.

Urinalysis can be a useful tool for assessing renal concentration capacity, infections, crystalluria, and proteinuria. The urine sediment test also detects exfoliated neoplastic cells, as in the case of transitional cell carcinoma. If chemotherapy is to be given, ruling out any silent urinary tract infections is important.

There are other optional tests that may be useful depending on the situation, such as blood pressure measurement, eye background examination and a complete oral examination, not forgetting rectal examination, especially in animals with hypercalcaemia.

Paraneoplastic Syndromes

Paraneoplastic syndromes are **secondary problems induced by a tumour that appear at a distant point to the tumour that causes them**.

Several have been described and some are more common than others. It is important to be aware of their possible presence and be able to recognise them when they appear, since some may need specific treatment in addition to anti-cancer treatment and others can cause significant morbidity. However, they can be useful in providing the key to the presence of a tumour before the tumour itself generates clinical signs. Later on, in the course of the disease, they can be useful markers of tumour recurrence, as with hypercalcaemia in lymphoma and adenocarcinoma of the apocrine glands.

The next chapter of this manual will review the different paraneoplastic syndromes in detail:

- gastrointestinal ulcers (mastocytoma) → H2/PPI antagonist +/- sucralfate
- hypercalcaemia → IV fluid therapy, calcitonin, furosemide
- hypoglycaemia → IV supplementation
- hyperglobulinaemia → plasmapheresis, medical
- erythrocytes → phlebotomy
- myasthenia → surgery.

Staging

Staging is the **evaluation of the degree of progression of the primary tumour and testing to identify if there are any metastasis or extent of the pathology** beyond the primary point of the tumour. It is a fundamental part of the diagnostic work-up in cancer patients and is of **great prognostic value** in many types of tumours, which provides information to make decisions concerning treatment and the willingness of clients to administer them.

Different types of neoplasms have different target organs to which they can metastasise, so it is important to obtain specific information about the biology of each specific tumour, in order to design an appropriate staging plan.

Staging of the Primary Tumour

The evaluation of the **size of the primary tumour, its anatomical location and adjacent structures** are important because this can be of prognostic value, as well as being essential in terms of planning treatment, particularly surgery.

An understanding of the anatomical structures surrounding the tumour can help decide whether it can be removed and whether removal is likely to have a curative effect (for example, that the muscle fascia below the tumour is intact or has reasonable margins of healthy tissue around it) or if only a programmed marginal excision is more useful, with the consequent debulking to a microscopic state followed by radiotherapy, or primary radiotherapy and chemotherapy may be more useful.

In many cases, simple physical examination allows a decision to be made directly (as in well-defined skin lesions that are not fixed), but it can be more complicated and require different imaging modalities in others (for example, an invasive thyroid tumour in the dog, feline sarcomas associated with a vaccine, invasive tumours of the abdominal wall or voluminous or infiltrative sarcomas), as well as in some anatomical locations where it is more difficult to plan a complete removal (cranial or oral cavity). Because of this, in highly infiltrative neoplasms and difficult anatomical locations, staging of the primary tumour often requires advanced imaging.

Staging: Looking for Metastasis

Lymph Nodes

Evaluation of a metastatic condition involves examination of the regional lymph nodes that drain the area where the tumour is, as well as obtaining thoracic and abdominal images.

Staging methods depend on the anatomical location and histology of the tumour, its grade, other possible prognostic factors, and will, of course, be dictated by the available imaging tools.

It is helpful to have a **good understanding of which regions are drained by which group of lymph nodes**, to ensure that the appropriate nodes are sampled during staging (Figures 1, 2 and 3):

- **head**: submandibular, retropharyngeal
- **base of the ear**: submandibular, prescapular
- **distal region of the forelimb**: prescapular
- **oral masses:** submandibular, as well as retropharyngeal, especially if they are in a caudal position within the oral cavity
- **proximal region of the forelimb**: axillary (may require ultrasound)
- **distal region of hindlimb**: popliteal
- **perineal, anogenital, rectal region**: inguinal, sublumbar
- **mammary glands**: can drain through the axillary, inguinal or iliac lymph nodes, depending on the species and the location of the neoplasm.

Not all lymph nodes are palpable on physical examination, even if they are enlarged. Also, not all metastatic lymph nodes are always enlarged. For this reason, in certain circumstances, **a diagnosis using imaging will be needed**, such as in order to examine the medial iliac lymph nodes (sublumbar nodes) or the deep cervical nodes, as well as the inguinal or axillary nodes, which cannot always be palpated during the physical examination.

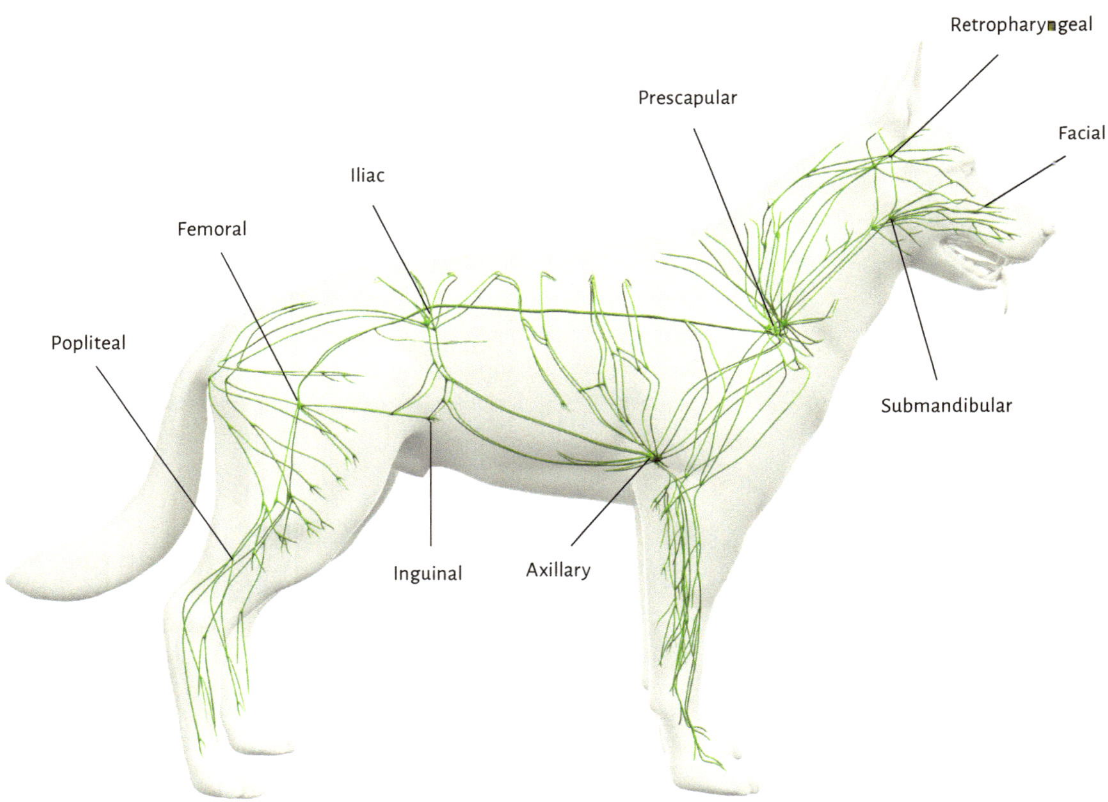

Figure 1. Diagram showing the main lymphatic vessels in the dog with the location of important superficial lymph nodes which can be palpated on physical examination.

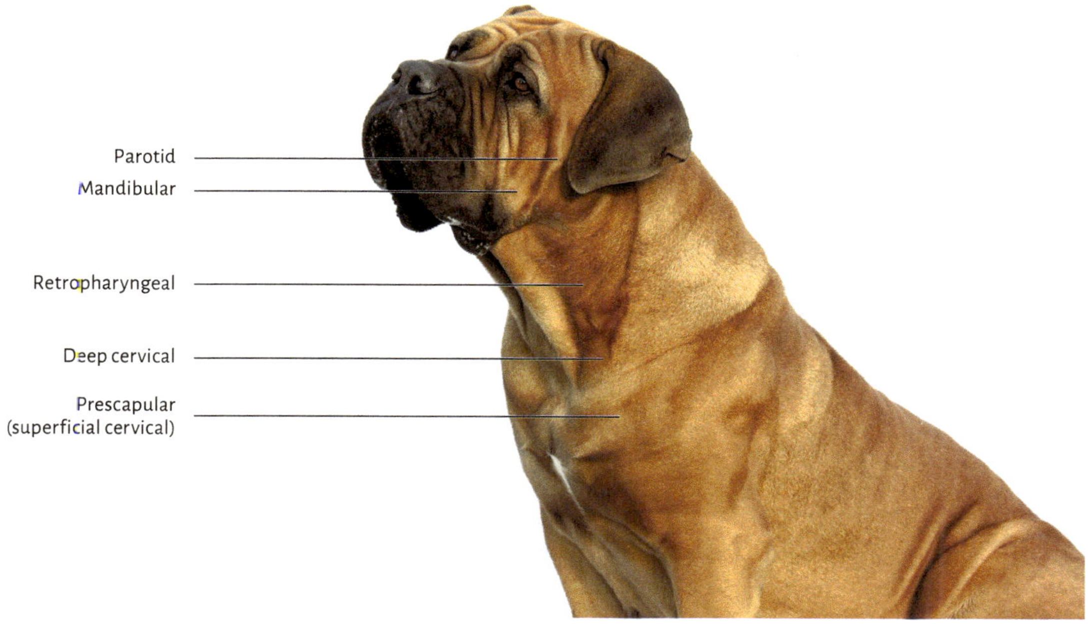

Figure 2. What is the approximate location of the main lymph nodes which should be examined if a patient has a neoplasm in the head or neck?

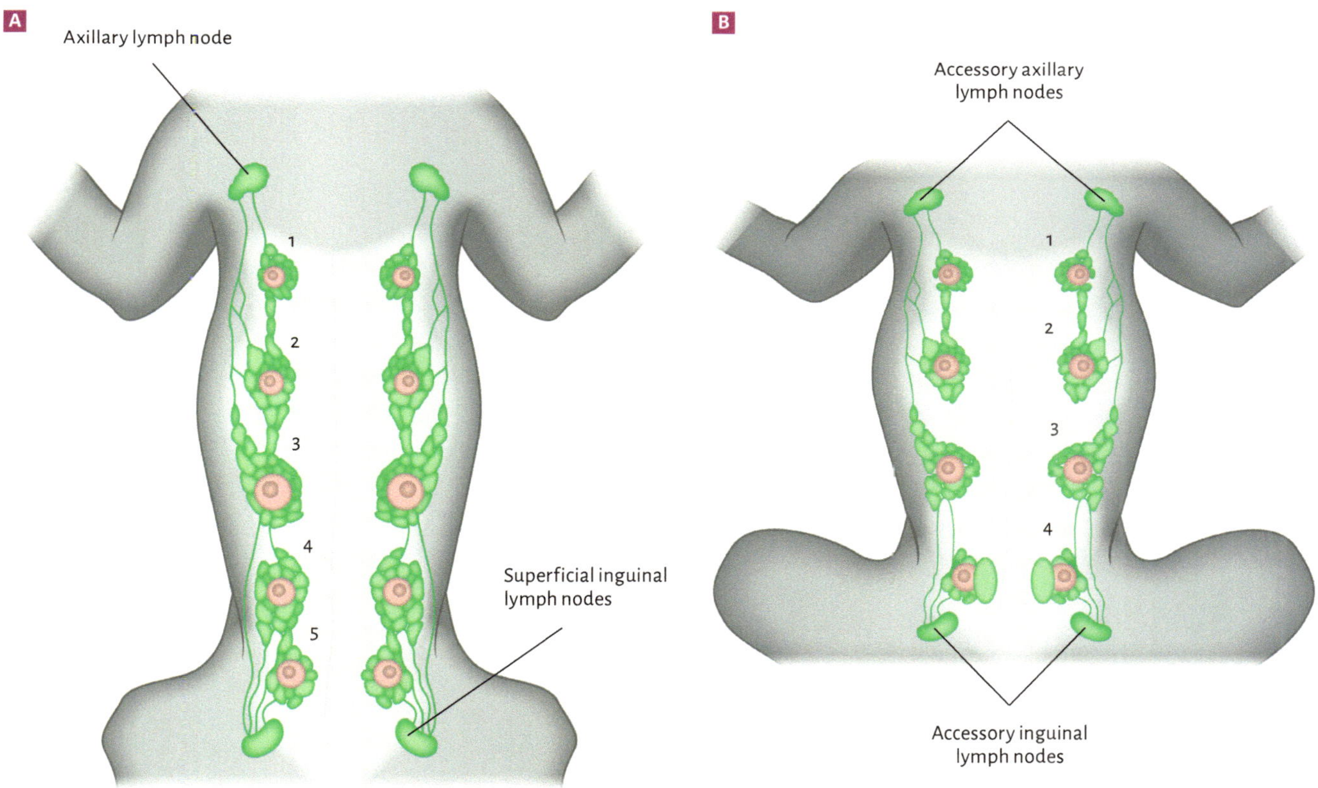

Figure 3. Lymphatic drainage of the mammary area in the bitch (**A**) and queen (**B**). In the bitch, mammary glands 1 and 2 drain into the axillary lymph node, 3 drains into the axillary or inguinal lymph node, meanwhile 4 and 5 only drain into the inguinal lymph node. In the queen, however, mammary glands 1 and 2 drain into the accessory axillary lymph nodes, 3 drains into these or the accessory inguinal lymph nodes, meanwhile 4 drains into only the accessory inguinal lymph nodes, or, on some occasions, into the medial iliac lymph nodes.

It is important to know whether a particular type of neoplasm tends to spread to the lymph nodes or not and, if it does, what its estimated rate of metastasis is, in order to decide how invasive clinical staging should be. For example, with a malignant oral melanoma that requires a maxillectomy for complete removal and has a metastatic rate of 90% sampling the submandibular and retropharyngeal nodes is warranted (which will require an ultrasound-guided aspiration biopsy), because performing an expensive intervention with some morbidity (maxillectomy) to later discover that it was not worth it because during the intervention a retropharyngeal lymph node that was affected was not removed is not advisable. On the other hand, an oral fibrosarcoma with a spread rate of around 20% usually to the lungs and less frequently to the lymph nodes, may not justify more than checking the lungs and submandibular nodes, at the most.

In any case, if a decision has been taken to sample the regional lymph nodes corresponding to the area of the malignant neoplasm, it should be done so regardless of their size. Many lymph nodes can **host metastatic cells and yet have a normal clinical appearance**. On the other hand, the lymph nodes may simply be enlarged in reaction to the condition. Therefore, it is common to both over and underestimate the presence of lymph node metastases when based only on palpation. In dogs, the presence of melanin-containing mast cells and macrophages in normal lymph node samples can make interpretation of mast cell tumours and melanocytic tumours difficult, respectively.

The other important aspect when biopsying lymph nodes as part of staging is that the **results can modify the treatment approach**, which often means that if there is a suspicion of metastasis or even if cytology confirms their existence, they can be removed immediately at the same time as the primary tumour. For example, the latest research on high-risk (high mitotic rate or rapidly evolving) mast cell tumours advocates removal of regional lymph nodes, because this has a positive effect on the overall prognosis, even if metastases are already present.

Another important consideration when staging uses advanced imaging techniques, such as computed tomography, is the possibility of applying techniques that allow **detection of sentinel lymph nodes**. For example, by injecting an iodinated contrast directly into the tumour. When a specific protocol is followed, this shows whether a particular malignant tumour drains to one or more lymph nodes and, importantly, if it also drains to the contralateral lymph nodes, as has been seen in some malignant tumours of the head and neck.

Diagnostic Imaging for Staging in an Animal with Cancer

Diagnostic imaging plays a **fundamental role in the diagnosis and treatment of cancer patients**.

It allows for diagnosis and localisation of primary neoplasms, as well as evaluation of their size and extension, with a higher sensitivity than physical examination or radiographs, in terms of local invasion and relationship with the surrounding structures. This information is essential for planning local treatment.

Diagnostic imaging is also of **fundamental importance for the staging of cancer patients**, to assess the extent to which the cancer may have spread throughout the body, allowing the evaluation of the presence or absence of metastases in the lymph nodes or other internal organs.

The imaging techniques used for the diagnosis and staging of cancer patients are radiography, ultrasound (which is also the fundamental tool for ultrasound-guided biopsies), computed tomography and magnetic resonance imaging. Other less commonly used techniques are positron emission tomography (PET) and CT.

All these techniques, their applications, advantages and disadvantages in the diagnosis of tumours are discussed in detail in chapter: "Diagnostic imaging of the cancer patient" of this book.

Palliative Care in the Pet with Cancer

Pain Management

Despite the fact that cancer pain is a described and known entity in pets and the fact that obvious pain associated with specific tumours such as osteosarcoma (OSA) has long been emphasised as a criterion for its diagnosis, there is very **little literature specifically investigating cancer pain in companion animals**.

Encouragingly, in recent years the first studies available on the subject have been published and started to analyse the mechanisms of cancer pain in companion animals. Not all tumours are painful, and the amount of pain is likely to vary considerably from animal to animal, even with similar tumour types. Using a conservative estimate, **30% of tumours in dogs and cats are associated with significant pain at the time of diagnosis**. Tumours most likely to be associated with pain include those of the oral cavity, bone, urogenital tract, eyes, nose, nerve roots, gastrointestinal tract, and skin.

In addition to that caused by the tumour itself, pain in cancer patients can also result from chemotherapy, radiation therapy, or surgery (perioperative pain, postoperative pain, and conditions such as the "phantom limb" associated with some amputations) and from concurrent conditions such as osteoarthritis, gingivitis and dermatological conditions.

General Approach to the Treatment of Cancer Pain

The incidence of pain in animals caused by cancer is very difficult to estimate, as is the effectiveness of analgesic therapy. Recent surveys have found that a significant number of animals in the operating environment were not receiving pain relief, although an overview of these studies seems to suggest that the situation is improving.

Analgesics are even less likely to be used for cancer pain. Glucocorticoids provide some analgesia, and their use may be more widespread, but specific treatment of cancer pain in animals is still likely to be suboptimal (Box 2).

Effective cancer treatment often involves a combination of pharmacological and non-pharmacological treatment, and good communication between all parties involved.

Box 2. Factors which mean the treatment of pain in animals with cancer is not optimum

- **Lack of appreciation that many cancers are associated with significant pain.**
- **Over focusing on the treatment of the cancer, instead of the comfort of the patient.**
- **Inability to evaluate pain in patients with cancer.**
- **Lack of knowledge of drugs, pharmacological treatment and other techniques to relieve pain.**
- **Lack of communication with clients and collaboration with clients in the evaluation and treatment phases.**
- **Under usage of nursing personnel for the evaluation and reevaluation of pain in patients with cancer.**

Evaluation of Pain Associated with Cancer

Assessing pain in animals is difficult, and yet extremely important. An individual animal's pain tolerance is likely to vary widely and is further complicated by the innate ability of dogs and cats to mask significant illness and pain. Physiological variables such as heart rate, respiratory rate, temperature, and pupil size are not accurate measures of acute perioperative pain in dogs and are unlikely to be helpful in chronic pain.

Changes in behaviour appear to be the **mainstay of pain assessment in cats and dogs suffering from cancer**. In general, if a tumour is considered painful in humans, it is appropriate to give an animal with a similar condition the benefit of the doubt and treat it for pain.

One of the most useful ways to determine if a tumour is painful is to **palpate the area and assess the animal's response**. Often this is not precisely correlated with the amount of pain the animal experiences spontaneously, but if a tumour is painful on handling or palpation, there is very likely spontaneous pain associated with it. As veterinarians measuring spontaneous pain is difficult. **Technicians, nurses, and other staff should be involved in pain assessment**, because they are generally the ones who spend the most time with patients in the hospital environment and may have the most time for relaxed and informal conversations with owners.

The most important people in the evaluation process are the owners. The vet should work closely with the owner to capture this information. Owners need to be educated as to what signs to look for and what particular behaviours are indicative of pain.

After **identifying and recording very specific changes in behaviour**, these can be used to monitor the effectiveness of analgesic therapy. In humans, quality of life (QOL) is a complex, abstract and multidimensional concept that defines an individual's satisfaction with life in areas that the individual considers important. The term HRQOL (health-related quality of life) reflects an attempt to restrict this complex concept to those aspects of life specifically related to the health of the individual and potentially modifiable through their care. **Both QOL and HRQOL have been used in veterinary medicine**: questionnaires have been developed to evaluate HRQOL in dogs and cats with cancer. Although pain certainly appears to be assessed with these tools, it is **not known how specific or sensitive** they are to ensure actions that reduce pain are exerted.

It is important to evaluate each of the following three aspects at each visit.

1. Palpation-induced pain.
2. Activity parameters.
3. Behavioural parameters.

Follow-up is important and evaluation of activity and behavioural parameters can be assessed over the phone.

Pharmacological Treatment

Drugs are the cornerstone of cancer pain management, although non-pharmacological complementary therapies are becoming increasingly important. The World Health Organization (WHO) has outlined a general approach to the treatment of cancer pain based on the use of the following groups of analgesics:

- non-opioid analgesics (for example, nonsteroidal anti-inflammatory drugs [NSAIDs] or acetaminophen)
- weak opioid drugs (such as codeine)
- strong opioid drugs (for example, morphine)
- adjuvant medications (such as corticosteroids, tricyclic antidepressants, anticonvulsants, N-methyl D-aspartate [NMDA] antagonists).

There is little information in medicine and practically none in veterinary medicine about which drugs are most effective for particular types of cancer pain. Many veterinary cancer patients present at an advanced stage of the disease and therefore already have moderate to severe pain. After pain has been present for a while, changes occur in the central nervous system (CNS) that alter the way pain signals are processed.

Classification of Pain Associated with Cancer

Pain is a multifactorial experience with **sensory** (feeling), **affective/emotional** (how does it make the subject feel) **and functional** (if the subject can still perform particular functions) components.

It can result from obvious causes (for example, an ulcerated skin tumour) and last for an estimated time. However, in many cases (such as pain after amputation), the pain persists after the original painful cancer has been removed or the surgical wound appears to have healed. In the past, pain was classified as acute or chronic based solely on duration; the latter is arbitrarily pain that lasts more than 3 to 6 months. However, it is now accepted that this classification is not useful.

It has been suggested that the terms adaptive and maladaptive be adopted:

- **adaptive pain** infers a normal response to tissue damage and involves an inflammatory component (e.g. a surgical incision) and is reversible over a relatively short time;
- **maladaptive pain** is the consequence of changes in the spinal cord and brain that result in abnormal sensory processing and is generally persistent. Maladaptive pain can result from poorly treated adaptive pain, and maladaptive pain can set in quickly in some circumstances. A key feature of maladaptive pain is central sensitisation: changes in the CNS (anywhere from the dorsal root ganglion cranially) that are likely initiated by cell coiling and result in amplification and facilitation of generation and transmission of nociceptive signals. **Until proven otherwise, cancer pain should be considered maladaptive**, with peripheral and central changes in pain processing contributing to its occurrence, in addition to the deleterious contribution of the cancer or pathologic area.

Ideally, pain would be classified by the underlying mechanism, e.g. inflammatory or neuropathic. However, many diseases are associated with overlapping "forms" of pain. Pain that occurs in different diseases or conditions would be classified by the underlying mechanisms in that particular disease and even in the patient. This could be called the **neurobiological signature of pain in a particular disease or patient**. Knowing this would better guide the professional in choosing an appropriate treatment. For example, a diagnosis of "cancer pain" is not very helpful, as the cause could be mechanical compression of a nerve, inflammation from tissue necrosis, mechanical distension of an organ, neuropathic pain, or a combination of all of these. However, a diagnosis of "transitional cell carcinoma bladder pain", with associated knowledge of peripheral sodium channel upregulation (e.g. NaV1.7), acid-sensing ion channel receptors (ASIC) central glial and nerve growth factor, cellular activity, and cyclooxy-genase-2 (COX-2) enzyme is much more informative in terms of guiding clinical treatment. Without this information, the treatment is empirical and is reduced to trial and error.

Early intervention is recommended to limit cell stimulation and prevent central sensitisation. In patients who experience persistent and long-lasting pain, which is common in cancer, changes may occur within the peripheral and central nervous systems. These changes (peripheral or central sensitisation) contribute to increased development of pain, separate from the initial cause that produced it. This should be considered in patients with pain who do not respond to first-line or conventional analgesics. Pain syndromes commonly associated with sensitisation include prolonged pain or pain experienced outside the immediately affected area, hyperalgesia (increased sensitivity to noxious stimuli), and allodynia (pain after non-noxious stimuli). Currently, the most important thing to remember in treating cancer pain is that in most situations, **multimodal therapy (use of more than one class of drug) is necessary for successful pain relief**.

Drugs and Strategies for Pain Management in Cancer Patients

There are no specific studies for most of the medications usually used to treat cancer pain in pets. Tables 4 and 5 show a series of treatments whose doses are the general doses used for painful conditions in dogs and cats, respectively, and the comments are based on the author's experience and pharmacological literature.

Nonsteroidal Anti-inflammatory Drugs

NSAIDs have been the foundation of therapy for chronic pain, especially osteoarthritis, and are an excellent first line of treatment for cancer pain:

- on a population basis, all NSAIDs are probably equally effective in relieving pain, but for a given patient, one

Table 4. Suggested analgesic doses to alleviate chronic pain associated with cancer in dogs.

Medication	Dose	Comments
Amantadine	· 4–5 mg/kg PO/day	Can cause diarrhoea at high doses. Do not use in patients with heart failure
Amitriptyline	· 0.5–2 mg/kg PO/day	Use with care if in combination with tramadol
Transdermal fentanyl patches	· 2–5 µg/kg/h	Very useful for short term control of pain, for example in pathological fractures. Limitation: patches need replacing every 4–7 days
Gabapentin	· 3–10 mg/kg PO/6–12 h	Can cause sedation. Useful for neuropathic pain
Pamidronate	· 1–1.5 mg/kg diluted in 4 ml/kg of saline solution (NaCl), slow IV infusion over 30 minutes to 2 h · Repeat every 4–6 weeks	Provide analgesia only for osteolytic lesions. Potential for nephrotoxicity at doses higher or more frequent than the recommended
Paracetamol (acetaminophen) + codeine (30 or 60 mg)	· 10–15 mg/kg de acetaminophen PO/12 h	Can cause sedation with doses of codeine over 2 mg/kg
Paracetamol (acetaminophen)	· 10–15 mg/kg PO/12 h	Can be combined with an NSAID to combat severe pain
Paracetamol (acetaminophen) + prednisolone	· 0.25–1 mg/kg PO/12–24 h · Reduce if possible every 48 h after 14 days	This combination is useful if there is a significant inflammatory component as part of the cause of pain. NSAIDs should not be administered with this combination
Prednisone	· 0,25–1 mg/kg PO/12–24 h · Reduce if possible every 48 h after 14 days	Useful corticoids when there is a severe inflammatory component as part of the pain or neoplasia in the peripheral nerves or CNS due to them crossing the haematocephalic barrier
Tramadol	· 4–5 mg/kg PO/6–12 h	Can be useful in visceral pain, but not for joint pain
Zoledronate	· 0.1–0.2 mg/kg in 50–100 ml 0.9% NaCl, IV in 15 min · Maximum of 4 mg per dog, can be repeated every 21–28 days	Only provides analgesia for osteolytic lesions

GI: gastrointestinal; NSAIDs: nonsteroidal anti-inflammatories; IV: intravenous; PO: oral.

Table 5. Suggested analgesic doses to alleviate chronic pain associated with cancer in cats.

Medication	Dose	Comments
Amantadine	· 3–5 mg/kg PO/24 h	Needs reformulation in capsules for cats
Amitriptyline	· 0.5–2 mg/kg PO/24 h	Can be combined with an NSAID
Buprenorphine	· 0.01–0.02 mg/kg sublingual/oral mucosa/8–12 h	Doses under 5–10 µg/kg can be used for long term administration, especially when combined with other drugs
Butorphanol	· 0.2–1 mg/kg PO/6 h	Considered to have little analgesic effect, has more effect in the case of visceral pain combined with other drugs
Gabapentin	· 10 mg/kg/12 h	Particularly effective when previous treatments seem to no longer work due to increased sensitivity
Ketoprofen	· 1 mg/kg PO/24 h	Used for chronic pain with a 5-day rest period between treatments or long term at 1 mg/kg every 3 days. Another regime is 0.5 mg/kg for 5 consecutive days and 2 rest days (weekend)
Meloxicam	· 0.1 mg/kg PO on day 1 and then 0.05 mg/kg daily indefinitely	The lowest dose evaluated which has been seen to have an effect on osteoarthritis is 0.035 mg/kg/day
Piroxicam	· 1 mg/cat PO daily for a maximum of 7 days	Usually administered on alternate days for long term treatment
Prednisolone	· 0.5–1 mg/kg PO/24 h	Useful in round cell tumours and when there is significant inflammation as the cause of pain. Do not combine with NSAIDs
Prednisone	· 0.5–1 mg/kg PO/24 h	Useful in round cell tumours and when there is significant inflammation as the cause of pain. Do not combine with NSAIDs
Robenacoxib	· 1–2 mg/kg/24 h	Useful for long term administration
Tramadol	· 1–2 mg/kg/12–24 h	Recent findings suggest that it can be effective against chronic pain in cats, but that the tablets can be very bitter
Transdermal fentanyl patches	· 2–5 µg/kg/h	The patch provides 5–7 days analgesia

GI: gastrointestinal; NSAIDs: nonsteroidal anti-inflammatories; IV: intravenous; PO: oral.

  - drug is often more effective than another;
- gastrointestinal side effects associated with NSAID use appear to be more common with drugs that preferentially block COX-1 over COX-2;
- there is no difference in kidney toxicity between COX-1 selective drugs and COX-2 selective drugs;
- hepatic toxicity can occur with any NSAID;
- there are no NSAIDs which are completely safe, but approved NSAIDs are significantly safer than older ones not approved for use in pets; and
- long-term or continuous use of NSAIDs appears to be more effective than short-term use. In relatively stable disease states, gradual dose reduction may be possible whilst maintaining efficacy.

Meloxicam is the only NSAID licensed for long-term administration approved in the European Union for the treatment of musculoskeletal pain in cats. However, several of these compounds can probably be used safely. The key to safe administration of NSAIDs in chronic conditions in cats is using the smallest effective dose and avoiding use or using reduced doses in cats with kidney disease.

The owner should be informed of the possible toxicity of NSAIDs, and which signs they may cause (lethargy, depression, vomiting, melaena, increased water intake). Patients on chronic NSAID therapy **should be monitored** with periodic check-ups (blood and urine tests) to assess kidney and liver function.

If pain relief with NSAIDs is inadequate, oral opioid medications such as morphine or tramadol may be administered (see below). Paracetamol/codeine combinations can often be used in conjunction with NSAIDs. Transdermal fentanyl can also be used. Fentanyl, morphine, or tramadol can be used in dogs that cannot be treated with NSAIDs. Other agents used to treat chronic pain include: amantadine (an NMDA antagonist), anticonvulsants like gabapentin, and tricyclic antidepressants like amitriptyline. All of these can be combined with NSAIDs, although the full extent of side effects or potential adverse interactions are unknown, especially in cancer patients who may be receiving other treatments.

Paracetamol

Paracetamol or acetaminophen is a **non-acidic NSAID**. With any chronic pain there are always CNS changes, so for what seems like a "peripheral" problem like many cancers, centrally acting pain relievers can be very effective. Although it is **highly toxic in cats, even in small amounts**, it can be used effectively in dogs to control pain in an acute context. There are no toxicity studies in dogs, but if toxicity was seen it would likely affect the liver and should be **used with caution in dogs with liver dysfunction**. It can be used alone or in combination with codeine and is initially dosed at approximately 10 to 15 mg/kg twice daily. The author often uses it as first-line analgesic therapy in dogs with compromised kidney function in which NSAIDs cannot be used or in dogs that appear to be intolerant to NSAIDs (from vomiting or gastrointestinal ulcers).

Opioids

Opioids are an effective part of cancer pain management, particularly when used as **part of a multimodal approach** (that is they include complementary NSAIDs or analgesics).

Side effects of opioids include diarrhoea, vomiting, sedation, and constipation with long-term use. Oral morphine, transdermal fentanyl, oral butorphanol, oral mucosal buprenorphine (cats only), and oral codeine are most commonly used for the relief of chronic cancer pain. None of these drugs have been fully evaluated for their clinical toxicity when administered long-term or for their efficacy against chronic cancer pain.

Dosing must be done on an individual basis, and dose adjustment to produce effective analgesia without undesirable side effects requires interaction and communication with clients. However, despite these suggestions, recent evidence has indicated that oral opioids may not achieve effective plasma concentrations in dogs when administered at levels currently recommended. There is currently no information on the long-term use of oral opioids for chronic pain in the cat.

There is **individual variation in the level of analgesia achieved with certain opioids**, especially in the case of acute pain with morphine and butorphanol. Buprenorphine appears to produce predictable analgesia when administered sublingually/orally and is well tolerated in cats. The small volume required (max. 0.066 ml/g [20 µg/kg]) simplifies administration. Based on clinical feedback from owners, this is an acceptable technique for home use. Loss of appetite can occur after several days of treatment, and sometimes lower doses (5 to 10 µg/kg) can overcome this problem. Simultaneous administration with other medications requires less frequent doses.

N-methyl D-aspartate Antagonists

The N-methyl D-aspartate (NMDA) receptor appears to be **key to the induction and maintenance of central sensitisation** and the use of NMDA receptor antagonists appears to offer benefit where central sensitisation has been established, that is, especially in chronic pain. Ketamine, tiletamine, and amantadine possess NMDA antagonist properties, among other actions.

Ketamine is not useful for the treatment of chronic pain due to the formulation available and the tendency to cause dysphoric side effects, even at low doses. Oral ketamine has not been evaluated in dogs or cats for long-term administration. Intraoperative microdoses of ketamine appear to provide beneficial effects for a variety of oncological surgical procedures, including limb amputations, which may decrease the incidence of chronic pain after surgery. Other studies suggest using low-dose perioperative ketamine, administered as a bolus (0.5 mg/kg IV) followed by an infusion (10 µg/kg/min) before and during surgical stimulation. A lower infusion rate (2 µg/kg/min) may be beneficial during the first 24 hours postoperatively and an even lower rate (1 µg/kg/min) over the next 24 hours. In the absence of an infusion pump, ketamine can be mixed in a bag of crystalloid solutions during anaesthesia at a rate of 10 ml/kg/h, 60 mg (0.6 ml) of ketamine should be added to a bag of 1 litre of crystalloid fluids to administer ketamine at 10 µg/kg/min.

Amantadine has been used for the treatment of neuropathic pain in humans and adding amantadine to the treatment in dogs that do not get complete pain relief with NSAIDs is believed to have advantages. Amantadine should be avoided in patients with congestive heart failure, a history of seizures, or those being administered with selegiline, sertraline, or tricyclic antidepressants.

Combination Analgesics

Tramadol is a synthetic derivative of codeine and is classified as an opioidergic, monoaminergic drug. The analgesic efficacy of tramadol is the result of complex interactions between the opiate, adrenergic, and serotonin receptor systems. Hepatic demethylation of tramadol produces the active metabolite, O-desmethyltramadol (M1). Different metabolites interact with different receptors, so efficacy in different species will likely depend on the metabolic characteristics in that particular species. Early research in dogs suggested that tramadol was sufficiently absorbed, producing levels that would theoretically provide analgesia. However, there is no published evidence of efficacy for canine pain.

Little is known about the side effects of tramadol in dogs and almost nothing is known about the side effects seen when tramadol is combined with other drugs in treatments for people or dogs. A recent study in rats evaluating the analgesic effects of various doses of rofecoxib and tramadol alone and in combination found that the combination of tramadol and rofecoxib with the most analgesic effects produced gastric lesions that were more severe than with rofecoxib or tramadol alone. Tramadol is metabolised differently in the cat and appears to have clinical efficacy when administered perioperatively intravenously and has shown antinociceptive activity when administered orally in an experimental setting.

Anticonvulsant Drugs

Many anticonvulsants, such as gabapentin, have been used to treat chronic pain. **Gabapentin and pregabalin are among the most effective drugs available for neuropathic pain in humans**, although the exact mechanism of action is unclear. One potential way by which they exert their analgesic effect is by binding to the α2-δ protein subunit of voltage-gated calcium channels, thus reducing the release of excitatory neurotransmitters through channel modulation or channel trafficking.

There is information on the availability of gabapentin in dogs and some information on its use as an anticonvulsant, but not on its use for the control of chronic or long-term pain. Information on the kinetics of gabapentin in cats is available but there are no scientific publications demonstrating its efficacy for long-term pain in this species. **The guidelines for gabapentin (and pregabalin) are unclear in veterinary patients**, although they appear to be helpful for cancer pain in some patients and are likely to be particularly effective in cancers with a neurogenic or nerve-destroying component.

Tricyclic Antidepressants

Tricyclic antidepressants have **been used for many years for the treatment of chronic pain syndromes in people** and are being used extensively for the modulation of behavioural disorders in animals.

Within the CNS, there are descending inhibitory serotonergic and noradrenergic pathways that reduce pain transmission in the spinal cord. Tricyclic antidepressants such as amitriptyline, clomipramine, fluoxetine, imipramine, maprotiline and paroxetine mainly inhibit the reuptake of several monoamines (serotonin for clomipramine, fluoxetine and paroxetine; noradrenaline for imipramine, amitriptyline and maprotiline).

Tricyclic antidepressants may also interact directly with 5-hydroxytryptamine (5-HT) and peripheral noradrenergic receptors and may also contribute to other actions, such as voltage-gated sodium channel blockade and reduced peripheral prostaglandin E2 (PGE2) activity or tumour necrosis factor (TNF).

The tricyclic antidepressant amitriptyline **appears to be effective in the cat for pain relief in interstitial cystitis** and many veterinarians report efficacy in other chronically painful conditions in the cat, including osteoarthritis. Amitriptyline has been used daily for periods of up to a year for interstitial cystitis and few side effects are reported. It probably should not be used simultaneously with other drugs that modify the serotonergic system, such as amantadine or tramadol, until more is known about drug interactions.

Sodium Channel Blockage

Alterations in the level of expression, cellular localisation, and distribution of sodium channels are observed in many pain states. These aberrantly expressed sodium channels produce **hyperexcitability and ectopic activity in peripheral and central nerves that encode nociceptive information**.

Low doses of **lidocaine and other sodium channel blockers produce pain relief**. Low dose IV lidocaine has been shown to be as effective as other commonly used medications for the treatment of neuropathic pain in humans and can be used to negatively regulate central sensitisation in animals with cancer. There is growing interest in the use of **transdermal lidocaine patches** for the treatment of cancer pain.

The potential systemic toxicity associated with lidocaine administration, including bradycardia, hypotension, cardiac arrest, muscle or facial spasms, tremors, seizures, nausea and vomiting, were **not observed in any study in dogs or cats**. Dosage guidelines have been suggested but their analgesic efficacy has not been evaluated in pets with cancer.

Corticosteroids

Corticosteroids have a **mild analgesic action**, can produce a state of euphoria, and are often used for these reasons to alleviate cancer and cancer pain in cats and dogs. They should not be used simultaneously with NSAIDs because the risk of side effects (especially gastrointestinal) increases dramatically.

Bisphosphonates

Malignant bone disease creates a unique pain state, with a different neurobiological signature to inflammatory and neuropathic pain. Pain associated with bone cancer is initiated and perpetuated by deregulated osteoclastic activity and the activation of nociceptors by prostaglandins, cytokines, and H^+ ions.

Therapies that block osteoclastic activity have the potential to reduce bone pain and may also mitigate other complications, such as pathological fractures and malignant hypercalcaemia. **Bisphosphonates** are synthetic pyrophosphate analogues and inhibit osteoclast activity, they accumulate in bone, and are released after osteoclast-mediated bone resorption, disrupting cellular functions, resulting in osteoclast death.

Oral absorption of bisphosphonates is poor, and **IV dosing** is the preferred route of administration. Possible adverse effects include potential nephrotoxicity at high doses and at higher than therapeutic frequencies, electrolyte abnormalities, and acute phase reactions. In vitro bisphosphonates can exert direct effects on cancer cells, including canine OSA and fibrosarcoma lines. Beneficial effects of IV pamidronate have been described in the treatment of malignant osteolysis associated with primary and secondary bone neoplasms. These studies have also suggested analgesic effects, but they have not been demonstrated using objective methods.

The dose of pamidronate is 1 to 2 mg/kg in a 1-hour infusion (diluted in saline) and this should be repeated at 3-to-5-week intervals. Other examples of bisphosphonates used in dogs are clodronate, alendronate, and zoledronate.

Radiotherapy

Radiation therapy is considered **to alleviate pain associated with secondary osteolysis in malignant canine bone lesions**. For this purpose, hypo fractionated radiotherapy regimens with weekly sessions of 8 to 10 Gy are used in the treatment of primary bone neoplasms and/or bone metastases.

Acupuncture

Acupuncture is applied by **positioning a needle or by positioning a needle combined with electrical stimulation** (high or low frequency, although most types of pain respond to low frequency stimulation).

The results of an experimental study in healthy dogs demonstrated a weak analgesic effect of electroacupuncture in anaesthetised patients, evaluated by a reduction in the minimum alveolar concentration (MAC) of the inhaled anaesthetic agent. Recent data using a rodent model suggests that electroacupuncture may have beneficial effects in treating pain associated with bone cancer. As of yet, there is **no evidence that acupuncture relieves pain in veterinary patients**.

Nutritional Approach to Cancer Patients

For years the role of nutrition and its relationship with the development, progression and prevention of various types of cancer has been studied, especially in medicine.

Unfortunately, although this is a very interesting field and is increasingly attracting more interest from owners, **scientific studies in veterinary medicine on this matter are very scarce** and it is very difficult to make exact recommendations for the veterinary cancer patient in relation to their nutrition.

Cancer Metabolism

Most neoplastic cells propagate more efficiently in a medium with a **high concentration of glucose**, probably due to a limited metabolism of fatty acids in combination with an increase in metabolic pathways that use glucose (Warburg effect). **Glycolysis is the main method of energy production in neoplastic cells**.

In addition, tumours participate in the Cori cycle: they consume glucose, produce a large amount of lactate that goes to the liver, where it is resynthesised into glucose, which the tumour cells will reuse. This also contributes to the **increase in resting energy requirements (RER) in cancer patients**.

Several metabolic disturbances have been observed in veterinary cancer patients:

- **in dogs diagnosed with lymphoma**, alterations in carbohydrate metabolism have been observed, such as increased serum lactate and insulin concentrations during the glucose tolerance test, as well as insulin resistance. Alterations in lipid metabolism, such as an increase in the basal concentration of triglycerides and cholesterol, have also been observed in these patients; and
- **in dogs diagnosed with osteosarcoma**, alterations in glucose metabolism, increased protein turnover and loss of protein in the urine were also observed. Likewise, an increase in the expenditure of energy while resting was observed in these dogs.

Anorexia

Anorexia is **common in cancer patients**. In some patients, the cause of anorexia may be related to the medical treatment of cancer: many chemotherapy drugs can cause gastrointestinal toxicity (for example, doxorubicin in dogs), leading to anorexia. These drugs can also cause alterations in the sense of taste and smell of patients. In fact, ageusia or dysgeusia can last for several months before regeneration of the olfactory bulb and/or the tongue.

Cachexia

In people, cachexia is usually diagnosed in association with various neoplasms and aggressive chemotherapy treatment. The mechanisms responsible for its appearance include excessive cytokine stimulation, which will lead to insulin resistance, extensive lipolysis and proteolysis of the tissue reserve. Tumour necrosis factor alpha (TNF-α), IL-1α, and IL-6 appear to promote proteolysis.

Cachexia does **not appear to be as common in canine cancer patients**, especially in cases of non-haematopoietic neoplasms.

Cachexia may be more common in cats. Approximately 56% of cats diagnosed with lymphoma or other solid tumours have a body mass index less than 5/9 (Figure 4). Results of one study showed that cats diagnosed with lymphoma and with a body mass index greater than 5/9 had a mean survival rate of 16.9 months compared to cats with lower body mass indexes, in which the median survival rate was less than 3.3 months in the same study.

Cats hospitalised for radiotherapy treatments may also suffer from reduced caloric intake due to prolonged hospitalisations and repeated anaesthesia that require fasting.

Epidemiology and Risk Factors

A complete and balanced diet is highly recommended. In people, two of the nutritional factors most closely associated with the development of cancer are excessive body weight and the consumption of fruits and vegetables. A western diet and consumption of small amounts of fruits and vegetables are associated with an increased relative risk of developing various types of cancer including colon, prostate and breast, as well as lymphomas and leukaemia.

Not much is known yet about the relationship between cancer development and different types of diet. There are also several confounding factors that can affect the results of the studies, such as the lifestyle of people and their pets, the inclusion, quality and digestibility of ingredients in different diets and the socioeconomic conditions of the owners. In addition, other factors such as the quality of health care, variation in different commercial diets, and environmental exposure can also greatly affect the results of epidemiological studies.

An epidemiological study in veterinary medicine that evaluated the eating habits of dogs diagnosed with mammary carcinomas showed that **dogs with a higher protein intake were linked to a higher survival rate**. In this study, the consumption of fat and carbohydrates had no impact on the median survival rate of these patients. Another study revealed that **dogs fed non-traditional, low-nutritional diets** (e.g. human food scraps) were at **higher risk of developing neoplasms**. In this study there was no association between serum selenium concentration and the likelihood of developing mammary carcinoma, but dogs diagnosed with mammary carcinomas were shown to have lower tissue retinol concentrations. The cause of this low concentration is unknown.

Scottish Terrier dogs have a genetic predisposition for the development of transitional cell carcinoma in the urinary bladder. A study that evaluated the eating habits of this breed of dog showed that the addition of vegetables to their diet was associated with a lower incidence of the development of transitional cell carcinoma of the urinary bladder.

Veterinary studies examining the relationship between obesity and the development of cancer are scarce. While the results of some of these did not show any association between the patients' body mass index and the development of cancer, in others it was shown that obesity is related. Some studies have shown that the risk of developing canine mammary carcinoma is higher in obese bitches and that obesity may also be an independent risk factor. Another study showed that bitches which were obese at one year of age and/or were obese one year before the diagnosis of mammary carcinoma were more likely to develop this neoplastic disease.

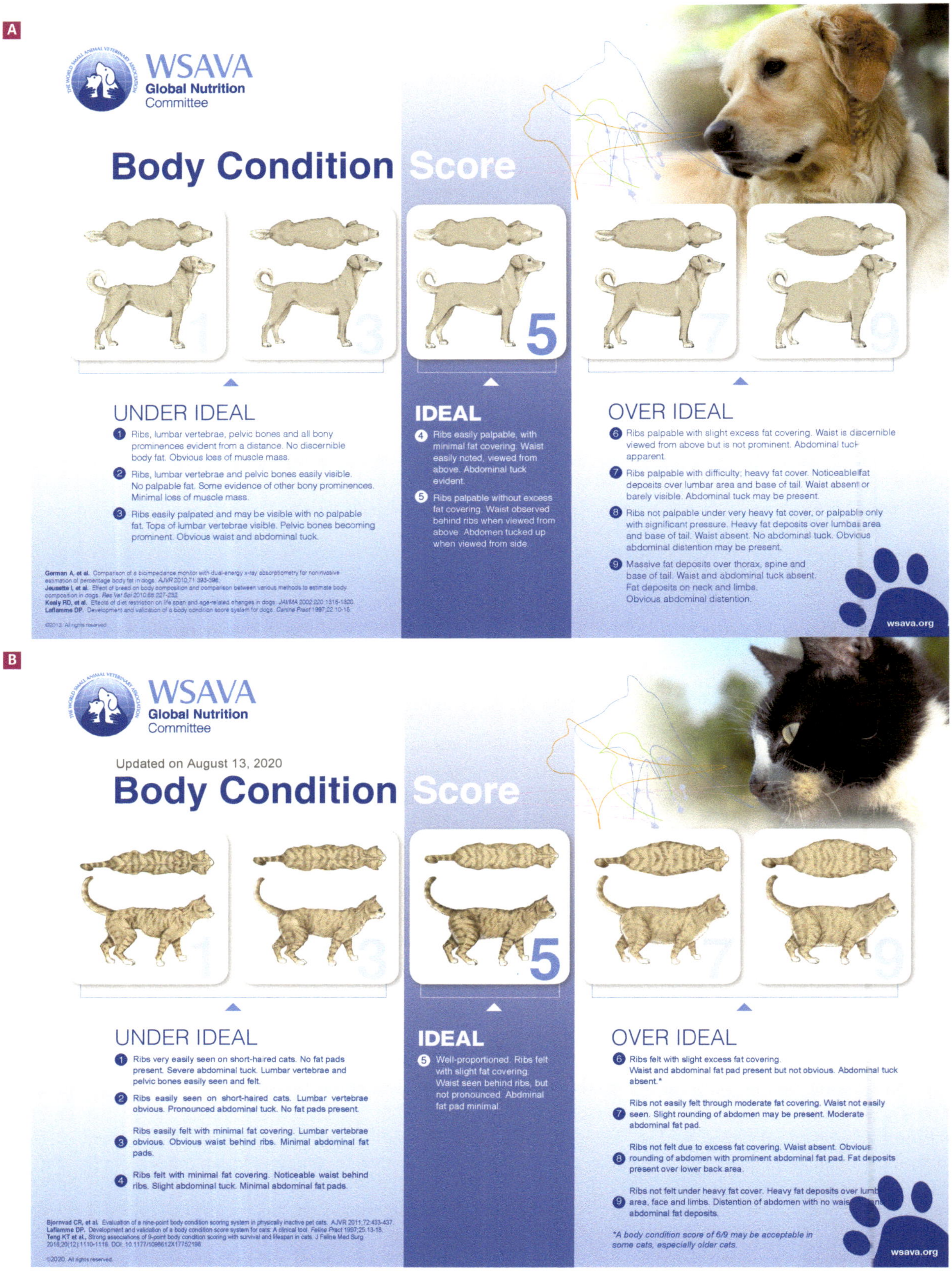

Figure 4. Body condition scoring in the dog (**A**) and cat (**B**). (Courtesy of the World Small Animal Veterinary Association, WSAVA. Toolkit for global nutrition from WSAVA available at: https://wsava.org/wp-content/uploads/2021/04/WSAVA-Global-Nutrition-Toolkit-English.pdf

Nutritional Evaluation

To fully evaluate the cancer patient, **obtaining a complete nutritional history is recommended**. Such information should include:

- body weight
- body mass index
- dietary history before and after anticancer treatment.

It is important that the clinician in charge is well informed about the type and amount of diet ingested by their patients and is also aware if they are receiving any form of nutritional supplement. This information also helps clinicians to feed their patients well during hospitalisation, if necessary, and to recognise any periods of hypophagia.

Evaluation of body weight is very important especially in cases of malnutrition. Malnutrition may be associated with **anorexia** (typically with loss of fat mass) and/or **cachexia** (typically with loss of fat and lean mass) that need treatment. Anorexia can usually be treated with nutritional and pharmacological interventions. Cachexia associated with cancer may require other types of treatments.

Likewise, it is important to consider the **history of seasonal deworming**, since a high parasite load in the gastrointestinal tract may also be associated with weight loss and patients with a depressed immune system due to some chemotherapeutic treatments may be more prone to gastrointestinal parasite infection.

The **body mass index from 1 to 9** (Figure 4) is the most widely used in veterinary medicine. In cats, which are animals where fat is usually deposited in larger quantities in the inguinal and abdominal area, the use of the muscle condition index is also recommended.

Physical examination of a patient can give us information about whether they are malnourished. Some clinical findings associated with malnutrition include poor quality hair, chronic gastrointestinal disorders, seborrhoea, lethargy, and paleness. The first signs of chronic nutritional deficiency in the case of anorexia and/or cachexia syndrome are manifested in regions of rapid cell turnover, including the skin and the gastrointestinal system, as well as with haematological alterations, especially in cases of prolonged anorexia. Chronic malnutrition can result in reduced haemoglobin and erythrocyte levels, hypoproteinaemia, and hypoalbuminaemia.

Owners using non-traditional diets should receive adequate training from a veterinary nutritionist. This type of diet has gained popularity in recent years and some of them may lack certain minerals such as calcium, iron and copper, which can result in haematological and bone disorders. Some home-made diets can also lack bone content and subsequently cause hyperparathyroidism and osteopaenia.

In dogs, obesity may be a bigger problem than malnutrition, although treating obesity is not usually a priority in most cancer patients. In one study, 68% of dogs lost weight during anticancer treatment, although this loss was less than 5% of their body weight, and 30% of dogs in this study were obese before starting anticancer therapy.

Feeding the Hospitalised Cancer Patient

The cancer patient may require hospitalisation in several cases, such as to treat adverse effects to chemotherapy (for example, gastrointestinal toxicity after administration of doxorubicin in a dog) or for radiotherapy (for example, in case of radiotherapy for an oral tumour in a cat).

The resting energy requirement (RER) is usually sufficient for the hospitalised cancer patient, but there are cases in which calculating the **disease energy requirement is recommended which can be between 1.1 to 2 times the RER**, for example in cases of transudate or exudate associated with the repair process and excessive protein loss.

When a patient is discharged, his RER usually increases as a result of increased activity, so this energy consumption should be adjusted to the RER at home.

Pharmacological and Affection Feeding Stimulation

Ensuring **adequate energy consumption** is very important in the cancer patient. However, this can be difficult in some situations, for example if the patient has a decreased appetite. Certain behaviours such as hand-feeding or feeding during family visiting hours can help canine and feline patients' feeding. In hospitalised cats, a covered food cage may be considered inside the hospitalisation cage away from the litter tray, where cats feel more secure and calm.

Addition of certain flavours can help: dogs have receptors for salt and sugar and cats have receptors for salt, although cats are often more likely to reject very salty foods. Adding protein to the diet can also increase appetite, as dogs tend to prefer foods that are high in protein and cats have lingual receptors for amino acids.

Supplementation with animal or vegetable fat can also be considered since it helps to make the food more palatable for animals, but it should be taken into account that an excessive amount of fat can decrease the nutritional value of the diet.

Offering other foods that the animal is not used to can also help a lot, but it is important to remember that one to two meals should be offered at a time, nothing more, since offering several meals at the same time can cause food aversion, especially if the animal is suffering from nausea.

A pharmacological approach to support enteral feeding may be necessary in some cases. The use of mirtazapine can increase appetite and decrease vomiting in cats, due to its anti-serotonergic action. Recent studies have shown that capromorelin can promote food consumption in hospitalised dogs due to its action as a ghrelin agonist. The action of capromorelin on the appetite in cats is currently being studied.

Assisted Enteral Feeding

In many cases, enteral nutritional support must be considered, particularly if a patient is not consuming adequate caloric requirements. Various techniques may be considered, such as syringe feeding, nasogastric tube placement, oesophagostomy tube, or gastric feeding tube.

Syringe feeding is the simplest method of performing assisted enteral feeding, although this can be quite difficult especially if the patient is nauseated and anosmic.

Nasogastric tubes are very useful for hospitalised patients, although they are limited to the administration of a liquid enteral diet due to their size, whereas **oesophagostomy tubes are ideal for medium to long-term enteral feeding** and are usually left in place for between two weeks and three months. Regarding **gastrostomy tubes, they should be considered when it is estimated that nutritional supplementation will be necessary for more than 6 to 8 weeks**. The advantages of these tubes are the direct delivery of nutrients to the stomach and the fact that in the case of emesis, this should not cause aversion to the tube.

Oesophagostomy and gastrostomy tubes allow for assisted enteral feeding of various diets. It is important to remember that some diets combined with water become a solution with less than 1 kcal per millilitre. Some veterinary prescription foods are higher in protein and fat and can be administered in smaller amounts when the patient is nauseated or cannot tolerate administration of large amounts of food. Some examples of these diets include Royal Canin Recovery RS, Hill's a/d, Purina CN, and Carnivore Care (Table 6).

Assisted Parenteral Feeding

If assisted enteral feeding is not feasible for a patient, assisted parenteral feeding should be considered.

There are two types of assisted parenteral feeding:

- **total assisted parenteral feeding**
- **partial assisted parenteral feeding**, which may also commonly be referred to as peripheral assisted parenteral feeding.

Veterinary studies on assisted parenteral feeding are limited and information on the usefulness of the three main substrate types (glucose, amino acids, and lipids) is unclear. One technique is to use glucose and lipid energy requirements and then add amino acids based on protein requirements per kg of patient bodyweight. Another technique is to just add the minimum required amount of protein in the form of amino acids as part of the RER. Protein requirements of the sick patient are not well understood, although slightly more protein than the required amount is usually added since protein turnover is faster during catabolic disease.

The addition of B-complex vitamins and cobalamin supplementation should also be considered, depending on the case. In addition, in cases of prolonged total assisted parenteral feeding, calcium supplementation should be considered.

Table 6. Examples of high calorie diets with elevated protein and fat content.

Diet	Calories	Protein	Fat	Water (ml) to be added to obtain 1 kcal/ml
Hill's a/d (156 g)	1.2 kcal/ml	9.2 g/100 kcal	6.3 g/100 kcal	30
Purina CN (156 g)	1.4 kcal/ml	8.0 g/100 kcal	7.5 g/100 kcal	53
Royal Canin Recovery RS (164 g)	1.1 kcal/ml	9.9 g/100 kcal	6.4 g/100 kcal	18

During the first day of total assisted parenteral feeding, it is recommended that only half of the caloric requirements be administered, mainly if the patient had a clinical history of anorexia, due to the possible development of refeeding syndrome. **Refeeding syndrome** is characterised by the development of hypophosphataemia, hypokalaemia, and hypomagnesaemia, due to rapid glucose metabolism when feeding is initiated after a prolonged period of anorexia. The patient's electrolytes should be assessed every 12 to 24 hours for the first 48 to 72 hours after implementing total assisted parenteral feeding.

Assisted parenteral feeding should be administered through a sterile catheter with its own multiple inlet line and the most distal inlet should be reserved for parenteral feeding. The administration of other medications along the same line should be avoided, since many medications are not compatible with parenteral feeding. Due to the high osmolality and pH of less than 7 of parenteral feeding, a vein of the largest possible calibre should be used to avoid the development of thrombophlebitis.

Some complications have been reported in animals receiving assisted parenteral feeding, including the development of hyperglycaemia, especially in cats. The development of sepsis in association with this type of feeding is a rare complication, although it can occur due to a transmigration of bacteria into the portal vein.

Nutritional Support for the Cancer Patient

The benefit of specific dietary regimes for the cancer patient continues to be studied and it is **not yet clear whether some types of diets can affect neoplasm progression**.

Neoplastic growth is glycolytic in nature and it has been hypothesised that there may be a benefit in limiting carbohydrate intake. However, more studies are needed to confirm this theory. If carbohydrates are limited, the energy source should be replaced by the addition of protein and/or fat. The addition of protein leads to an increase in the activity of deaminases and transaminases, which will cause conversion of protein into glucose and glucose carbon precursors, or synthesis of fatty acids, which means serum glucose concentration and glucose delivery to neoplastic cells are kept constant.

Results from one study showed that a diet rich in polyunsaturated fat (rich in ω-3 fatty acids) and arginine was associated with a higher median survival and remission rate in dogs with lymphoma. Another study regarding xenograft tumours in rodents showed that a diet rich in protein (50%) and low in carbohydrates reduced tumour growth. As the protein concentration in this diet was high, it may be that the benefit of the diet on tumour growth in this study was due to the protein concentration.

In cats there may be a benefit to using a protein-rich diet to increase muscle mass when these patients have a weakened lean mass.

If appetite is reduced, a diet rich in protein and fat increases palatability and caloric density.

However, in summary, there are currently no specific nutritional recommendations for the veterinary cancer patient and more studies and clinical trials are needed. Each patient should be evaluated individually based on their body condition, type of neoplastic disease and type of anticancer treatment. The most important thing is to provide a complete and balanced nutrition to prevent weight loss and always ensure a good quality of life for the animal.

Amino Acids

Amino acids can have an **inhibitory effect on neoplastic cell proliferation** and a high protein mixed diet is usually recommended to promote enterocyte health and mucosal barrier function.

Low millimolar concentrations of arginine have been shown to be capable of altering cell cycle progression and inhibiting proliferation of various neoplastic cells. Results from one study showed that dogs diagnosed with lymphoma that were fed a diet rich in arginine and ω-3 fatty acids had a higher median survival and remission rate. However, the addition of arginine to the diet requires further study. There are also some drawbacks with arginine supplementation: the required dose of arginine exceeds 100 mg/kg of body weight, its taste is quite bitter, and there is the possibility of causing amino acid imbalance if arginine is administered long-term.

There are also some studies on the usefulness of glutamine supplementation, although its real effect is not clear, since the use of glutamine by enterocytes and first-pass hepatic metabolism do not allow it to have any significant effect on fat mass.

Polyunsaturated Fats

The use of fat in the diet is **very useful to improve its palatability and caloric density**. Results of some studies in humans and rodents suggest that the consumption of high concentrations of ω-3 fatty acids, such as eicosapentaenoic acid (EPA) and docosahexaenoic acid (DHA), can produce changes in lean body mass and reduce the rate of neoplastic growth.

A study in dogs with cancer that received a diet rich in ω-3 fatty acids from fish showed a small improvement in the median survival rate of these patients. However, the data collected in this study is difficult to interpret, since other variables such as the addition of arginine could have affected the results.

At the moment, veterinary studies on the benefit of supplementing the diet with ω-3 fatty acids are very limited, but there are probably few disadvantages to increasing the consumption of ω-3 fatty acids in the diet of cancer patients. However, due to the lack of studies, the recommended dose of ω-3 fatty acids in these cases remains unclear. It is important to note that in cats dietary supplementation with ω-3 fatty acids can be associated with platelet disorders and alterations in clotting times, although this also requires further studies.

Vitamins and Minerals

Supplementation in the cancer patient with vitamins and minerals is **an area of great interest in medicine**, with special attention to the study of vitamins A, D and selenium. In some preclinical models, the use of some vitamins was associated with a reduction in cell proliferation. Many studies are being performed in this area of medicine.

Various studies have shown that dogs diagnosed with lymphomas and mast cell tumours have lower vitamin D levels than healthy dogs, making vitamin D status a very interesting area of study.

A recent clinical trial in dogs diagnosed with mast cell tumours that received treatment with high doses of calcitriol, showed that most of these patients developed toxicity and clinical signs of hypercalcaemia, loss of appetite and vomiting associated with administration, so more studies are necessary in this area.

Antioxidants

Most veterinary oncology referral centres do not usually recommend the use of antioxidants, herbal supplements and home-made or raw diets, due to the lack of clinical studies that justify their use and guarantee their safety.

According to one study, approximately 65% of the owners of veterinary patients are using some type of alternative treatment and approximately 30% are administering oral supplements. Furthermore, approximately 50% of the veterinarians of these patients approve of the use of these treatments. Another study also showed that more than 50% of pet owners start offering some type of non-traditional diet if they are diagnosed with cancer. About 39% supplement their pets' diet.

In tumour tissues there is an imbalance between oxidising and antioxidant substances. In theory, the administration of antioxidant substances would make sense, although it must be taken into account that some of these substances may have pro-oxidant properties in some cases.

There are several in vitro studies of the efficacy of different antioxidants in the treatment of neoplastic cells: isoflavones appear to induce apoptosis of mitochondria in canine lymphoma cells. Rosemary and turmeric extracts showed antineoplastic activity and synergistic action when administered at doses higher than the expected physiological dose in epithelial, round and mesenchymal neoplastic cells. However, the results of a more recent study contradicted these findings.

Although most antioxidant supplements may not have detrimental effects on cancer patients, nor a negative impact on the results of cancer treatment, there are other aspects to consider about their use as well, including absorption, hepatic metabolism and obtaining in vivo concentrations similar to in vitro study concentrations. It must also be taken into account that in most cases it is not known whether certain nutritional supplements can cause some type of negative synergy in combination with some conventional anticancer treatments or increase the probability of developing toxicities associated with the treatments. More clinical studies are necessary to study the necessary doses and the efficacy and safety of the different types of antioxidants.

Bibliography

The Aetiology of Cancer

■ Adams, V.J., Evans, K.M., Sampson, J. et al. (2010) Methods and mortality results of a health survey of purebred dogs in the UK. *J Small Anim Pract*, 51, 512–524.

■ B Melin, M., Rivera, P., Arendt, M. et al. (2016) Genome-wide analysis identifies germ-line risk factors associated with canine mammary tumours. *PLoS Genet*, 12:e1006029.

■ Balmain, A., Gray, J., Ponder, B. (2003) The genetics and genomics of cancer. *Nature Genetics*, 33:238.

■ Breen, M, Modiano, J.F. (2008) Evolutionarily conserved cytogenetic changes in hematologic malignancies of dogs and humans—man and his best friend share more than companionship. *Chromosome Res*, 16:145–54.

■ Devita V.T., Hellman, S., Rosenberg, S.A. (2005) *Cancer: principles and practice of oncology*, ed 7. Philadelphia: Lippincott Williams & Wilkins.

■ Fidler, I.J (2003) The pathogenesis of cancer metastasis: the 'seed and soil' hypothesis revisited. *Nat Rev Cancer*, 3:453–458.

■ Gollin, S.M. (2005) Mechanisms leading to chromosomal instability. *Semin Cancer Biol*, 15:33–42.

■ Golub, T.R., Slonim, D.K., Tamayo, P. et al (1999) Molecular classification of cancer: class discovery and class prediction by gene expression monitoring. *Science*, 286:531–37.

■ Grivennikov, S.I., Greten, F.R, Karin, M (2010) Immunity, inflammation, and cancer. *Cell*, 140:883–899.

■ Hanahan, D., Weinberg, R.A. (2000) The hallmarks of cancer. *Cell*, 100:57.

■ Johnson, C.D., Esquela-Kerscher, A., Stefani, G. et al (2007) The let-7 microRNA represses cell proliferation pathways in human cells. *Cancer Res*, 67:7713–22.

■ Lapidot, T., Sirard, C., Vormoor, J. et al (1994) A cell initiating human acute myeloid leukaemia after transplantation into SCID mice. *Nature*, 367:645–48.

■ Modiano, J.F., Ritt, M.G., Wojcieszyn, J. et al (1999) Growth arrest of melanoma cells is differentially regulated by contact inhibition and serum deprivation. *DNA Cell Biol*, 18:357–367.

■ Moore, G.E., Burkman, K.D., Carter, M.N. et al (2001) Causes of death or reasons for euthanasia in military working dogs: 927 cases (1993–1996). *J Am Vet Med Assoc*, 219:209–214.

■ Nowell, P.C. (1976) The clonal evolution of tumour cell populations. Science, 194:23–28.

■ O'Brien, C.A., Kreso, A., Jamieson, C:H. (2010) Cancer stem cells and self- renewal. *Clin Cancer Res*, 16:3113–3120.

■ Pang, L.Y., Argyle, D.J. (2009) Using naturally occurring tumours in dogs and cats to study telomerase and cancer stem cell biology. *Biochim Bio-phys Acta*, 1792:380–391.

■ Pelangaris, S., Khan, M. (2006) *The molecular biology of cancer*. Malden: Blackwell Publishing.

■ Rajagopalan, H., Lengauer, C. (2004) Aneuploidy and cancer. *Nature*, 432:338–341.

■ Sjöblom, T., Jones, S., Wood, L.D. et al (2006) The consensus coding sequences of human breast and colorectal cancer. *Science*, 314:268–74.

■ Tannock, I.F., Hill, R.P., Bristow, R.G., Harrington, L. (2005) *The basic science of oncology*, ed 4. New York: McGraw-Hill.

■ Thomas, R., Borst, L., Rotroff, D. et al (2014) Genomic profiling reveals extensive heterogeneity in somatic DNA copy number aberrations of canine hemangiosarcoma. *Chromosome Res*, 22:305–319.

■ Tomasetti, C., Li, L., Vogelstein, B. (2017) Stem cell divisions, somatic mutations, cancer etiology, and cancer prevention. *Science*, 355:1330–1334.

Carcinogenesis: Physical, Chemical and Hormonal Factors

■ Bertone, E.R., Snyder, L.A., Moore, A.S. (2002) Environmental tobacco smoke and risk of malignant lymphoma in pet cats. *Am J Epidemiol*, 156:268.

■ Bryan, J.N., Henry, C.J., Hahn, A.W., Caldwell, C.W. (2007) A population study of neutering status as a risk factor for canine prostate cancer. *Prostate*, 67:1174.

■ Glickman, L.T., Raghavan, M. Knapp, D.W. et al. (2004) Herbicide exposure and the risk of transitional cell carcinoma of the urinary bladder in Scottish Terriers. *J Am Vet Med Assoc*, 224:1290.

■ Hayes, H.M., Tarone, R.E., Cantor, K.P. et al. (1991) Case-control study of canine malignant lymphoma: positive association with dog owner's use of 2,4-dichlorophenoxyacetic acid herbicides. *J Natl Cancer Inst*, 83:1226.

■ Mcentee, M.C., Page, R.L., Theon, A. et al. (2004) Malignant tumour formation in dogs previously irradiated for acanthomatous epulis. *Vet Radiol Ultrasound*, 45:357.

■ Overley, B., Shofer, F.S., Goldschmidt, M.H. et al. (2005) Association between ovariohysterectomy and feline mammary carcinoma. *J Vet Intern Med*, 19:560.

■ Schneider, R., Dorn, C.R., Taylor, D.O.N (1969) Factors influencing canine mammary tumour development and postsurgical survival. *J Nat Cancer Inst*, 43:1249.

Principles of Tumour Biology and General Pathology of Neoplasms

■ Aitken, M.L., Patnaik, A.K. (2000) Comparison of needle-core (Trucut) biopsy and surgical biopsy for the diagnosis of cutaneous and subcutaneous masses: a prospective study of 51 cases. *J Am Anim Hosp Assoc*, 36:153–157.

■ Ehrhart, E.J., Powers, B. (2013) The Pathology of neoplasia. In: Withrow SJ, Vail DM (eds): *Withrow and MacEwen's Small Animal Clinical Oncology*, 5th Ed. St Louis: Saunder-Elsevier, p. 54–67.

■ Ehrhart, N. (1998) Principles of tumour biopsy. *Clin Tech Small Anim Pract*, 13:10–16.
■ Meuten, D.J. (2002) *Tumors in domestic animals*, ed 4. Ames: Iowa State University Press.
■ Ramos-Vara, J.A. (2005) Technical aspects of immunohistochemistry. *Vet Pathol*, 42:405.
■ Reimer, B.S., Séguin, B., Decock, H.E. et al. (2005) Evaluation of the effect of routine histologic processing on the size of skin samples obtained from dogs. *Am J Vet Res*, 66:500–505.
■ Seitz, S.E., Foley, G.L., Marretta, S.M. (1995) Evaluation of marking materials for cutaneous surgical margins. *Am J Vet Res*, 56:826–833.

Diagnosis in the Cancer Patient

■ Couto, C.G. (2014) Principles of cancer treatment. In: Nelson, R., Couto, C.G. editors. *Small animal internal medicine*, ed. 5. St. Louis: Elsevier, p. 1134.
■ Owen, L.N. (ED) (1980) *TNM Classification of Tumours in Domestic Animals*. World Health Organization, Geneva.
■ Wilthrow, S.J., Susaneck, S.J., Macy, D.W. et al. (1985) Aspiration and punch biopsy techniques for nasal tumours. *Journal of the American Animal Hospital Association*, 21:551–554.
■ Wrigley, R.H. (1991) Ultrasonography of the spleen. Life-threatening splenic disorders. *Problems in Veterinary Medicine*, 3:574–581.

Palliative Care in the Pet with Cancer

■ Biller, B., Berg, J., Garrett, L. et al. (2016) AAHA Oncology guidelines for dogs and cats. *J Am Anim Hosp Assoc*, 52:181–204.
■ Duncan B, Lascelles X, McFarland JM, et al. (2005) Guidelines for safe and effective use of NSAIDs in dogs. *Vet Ther* 6:237–251.
■ Egger, C.M., Glerum, L., Haag, K.M. et al. (2007) Efficacy and cost- effectiveness of transdermal fentanyl patches for the relief of postoperative pain in dogs after anterior cruciate ligament and pelvic limb repair. *Vet Anaesth Analg*, 34:200–208.
■ Fan, T.M., De Lorimier, L.P., Charney, S.C. et al. (2005) Evaluation of IV pamidronate administration in 33 cancer-bearing dogs with primary or secondary bone involvement. *J Vet Intern Med*, 19:74–80.
■ Fan, T.M., Lorimier, L.P.DE, Garrett, L.D. et al. (2008) The bone biologic effects of zoledronate in healthy dogs and dogs with malignant osteolysis. *J Vet Intern Med*, 380–387.
■ Giorgi, M., Saccomanni, G., Łebkowska-Wieruszewska, B. et al. (2009) Pharmacokinetic evaluation of tramadol and its major metabolites after single oral sustained tablet administration in the dog: a pilot study. *Vet J*, 180:253–255.
■ Lascelles B.D.X., Court, M.H., Hardie, E.M. et al. (2007) Non-steroidal anti-inflammatory drugs in cats: a review. *Vet Anaesth Analg* 34:4, 228.
■ Lascelles B.D.X, Robertson, S.A., Taylor, P.M. et al. (2003) Comparison of the pharmacokinetics and thermal antinociceptive pharmacodynamics of 20 μg kg^{-1} buprenorphine administered sublingually or intravenously in cats. *Vet Anaesth Analg*, 30:99–119.
■ Lascelles B.D.X. (2012) Surgical pain: pathophysiology, assessment and treatment strategies. In: Tobias, K.M.J.S. editor. *Veterinary surgery small animal*. St. Louis: Elsevier, pp. 237–247.
■ Lynch, S., Savary-Bataille, K., Leeuw, B. et al. (2011) Development of a questionnaire assessing health-related quality-of-life in dogs and cats with cancer. *Vet Comp Oncol*, 9:172–182.
■ Mellanby, R.J., Herrtage, M.E., Dobson, J.M. (2003) Owners' assessments of their dog's quality of life during palliative chemotherapy for lymphoma. *J Small Anim Pract*, 44:100–103.
■ Monteiro-Steagall, B.P., Steagall, P.V.M., Lascelles, B.D.X (2013) Systematic review of non-steroidal anti-inflammatory drug-induced adverse effects in dogs. *J Vet Intern Med*, 27:1011–1019.
■ Pypendop, B.H., Siao, K.T., Ilkiw, J.E. (2010) Thermal antinociceptive effect of orally administered gabapentin in healthy cats. *Am J Vet Res*, 71:1027–1032.
■ Radulovic, L.L., Türck, D., Von Hodenberg, A. et al. (1995) Disposition of gabapentin (neurontin) in mice, rats, dogs, and monkeys. *Drug Metab Dispos*, 23:441–448.
■ Sabino M.A.C., Mantyh, P.W. (2005) Pathophysiology of bone cancer pain. *J Support Oncol*, 3:15–24.
■ Tzanness, S., Hammond, M.F., Murphy, S. et al. (2008) Owners "perception of their cats" quality of life during COP chemotherapy for lymphoma. *J Feline Med Surg*, 10:73–81.
■ Weinstein, J.I., Paynes, S., Poulson, J.M. et al. (2009) Use of force plate analysis to evaluate the efficacy of external beam radiation to alleviate osteosarcoma pain. *Vet Radiol Ultrasound*, 50:673–678.

Nutritional Approach to Cancer Patients

■ Baez, J.L., Michel, K.E., Sorenmo, K., Shofer, F.S. (2007) A prospective investigation of the prevalence and prognostic significance of weight loss and changes in body condition in feline cancer patients. *J Feline Med Sur*, 9:411–417.
■ Chan, D.L., Freeman, L.M., Labata, M.A. et al. (2002) Retrospective evaluation of partial parenteral nutrition in dogs and cats. *J Vet Int Med*, 16:440–445.
■ Chandler, M.L., Payne-James, J.J. (2006) Prospective evaluation of a peripherally administered three-in-one parenteral nutrition product in dogs. *J Am An Hosp Assoc*, 47:518–523.
■ Crabb, S.E., Freeman, L.M., Chan, D.L. et al. (2006) Retrospective evaluation of total parenteral nutrition in cats: 40 cases (1991–2003). *J Vet Emer Crit Care*, 16:S1–S26.
■ Koppenol, W.H., Bounds, P.L., Dang, C.V (2011) Otto Warburg's contributions to current concepts of cancer metabolism. *Nat Rev*, 11:325–337.
■ Mazzaferro, E.M., Hackett, T.B., Stein, T.P. et al. (2001) Metabolic alterations in dogs with osteosarcoma. *Am J Vet Res*, 62:1234–1239.

■ Ogilvie, G.K., Fettman, M.J., Mallinckrodt, C.H. et al. (2000) Effect of fish oil, arginine, and doxorubicin chemotherapy on remission survival time for dogs with lymphoma: a double-blind randomized placebo-controlled study. *Cancer*, 88:1916–1928.

■ Ogilvie, G.K., Vail, D.M., Wheeler, S.L. et al. (1992) Effects of chemotherapy and remission on carbohydrate metabolism in dogs with lymphoma. *Cancer*, 69:233–238.

■ Ogilvie, G.K., Vail, D.M (1990) Nutrition and cancer – recent developments. *Vet Clin North Am Small Anim Pract* 20:969–985.

■ Ogilvie, G.K., Walters, L.M., Fettman, M.J. et al. (1993) Energy expenditure in dogs with lymphoma fed two specialized diets. *Cancer*, 71:3146–3152.

■ Ogilvie, G.K., Walters, L.M, Salman, M.D. et al. (1997) Alterations in carbohydrate metabolism in dogs with non- hematopoietic malignancies. *Am J Vet Res*, 58:277–281.

■ Ogilvie, G.K., Walters, L.M, Salman, M.D. et al. (1996) Resting energy expenditure in dogs with non-hematopoietic malignancies before and after excision of tumours. *Am J Vet Res*, 57:1462–1467.

■ Pérez Alenza, D., Rutteman, G.R., Peña, L. et al. (1998) Relation between habitual diet and canine mammary tumours in a case-control study. *J Vet Inten Med*, 12:132–139.

■ Pyle, S.C., Marks, S.L., Kass, P.H. (2004) Evaluation of complications and prognostic factors associated with administration of total parenteral nutrition in cats: 75 cases (1994–2001). *J Am Vet Med Assoc*, 225:242–250.

■ Raghavan, M., Knapp, D.W., Bonney, P.L. et al. (2005) Evaluation of the effect of dietary vegetable consumption on reducing risk of transitional cell carcinoma of the urinary bladder in Scottish Terriers. *J Am Vet Med Assoc*, 227:94–100.

■ Rajagopaul, S., Parr, J.M., Woods, J.P. et al. (2016) Owners' attitudes and practices regarding nutrition of dogs diagnosed with cancer presenting at a referral oncology service in Ontario, Canada. *J Small Anim Pract*, 57:484–490.

■ Rassnick, K.M., Muindi, J.R., Johnson, C.S. et al. (2011) Oral bioavailability of DN101, a concentrated formulation of calcitriol, in tumour-bearing dogs. *Cancer Chemother Pharmacol*, 67;165–171.

■ Selting, K.A., Sharp, C.R., Ringold, R. et al. (2016) Serum 25-hydroxyvitamin D concentration in dogs – correlation with health and cancer risk. *Vet Comp Oncol*, 14:295–305.

■ Shofer, F.S., Sonnenschein, E.G., Goldschmidt, M.H. et al. (1989) Histopathologic and dietary prorgnostic factors for canine mammary carcinoma. *Breast Cancer Res Treat*, 13:49–60.

■ Sonnenschein, E.G., Glickman, L.T., Goldschmidt, M.H. et al. (1991) Body conformation, diet and risk of breast cancer in pet dogs: a case-control study. *Am J Epidemiol*, 133:694–702.

■ Szczubial, M., Kankofer, M., Lopuszynski, W. et al. (2004) Oxidative stress parameters in bitches with mammary gland tumours. *J Vet Med*, 51:336–340.

■ Vail, D.M., Ogilvie, G.K., Wheeler, S.L. et al. (1990) Alterations in carbohydrate metabolism in canine lymphoma. *J Vet Int Med*, 4:8–11.

■ Wakshlag, J.J., Rassnick, K.M., Malone, E.K. et al. (2011) Cross sectional study to investigate the association between serum vitamin D and cutaneous mast cell tumours in Labrador retrievers. *Br J Nutr*, 106:S60–S63.

■ Wheet, L.P., Fascetti, A.J., Kass, P.H. et al. (2007) Prevalence of obese dogs in a population of dogs with cancer. *Am J Vet Res*, 68:389–398.

■ Winter, J.L., Barber, L.G., Freeman, T.M. et al. (2009) Antioxidant status and biomarkers of oxidative stress in dogs with lymphoma. *J Vet Int Med*, 23:311–316.

■ Withrow, S.J., Vail, D.M. (ED) (2007) *Withrow & MacEwen's Small Animal Clinical Oncology*. St. Louis, Mo.: Saunders Elsevier.

■ Zollers, B., Wofford, J.A., Heinen, E. et al. (2016) A prospective, randomized, masked, placebo-controlled clinical study of capromorelin in dogs with reduced appetite. *J Vet Intern Med*, 30:1851–1857.

Test

Answers on Page 34

1. **What is the Warburg effect?**
   a. Cancer cell aneuploidy is necessary for carcinogenesis.
   b. Many tumour cells preferentially use the lactate-generating anaerobic glycolytic pathway to generate energy even when oxygenation conditions are appropriate.
   c. The ability of tumour cells to travel from the site of the primary tumour through blood or lymph to other locations in the body.
   d. Tumour cells possess intracellular vesicles called autophagosomes that can fuse with lysosomes and intracytoplasmic organelles to form new molecules that provide the cellular energy-producing machinery.

2. **Which of the following statements is untrue?**
   a. Some epigenetic changes in cancer cells can be inherited.
   b. Hereditary cancer syndromes account for 5–10% of cancers in humans.
   c. Tumour stem cells retain or acquire the capacity for self-renewal and are capable and responsible for initiating the process of tumour genesis, as well as keeping the neoplasm alive.
   d. Epigenetic changes and gene silencing are the mechanisms that the immune system uses to fight tumour cells.

3. **What does the intrinsic resistance of tumours to chemotherapy treatments consist of?**
   a. Tumour stem cells acquire resistance mechanisms to cytotoxic drugs and pass them on to their clones.
   b. The tumour cell acquires a drug-resistant phenotype by random mutation and transmits it to its offspring.
   c. Stem cells and cells of variable differentiation have inherent drug resistance, so treatments are ineffective, leading to tumour growth.
   d. Intrinsic resistance does not exist, all forms of tumour cell resistance come from adaptation by genetic mutations.

4. **The terms tumour, neoplasm, and cancer are often used incorrectly as synonyms. Which of the following definitions is correct?**
   a. A neoplasm is the abnormal growth of a tissue causing a mass, which can be benign or malignant, and which does not respond to the usual control mechanisms.
   b. A cancer is the abnormal growth of a tissue causing a mass, which can be benign or malignant, and which does not respond to the usual control mechanisms.
   c. A tumour is the abnormal growth of a tissue causing a mass, which can be benign or malignant, and that does not respond to the usual control mechanisms.
   d. None of the above is correct.

5. **Different characteristics of neoplasms should be focused upon to determine their degree of malignancy. What are they?**
   a. Degree of differentiation, amount of necrosis and size of nucleoli.
   b. Mitotic index, degree of cellular polymorphism and overall cellularity.
   c. Invasiveness, stromal reaction, and lymphatic response.
   d. All of the above.

6. **Regarding tumour margins after surgery, which answer is correct?**
   a. In feline injection site sarcomas, the recurrence rate reaches 80% even if the surgical margins are clean.
   b. Clean surgical margins guarantee that there will be no recurrence in the six months following the operation.
   c. Observation of surgical margins is something objective that follows certain rules, it does not depend on factors such as the type of sample, the dissection method or the surgeon.
   d. Shrinkage of the tissues after processing to send samples to the laboratory is negligible and does not influence the diagnosis.

7. What answer is true when talking about the diagnosis of a patient with neoplasms?

a. The clinical history and anamnesis are of very little importance since the owners lie and the data that can be collected is misleading rather than helpful.
b. If the tumour is very obvious, the clinician should focus on it and not waste time with more routine tests that will only increase the bill and dangerously delay the start of treatment.
c. A careful palpation of the regional lymph nodes must be carried out to see whether they are affected or not and obtain cytological samples of these if it is considered necessary.
d. The first thing to do, if this diagnostic tool is available, is an MRI of the thorax and abdomen to detect possible metastases.

8. When talking about cancer-associated pain, what is the wrong answer?

a. The key to pain assessment in cats and dogs with cancer are behavioural changes.
b. Owners are not an important part in assessing a pet's pain because they are not objective with their observations.
c. To evaluate pain, at each patient visit, the pain induced by palpation, the patient's activity parameters and their behaviour should be monitored.
d. Drugs are the basis for treating cancer pain.

9. Regarding nutritional disorders that occur in cancer patients, what is the correct answer?

a. Anorexia and cachexia are synonymous terms.
b. Cachexia is more common in canine cancer patients than in felines.
c. Cachexia is more common in feline cancer patients than in canines.
d. Ageusia or dysgeusia resulting from chemotherapy treatment never lasts more than a couple of weeks.

10. Assisted feeding may be necessary in many cancer patients. Which of the following answers is incorrect?

a. Oesophagostomy tubes are ideal for medium to long-term assisted enteral feeding.
b. A gastrostomy tube should be used if nutritional supplementation is expected to be necessary for more than 6 to 8 weeks.
c. If assisted enteral feeding is not feasible for a patient, parenteral feeding should be considered.
d. One of the most frequent complications of assisted parenteral feeding is the development of sepsis due to migration of bacteria into the portal vein.

Correct Answers:

1. b
2. d
3. c
4. a
5. d
6. a
7. c
8. b
9. c
10. d

Notes

Paraneoplastic Syndromes

Sofia Carvalho

Paraneoplastic syndromes are cancer-associated conditions that cause clinical disorders but that are **not necessarily directly related to the physical effects of the primary or metastatic neoplasia**.

Paraneoplastic syndromes are usually caused by molecules produced by tumour cells which are released into the circulation. These can include hormones, cytokines and/or peptides. These syndromes may also result from a reduction in the concentration of certain circulating molecules due to the presence of the neoplasm or may also result from immune-mediated responses.

A paraneoplastic syndrome **may be the first clinical sign of oncological disease**. It is also common that if at time of diagnosis of a neoplasia presents with a paraneoplastic syndrome, when that neoplasm progresses or recurs after having been positively treated, the patient may develop and is sometimes likely to develop the same paraneoplastic syndrome. Moreover in many cases the paraneoplastic syndrome precedes the clinical detection of neoplastic disease. This can prove helpful in diagnosing a possible disease relapse or recurrence earlier.

Paraneoplastic syndromes can be associated with several tumours and they can have a very negative effect on the quality of life of cancer patients. A correct understanding and identification of the different paraneoplastic syndromes and neoplasms that can cause them is very important to allow an early cancer diagnosis and ensure anti-cancer treatment is started as quickly as possible. **In most cases successful treatment of the neoplasm resolves the paraneoplastic syndrome**.

However, this is not true for all neoplasms and their associated paraneoplastic syndromes, as **some will remain present despite successful anticancer treatments**. There are cases when the paraneoplastic syndrome needs to be treated directly too to improve the patient's quality of life, for example when the anti-cancer treatment was not successful or/nor pursued for other reasons.

Haematological Paraneoplastic Syndromes

Anaemia

Anaemia is the **most common paraneoplastic syndrome in veterinary cancer patients**.

Paraneoplastic anaemia occurs in approximately 30–43% of dogs and 43–58% of cats diagnosed with lymphoma. The presence of paraneoplastic anaemia is also considered a negative prognostic factor in dogs and cats diagnosed with lymphoma.

Other tumours such as leukaemia and haemangiosarcoma can also cause paraneoplastic anaemia, and in dogs it can commonly occur in cases of disseminated mast cell tumours and histiocytic sarcomas (Figure 1).

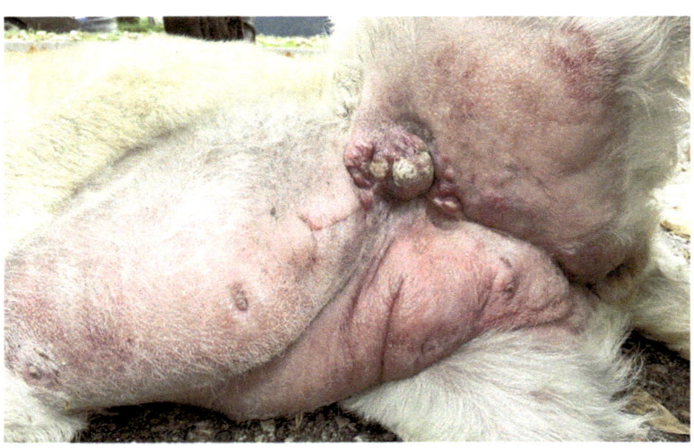

Figure 1. High-grade canine mast cell tumour in the left inguinal area, with evidence of tumoural necrosis in the centre of the mass. The presence of significant oedema and peritumoural inflammation can be seen as well as peritumoural satellite nodules. This mass had also suffered various episodes of chronic intermittent haemorrhage. These aggressive mast cell tumours tend to release histamine, heparin and other vasoactive enzymes, which affect the clinical presentation of the patient. (Image: Ignasi Rodriguez, DVM, PhD, MVetMed, Dip. ACVIM Oncology).

The **pathogenesis of paraneoplastic anaemia is multifactorial** and includes several types of anaemia: anaemia due to inflammation or chronic disease, anaemia due to haemorrhage, anaemia due to destruction of erythrocytes and/or anaemia due to decreased production of erythrocytes.

- **Anaemia due to inflammation** or chronic disease. The inflammatory cytokines IL-1, IL-5, IL-6, interferon gamma (IFN-γ), and tumour necrosis factor alpha (TNF-α) reduce the production of endogenous erythropoietin when there is hypoxia, and suppress the erythroid progenitor responde to erythropoietin. IL-6 also causes increased production of hepcidin in the liver, which increases degradation of ferropoietin, causing the sequestration of iron, decreasing its availability to erythrocytes.
- **Anaemia due to haemorrhage** can be acute and severe and is commonly seen in cases of haemorrhagic splenic haemangiosarcoma or other splenic tumours. Anaemia due to haemorrhage may also be seen in patients with cortical or medullary adrenal carcinomas, hepatocellular carcinomas, and thyroid carcinomas, as well as other neoplasms that cause bleeding. In some cases, paraneoplastic anaemia due to haemorrhage can be chronic and low-grade, such as that seen in patients with gastrointestinal tumours (for example, cats with gastrointestinal lymphoma), tumours of the nasal cavity, urinary bladder, or tumours that cause a gastrointestinal ulceration such as mastocytomas and gastrinomas.
- **Immune-mediated haemolytic anaemia** is more common in cases of canine and feline lymphoma. In cats, immune-mediated haemolytic anaemia can be secondary to feline leukaemia virus.
- **Non-immune-mediated anaemia** can occur secondary to microangiopathy, neoplastic erythrophagocytosis, or due to oxidative damage to erythrocytes.
  - **Haemolytic microangiopathic anaemia** is quite common in cases of haemangiosarcoma that present with disseminated intravascular coagulation caused by abnormalities in the vascular system.
  - **Erythrophagocytic anaemia** is seen more frequently in patients with haemophagocytic histiocytic sarcoma. Erythrophagocytosis can also occur in patients with lymphoma, plasma cell tumours, acute megakaryoblastic leukaemia, and in cats with lymphoma or mastocytoma.
  - **Oxidative damage to red blood cells** is frequently seen in lymphoma patients.
- **Non-regenerative paraneoplastic anaemia** is also common. This anaemia can occur due to myeloptysis due to neoplastic infiltration, which is most commonly seen in association with haematopoietic neoplasms such as lymphoma, acute leukaemia, multiple myeloma, mast cell tumours, and histiocytic sarcoma.
- **Aplastic anaemia** occurs in cases of paraneoplastic hyperoestrogenism.

Erythrocytosis

Paraneoplastic erythrocytosis can be seen in dogs diagnosed with renal carcinoma and adenocarcinoma, renal fibrosarcoma, renal lymphoma, nasal fibrosarcoma, caecal leiomyosarcoma, and spinal cord schwannoma. In cats, paraneoplastic erythrocytosis has been observed in cases of renal adenocarcinoma. Paraneoplastic erythrocytosis is associated with **increased levels of erythropoietin**, which is produced by tumour cells, and/or due to **hypoxia of local tissues due to damage to renal blood flow**.

Surgical excision of the neoplasm responsible for paraneoplastic erythrocytosis usually results in the resolution of this syndrome. In some cases that also present with hyperviscosity syndrome, stabilisation of the patient with medical treatment of this syndrome is recommended before carrying out any surgery.

Thrombocytopaenia

Paraneoplastic thrombocytopaenia is most commonly associated with haematopoietic and vascular tumours. Causes for the development of paraneoplastic thrombocytopaenia include **decreased platelet production** (due to myeloptysis or hyperoestrogenism), **increased platelet destruction** (most commonly due to microangiopathy), **increased platelet sequestration, and increased platelet consumption** (for example due to bleeding or hypercoagulability associated with cancer).

Approximately 13–26% of dogs with cancer suffer from thrombocytopaenia at time of diagnosis of cancer and approximately 39% of cats that present with thrombocytopaenia are diagnosed with cancer. Paraneoplastic immune-mediated thrombocytopaenia is most commonly associated with the diagnosis of lymphoma, multiple myeloma, histiocytic sarcoma, haemangiosarcoma, mammary carcinoma, mastocytoma, nasal adenocarcinoma, and fibrosarcoma.

Platelet sequestration can occur in cases of splenomegaly due to neoplasia, which can occur in cases of splenic lymphoma, haemangioma, haemangiosarcoma, and in feline splenic mast cell tumours.

Leucocytosis

Paraneoplastic leucocytosis **usually has mild clinical implications**. Mild to moderate neutrophilia is common in dogs and cats with cancer and can generally be associated with the presence of inflammation and/or tissue necrosis associated with the neoplasia. In some cases, neutrophilia can be severe (greater than 70 000 x 10^9/l) and associated with a left shift, monocytosis, and eosinophilia. These cases can be seen in dogs with pulmonary carcinoma, renal tumours, intestinal T-cell lymphoma, metastatic fibrosarcoma, and adenomatous rectal polyps. In cats, these cases can be seen in animals diagnosed with squamous cell pulmonary carcinoma and tubular adenocarcinoma of the dermis.

Paraneoplastic leucocytosis occurs due to production of granulocyte colony-stimulating factor (G-CSF) and/or granulocyte-macrophage colony-stimulating factor (GM-CSF) by the tumour cells.

Paraneoplastic eosinophilia is rare in veterinary oncology, and the tumours most commonly associated with this syndrome include canine and feline mastocytomas and T-cell lymphomas. Mast cell tumours produce eosinophilic interleukin 5 (IL-5) as well as other chemotactic factors that attract eosinophils.

Other tumours such as oral fibrosarcoma, mammary carcinoma and leiomyosarcoma can also cause paraneoplastic eosinophilia in dogs and the same can occur in cats with oral squamous cell carcinoma and transitional cell carcinoma of the urinary bladder.

Hyperglobulinaemia

Monoclonal gammopathies are commonly seen in patients diagnosed with multiple myeloma or associated with other myeloma-related disorders, including solitary plasmacytoma of bone, cutaneous and non-cutaneous extramedullary plasmacytoma, IgM macroglobulinaemia, plasmacytic leukaemia, IgG-secreting lymphoma, and chronic immunoglobulin secreting lymphocytic leukaemia.

The neoplastic cells of plasma cell disorders produce an overabundance of a portion or a single type of immunoglobulin, which is referred to as the M component. This abnormality is most commonly seen in the immunoglobulin gamma region, although in rare cases it can also be seen in the beta region.

Gammopathies are usually monoclonal, although there are also reported cases of biclonal gammopathies. The M component can interfere with clotting and also result in hyperviscosity syndrome.

Bence Jones Proteinuria

Similar to what happens with paraneoplastic gammopathies, Bence Jones proteinuria is **frequently associated with myeloma-related disorders**.

Bence Jones proteinuria occurs when there is an excess of immunoglobulin light chains excreted in the urine. This can lead to the development of interstitial nephritis and ultimately kidney failure. Bence Jones proteinuria syndrome is diagnosed using urine electrophoresis, since light chain immunoglobulins are not identified using urine dipstick analysis.

Hyperviscosity Syndrome

This syndrome is the result of excessive blood viscosity, which reduces blood flow in small blood vessels, affecting cellular delivery of oxygen and nutrients and causing clotting problems.

Patients suffering from hyperviscosity syndrome present with neurological symptoms: stupor, ataxia, and seizures. These patients also present with ocular symptoms that include enlarged and tortuous retinal vessels, haemorrhages, and retinal detachment. Likewise, patients with hyperviscosity syndrome may present with susceptibility to bleeding, hypertrophic cardiomyopathy, and congestive heart failure.

Hyperviscosity syndrome **occurs more frequently in patients with myeloma-related disorders, most commonly in cases of IgM macroglobulinaemia**. The syndrome can also occur in patients diagnosed with polycythaemia vera and paraneoplastic erythrocytosis.

In severe cases of hyperviscosity syndrome, emergency treatment is recommended. Plasmapheresis is indicated when the hyperviscosity syndrome results from an increase in serum proteins. Phlebotomy and intravenous fluid therapy are recommended when hyperviscosity syndrome is caused by erythrocytosis.

Coagulopathies

Hypercoagulability is common in cancer patients and has been reported in approximately 50% of canine patients diagnosed with cancer and in approximately 56% of canine patients diagnosed with lymphoma. Many patients with hypercoagubility do not necessarily present any symptoms associated with this. According to one study, cancer has been identified in 27% of dogs with portal vein thrombosis, in 30% of dogs with pulmonary embolism, and in 54% of dogs with splenic vein thrombosis.

Hypocoagulability can be caused by thrombocytopaenia and abnormal platelet function, secondary to paraproteinaemia.

Cancer patients may also be predisposed to bleeding if they suffer from hyperviscosity syndrome.

The most common clotting factor dysfunction in veterinary cancer patients is associated with cases of mast cell tumours due to the release of heparin by mast cells, which acts as a co-factor for antithrombin III and inactivates clotting factors IX, X, XI and XII.

Disseminated Intravascular Coagulation

Cancer is one of the most common causes for the development of disseminated intravascular coagulation. It is estimated that approximately 10% of dogs diagnosed with cancer suffer from disseminated intravascular coagulation.

Disseminated intravascular coagulation activates coagulation and leads to the development of microthrombosis. Subsequently, consumption of platelets and clotting factors leads to uncontrollable bleeding. **Haemangiosarcoma is the neoplasm most commonly associated with the development of disseminated intravascular coagulation**. It is estimated that approximately 50% of patients diagnosed with haemangiosarcoma present with disseminated intravascular coagulation.

Other tumours also associated with the development of this syndrome include mammary adenocarcinoma, especially inflammatory mammary carcinoma, and pulmonary carcinomas.

Gastrointestinal Paraneoplastic Syndromes

Cancer-associated Anorexia and Cachexia

Hyporexia and anorexia are common in cancer patients, especially if the oncologic disease is advanced. Inflammation and the cytokines, interleukin 1 and 6 (IL-1 and IL-6), affect anorexigenic and orexigenic signals and are, in part, responsible for paraneoplastic hyporexia and anorexia.

Cancer-associated cachexia is characterised by severe muscle weakness, sometimes with loss of fat mass, and abnormal fat and carbohydrate metabolism, despite adequate nutrient intake.

Tumour necrosis factor alpha (TNF-α), IL-1 and IL-6 induce anorexia, cause an increase in energy metabolism, and accelerate the loss of lean body mass. TNF-α also exerts effects on the protein myostatin, which inhibits muscle growth and differentiation, and interferes with the anabolic effects of growth hormone and insulin-like growth factor (IGF-1).

Approximately 35% of canine cancer patients suffer from muscle weakness and about 44% of feline cancer patients have a body mass index less than 5.

Lymphoma and oral squamous cell carcinoma are common in feline cancer patients and these tumours can affect food intake and nutrient absorption, which will affect the body mass index of patients.

Low body weight along with a low body mass index are proven to be factors that can have a negative impact on the prognosis of some patients (for example, in cases of feline lymphoma).

Gastrointestinal Ulceration

The tumour most frequently associated with the development of paraneoplastic gastrointestinal ulceration is the **mastocytoma**.

Mast cells produce high levels of histamine. Histamine binds to histamine H2 receptors on parietal gastric cells, which stimulate gastric acid secretion. Histamine also has a direct effect on the gastric mucosa causing increased vascular permeability, local protein exudation, and increased blood flow in the gastric mucosa.

The release of histamine by mast cells can be spontaneous or triggered by physical manipulation of the mast cell or treatment with chemotherapy and/or radiotherapy.

Although plasma histamine concentrations are increased in cases of macroscopic and/or metastatic mast cell tumours, this concentration does not predict the development of symptoms of gastrointestinal ulceration.

Symptomatic therapies for paraneoplastic gastrointestinal ulceration associated with a diagnosis of mastocytoma include H2 antihistamines, proton pump inhibitors (such as omeprazole), misoprostol, sucralfate, and clinical rehydration when deemed necessary.

In patients with advanced mast cell disease or in patients who have large macroscopic mast cell tumours and/or metastatic disease, prophylactic treatment for gastrointestinal ulceration is also recommended.

Another tumour associated with paraneoplastic gastrointestinal ulceration is the **gastrin-secreting pancreatic tumour**, which originates from pancreatic D cells, although these tumours are quite rare in veterinary patients. Zollinger-Ellison syndrome has also been reported in veterinary medicine, which is defined as a triad of hypergastrinaemia, a neuroendocrine pancreatic tumour that does not originate in the β cells of the pancreas, and gastrointestinal ulceration.

Endocine Paraneoplastic Syndromes

Hypercalcaemia

Hypercalcaemia is **diagnosed in approximately 60% of canine cancer patients and 30% of feline cancer patients**.

Various mechanisms are responsible for the development of **malignant hypercalcaemia**: neoplastic cells usually release substances into the circulation that act on the kidneys and bone using endocrine and paracrine signals, a phenomenon known as **humoral malignant hypercalcaemia**. The parathyroid hormone-related protein (PTHrP) is the substance most frequently involved in this process. PTHrP is very similar to parathyroid hormone (PTH) and therefore, when PTHrP is released into the circulation by neoplastic cells, it is able to bind to PTH receptors on osteoblasts and renal tubular cells. Other substances involved in the development of malignant hypercalcaemia are interleukins 1 and 6 (IL-1, IL-6), tumour necrosis factor (TNF) and calcitriol.

Malignant hypercalcaemia can **also be a consequence of osteolysis** when there is tumour invasion in the bone system. The number and activity of osteoclasts can also increase with the release of IL-1, IL-6, TNF, receptor activator of nuclear factor kappa-B ligand (RANKL), TGF-α, TGF-β and prostaglandins.

Dogs with hypercalcaemia usually present with polyuria, polydipsia, anorexia, vomiting, weakness, and muscle spasms. In cats, polyuria and polydipsia are less common and these patients present more often with anorexia and vomiting.

Polyuria and polydipsia result from an abnormality in the action of antidiuretic hormone (ADH) on the tubular cells of the collecting duct. Dehydration is common, and kidney damage results from renal vasoconstriction, tubular degeneration and necrosis, interstitial fibrosis, and mineralisation of the renal tubules, basement membranes, and interstitium. The resulting azotaemia may or may not be reversible, depending on its cause.

Measurement of ionised calcium is much more accurate than measurement of total calcium and it is recommended that ionised calcium is always analysed when diagnosing and monitoring malignant hypercalcaemia. The serum phosphate value in a dog or cat with humoral hypercalcaemia that is neither azotaemic nor dehydrated should be low or low-normal.

Whenever the clinician suspects malignant hypercalcaemia based on the clinical history, symptoms, and initial blood tests, further diagnostic tests should be performed.

- A detailed physical examination should be performed, including evaluation of peripheral lymphadenopathy, nodules/masses in the anal glands, or cervical nodules.
- Further diagnostic tests are recommended as soon as possible, including a complete blood count with blood smear evaluation (for example, to identify any circulating neoplastic cells), detailed biochemistry profile, urinalysis, thoracic radiographs and abdominal ultrasound.
- Depending on the results of the previous tests, further diagnostic tests should be performed, mainly if a clinical diagnosis for the cause of malignant hypercalcaemia has not been identified. These tests may include ultrasound of the cervical region (for example, to look for a parathyroid gland injury), orthopaedic radiographs, bone marrow aspiration, and/or measurement of PTH, PTHrP, and calcitriol values. In cases of malignant hypercalcaemia, PTHrP should be high (or normal) and PTH should be low (due to negative feedback) in most cases. Calcitriol is usually normal, although it may also be high or low depending on the case.

The tumour most commonly associated with malignant hypercalcaemia in dogs is T-cell lymphoma. Hypercalcaemia occurs in 35–55% of dogs with this type of neoplasm. Another canine tumour in which patients commonly present with malignant hypercalcaemia is anal sac gland carcinoma, whereas malignant hypercalcaemia can occur in 25% of the patients. Paraneoplastic hypercalcaemia can occur in association with the following diagnoses: malignant lymphocytic leukaemia, clitoral adenocarcinoma, hepatocellular carcinoma, nasal carcinoma, penile adenocarcinoma, pulmonary carcinoma, thymoma, osteosarcoma, mammary carcinoma, melanoma, multiple myeloma, pheochromocytoma, renal angiomyxoma, renal cell carcinoma, thyroid and parathyroid adenoma (or adenomatous parathyroid hyperplasia).

The tumours most commonly associated with malignant hypercalcaemia in cats are lymphoma, oral squamous cell carcinoma, and multiple myeloma. Other neoplasms associated with the development of malignant hypercalcaemia in cats include fibrosarcoma, acute leukaemia, osteosarcoma, pulmonary carcinoma, renal carcinoma, thyroid carcinoma, undifferentiated sarcomas, and parathyroid adenoma (or adenomatous parathyroid hyperplasia).

The **treatment for malignant hypercalcaemia is based on treating the underlying neoplasia** responsible for the hypercalcaemia. Depending on the neoplasm, treatment may include a combination of surgery, chemotherapy, and/or radiotherapy. Concurrent medical treatment of hypercalcaemia is recommended if the concentration of calcium in the serum is greater than 16 mg/dl, if the sum of calcium and phosphate is greater than 60, if the patient is azotaemic or ill or in patients for whom there is no effective therapy for the underlying cancer such as surgery, chemotherapy, or radiation therapy.

The medical treatment of hypercalcaemia should begin with the administration of intravenous fluid therapy with 0.9% NaCl. The goal is to correct the initial dehydration and then increase the glomerular filtration rate and filter calcium. When the patient is already hydrated, furosemide can be administered to promote urinary calcium excretion. In more refractory cases, bisphosphonates that inhibit osteoclast-mediated bone resorption can be administered and their use can have a prolonged effect. Salmon calcitonin is used for cases that require rapid restoration of hypercalcaemia, due to its rapid effect, although resistance to this treatment also rapidly develops. It is important to administer the different therapies consecutively and to monitor the serum concentration of ionised calcium very regularly.

Glucocorticoids can induce a rapid reduction in calcium levels, however these should never be administered to patients with malignant hypercalcaemia if a definitive diagnosis for the underlying hypercalcaemia has not been achieved, since early administration of glucocorticoids can have a negative impact on the efficacy of treatment and the prognosis of the patient, mainly in the case of lymphoma and other haematopoietic neoplasms. Furthermore, the early administration of glucocorticoids in these cases can also make it difficult to confirm the diagnosis or cause resistance to medical antineoplastic therapy, reducing the probability of achieving remission of the cancer and decreasing the median survival rate. Each case of hypercalcaemia should be treated individually, depending on the clinical presentation of the patient.

Hypoglycaemia

The **most common cause of paraneoplastic hypoglycaemia is insulinoma**, a pancreatic β-cell tumour that usually produces excess insulin. In rarer cases, the insulinoma can also produce an excess of IGF-1 and IGF-2 (insulin growth factors type 1 and 2).

There are also other non-pancreatic tumours that can frequently cause paraneoplastic hypoglycaemia, generally due to excessive IGF-2 production from their cells. These neoplasms include hepatocellular adenomas and carcinomas, as well as leiomyomas and leiomyosarcomas of the liver, stomach, duodenum, and jejunum. Other tumours that can more rarely cause paraneoplastic hypoglycaemia are haemangiosarcoma, lymphoma, lymphocytic leukaemia, mammary gland carcinoma, melanoma, plasma cell tumuors, renal adenocarcinoma, and salivary gland adenocarcinoma.

Other mechanisms that cause the development of paraneoplastic hypoglycaemia include an excess production of somatomedins, glucose hypermetabolism, production of substances that stimulate insulin release, production of the hepatic glucose inhibitor, proliferation of the insulin receptor, binding of a monoclonal immunoglobulin to insulin and ectopic insulin production.

The **treatment of choice for insulinoma is surgery for tumour excision and metastasis whenever possible**. Medical treatment can be recommended after surgery in cases with persistent metastatic disease and/or hypoglycaemia, as an alternative to surgery in cases with advanced metastatic disease or also to stabilise patients before surgery.

Hyperoestrogenism

The tumour that is most frequently associated with the development of paraneoplastic hyperoestrogenism is the **Sertoli cell tumour**, and hyperoestrogenic syndrome occurs in approximately 25–50% of patients with this disease. Approximately 50% of Sertoli cell tumours occur in dogs with cryptorchid testes, and paraneoplastic hyperoestrogenism is also more common if the tumour occurs in the cryptorchid testes.

Sertoli cell tumour patients have elevated plasma oestradiol-17B levels and lower expression of type 1 5-alpha reductase and plasma testosterone.

Paraneoplastic hyperoestrogenism can also develop in patients with seminomas, interstitial cell tumours, and ovarian granulosa cell tumours.

Symptoms associated with hyperoestrogenism include symmetrical bilateral alopecia, hyperpigmentation of the skin, thinning of the epidermis, gynecomastia, galactorrhoea, pendulous prepuce, penile atrophy, contralateral testicular atrophy, prostate atrophy or prostatomegaly, and attraction of other males.

Oestrogen is myelotoxic and initially causes transient neutrophilic leucocytosis, followed by hypoplasia or aplasia of the bone marrow, which causes non-regenerative anaemia, thrombocytopaenia, and leucopaenia.

The treatment of choice for paraneoplastic hyperoestrogenism is surgical excision of the tumour. The symptoms associated with hyperoestrogenism usually resolve with tumour excision, although this may take several months. Mortality in patients with myelotoxicosis and severe pancytopaenia is high.

Acromegaly

Feline acromegaly results from excessive secretion of growth hormone from a pituitary adenoma of somatotrophic cells (hypersomatotropism). Growth hormone reduces the number of insulin receptors and antagonises the effect of insulin.

Cats diagnosed with acromegaly often present with diabetes mellitus, and insulin resistance is common. With the progression of the disease, cats develop excessive growth of connective tissues, bones, and viscera, presenting with wide facial characteristics, lower prognathism, diffuse thinning of the oropharyngeal tissues, hepatomegaly, renomegaly, adrenomegaly, hypertrophic cardiomyopathy, enlargement of the legs and distal part of the limbs and degenerative arthropathy.

Canine acromegaly is usually caused by excessive progestin secretion by growth hormone-induced mammary duct epithelium cells.

Ectopic Adrenocorticotropic Hormone Syndrome

Ectopic adrenocorticotropic hormone syndrome is **very rare** in veterinary medicine and only a few cases have been recorded in dogs. Tumours where the occurrence of this syndrome has been reported include primary pulmonary neoplasia, metastatic pancreatic neuroendocrine tumour, and hepatic carcinoid.

Patients with adrenocorticotropic hormone syndrome generally present with typical symptoms of hyperadrenocorticism since this syndrome results from an expression of the proopiomelanocortin gene, which contains ACTH. This gene also determines the production of the melanocyte-stimulating hormone, lipocortin, endorphins, and enkephalins, so patients with ectopic adrenocorticotropic hormone syndrome can also present with other symptoms, such as hyperpigmentation.

Renal Paraneoplastic Syndromes

Paraneoplastic syndromes associated with the renal system are rare. Only **two cases of paraneoplastic glomerular disorder have been reported** in the veterinary literature. These include a dog with primary erythrocytosis and a dog with lymphocytic leukaemia.

Glomerular disorder is thought to be the consequence of a deposit of tumour antigens in the glomerulus that, consequently, bind to antibodies forming an immune complex that activates the complement system. In human patients, membranous nephropathy is the most commonly observed glomerular disorder as a renal paraneoplastic syndrome and is often associated with solid tumours.

Polyuria and polydipsia are frequently observed in association with malignant hypercalcaemia, which can sometimes result in kidney damage. Polyuria and polydipsia can also be seen in some cases of ectopic adrenocorticotropic hormone syndrome, although this is very rare in veterinary patients. Diabetes insipidus has been observed in a dog with intestinal leiomyosarcoma.

Neurological Paraneoplastic Syndromes

Peripheral Neuropathy

Peripheral paraneoplastic nerve injuries are relatively common. The most commonly observed neural lesions include paranodal or segmental demyelination, remyelination, and axonal degeneration. These alterations have been described in cases of bronchogenic carcinoma, mammary adenocarcinoma, melanoma, insulinoma and osteosarcoma, although patients do not always present with symptoms of localised or diffuse neuropathy, and even this seems to be rare.

Paraneoplastic polyneuropathies are usually characterised by diffuse lower motor neuron symptoms, although these are not very common. Paraneoplastic polyneuropathies have been described in a number of neoplasms including insulinoma, multiple myeloma, lymphoma, fibrosarcoma, leiomyosarcoma, anaplastic sarcoma, pancreatic adenocarcinoma, prostatic adenocarcinoma, mixed combined mammary adenoma, pulmonary adenoma, combined pulmonary carcinoma, metastatic feline renal haemangiosarcoma.

Myasthenia Gravis

Myasthenia gravis is **usually seen in association with canine and feline thymoma**. Other neoplasms associated with myasthenia gravis syndrome in dogs also include osteosarcoma, cholangiocellular carcinoma, oral sarcoma, and non-epitheliotropic cutaneous lymphoma.

Paraneoplastic myasthenia gravis is an immune-mediated disease: antibodies against nicotinic acetylcholine receptors are formed in the postsynaptic sarcolemma of the neuromuscular junction.

Patients with generalised myasthenia gravis present with appendicular muscle weakness that is usually induced by exercise. They can also present with megaoesophagus and weakness of the muscles of the face, pharynx, and larynx. If myasthenia gravis is focal, the muscle weakness most commonly affects the muscles of the oesophagus.

The treatment of paraneoplastic myasthenia gravis consists of **reducing the levels of antibodies against the acetylcholine receptor**. The goal of treatment is to reduce the tumour burden. In the case of thymomas, surgical resection of the tumour and/or radiation therapy is recommended and, although it is common for excision of the tumour to result in resolution of myasthenia gravis, this is not guaranteed in all cases.

Patients presenting with myasthenia gravis or paraneoplastic megaoesophagus associated with thymoma do not necessarily appear to have a worse prognosis. However, these same patients are predisposed to develop complications associated with megaoesophagus, such as aspiration pneumonia.

Dermatological Paraneoplastic Syndromes

Nodular Dermatofibrosis

Patients with nodular dermatofibrosis syndrome present with multiple, slow-growing, cutaneous collagen nodules that are associated with the diagnosis of cystadenocarcinoma or renal cystadenoma. This syndrome is of **autosomal dominant inheritance and is seen almost exclusively in German Shepherd dogs** The mutation responsible is identified on the Birt-Hogg-Dubé gene on chromosome 5, which encodes the protein folliculin. This same gene is related to the Birt-Hogg-Dubé syndrome associated with renal cancer in humans.

Nodular paraneoplastic dermatofibrosis syndrome generally presents with the presence of multiple firm skin nodules, which are usually itchy and not painful. The lesions are mainly found on the limbs, head, and trunk. Nodular dermatofibrosis almost always precedes the appearance of renal failure induced by renal neoplasia and/or the presence of metastases. Microscopic renal alterations can occur from an early age, but it may take months or years for the development of renal failure associated with neoplasia and/or development of metastatic disease. Affected female canines often suffer concurrently from uterine leiomyomas, although these are not usually of great clinical significance.

Patients diagnosed with cystadenocarcinomas or renal cystadenomas usually present with bilateral and multiple tumours, making surgery difficult in most cases. Unfortunately, effective medical treatment is not currently available. Nodular dermatofibrosis nodules can be removed palliatively if they impact the quality of life of patients. The median survival rate for patients presenting with nodular dermatofibrosis is approximately two and a half years from the appearance of the first symptoms of dermatofibrosis.

Necrolytic Superficial Dermatitis

Patients with paraneoplastic necrolytic superficial dermatitis present with erosions, ulcerations, alopecia, exudation, and scabs on the flank, perineal area, face, facial mucocutaneous junctions, oral cavity, legs, and pressure areas such as the elbow or calcaneal tuberosity. The lesions are painful and itchy, and patients also suffer from hyperkeratosis and fissures on the pads.

Superficial necrolytic paraneoplastic dermatitis is **seen in patients with glucagon-secreting neoplasms of the pancreas and liver**. This syndrome can also be seen in patients with liver disease, which is commonly referred to as hepatocutaneous syndrome.

Hypoaminoacidaemia is often associated with necrolytic superficial dermatitis syndrome and is thought to result from elevated glucagon levels that support gluconeogenesis and amino acid catabolism. These processes lead to protein depletion and subsequent keratinocyte necrolysis.

Unfortunately, many of the neoplasms associated with the development of paraneoplastic necrolytic dermatitis present themselves at an already advanced stage and medical treatment options are scarce in most cases. However, if the disease is local, surgical excision of the tumour can result in resolution of the necrolytic dermatitis. There is also a report of a dog which was successfully treated with octreotride (somatostatin analogue).

Feline Paraneoplastic Alopecia

Cats with paraneoplastic alopecia present with a progressive non-pruritic symmetrical alopecia that mainly affects the ventral abdomen and the medial aspect of the limbs. The pads may also be affected and are often painful, dry, cracked, and crusted, or sometimes moist and erythematous. The hairs are easily epilated, and the skin becomes shiny, fine and loses its elastic properties.

Neoplasms associated with the development of paraneoplastic alopecia include **pancreatic carcinoma and biliary carcinoma**. Unfortunately, these neoplasms are usually quite aggressive, and many cats present with clinically advanced metastatic disease and are only treated palliatively. However, if the disease is localised, surgical excision of the tumour can result in resolution of the paraneoplastic alopecia.

Feline Thymoma-associated Exfoliative Dermatitis

Cats with thymoma-associated exfoliative dermatitis initially present with small scabs and mild erythema on the head, trunk, and limb areas. These lesions progress and alopecia develops. Keratosebaceous material also usually accumulates between the digits, in the nail beds and in the ear canal, where scabs and ulcers can also develop.

Paraneoplastic exfoliative dermatitis appears to have an immune-mediated component.

Surgery to remove the thymoma is the treatment of choice and the dermatitis should resolve after tumour excision, although as exfoliative dermatitis associated with feline thymoma is a rare paraneoplastic syndrome, there are not many reports on this topic in the veterinary literature.

Other Paraneoplastic Syndromes

Fever

The development of paraneoplastic fever may be **related to an innate immune response against tumour antigens, or it may also be related to the presence of tumour necrosis**. Fever is primarily mediated by TNF-α and interleukins IL-1 and IL-6 in the hypothalamus. These cytokines activate the arachidonic acid cascade, stimulating the production of prostaglandin E2 that will act in the thermoregulatory centre of the hypothalamus.

Haematopoietic neoplasms are the neoplasms most commonly associated with the development of paraneoplastic fever. In a veterinary study of cases of fever of unknown cause, the presence of paraneoplastic fever was diagnosed in less than 10% of cases, and haematopoietic neoplasms were the most frequently diagnosed cancer.

It is important for other causes of fever to be excluded as the fever may be associated with other factors, such as the presence of a concurrent or secondary infection to the tumour, the presence of large areas of necrosis, or tumour ulceration.

Depending on the location and type of tumour which is diagnosed, fever can be caused by various factors. Tumours of the gastrointestinal tract can cause perforations of the gastrointestinal tract, which can result in septic peritonitis. Sepsis secondary to the presence of severe leucopaenias can also occur, as in cases of haematopoietic neoplasms (e.g. acute lymphocytic leukaemia). Other infections may also be related to anticancer treatment, such as postoperative healing complications, severe neutropaenias associated with chemotherapy, and sepsis or vomiting associated with gastrointestinal toxicity from chemotherapy and subsequent development of aspiration pneumonia.

As in most paraneoplastic syndromes, paraneoplastic fever usually resolves after successful treatment of the underlying neoplasm. However, in clinical cases where successful tumour treatment is not possible, symptomatic treatment should be administered to improve the patient's quality of life (for example, with nonsteroidal anti-inflammatory drugs).

Hypertrophic Osteopathy

Hypertrophic osteopathy (Figure 2) is a disorder of the periosteum that affects the long bones of the limbs. It usually begins in the toes and progresses proximally. The lesions are typically bilateral and symmetrical and usually affect all four limbs.

The neoplasms most commonly associated with the development of paraneoplastic hypertrophic osteopathy in dogs are primary pulmonary neoplasms and neoplasms causing metastatic pulmonary disease. In fact, **metastatic pulmonary disease is the one most frequently associated with the development of hypertrophic osteopathy**, and canine osteosarcoma is the tumour most commonly associated with this syndrome when there are pulmonary metastases. Other canine tumours that have been reported in association with hypertrophic osteopathy syndrome include canine transitional cell renal carcinoma, nephroblastoma, botryoid rhabdomyosarcoma of the urinary bladder, hepatocellular carcinoma, adenocarcinoma of the oesophagus, and schwannoma of the vagus nerve. In cats, the paraneoplastic syndrome associated with hypertrophic osteopathy has been reported in cases of adrenocortical carcinomas and renal adenomas.

Hypertrophic osteopathy has also been observed in non-neoplastic diseases, such as inflammatory or infectious diseases of the lung parenchyma, *Dirofilaria immitis* infections, bacterial endocarditis, patent ductus arteriosus with right-to-left shunt, oesophageal granulomas due to *Spirocerca lupi*, oesophageal foreign bodies and in cases of congenital megaoesophagus. Cases of idiopathic paraneoplastic hypertrophic osteopathy have also been observed in cats.

Patients with paraneoplastic hypertrophic osteopathy present clinically with lameness and difficulties moving. During the clinical examination, swelling and oedema of the distal part of the limbs and pain on palpation of the affected area are usually found, which is also usually warm. On many occasions, patients also present with bilateral serous-mucopurulent ocular discharge and episcleral congestion. Less than 50% of patients present with pulmonary symptoms, according to data from one study.

Radiographic signs of hypertrophic osteopathy include formation of new periosteal bone that appears nodular and spiculated and normally grows at a 90 degree angle to the longitudinal axis. Evidence of swelling and oedema of the adjacent soft tissues is also seen in many cases.

The pathophysiological alterations of hypertrophic osteopathy include increased peripheral blood circulation, proliferation of vascular connective tissue, and consequent formation of bone spicules. A neural reflex originating in the thorax and carried by vagal afferent fibres may occur, and cases have been observed in which a vagotomy has resulted in the regression of hypertrophic osteopathy. Elevated levels of vascular endothelial growth factor (VEGF) and platelet-derived growth factor (PDGF) have been observed in people diagnosed with lung cancer and paraneoplastic hypertrophic osteopathy. This may have important therapeutic implications, although in veterinary patients information regarding this is not yet available.

The treatment of hypertrophic pulmonary osteopathy consists primarily of treating the cancer responsible for the development of the syndrome, if possible. This may include surgical resection of the primary lung tumour or metastectomy of some metastatic lung lesions, depending on the clinical case and the causative neoplasm. Chemotherapy may also be considered in cancers susceptible to medical treatment. In people, treatment with bisphosphonates (zolendronate and pamidronate) has been shown to be effective in controlling the pain associated with hypertrophic osteopathy in a palliative manner. It is not known if such an effect also occurs in veterinary patients, although this treatment is commonly used in these cases.

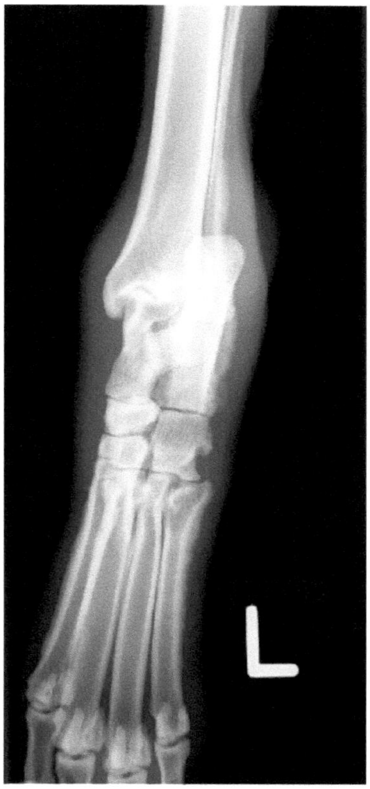

Figure 2. Hypertrophic osteopathy in the distal part of the hindlimb of a dog with metastatic pulmonary osteosarcoma. The formation of new periosteal bone with a spiculated appearance can be seen with a radiation of 90 degrees from the long axis of the calcaneal and fourth tarsal bones. There is also evidence of oedema in the soft tissue. (Image: Charlotte Johnston, DVM, MVetSc, MRCVS, DipACVIM Oncology)

Bibliography

- Abbo, A.H., Lucroy, M.D. (2007) Assessment of anemia as an independent predictor of response to chemotherapy and survival in dogs with lymphoma. *J Am Vet Med Assoc*, 231:1836–1842.
- Baez, J.L., Michel, K.E., Sorenmo, K. et al. (2007) A prospective investigation of the prevalence and prognostic significance of weight loss and changes in body condition in feline cancer patients. *J Feline Med Surg*, 9:411–417.
- Barrs, V.R., Martin, P., France, M. et al. (1999) What is your diagnosis? Feline paraneoplastic alopecia associated with pancreatic and bile duct carcinomas. *J Small Anim Pract*, 40(559):595–596.
- Braund K.G., McGuire, J.A., Amling, A.K. et al. (1987) Peripheral neuropathy associated with malignant neoplasms in dogs. *Vet Pathol*, 24:16–21.
- Celio L.M., Dennis, J. (2005) Canine superficial necrolytic dermatitis. *Compend Contin Ed Small Anim Pract*, 27:820–825.
- Childress, M.O. (2012) Hematologic abnormalities in the small animal cancer patient. *Vet Clin North Am Small Anim Pract*, 42: 123–155.
- Fox, L.E., Rosenthal, R.C., Twedt, D.C. et al. (1990) Plasma histamine and gastrin concentrations in 17 dogs with mast cell tumors. *J Vet Intern Med*, 4:242–246.
- Giraudel, J.M., Pagès, J.P., Fuilfi, J.F. (2002) Monoclonal gammopathies in the dog: a retrospective study of 18 cases (1986–1999) and literature review. *J Am Anim Hosp Assoc*, 39: 135–147.
- Goutal, C.M., Brugmann, B.L., Ryan, K.A. (2012) Insulinoma in dogs: a review. *J Am Anim Hosp Assoc*, 48:151–163.
- Griffiths, I.R., Duncan, I.D., Swallow, J.S. (1977) Peripheral polyneuropathy in dogs: a study of five cases. *J Small Anim Pract*, 18:101–106.
- Grindem, C.B., Breitschwerdt, E.B., Corbett, W.T. et al. (1994) Thrombocytopenia associated with neoplasia in dogs. *J Vet Intern Med*, 8:400–405.
- Hammer, A.S., Couto, C.G. (1994) Complications of multiple myeloma. *J Am Anim Hosp Assoc*, 30:9–14.
- Helfand, S.C., Couto, C.G., Madewell, B.R. (1985) Immune-mediated thrombocytopenia associated with solid tumours in dogs. *J Am Anim Hosp Assoc*, 21:787–794.
- Hurry, C.A., Flatland, B. (2005) Feline acromegaly, a review of the syndrome. *J Am Anim Hosp Assoc*, 41:292–297.
- Ishiguro, T., Kadosawa, T., Takagi, S. et al. Relationship of disease progression and plasma histamine concentrations in 11 dogs with mast cell tumors. *J Vet Intern Med*, 17:194–198.
- Lainesse, M.F.C., Taylor, S.M., Myers, S.L. et al. (1996) Focal myasthenia gravis as a paraneoplastic syndrome of canine thymoma: improvement following thymectomy. *J Am Anim Hosp Assoc*, 32: 111–117.
- Lingaas, F., Comstock, K.E., Kirkness, E.F. et al. (2003) A mutation in the canine BHD gene is associated with hereditary multifocal renal cystadenocarcinoma and nodular dermatofibrosis in the German shepherd dog. *Hum Mol Genet*, 12:3043–3053.
- Liptak, J.M., Monnet, E., Dernell, W.S. et al. (2004) Pulmonary metastectomy in the management of four dogs with hypertrophic osteopathy. *Vet Comp Oncol*, 2:1–12.
- Lucas, P., Lacoste, H., deLorimier, L-P et al. (2007) Treating paraneoplastic hypercalcemia in dogs and cats. *Vet Med*, 314–330.
- MacEwen, G.E., Hurvitz, A. (1977) Diagnosis and management of monoclonal gammopathies. *Vet Clin North Am*, 7:119–132.
- Madewell, B.D., Feldman, B.F., O'Neil, S. (1980) Coagulation abnormalities in dogs with neoplastic disease. *Thromb Haemost*, 44:35–38.
- Madewell, B.R., Feldman, B.F. (1980) Characterization of anemias associated with neoplasia in small animals. *J Am Vet Med Assoc*, 176:419–425.
- Madewell, B.R. (1986) Hematological and bone marrow cytological abnormalities in 75 dogs with malignant lymphoma. *J Am Animal Hosp Assoc*, 22:235–240.
- McCandlish, I.A., Munro, C., Breeze, R.G et al. (1979) Hormone producing ovarian tumours in the dog. *Vet Rec*, 105:9–11.
- McNiel, E.A., Ogilvie, G.K., Fettman, M.J. et al. (1997) Platelet hyperfunction in dogs with malignancies. *J Vet Intern Med* 11:178–182.
- Michel, K.E., Sorenmo, K., Shofer, F.S. (2004) Evaluation of body condition and weight loss in dogs presented to a veterinary oncology service. *J Vet Intern Med* 18:692–695.
- Miller, A.G., Morley, P.S., Rao, S. et al. (2009) Anemia is associated with decreased survival in dogs with lymphoma, *J Vet Intern Med*, 23:116–122.
- Mischke, R., Meurer, D., Hoppen, H.O. et al. (2002) Blood plasma concentrations of oestradiol-17B, testosterone, and testosterone/estradiol ratio in dogs with neoplastic and degenerative testicular diseases. *Res Vet Sci*, 73: 267–272.
- Murayama, H., Miura, T., Sakai, M. et al. (2004) The incidence of disseminated intravascular coagulation in dogs with malignant neoplasia. *J Vet Med Sci*, 66:573–575.
- Nitsche, E.K. (2004) Erythrocytosis in dogs and cats: diagnosis and management. *Compend Cont Ed Small Anim Pract*, 26:104–118.
- Pascal-Tenorio, A., Olivry, T., Gross, T.L. et al. (1997) Paraneoplastic alopecia associated with internal malignancies in the cat. *Vet Dermatol*, 8:47–51.
- Reif, J.S., Brodey, R.S. (1969) The relationship between cryptorchidism and canine testicular neoplasia. *J Am Med Assoc*, 155:2005–2010.
- Rosol, T.J., Nagode, L.A., Couto, C.G. et al. (1992) Parathyroid hormone (PTH)-related protein, PTH, and 1,25-dihydroxyvitamin D in dogs with cancer-associated hypercalcemia. *Endocrinology*, 131:1157–1164.
- Tobin, R.L., Nelson, R.W., Lucroy, M.D. et al. (1999) Outcome of surgery versus medical treatment of dogs with beta cell neoplasia: 39 cases *(1990–1997)*. *J Am Vet Med Assoc*, 215: 226–230.
- Turek, M. (2003) Cutaneous paraneoplastic syndromes in dogs and cats: a review of the literature. *Vet Dermatol*, 14:279–296.

■ Vasilopulos, R.J., Mackin, A. (2003) Humoral hypercalcemia of malignancy: diagnosis and treatment. *Compend Cont Ed Sm Anim Pract*, 25:129–137.
■ Weaver, A.D. (1983) Survey with follow-up of 67 dogs with testicular Sertoli cell tumours. *Vet Rec*, 113:105–107.
■ Withers, S.S., Johnson, E.G., Culp, W.T.N. et al. (2015) Paraneoplastic hypertrophic osteopathy in 30 dogs. *Vet Comp Oncol*, 13:157–165.
■ Withrow, S.J., Vail, D.M. (ed) (2007) *Withrow & MacEwen's Small Animal Clinical Oncology*. St. Louis, Mo., Saunders Elsevier.

Test

1. **Which of the haematological paraneoplastic syndromes is most commonly seen in veterinary cancer patients?**
   a. Thrombocytopaenia.
   b. Eosinophilia.
   c. Anaemia.
   d. Hyperviscosity syndrome.

2. **Which neoplasm is associated with the development of a paraneoplastic gastrointestinal ulceration?**
   a. Feline histiocytic sarcoma.
   b. Canine gastrinoma.
   c. Canine epitheliotropic lymphoma.
   d. Feline hepatocellular carninoma.

3. **In cases of malignant hypercalcaemia, what could be expected in terms PTHrP/PTH concentrations?**
   a. High PTHrP, low PTH.
   b. High PTHrP, high PTH.
   c. Low PTHrP, low PTH.
   d. Low PTHrP, high PTH.

4. **What initial symptomatic treatment would be recommended for a patient diagnosed with malignant hypercalcaemia who is not azotaemic?**
   a. Furosemide 1 mg/kg IV every 8 hours.
   b. Intravenous fluid therapy with 0.9% NaCl.
   c. Intravenous fluid therapy with lactated Ringer's.
   d. Prednisolone 0.5 mg/kg BID.

5. **What neoplasm can be related to the development of paraneoplastic hyperoestrogenism?**
   a. Sertoli cell tumour.
   b. Seminoma.
   c. Granulosa cell tumour of the ovary.
   d. All of the above.

6. **Nodular dermatofibrosis syndrome is associated with the diagnosis of renal cystadenocarcinoma or cystadenoma mainly in the German Shepherd, due to a mutation in the:**
   a. Birt-Hogg-Dubé gene on chromosome 4.
   b. Birt-Hogg-Dubé gene on chromosome 5.
   c. Birt-Hogg-Dubé gene on chromosome 10.
   d. Birt-Hogg-Dubé gene on chromosome 12.

Answers on Page 50

7. **What paraneoplastic syndromes can be seen in cats diagnosed with thymoma?**
   a. Myasthenia gravis and feline paraneoplastic alopecia.
   b. Myasthenia gravis and feline exfoliative dermatitis.
   c. Myasthenia gravis and nodular dermatofibrosis.
   d. Hyperviscosity syndrome.

8. **Paraneoplastic fever is mediated in the hypothalamus by:**
   a. TGF-β (growth factor beta), IL-2 and IL-9.
   b. TGF-β and prostaglandin E2.
   c. IL-5 and prostaglandin E2.
   d. TNF-α (tumour necrosis factor alpha), IL-1 and IL-6.

9. **What is the neoplasm most commonly associated with the development of paraneoplastic hypertrophic osteopathy?**
   a. Canine appendicular osteosarcoma with pulmonary metastases.
   b. Feline appendicular osteosarcoma with pulmonary metastases.
   c. Primary osteosarcoma of the jaw in the dog.
   d. Primary chondrosarcoma of the rib in the dog.

10. **What would be the treatment of choice for a patient diagnosed with a single 2 cm lung mass (cytology consistent with osteosarcoma) and paraneoplastic hypertrophic osteopathy, three months after a left forelimb amputation due to humeral osteosarcoma?**
   a. Doxorubicin 30 mg/m² every 14 days.
   b. Doxorubicin 30 mg/m² every 21 days.
   c. Surgical resection of the pulmonary mass.
   d. Carboplatin 300 mg/m² every 21 days.

Clinical Case

An 8-year-old female neutered dog was taken to the clinic with a two-week history of inappetence, slight lethargy, polyuria, and polydipsia. Otherwise, the dog was reported to be well.

On physical examination, the body mass index was 4/9 and no other abnormalities were found.

Blood tests were performed. The results appear in Tables 1 and 2.

Table 1. Complete blood count.

Parameter	Value	Reference values
Total leucocytes (x10³/µl)	10.90	6.00–17.00
Neutrophils (x10³/µl) (%)	8.27 (75.9)	3.62–12.3 (52.0–81.0)
Lymphocytes (x10³/µl) (%)	1.30 (11.9)	0.8–5.1 (12.0–33.0)
Monocytes (x10³/µl) (%)	1.17 (10.7)	0.0–1.8 (2.0–13.0)
Eosinophils (x10³/µl) (%)	0.16 (1.5)	0.04–1.62 (0.5–10.0)
Basophils (x10³/µl) (%)	0.00 (0.0)	0.00–0.12 (0.0–1.3)
Erythrocytes (x10⁶/µl)	4.76	5.10–8.50
Haemoglobin (g/dl)	112	110–190
Haematocrit (%)	30.7	33.0–56.0
MVC (fl)	64.4	60.0–76.0
MCH (pg)	23.6	20.0–27.0
MCHC (g/dl)	366	300–380
RDW-CV (%)	15.7	12.5–17.2
RDW-SD (fl)	45.7	33.0–46.3
Platelets (x10³/µl)	532	117–490
MPV (fl)	7.0	8.0–14.1
PDW (10GSD)	15.1	12.0–17.5
PCT (%)	0.374	0.090–0.580

Table 2. Serum biochemistry.

Parameter	Value	Reference values
Total protein (g/dl)	6.1	5.0–7.2
Albumin (g/dl)	3.0	2.6–4.0
ALP (IU/l)	56	13–83
Glucose (mg/dl)	108	75–128
Total bilirubin (mg/dl)	0.2	0.1–0.5
Phosphorus (mg/dl)	2.1	1.9–5.0
Total cholesterol (mg/dl)	230	111–312
GGT (IU/l)	10	5–14
ALT (IU/l)	115	17–78
Total calcium (mg/dl)	15.4	9.4–11.8
Ionised calcium (mmol/l)	1.7	1.12–1.4
Creatinine (mg/dl)	1.6	0.4–1.4
BUN (mg/dl)	39	9.2–29.2
Globulins	3.1	1.6–3.7

Based on the clinical history, physical examination, and test results:

1. **What would the next step be?**
2. **Which diagnostic tests should be performed next to reach a diagnosis in this patient?**
3. **What are the most likely differential diagnoses?**

Correct Answers:

Test

1. c
2. b
3. a
4. b
5. d
6. b
7. b
8. d
9. a
10. c

Clinical Case

1. **What would the next step be?**
   Hypercalcaemia is considered a medical emergency in many cases. As soon as a patient is diagnosed with hypercalcaemia, steps should be taken to identify its cause, guide additional complementary diagnostic tests, and implement treatment.

   A thorough and detailed physical examination is essential, including examination of the anal sac glands and palpation of the peripheral lymph nodes.

   Given the hypercalcaemia in this patient together with clinical symptoms, starting medical treatment for hypercalcaemia as soon as possible is recommended with the administration of intravenous fluid therapy with 0.9% NaCl, while performing diagnostic tests. The goal is to correct initial dehydration, increase glomerular filtration rate, and filter calcium. The duration of supportive medical therapy will depend on the duration of the hypercalcaemia and treatment of its underlying cause. In addition, depending on the progression of hypercalcaemia and the clinical status of the patient, other therapeutic measures (for example, administration of furosemide or bisphosphonates) can be initiated depending on the results of further diagnostic tests.

2. **Which diagnostic tests should be performed next to reach a diagnosis in this patient?**
   The next diagnostic tests should include urinalysis (dipstick, sediment, USG, and culture), thoracic radiographs, abdominal ultrasound, and fine needle aspirations, and cytology of any lesions found (e.g. peripheral lymph nodes, an anal sac mass). Depending on the results of these tests, other diagnostic tests may be necessary such as ultrasound of the neck (for example, to look for a lesion in the parathyroid gland), orthopaedic radiographs, bone marrow aspiration and/or measurement of the PTH, PTHrP and calcitriol values.

3. **What are the most likely differential diagnoses?**
   Approximately 60% of canine patients who present with hypercalcaemia are diagnosed with cancer. The tumour most commonly associated with malignant hypercalcaemia in dogs is T-cell lymphoma. Other neoplasms associated with the development of malignant hypercalcaemia in dogs include malignant lymphocytic leukaemia, anal sac gland carcinoma, clitoral adenocarcinoma, hepatocellular carcinoma, nasal carcinoma, penile adenocarcinoma, pulmonary carcinoma, thymoma, osteosarcoma, mammary carcinoma, melanoma, multiple myeloma, pheochromocytoma, renal angiomyxoma, renal cell carcinoma, thyroid carcinoma, and parathyroid adenoma (or adenomatous parathyroid hyperplasia). Other non-neoplastic causes of hypercalcaemia in dogs include kidney failure, primary hyperparathyroidism, Addison's disease, osteolytic disorders, granulomatous-type inflammatory diseases, and vitamin D poisoning.

Notes

Diagnostic Imaging of the Cancer Patient

Audrey Petite

External organ neoplasia is often identified during a physical clinical examination, but internal neoplastic lesions are more difficult or almost impossible to identify on physical examination of the patient. Hence **diagnostic imaging is often the first line of diagnostic investigation when a cancer (benign or malignant) is suspected in veterinary patients**. Unlike in human medicine, where the majority of cancer search is by preventive screening, in veterinary medicine there is usually already a strong suspicion of neoplasia when the patient is presented for diagnostic imaging.

The aim of imaging investigations are primarily to help identify the origin of the tumour (primary organ affected), as well as the effect on the adjacent structures. They also aid in establishing a prioritised list of differential diagnoses, obtaining a definitive diagnosis through guided biopsies for cytology or histopathology, assisting in patient staging, as well as providing invaluable information for treatment planning. This may include surgery, radiotherapy, chemotherapy, or any combination of these modalities. Up to 3% of cancer patients have been reported to present with an additional unrelated tumour. Diagnostic imaging also helps to identify these patients, as it may have a significant impact on both the choice of treatment and prognosis. To work these patients up, it is essential to know the advantages and disadvantages of each imaging tool available, its best applications for diagnosis of both primary and secondary lesions, and its limitations.

Advantages and Disadvantages of the Different Methods of Diagnostic Imaging

Historically, radiography and thereafter ultrasonography have been the first techniques used, both due to their wide availability, and their cost efficiency. Most of these examinations can be conducted on conscious or sedated patients, avoiding the need for general anaesthesia. In the last couple of decades, new and more advanced imaging modalities have become more widely available in veterinary practices and referral centres, mainly the tomographic techniques, including computed tomography (CT) and magnetic resonance imaging (MRI). These imaging modalities have revolutionised both the diagnostic and the staging approach for cancer. They provide a vastly superior imaging resolution, and the tomographic nature of these techniques allows for three dimensional investigations and reconstruction, which provide invaluable support to clinicians both for lesion detection and assessment, and for treatment planning.

Currently, **complete assessment of a cancer patient often involves more than one imaging technique**. It remains important

Table 1. Availability, cost, sensitivity, and specificity of the different diagnostic imaging modalities for the diagnosis of neoplasia, according to the region of interest.

Body part \ Imaging modality		RADIOGRAPHY Availability: high Cost: low	ULTRASONOGRAPHY Availability: high Cost: low	CT Availability: moderate Cost: moderate	MRI Availability: low Cost: high
Skeletal structures	Sensitivity	high	low	high	moderate
	Specificity	high	low	high	moderate
Head and neck	Sensitivity	low	moderate	high	high
	Specificity	low	moderate	moderate	high
Nervous structures	Sensitivity	low	low	moderate	high
	Specificity	low	low	low	high
Thoracic structures	Sensitivity	low	low to moderate	high	low
	Specificity	low	moderate	moderate	moderate
Abdominal structures	Sensitivity	low	high	high	high
	Specificity	low	high	moderate	high
Staging	Sensitivity	low	high	high	moderate
	Specificity	low	high	moderate	moderate

to carefully consider the balance between the diagnostic yield of an imaging study, and its cost, to avoid unnecessary procedures. Due to the inherent technological advances applied to diagnostic imaging, it is to be expected that progress in this field will continue to provide more applications relevant to the diagnosis and of benefit to the treatment of veterinary cancer patients.

Choice of the imaging modality depends on multiple criteria. The most obvious one would be the relative **availability** of imaging techniques to a practitioner, as well as their personal **ability** to use the technique and **expertise** in interpreting the obtained images. It will also depend on the **organ/region** of the body under investigation and the **type of primary neoplastic condition** suspected. The **needs for sedation/anaesthesia** as well as **owners' financial constraints** are further important factors for consideration (Table 1).

For **detection of metastatic disease**, good knowledge of the neoplastic behaviour of the lesion being investigated is essential. Some neoplasia will tend to only be locally invasive, while others will spread preferentially to lungs, liver, spleen and/or to the regional lymph nodes. Hence the imaging modality used should be chosen accordingly. Excellent knowledge of the lymphosomes (lymphatic drainage territories) is necessary, as organs can be drained by several lymph nodes, and one lymph node may drain several organs (Table 2).

The imaging technique used to follow-up and monitor the response to the implemented treatment may also affect the choice of imaging technique. This may vary for the different techniques used to achieve the primary diagnosis or for staging purposes.

Regardless of the imaging modality used, the interpretative principles are broadly the same for primary neoplasia, relying on the **identification of organ enlargement or presence of a mass lesion**, as well as the secondary changes that may be induced by the primary lesion. These include displacement, compression, destruction or obstruction of adjacent structures, accumulation of fluid and intra- or extralesional bleeds.

Table 2. Superficial and deep lymph nodes and their corresponding drained areas (lymphosome). Note that a large overlap is present as well as individual variations.

Lymph node	Lymphosome
Superficial lymph nodes	
Cervical (cranial, mandibular, tonsillar, parotid, retropharyngeal)	Head
Prescapular	Neck, cranial thorax, anterior aspect of the forelimbs
Axillary	Superficial structures of the thoracic dorsum, posterior aspect of the forelimbs, thoracic and cranial abdominal mammary glands
Inguinal	Superficial structures of the abdominal dorsum, abdominal and inguinal mammary glands, back end
Popliteal	Distal third of the hindlimbs
Deep lymph nodes	
Craniomediastinal	Caudal cervical vertebrae, thoracic vertebrae, trachea, oesophagus, heart
Presternal	Sternum, ribs, thymus, peritoneal cavity, mammary glands
Tracheobronchial	Lungs, bronchi, trachea, oesophagus, aorta, heart, diaphragm
Hepatic	Liver, stomach, duodenum, pancreas
Splenic	Spleen, liver, oesophagus, stomach, duodenum, pancreas, omentum
Gastric	Diaphragm, liver, oesophagus, stomach, duodenum, pancreas, peritoneum
Pancreaticoduodenal	Duodenum, pancreas, omentum
Mesenteric	Jejunum, ileum, pancreas
Colic	Ileum, caecum, colon
Lumbar, aortic, renal	Lumbar vertebrae, caudal ribs, lumbar muscles, aorta, abdominal wall, peritoneum, kidneys, adrenal glands, urinary bladder, uterus, prostate, ovaries or testicles
Medial iliac, hypogastric, sacral	Ureters, urinary bladder, uterus, prostate, ovaries or testicles, pelvic region, abdominal wall

Conventional Radiography: Principles and Interpretation of Clinical Cases

Radiography relies on the differential absorption of X-rays by the structures under investigation. This differential absorption results in a two dimensional projected image of the area, with a range of grey shades varying from almost white for the highly absorbing structures (high density, such as cortical bone) to almost black for poorly absorbing structures (low density, such as gas/air). **The main disadvantage of radiography is that all organs included in the projection**

are superimposed on each other, rendering the interpretation more complex.

As it provides a general overview of the area under investigation, **it is used as a screening modality**, usually opening the path for further diagnostic imaging modalities for better definition of the tumour extent and behaviour.

Skeletal Structures

The **strong point of conventional radiography is imaging of the skeletal structures**, mainly the appendicular structures.

Radiographic features of bone malignancy are well described both in terms of bone loss and bone production. **Bone loss needs to reach approximately 30% of the mineralised matrix to be radiographically detectable**; therefore, early changes may not be visible on conventional radiographs. When assessing bone lesions, the most aggressive radiographic feature should be considered to reflect the aggressiveness of the overall lesion. Associated soft tissue changes can also be assessed radiographically, including muscle wastage, soft tissue swelling and/or joint effusion.

Primary bone neoplasia has a predilection distribution to the proximal humerus, distal radius, distal femur, and proximal tibial metaphysis. It is usually monostotic (affecting only one bone) and does not cross over joint spaces. These lesions present a wide range of radiographic signs depending on the osteoblastic versus osteoclastic behaviour of the lesion. These signs may include an expansile lytic lesion and/or disruption of the cortical bone with presence of irregular periosteal reaction. The transition between the abnormal bone and the normal bone is usually long and irregular, without a clear sclerotic margin (Figure 1). Disruption of the cortical bone may lead to pathological fractures. Elevation of the periosteum may lead to the formation of a triangle of new bone called "Codman's triangle". None of these features are pathognomonic for primary bone neoplasia. **Orthogonal projections of the area of concern should be obtained**.

Multiple myeloma may also present as lytic lesions, described as "punched out", anywhere along the skeletal structures, but with a predilection for the ribs, sternebrae and vertebrae (Figure 2).

Occasionally, palisading periosteal reaction is identified along the diaphysis of the long bones, often starting on the digits, and extending proximally, more on the abaxial cortices, often symmetrically. **Hypertrophic osteopathy** (also called Marie's disease) is most commonly associated with intrathoracic mass lesions but can also occasionally be associated with intra-abdominal mass lesions. Hence **this is a warning sign for primary neoplastic lesions elsewhere in the body cavities**, and these should be investigated accordingly.

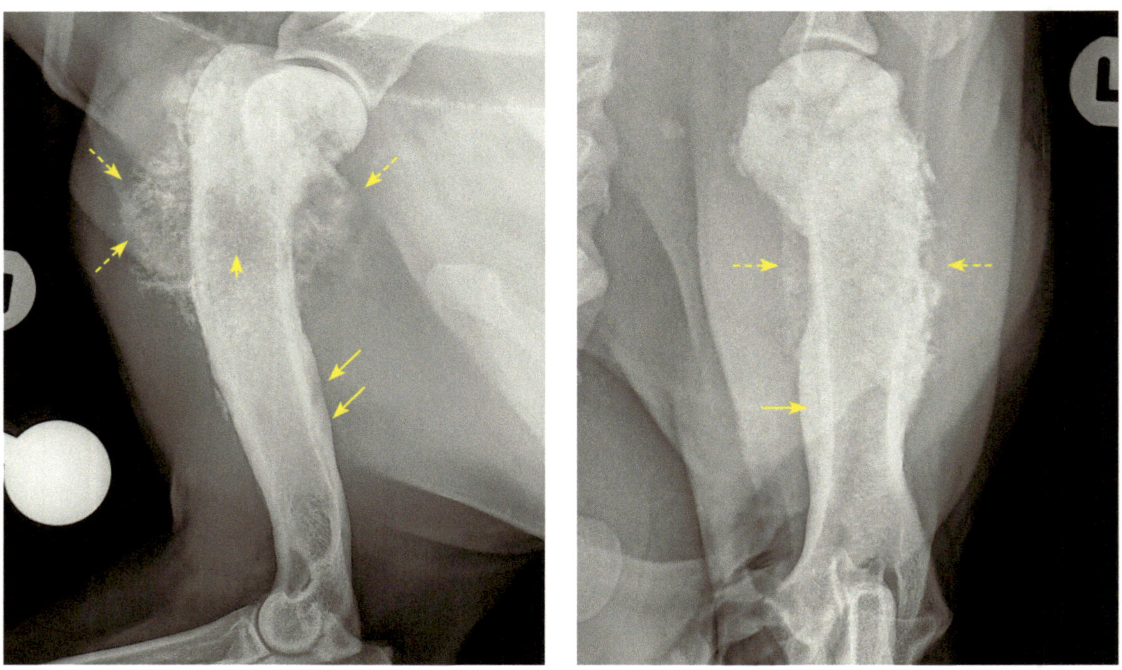

Figure 1. Orthogonal projections of the humerus, showing an area of lysis (arrowhead), cortical thickening (arrows) and an amorphous periosteal reaction (dotted arrows), associated with a primary osteosarcoma.

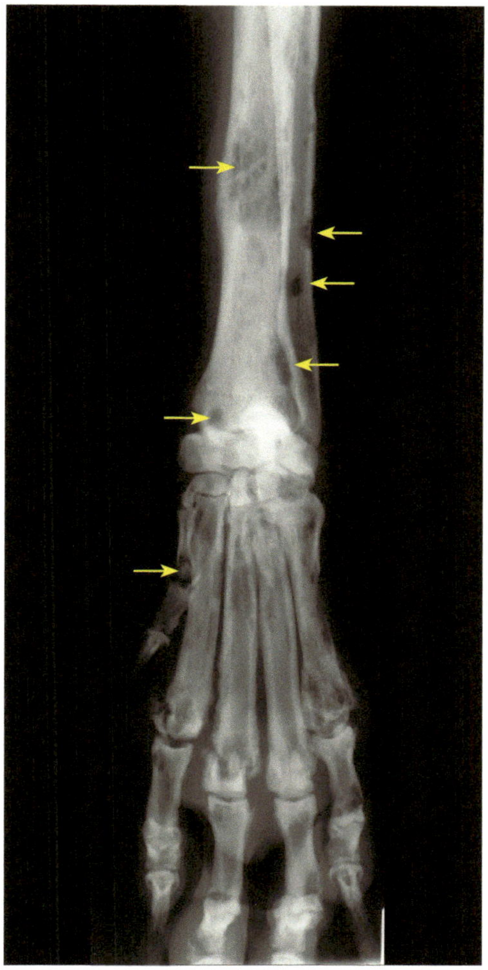

Figure 2. Dorsopalmar projection of the antebrachium showing multiple round focal lytic bone lesions (arrows) in a confirmed case of multiple myeloma.

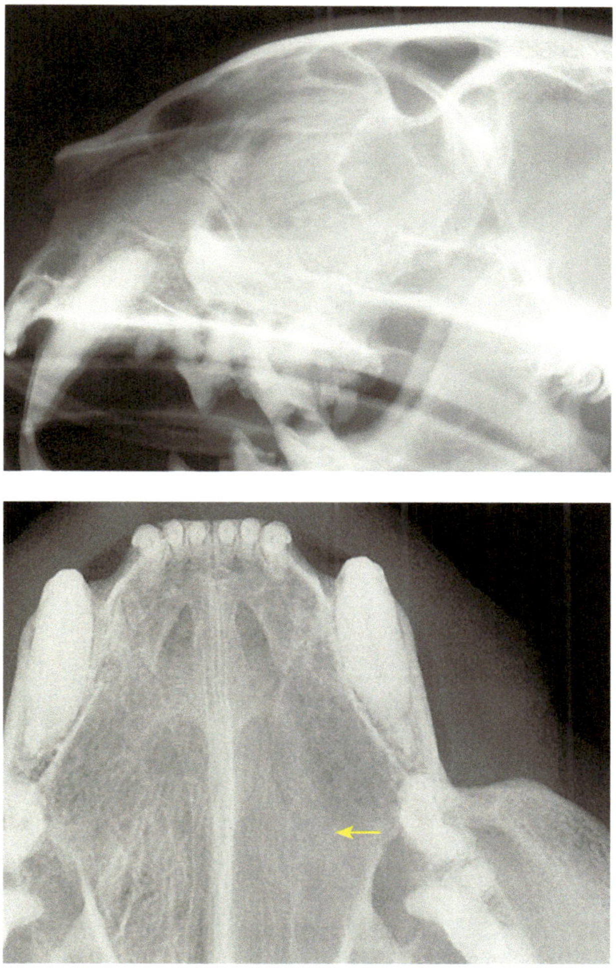

Figure 3. Lateral and intraoral projections of nasal lymphoma in a feline patient. Complete effacement of the turbinate pattern is present in the left nasal cavity (arrow). Note the lack of information provided by the lateral projection only, it should always be associated with several other projections.

Head and Neck

Due to the complexity of the head structures and their superimposition over each other, **use of radiography is limited to assessing bony involvement of cancerous lesions**, whether of primary bone or soft tissue origin. The principles of interpretation are the same as those used for the remainder of the skeleton.

For the skull, the superimposition of such fine and complex structures makes interpretation difficult. Nevertheless, it remains a good screening tool in most practices for nasal and oral cavities, providing that an appropriate radiographic protocol is used. For the nasal cavities and sinuses this should include, but not be limited to, an intraoral dorsoventral projection or a ventrodorsal oblique open mouth projection to visualise the nasal cavities and the cribriform plate with as little superimposition as possible. Other essential projections are lateral and dorsoventral projections of the skull, and if necessary, a craniocaudal skyline projection of the sinuses may be added. Presence of soft tissue material in the nasal chambers, associated with turbinate or bony case destruction is suggestive of tumours (Figure 3). Differential diagnoses include destructive rhinitis, particularly of fungal origin.

Oral destructive lesions can also be identified on radiographs, and oblique projections of the mandible will provide a reasonable idea of the extent of the bone involvement. Unfortunately, **radiography will only provide limited information in cases of tumours not involving any bony structure**, showing at best a space occupying soft tissue mass.

Thoracic Structures

The **second main application of conventional radiography is investigation of the thoracic structures, the lungs**.

Lung Tumours

The differential absorption between the air contained in the pulmonary alveoli and a potential soft tissue pulmonary mass lesion/lobar consolidation is high. The radiographic protocol for detection of pulmonary masses should include **right and left lateral recumbency projections** acquired at full inflation at the peak of the inspiratory phase. A **dorsoventral or ventrodorsal** projection should then be added depending on the dorsal or ventral location of the lesion.

Radiographic changes associated with primary pulmonary tumours are most commonly reported to be a focal mass lesion or lobar consolidation. Although a minimal size of 2–3 cm in diameter is needed, radiographic detection and accurate localisation is possible in most cases, both in dogs and cats (Figure 4). About one third of patients will present with more than one lobe involved. When an entire lobe is consolidated, the lobe is usually enlarged, rounded, and causes a mediastinal shift away from the affected lobe. Compression of the adjacent bronchi or pleural effusion may also be present. Pleural thickening or widening can be identified radiographically as a thickening of the interlobar fissures.

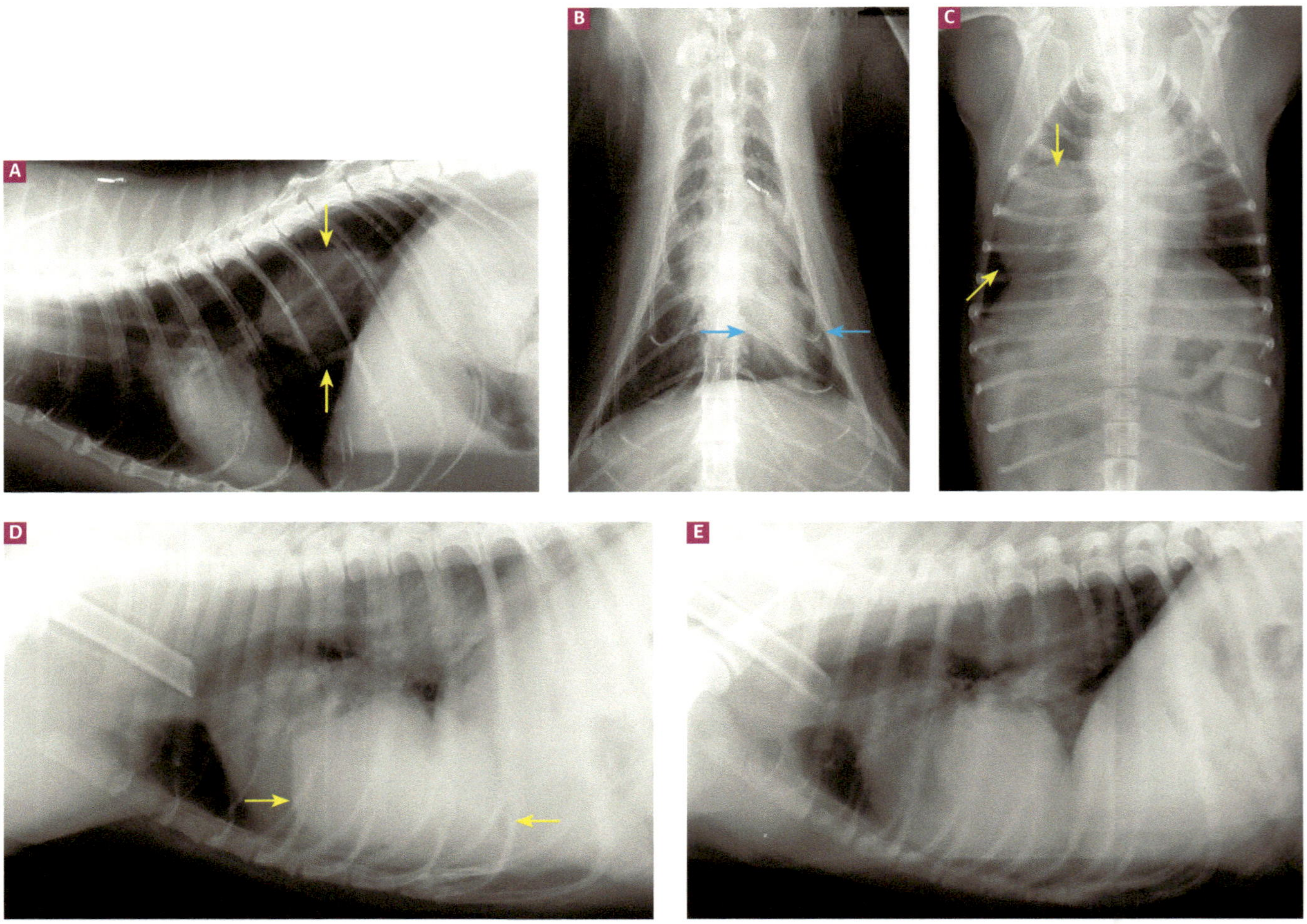

Figure 4. Orthogonal projections of a feline patient presenting a confirmed pulmonary carcinoma in the left caudal lung lobe (**A** and **B**). Three projections of a canine patient with the same condition affecting the right cardiac lobe (arrows) (**C, D** and **E**). Note the displacement of the cardiac silhouette to the left side and the much better appreciation of the lesion in the left lateral recumbency projection (**D**) than in right lateral recumbency (**E**).

Mediastinal Tumours

The mediastinum is the midline space of the thoracic cavity and runs slightly oblique from cranial right to caudal left of the thoracic cavity. It is continuous, with the caudal neck cranially and with the retroperitoneal space caudally. It contains the thoracic trachea, the thoracic oesophagus, the thymus, lymph nodes, nerves, the great vessels, and the heart. Depending on the amount of surrounding fat contained in the mediastinum, these structures will be more or less visible radiographically.

It is important to recognise the normal variation of mediastinal width according to the type of chest radiographed; deep chested patients usually present with a narrow mediastinum, with a small amount of mediastinal fat, while barrel-chested dogs tend to have more mediastinal fat leading to a wider mediastinum. Presence of malignancy affecting these structures will result in a widening of the corresponding region of the mediastinum and displacement of adjacent structures. This will be more readily visible on dorsoventral or ventrodorsal projections, but superimposition of the spine may hinder the radiographic interpretation.

The differential diagnosis of mediastinal tumours is summarised in Table 3, according to the enlarged area of the mediastinum. Note that haemangiosarcoma, lipoma, liposarcoma and histiocytic sarcoma may affect any area of the mediastinum.

Table 3. Differential diagnosis of mediastinal tumours according to their location.

Mediastinal area enlarged	Differential diagnosis
Cranioventral	Lymphoma, thymoma (Figure 5), thymic lymphoma
Craniodorsal	Neural or neuroendocrine tumours, paravertebral tumours, oesophageal tumours
Perihilar	Lymphoma, heart-based tumours, oesophageal tumours
Caudoventral	Diaphragmatic tumours
Caudodorsal	Oesophageal tumours, diaphragmatic tumours, neural tumours

Thoracic Wall Tumours

The **last thoracic structure to assess radiographically for tumours is the thoracic wall**. Tumours of the thoracic wall can arise both from skeletal and soft tissue structures, the former being much more common. Both are likely to produce a mass effect, with or without associated rib destruction, causing an "extrapleural sign". This is recognised as a broad-based lesion on the thoracic wall side, and an intrapleural bulge.

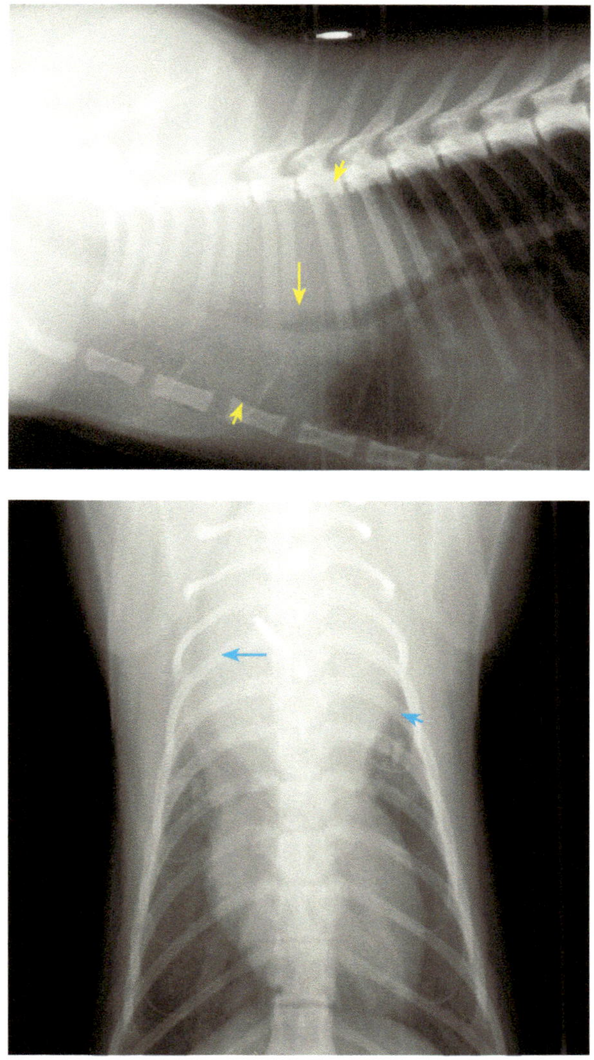

Figure 5. Orthogonal projections of a young British Shorthair with confirmed thymoma. A large soft tissue mass is identified cranial to the cardiac silhouette (arrowheads). On the dorsoventral projection, widening of the cranial mediastinum and displacement of the trachea ventrally and to the right can be observed (arrows).

Thoracic wall tumours may also cause widening/displacement of the normally regular rib spacing.

Abdominal Structures

Radiography for detection of intra-abdominal tumours is **limited to the detection of mass lesions**. The natural contrast provided by abdominal fat and gastrointestinal gas guides interpretation. Contrast studies with barium for the gastrointestinal tract or with iodine products for the urinary tract have been replaced by ultrasonographic examination.

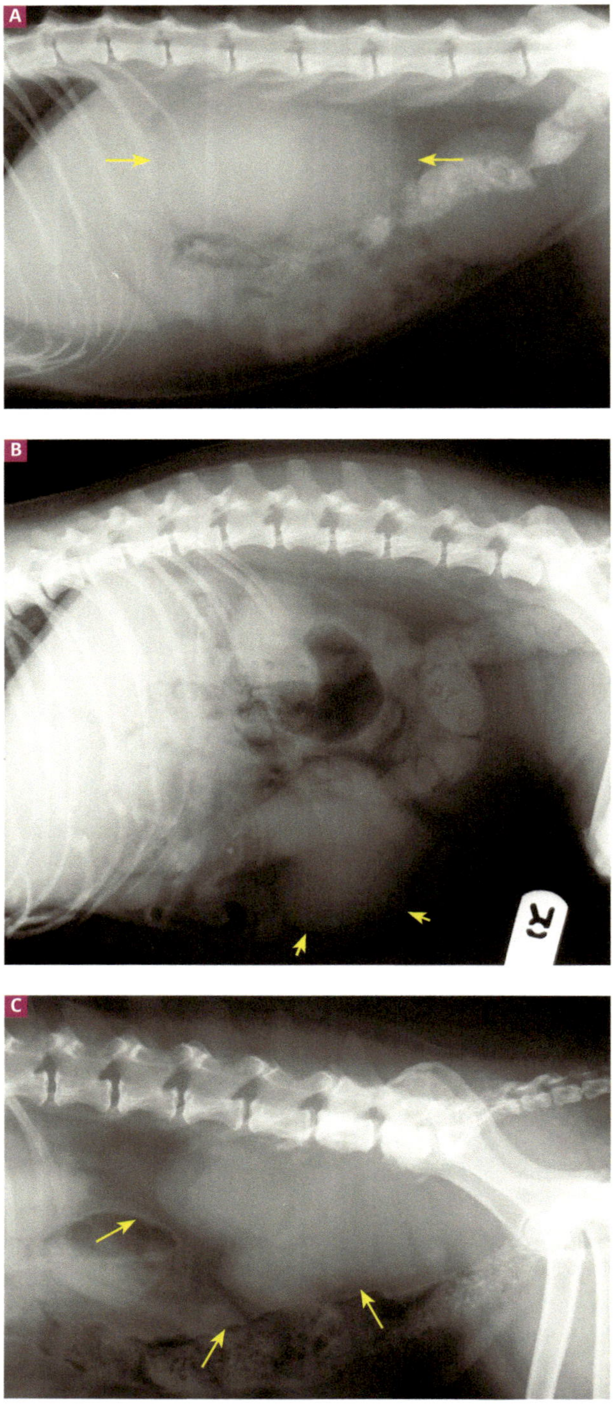

Figure 6. Three lateral radiographs of patients with masses in different abdominal areas. **A**. Feline patient with confirmed renal lymphoma (arrows). Note the mass effect in the mid-dorsal abdomen. **B**. Canine patient with splenic haemangioma, the mass is located in the midventral abdomen (arrowheads). **C**. Canine patient with severe iliac/hypogastric metastatic lymphadenomegaly from an anal sac carcinoma. They are located in the caudodorsal abdomen (arrows). Note the changes on the ventral aspect of the last two lumbar vertebral bodies suggestive of spinal involvement.

Displacement of abdominal structures should provide a good indication of the organ involved (Figure 6). As for the mediastinum, a differential list of the potentially affected organs can be established according to the location of the mass detected (Table 4). Complementary imaging studies are usually required to establish the affected organ and determine the extent of the tumour.

Table 4. Organs possibly affected according to mass effect localisation.

Abdominal area enlarged		Organs possibly affected
Cranioventral	Right	Liver, pylorus
	Left	Liver
Craniodorsal	Right	Liver
	Left	Liver, spleen
Midventral	Right	Liver, pylorus, duodenum, pancreas, spleen, mesenteric lymph nodes
	Left	Liver, spleen, small intestinal tract, pancreas, mesenteric lymph nodes
Mid-dorsal	Right	Liver, right kidney, right adrenal, right ovary
	Left	Liver, stomach, spleen, left kidney, left adrenal, left ovary
Caudoventral		Small intestinal tract, mesenteric lymph nodes, bladder, prostate
Caudodorsal		Sublumbar, iliac and hypogastric lymph nodes, uterus, colon, rectum, anal glands

Nervous System

Radiography provides poor discrimination of nervous structures and only allows detection of secondary signs such as muscle wastage. It has therefore been largely superseded by tomographic imaging techniques; computed tomography and magnetic resonance imaging.

Metastatic Disease

With its wide availability and low cost, **radiography is a good modality for detection of metastatic lesions affecting skeletal structures and lungs**.

Although not common, metastatic bone lesions can be found anywhere along the skeletal structures but are more likely to be found in the diaphysis of long bones, in the vertebrae or the pelvic bones. Metastatic lesions are usually more lytic than proliferative, except for urogenital tract carcinomas, which may produce irregular new bone along the ventral aspect of the lumbar or coccygeal vertebrae, or along the pelvic bones.

Lung Metastasis

The lungs are one of the most common locations for metastatic disease, but metastatic spread may not be limited to the lungs and may also develop on the pleura, the pleural space, the lymph nodes or even in the skeletal structures of the chest.

The basic radiographic protocol for detection of thoracic metastatic disease should include a minimum of **three projections obtained at the peak of the inspiratory phase, or under manual inflation of the lungs**. Usually both lateral recumbent projections and a dorsoventral projection are obtained.

Soft tissue pulmonary parenchymal nodules are the most common presentation of pulmonary metastases. The nodules usually represent a homogeneous population of well-circumscribed lesions of similar opacity (Figure 7). Occasionally, associated with highly aggressive primary lesions, nodular lesions may be present in large numbers, and with a smaller diameter, called **miliary metastases**. Some metastatic lesions can become cavitated, leaving only a round air-filled lesion with a more or less thick rim. This happens when the content of the lesion becomes necrotic and empties into an adjacent bronchus.

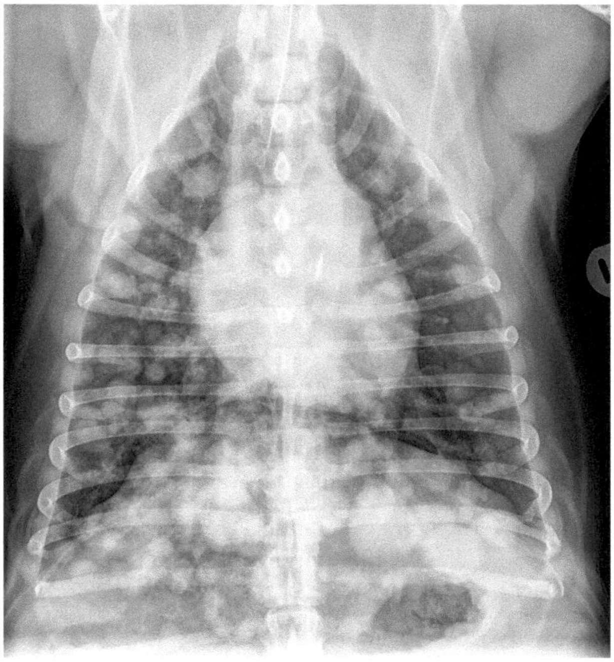

Figure 7. Dorsoventral projection of the thorax of a patient with pulmonary metastatic disease. Note the homogeneous population of interstitial nodular lesions.

These lesions can be difficult to differentiate from small lung bullae. Nodular lesions need to be 7 mm or more in diameter to be radiographically visible. If the metastatic process involves a lymphatic path, metastatic lesions are more likely to present as a more diffuse parenchymal infiltrate. **Sequential radiographic studies** are a reasonable way of monitoring the rate of growth of pulmonary metastases, which is a useful indicator of response to chemotherapy treatment.

Pleural metastatic disease can be difficult to identify on radiographs unless a significant volume of effusion has accumulated in the pleural space. After which the interlobar fissures become visible and thickened on radiographs.

Lymphatic Spread

Lymphatic spread of metastatic cells may lead to **lymphadenopathy**. Depending on the location of the draining lymph nodes, they may or may not be radiographically detectable.

With the exception of the popliteal lymph nodes, the superficial lymph nodes are poorly visible radiographically. Unless grossly enlarged, they are difficult to differentiate from the surrounding soft tissue structures, in which case they are readily palpable on physical examination.

Several distinct networks of lymph nodes are located along or inside the chest. Three deep lymph node networks are present in the thorax. All three may be seen radiographically, if they are significantly enlarged.

- The **presternal lymph node(s)** (one or two lymph nodes in the dog, only one in the cat) is/are located in the cranial mediastinum, lying just dorsal to sternebrae 2 and 3. They are usually more noticeable on lateral projections when enlarged, but are difficult to visualise on the dorsoventral projection as they are superimposed over the cranial mediastinal structures (Figure 8). As noted in Table 2, although intrathoracic, these lymph nodes also drain the peritoneal cavity as well as the mammary glands, hence when enlarged, a primary lesion should also be sought in these regions.
- **The cranial mediastinal lymph nodes** are located ventral to the trachea, along the main vessels. A significant enlargement of these lymph nodes will induce a dorsal deviation of the trachea on lateral projections and widening of the cranial mediastinum on the dorsoventral projection. It is important to note that there are no lymph nodes in the caudal mediastinum.
- **The tracheobronchial lymph nodes** are located along the distal portion of the trachea, around the carina. Two are located laterally to the main stem bronchi and one is located between them. Again, these need to be significantly enlarged to be visible radiographically and are usually best assessed on the lateral projections. They are

only visible due to the difference in radiopacity between them (soft tissue opacity) and the surrounding pulmonary gas. Presence of a pulmonary primary mass may therefore hinder their radiographic visibility.

The only **abdominal lymph nodes** reliably visible radiographically are the lumboaortic, the medial iliac, and hypogastric lymph nodes. Again, they need to be significantly enlarged to be visible. Due to their localisation, they are mainly visible on lateral projections with the help of the perinodal fat, which provides the radiographic contrast in the retroperitoneal space. If sufficiently enlarged, they may displace the adjacent peritoneal organs ventrally. Other abdominal lymph nodes, if sufficiently enlarged, may cause a radiographically visible mass effect, but this is poorly specific for determination of the origin of the mass and leads to a wide differential list.

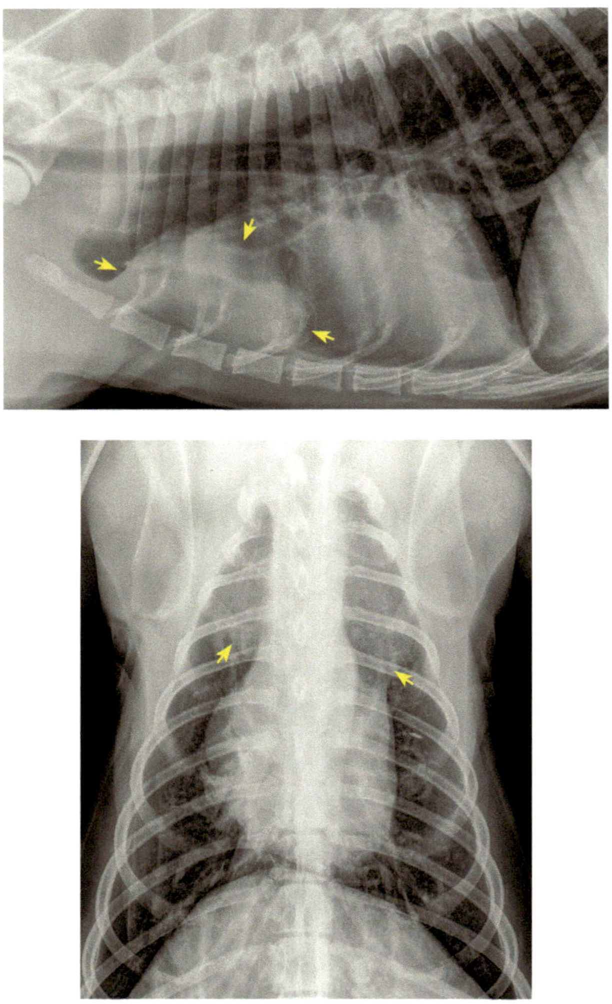

Figure 8. Right lateral and dorsoventral projections of the thorax of a canine patient with presternal lymphadenopathy (arrowheads). Note the superimposition of the lymph nodes over the spine, confirming a mediastinal location.

Ultrasound: Principles and Interpretation of Clinical Cases

Ultrasound relies on the acoustic impedance (product of the physical density and the velocity of sound through the tissue) of the different tissues that will reflect or absorb the sonic waves travelling through them. The reflected waves and the time they take to travel back and forth from the probe to the tissue and back to the probe are then processed into a two-dimensional image by a software system. The images produced are a slice representation in a gradient of greys through the organs observed, with fluids being blacker, whilst denser structures and gas are whiter.

Ultrasound has become the **first line imaging modality for assessment of the abdominal organs**, both for primary neoplastic lesions and for staging purposes. Ultrasound waves are unable to travel through cortical bone or through gas, meaning assessment of skeletal and pulmonary structures is limited to their interface unless they are altered. Ultrasound waves travel particularly well in fluids, making ultrasound highly superior to radiography in case of effusion, both pleural and peritoneal, which decreases the natural radiographic contrast between organs.

Primary neoplastic lesions are most often recognised as nodular or mass lesions with alteration of the normal echostructure of the affected organ. Round cell tumours are an exception though and may present as diffuse changes infiltrating the affected organ. Although detection of the changes is relatively easy, they are often non-specific and differentiation between benign and malignant lesions remains challenging. In the last decade, research has largely focused on this aspect of imaging.

Doppler ultrasound can provide essential information on the vascularisation of a particular lesion, with an **increase of the peripheral arterial supply being more suggestive of a malignant lesion**. In these cases, arteries are often more tortuous with an increased flow velocity due to the active angiogenesis associated with tumour growth.

The use of ultrasound contrast agents and harmonics remain areas of ongoing investigations. The contrast agents consist of microbubbles injected intravenously. These bubbles are designed to travel through tissular organs. The arterial perfusion time ("wash-in") and the venous drainage time ("wash-out") are recorded. In human medicine, characteristic timing differences have been demonstrated when comparing malignant tumours to benign lesions, but so far, veterinary studies have proven to be frustrating, due to the large overlap of the different timing results.

Skeletal Structures

Due to the high acoustic impedance of cortical bone, ultrasounds are unable to travel through bony structures meaning **assessment of skeletal structures is limited to their interface, unless they are altered**. Normal bone interface consists of a hyperechoic interface, casting a hypoechoic shadow. Therefore, expansile bone lesions, and periosteal reaction as commonly found in primary bone tumours, may be ultrasonographically visible as an interruption or an irregular pattern of this hyperechoic interface and disruption of the normal shadowing artefact. This allows guidance of biopsy needles into the periphery of the lesions where a better yield is expected for cytological/histological examination.

Head and Neck

Ultrasound is a **very useful imaging tool for the soft tissue neoplastic conditions of the head and the neck** if adequate equipment is available. A high frequency linear probe is necessary for assessing superficial structures such as eyes, orbits, salivary glands, larynx, thyroid, and parathyroid glands.

In ocular assessment, ultrasound plays a key role, allowing investigation of the deep intraocular structures despite the presence of opaque media such as cataract. Fine needle samples can even be performed in some peripheral nodular lesions through the sclera, to achieve a cytological diagnosis (Figure 9).

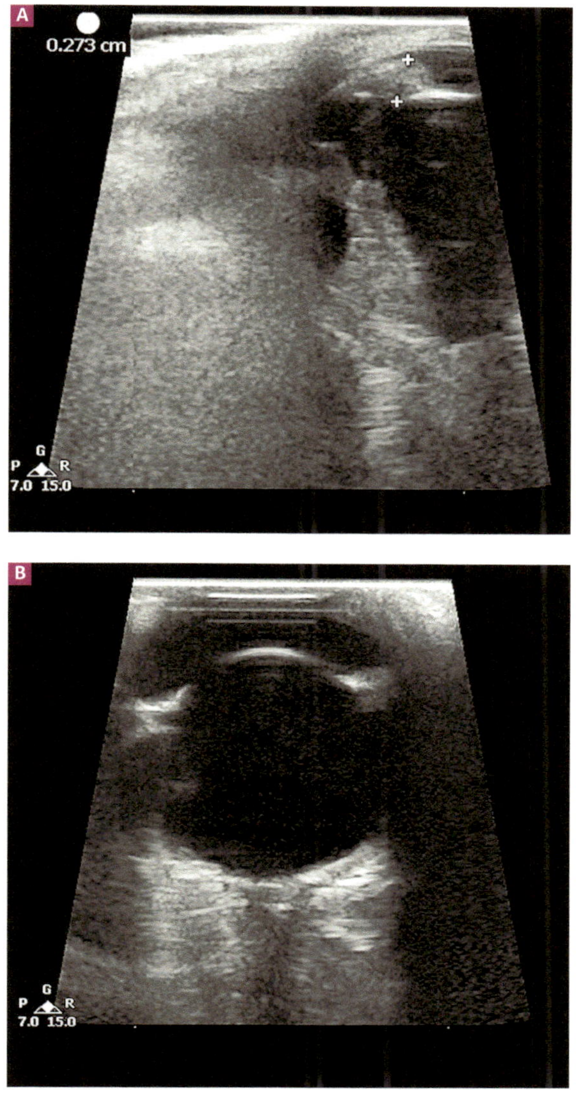

Figure 9. A. Ultrasound image of a small ciliary body mass, a confirmed melanoma. **B**. Ultrasound image of the other eye of the same patient for comparison.

For the neck, comparison between sides is helpful. Enlargement of a thyroid with increased vascularisation and mineralised foci is highly suggestive of carcinoma. Parathyroid glands can be identified by experienced operators as hypoechoic nodular structures. A normal parathyroid should measure approximately 2 mm, while a parathyroid over 4 mm is likely neoplastic, either an adenoma or an adenocarcinoma (Figure 10).

Thoracic Structures

Due to the low acoustic impedance of gas/air, ultrasounds are unable to travel through gas containing structures (such as lungs and gastrointestinal tract), limiting **assessment of pulmonary structures to their interface, unless altered**. Therefore, nodular lesions present at the periphery of the lungs can be identified as a hypoechogenic interruption of the normally smooth hyperechoic pulmonary surface. This will only be visible through an intercostal window.

Most commonly a pulmonary nodule/mass is initially identified radiographically or on CT. **If in contact with the thoracic wall, the lesion is readily visible with ultrasound** (Figure 11). If the nodular/mass lesion does not contact the wall, the gas contained in the lungs around the lesion will hinder visualisation of the lesion on ultrasound. The patient can be positioned on the affected side for a few minutes, causing some atelectasis of the lungs between the lesion and the thoracic wall. This technique can be used to allow visualisation and ultrasound guidance of a needle biopsy into the lesion.

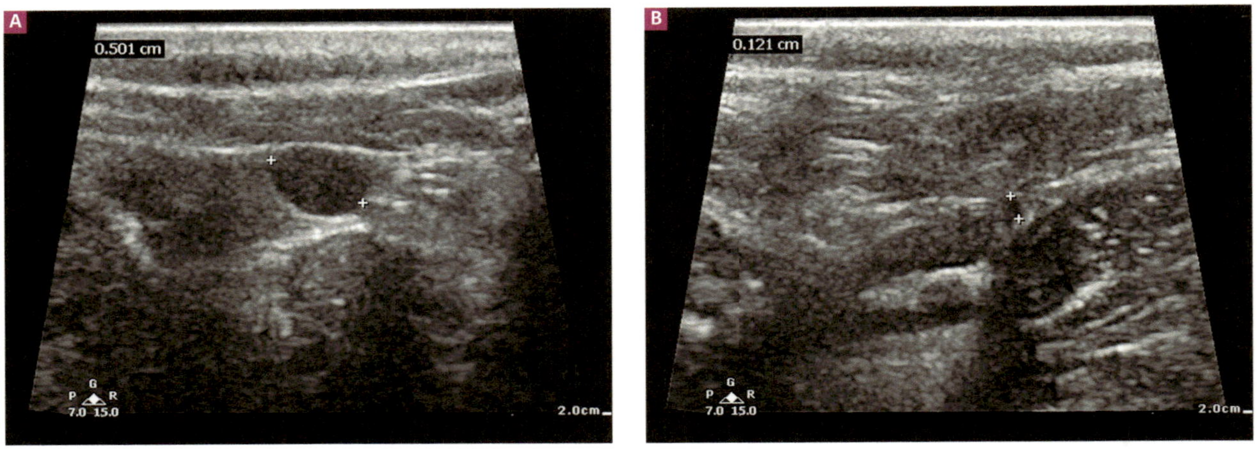

Figure 10. A. Ultrasound image of the left cranial parathyroid gland of a canine patient presented with severe hypercalcaemia. The size was suggestive of a neoplastic process, which was confirmed as a carcinoma. **B**. Contralateral side with normal measurements.

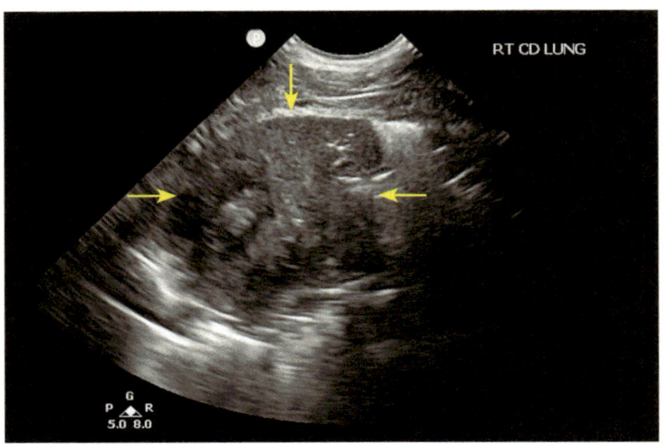

Figure 11. Ultrasound image of the right caudal lung lobe through an intercostal window in a canine patient. A focal area of consolidation (arrows) is easily identified as an area of low echogenicity contacting the thoracic wall and replacing the normal aerated lungs as seen caudal to the lesion. Fine needle aspirates confirmed a pulmonary carcinoma.

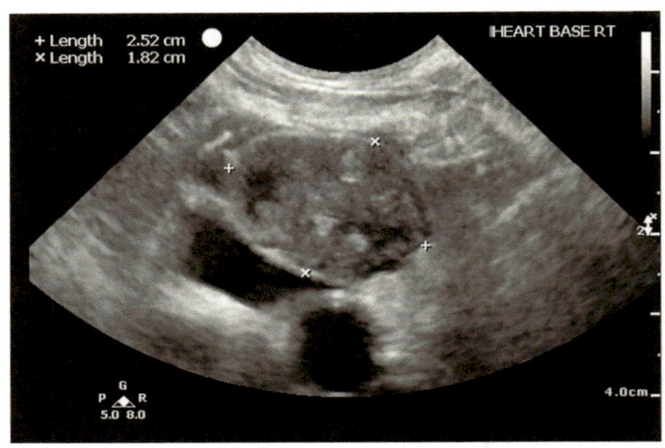

Figure 12. Ultrasound image of a right atrial mass.

Cranial mediastinal tumours are accessible to ultrasound assessment through the thoracic inlet and a cranioventral parasternal window. **Heart-based tumours** can be assessed through a cardiac window (Figure 12). This is limited by the surrounding gas filled structures, the lungs, but also the trachea and the oesophagus. **Lymphoma** (Figure 13) and **thymoma** are the most common mediastinal tumours and differentiation between the two can be challenging. Ultrasound-guided biopsies play an essential role in differentiating these entities for treatment considerations. Unfortunately, even when ultrasonographically visible, sampling of heart-based tumours remains challenging and should be reserved for experienced ultrasonographers.

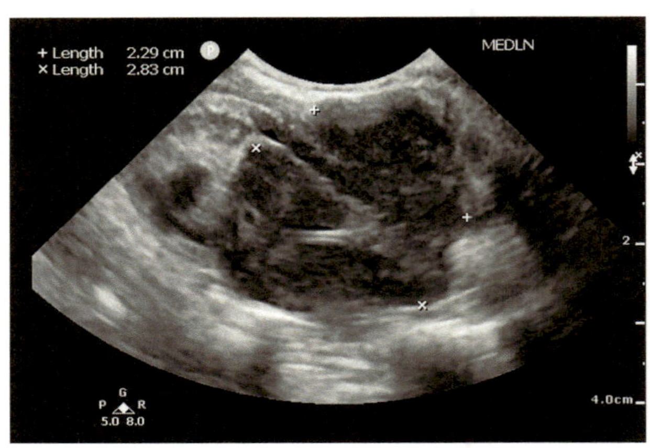

Figure 13. Ultrasound image of enlarged cranial mediastinal lymph nodes in a feline patient with confirmed lymphoma.

Ultrasound waves travel particularly well in fluids, **making ultrasound largely superior to radiography in cases of effusion**, which decreases the natural radiographic contrast between organs. Therefore, ultrasonography is excellent for visualisation of pleural, pericardial, and mediastinal fluid, to assess its echogenicity, and obtain a sample. **Transudate should be anechoic, while modified transudate and exudate will be more or less echogenic.** Neoplastic effusions may or may not contain tumour cells, which is why sampling can provide precious diagnostic information. Ultrasound guidance also allows drainage of these cavities when the volume of effusion becomes life threatening, compromising either the respiratory or cardiac functions.

Abdominal Structures

Ultrasound has become the **first line imaging modality to assess the abdominal organs for primary tumours**. As described above, radiography at best provides confirmation of the presence of an organomegaly or of a mass lesion but fails to provide reliable information on which organ is affected and the extent of the tumour invasion. Like all imaging modalities ultrasound will not provide a definitive diagnosis but it will allow accurate localisation of the primary tumour, provide information about the extent of the lesion and extension to adjacent structures, which will influence treatment options.

Colour Doppler ultrasonography is useful to assess the vascularisation of the tumour. Aggressive tumours are often associated with increased arterial vascularisation, and this arterialisation leads to tortuous shaped vessels. Colour Doppler also allows assessment of adjacent vessels for vascular invasion or presence of thrombi due to the modification in blood flow.

Liver and Spleen Tumours

Primary parenchymal neoplastic lesions such as in hepatic and splenic tumours will most commonly present as solitary nodular or mass lesions affecting an area of an organ/system (Figure 14).

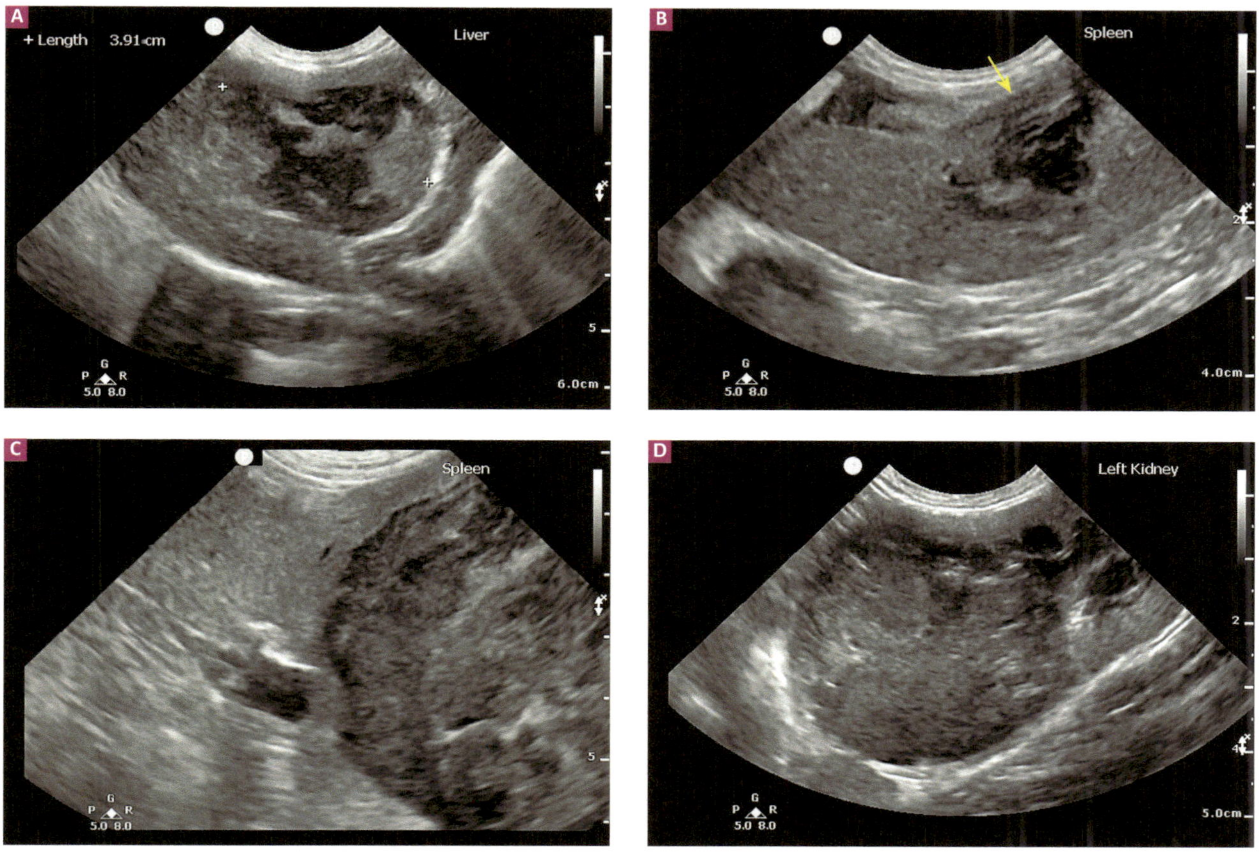

Figure 14. A. Ultrasound image of a confirmed hepatic carcinoma in a cat. The mass has a heterogeneous echostructure and is well circumscribed. **B.** Splenic haemangiosarcoma with capsular disruption and intra-abdominal bleeding in a canine patient (arrow). **C.** Large poorly defined splenic sarcoma in a canine patient. Note the clear continuity between the normal splenic parenchyma and the large mass lesion. **D.** Renal carcinoma in a canine patient. Note the normal echostructure of the caudal pole that confirms the renal localisation.

A nodule becomes a mass when it reaches 3 cm in diameter. As these lesions are space occupying, the adjacent structures, in particular the blood vessel may be contouring the lesion, seeming to "wrap" around the lesion. The echostructure of the lesion is usually different to the adjacent normal echostructure of the organ. It may be homogeneously hyper- or hypoechoic or have a heterogeneous echostructure. Intralesional cavitation may be present, and this may indicate a degree of intralesional bleeding or necrosis, as seen in haemangiosarcoma common in the liver and the spleen.

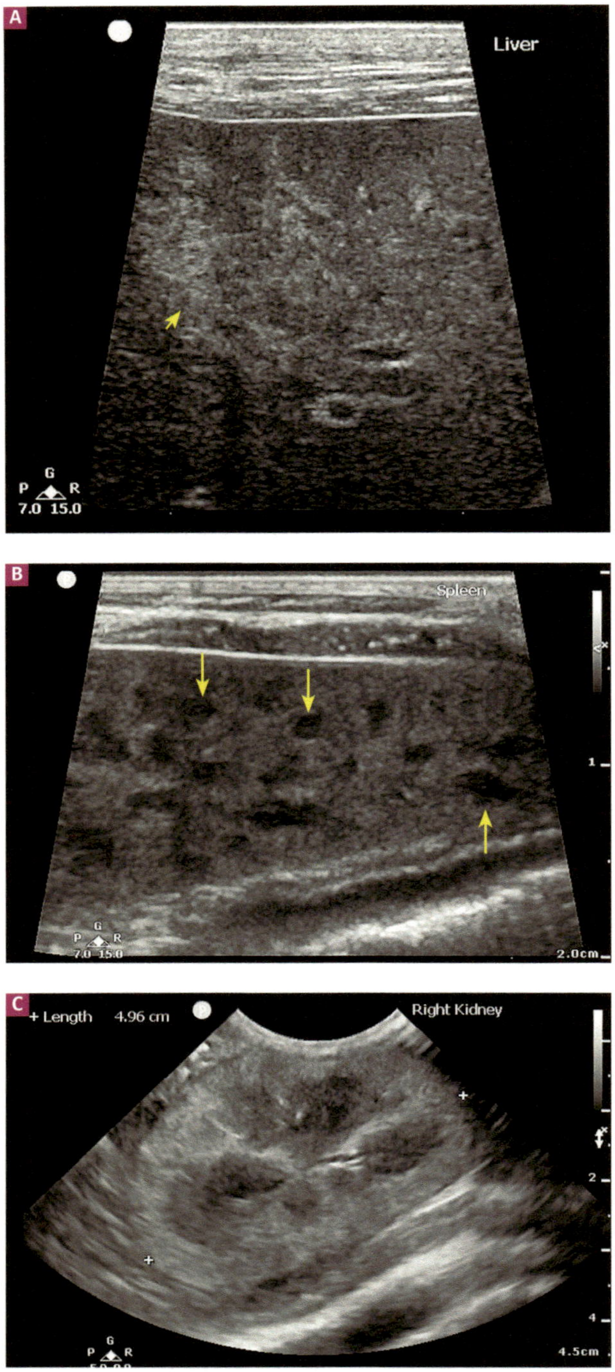

Figure 15. Various ultrasonographic presentations of lymphoma: **A**. Irregular patches of increased echogenicity of the parenchyma in the liver (arrowheads). **B**. Multifocal rounded hypoechoic splenic lesions also called "Swiss cheese" pattern (arrows). **C**. Renomegaly with a small volume of perirenal effusion.

Cystic components can be identified with anechoic material as seen frequently in **hepatic or biliary cystadenoma** or **cystadenocarcinoma**, which are common in cats. Disruption of an organ capsule associated with intra-abdominal bleeding is suggestive of a neoplastic process, although haemoabdomen can occur in benign lesions, particularly associated with the spleen. Myelolipomas are commonly found in the spleen and have a characteristic hyperechoic irregular shape, with a perivascular or subcapsular distribution. Although this is a benign tumour, in the dog, they can become very large in size.

Diffuse round cell tumours such as lymphoma, mast cell tumour or histiocytic sarcomas often, but not always, present as a diffuse process, which can affect part/or an entire organ or system. In these cases, a variable degree of organomegaly will be present, with or without modification of the echostructure of the organ (Figure 15). Lymphoma affecting the spleen may present with multifocal small hypoechoic lesions, also called "Swiss cheese" echostructure, easily recognised on ultrasound. These are highly suggestive, but not pathognomonic for lymphoma. Presence of regional lymphadenopathy will also raise/support a suspicion of round cell tumours. Occasionally these tumours may present with no ultrasonographically detectable changes.

Pancreatic Tumours

Pancreatic tumours can be difficult to identify ultrasonographically even for experienced operators, as they can cause significant clinical signs when only very small in size as in cases of insulinoma or gastrinoma. Carcinoma is more easily visible on ultrasound as it usually reaches a larger size and they are usually irregular and hypoechoic. Dependant on their location in the pancreas they may cause a mass effect, compressing the common bile duct, causing dilation of the biliary system. They are usually associated with signs of a hyperechoic peritoneum due to severe regional inflammation.

Gastrointestinal Tract Tumours

Ultrasound has become the preferred imaging modality for the gastrointestinal tract (Figure 16). Although small gastric tumours can be overlooked with ultrasound due to the presence of gas, large mass lesions protruding into the lumen with or without disruption of the layering can be identified.

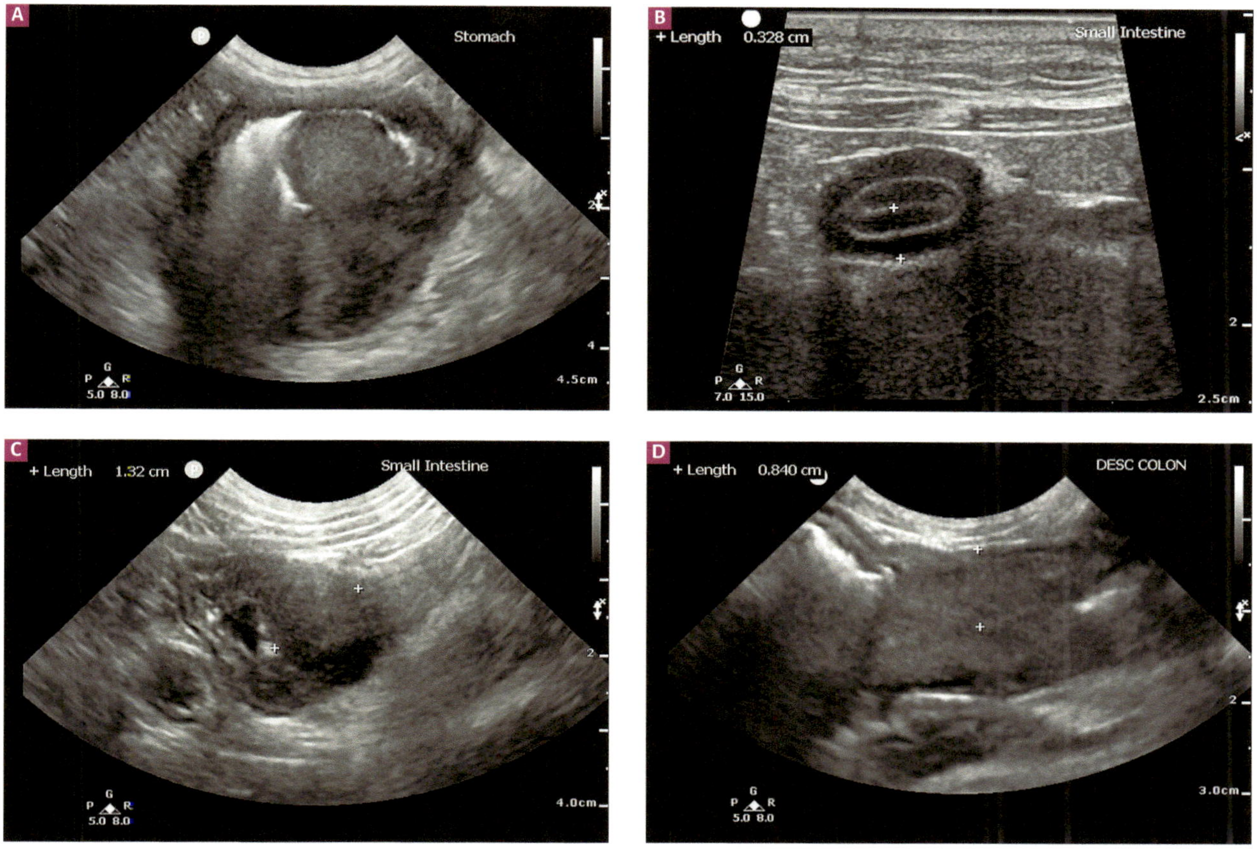

Figure 16. Ultrasound images of gastrointestinal tumours. **A**. Gastric lymphoma causing an asymmetrical thickening of the wall with loss of normal layering. **B**. Small intestinal lymphoma causing annular diffuse thickening of the muscularis layer. **C**. Small intestinal carcinoma in a feline patient, causing asymmetrical mural thickening with loss of layering. **D**. Colic lymphoma with colic wall thickening and loss of layering.

Depending on their location, they may cause some outflow obstruction causing significant distension of the gastric lumen. **Carcinoma** and **leiomyoma/sarcoma** cannot be differentiated. Lymphoma tends to cause a more diffuse wall thickening. Layering may be absent or retained, but the relative thickness of the layers may be altered.

Intestinal tumours are associated with a focal thickening of the wall of the affected segment, with or without disruption of the layering. The lesion can be circumferential or asymmetrical. Carcinoma and leiomyosarcoma tend to present as large irregular masses and they can cause partial or complete secondary obstruction, causing dilation of the segments proximal to the lesion. They can have a very ulcerated mucosal surface causing irregular gas artefacts representing the irregular luminal interface. **Round cell tumours** tend to present with an annular distribution, with a variable degree of effacement of the normal layering. Thickening of the muscularis layer is also a common presentation of **lymphosarcoma**. It can be associated with a variable degree of enlargement of the regional lymph nodes, which in extreme cases may become hypoechoic, cavitated and associated with a hyperechoic rim of reactive fat. These changes are unfortunately non-specific and still require sampling, which can be performed under ultrasound guidance. **Caecal and colic tumours** can be identified with ultrasound and may be associated with regional lymphadenopathy.

Adrenal, Kidney and Urinary Tract Tumours

Benign adrenal tumours such as adenoma, lymphoma and myelolipoma tend to remain contained in the gland capsule. They will reach a moderate size and usually have a homogeneous echostructure. To the contrary **malignant adrenal tumours** have the potential to reach a large size and volume and are likely to have a heterogeneous echostructure (Figure 17). Dystrophic mineralisation is a common feature of carcinomas, and this is identified on ultrasound as foci with a hyperechoic interface casting shadowing artefact within a suspected lesion. Adrenal tumours are also well recognised for invading adjacent vessels (renal vein or caudal vena cava), in particular carcinoma and pheochromocytoma. It can be difficult to clearly decide what is tumour invading the vessel or thrombus formation, and often it is a combination of both.

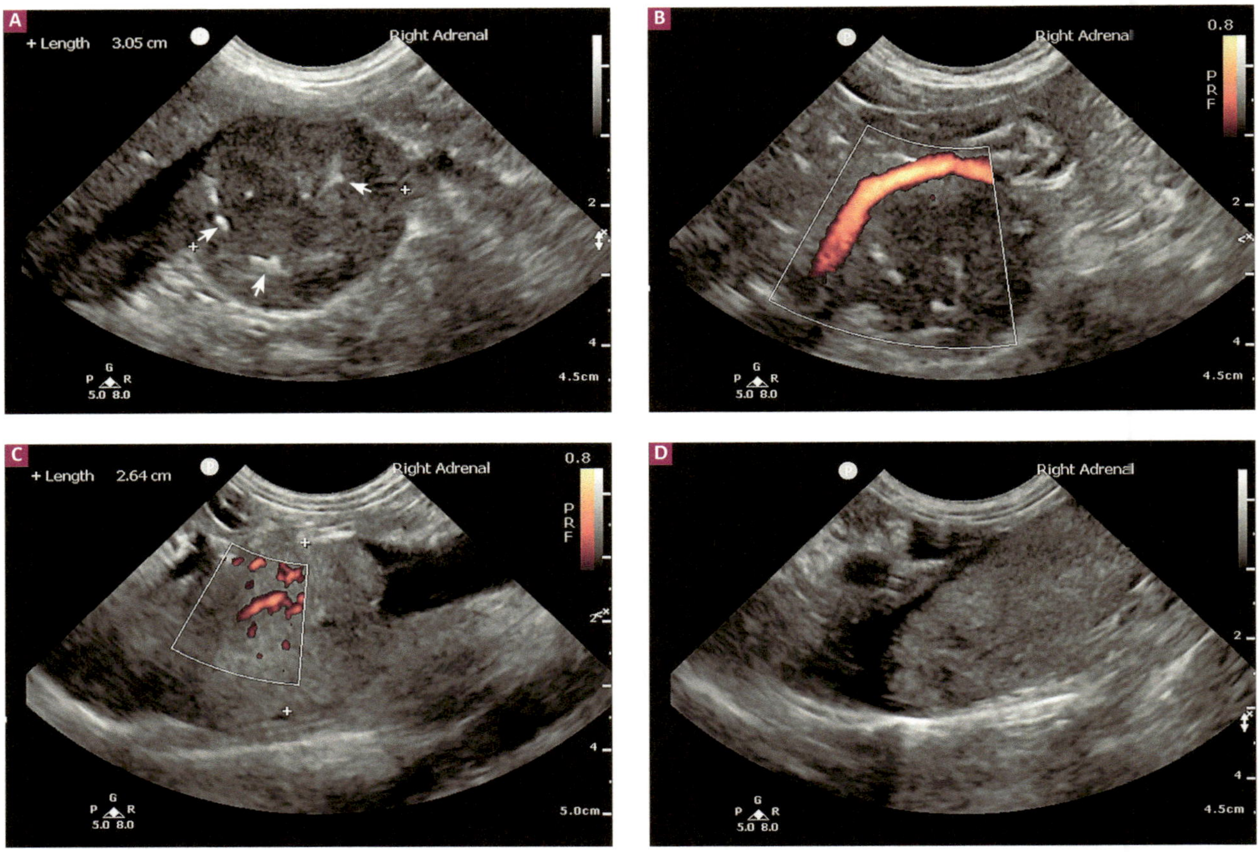

Figure 17. Ultrasound images of two canine patients with adrenal tumours. **A.** and **B.** A case of adrenal carcinoma, presenting a round mass with small parenchymal mineralisations (arrowheads), displacing the adjacent vessel. **C.** and **D.** A case of pheochromocytoma, presenting as a more irregularly shaped mass, highly vascularised, extending through the wall of the caudal vena cava. Material is identified extending cranially inside the caudal vena cava (CVC), partly neoplastic tissue, partly thrombus.

Renal tumours present as solitary masses often hyperechoic or isoechoic to the renal parenchyma, replacing the normal echostructure of the affected kidney. They can be of varying size at the time of diagnosis and can become challenging to clearly relate to the original kidney when they become large in size. Identification of half to one third of normal renal architecture adjacent to a 15 cm diameter mass lesion can be challenging. Lesions can also have a heterogeneous echostructure when the mass is associated with necrotic or cystic components. For small hypoechoic lesions, Doppler can be very helpful for their detection, as an increased flow velocity can be observed in the affected parenchyma. Unfortunately, this has proven to remain non-specific in terms of type of tumour. **Renal lymphoma** most commonly presents as generalised renomegaly, usually bilateral. The corticomedullary demarcation may be decreased, mild pyelectasis may be present and subcapsular effusion is occasionally identified. Although this is the most common presentation, renal lymphoma can also affect the kidney in a very irregular pattern, causing a mass lesion and/or causing a radiating internal pattern. Fine needle aspiration is key to confirm the diagnosis.

Good assessment of the bladder is possible when the bladder is sufficiently distended. When empty, the wall becomes thicker as a normal feature and detection of wall abnormalities is more difficult. The **most common bladder neoplasia is transitional cell carcinoma**. They most commonly affect the trigone region of the bladder, as a broad-based mass lesion of irregular luminal outline (Figure 18). If the mass lesion involves the ureterovesical junction, it may cause ipsilateral hydronephrosis due to obstruction of the papilla. They can spread locally inside the bladder to locations distant from the initial lesion. They can also spread caudally into the urethra, although they can also originate from the urethra and progress cranially into the bladder. They have been reported to seed along the needle tract if sampled transabdominally. Therefore, performing ultrasound-guided sampling placing a urinary catheter next to the lesion on an empty bladder and applying strong suction with a large volume syringe to aspirate fragments of tissue that can be sent for histological examination is preferred. Other bladder tumours are also reported, and **mesenchymal tumours** are reported to present with a smoother luminal outline.

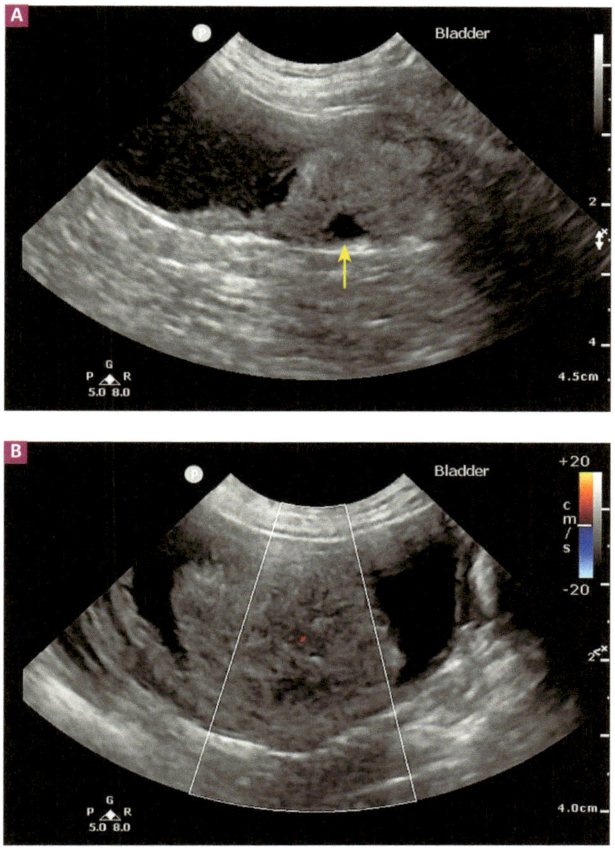

Figure 18. Ultrasound images of urinary bladder neoplasia. **A**. Classical case of transitional cell carcinoma (TCC), in the trigone location, involving the ureteric papillae (arrow). **B**. Patient with a leiomyoma, note the more cranial position of the mass, with a more discrete outline than the TCC.

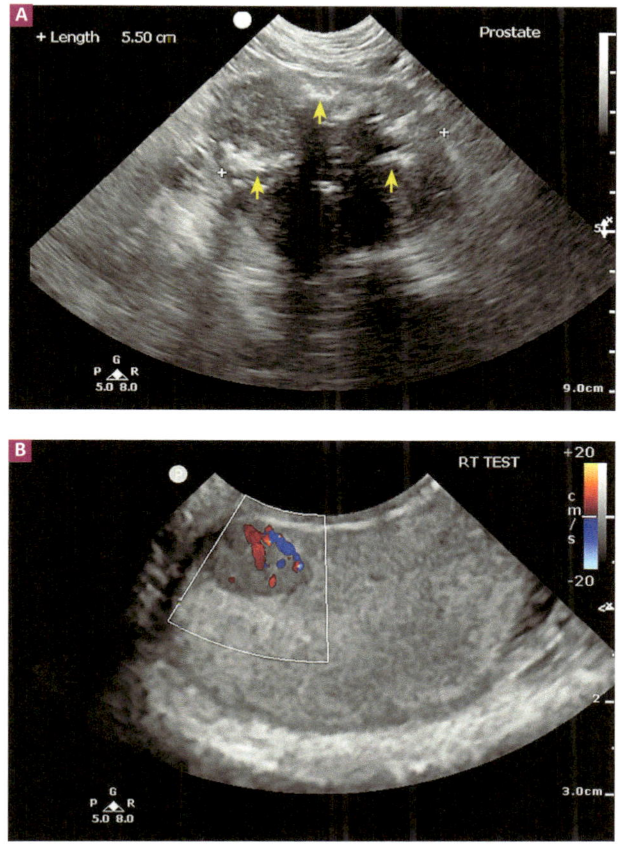

Figure 19. Ultrasound of genital tract tumours in male patients. **A**. Moderately enlarged prostate with shadowing parenchymal mineralisations (arrowheads) in a confirmed case of prostatic carcinoma. **B**. Ultrasound image of a testicle presenting a small focal but well vascularised lesion, confirmed as testicular interstitial cell tumour.

Genital Tract Tumours

Ultrasound is largely used for assessment of the genital tract. In female patients, **ovarian tumours** are identified as mass lesions caudal to the ipsilateral kidney and it is not uncommon for both ovaries to be affected. These lesions can vary from a solid mass, to a partially cavitated lesion causing a heterogeneous echostructure. They can reach a large size and may lead to secondary pyometra or hyperplastic endometriosis. When large enough they are usually found more ventrally than the kidneys.

Neoplasia of the uterus itself is rare but will present as a mural thickening or a mass projecting into the lumen of the affected uterine segment. **Intrapelvic segments of the genital tract cannot be examined with ultrasound** and the vagina and vestibule are therefore better assessed with retrograde radiographic or CT vaginography.

Prostatic carcinoma is the most common tumour affecting the genital tract of male dogs. Ultrasonographic findings include a variable degree of prostatomegaly with either a focal mass lesion causing asymmetry of the prostatic lobes, or a more diffuse disruption of the prostatic parenchyma often associated with foci of dystrophic mineralisations. Cystic areas may also be present in variable number and size (Figure 19). In neutered patients, it is helpful to know the age of neutering as late neutering may result in a larger sized prostate than in a patient neutered at a very young age. The changes can extend along the urethra into the bladder neck. As with bladder carcinomas, seeding along the sample needle is reported and therefore ultrasound-guided catheter sampling with prostatic wash is the preferred method to achieve a definitive diagnosis. Although the regional lymph nodes are easily assessed with ultrasound, **these carcinomas tend to spread to bone**, in particular along the lumbar, sacral and even coccygeal vertebral bodies as well as to the pelvic bones and therefore, further imaging is particularly recommended to stage these patients.

Although normally not intra-abdominal, **testicles are included in the routine ultrasonographic examination of the**

abdomen of entire male patients. Testicular tumours usually present as unilateral or bilateral nodular lesions of various sizes. They can be heterogeneous and may displace or efface the mediastinum testis. If one testicle is affected with a Sertoli cell tumour the other one may be atrophied. Retained testicles are significantly more at risk of developing a tumour. They can become large and heterogeneous with intralesional bleeding. Like large ovarian tumours, they may be found ventrally to the kidneys.

Nervous System

Due to the poor penetration of ultrasound waves through bony structures, **primary tumours of the nervous system are poorly amenable to ultrasonographic assessment**, as they are well protected in the skull and the spine. Only peripheral nerve tumours can be identified, and this is mainly for sampling guidance. Advanced tomographic modalities have largely taken the lead with respect to this type of tumour.

Metastatic Disease

Ultrasound also plays a key role in patient staging for all types of tumours. It is superior to radiography in detection of lymphadenopathies, except for the deep thoracic lymph nodes, in particular tracheobronchial lymph nodes. Although it is not possible to differentiate reactive inflammatory from metastatic lymphadenopathies, a rounded shape, with decreased or heterogeneous echostructure, modification from hilar to peripheral blood supply and increased perinodal fat echogenicity are important clues to suspect neoplastic involvement (Figure 20).

Metastatic disease is not limited to lymphadenopathy and may also appear in any organ. **Lungs**, liver, and spleen are the most commonly targeted organs for staging purposes. As explained above, despite the inherent poor amenability of pulmonary structures to ultrasound, the pulmonary interface can be explored. The presence of multiple hypoechoic nodules interrupting the hyperechoic interface of the

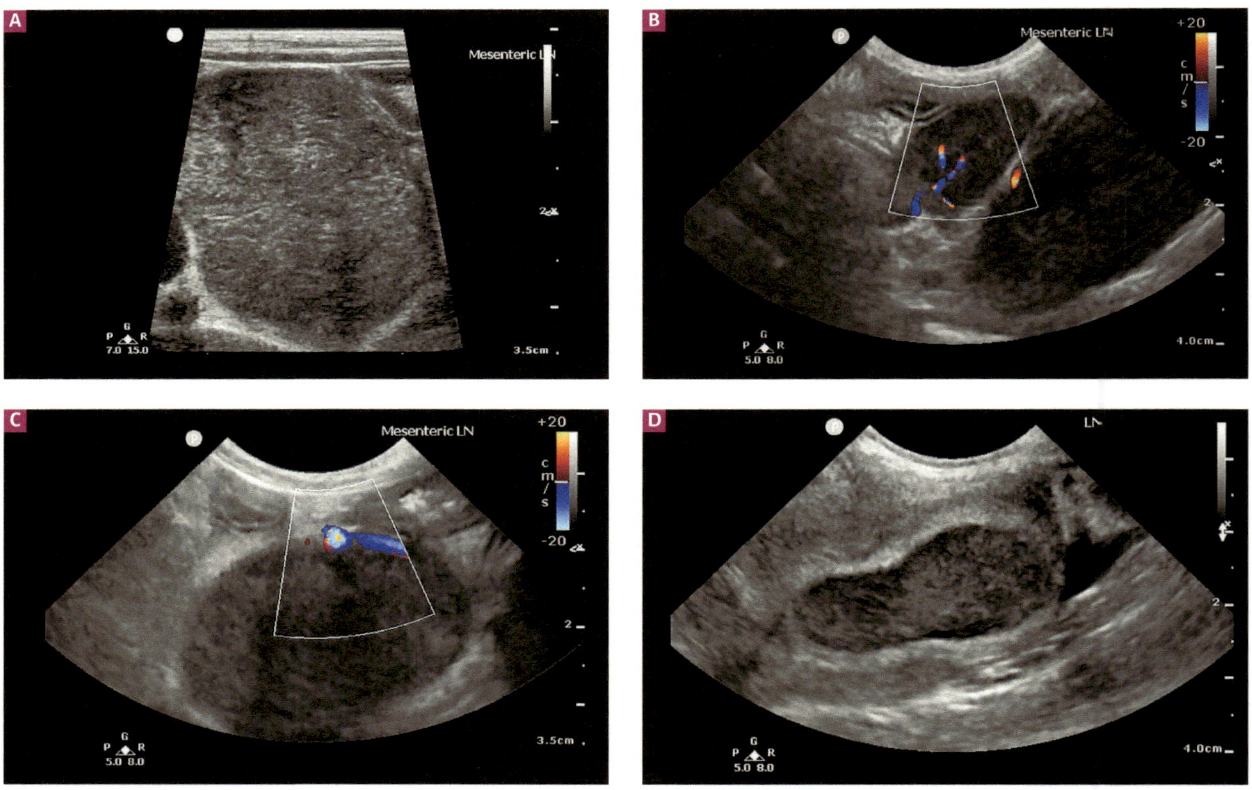

Figure 20. Ultrasound images of lymph nodes with confirmed neoplastic disease, showing criteria of malignancy. **A**. Enlarged, rounded and hypoechoic mesenteric lymph node. B and C. Lymph nodes in the same patient, some of them presenting hilar vascularisation (**B**) and some with a modified peripheral vascularisation (**C**). Hyperechoic perinodal hyperechoic fat (**D**).

lungs should raise the suspicion of multifocal nodular disease, which in the presence of a primary tumour is highly suggestive, but not pathognomonic, of pulmonary metastatic disease (Figure 21).

Metastatic disease affecting **the liver and the spleen** may present as diffuse or multifocal changes. Occasionally, presence of metastatic disease may remain undetectable ultrasonographically, and depending on the grade in tumours such as mast cell tumours, sampling may be advised despite the absence of any suggestive ultrasonographic modifications. "Target lesions" on ultrasound have a high predictive value for neoplastic lesions (Figure 22). When more than one lesion is noted, metastatic disease is most likely. Lesions are most commonly found in the hepatic or splenic parenchyma. They are described as nodular parenchymal lesions with a typical hyperechoic or isoechoic centre surrounded with a hypoechoic rim. Differential diagnoses for these lesions includes benign hyperplasia, as well as multiple types of hepatitis, and therefore ultrasound sampling remains mandatory for definitive diagnosis.

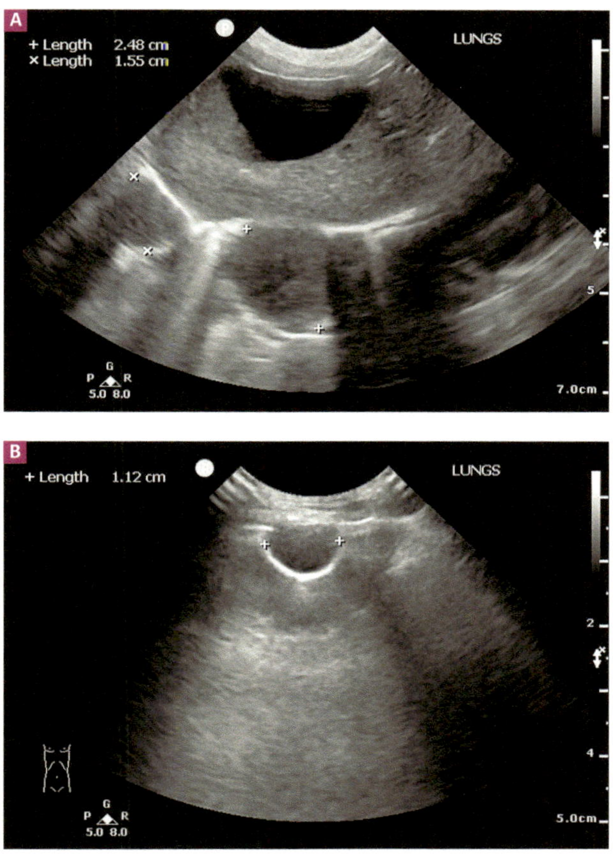

Figure 21. Ultrasound images of pulmonary metastatic lesions from a renal carcinoma. **A**. Transhepatic window. **B**. Thoracic window. Note the very clear interface between the rounded lesions and the surrounding gas filled lungs.

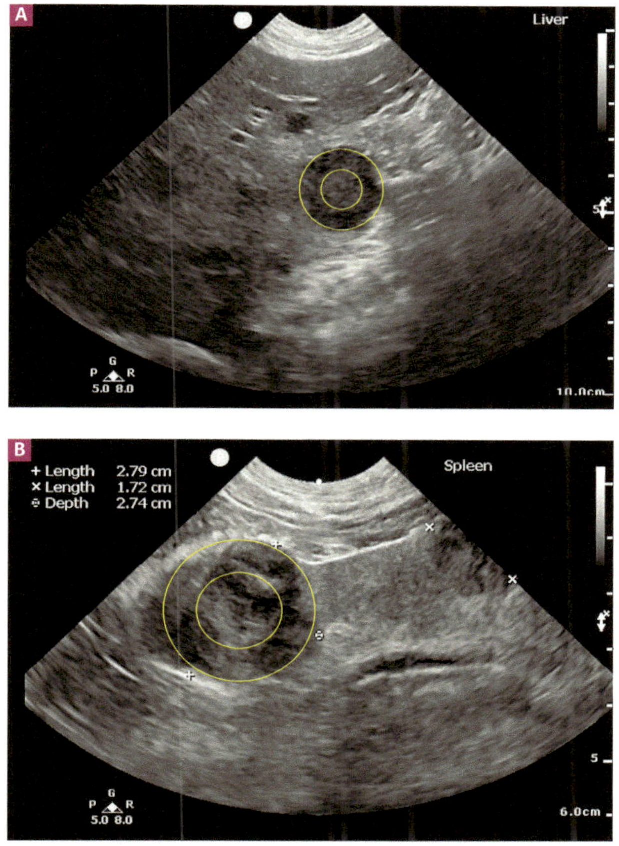

Figure 22. Ultrasound images of target lesions in a patient with confirmed histiocytic sarcoma. **A**. In the liver. **B**. In the spleen.

Ultrasound-guided Biopsies

As mentioned, multiple times above, **the ability to perform guided sampling of the lesions is one of the key features of ultrasonography**. It is a cost effective and minimally invasive way to obtain definitive cytological or histopathological diagnoses (Figure 23). The diagnostic yield of **FNAs** (**fine needle aspirations**) depends on the ability of the lesion to exfoliate. Hence **FNA may be the technique of choice for round cell tumours**, which tend to exfoliate more readily than sarcomas. For the latter, a biopsy is therefore preferred. In both cases, adequate equipment and technique should be used to optimise the samples' yield.

Patient preparation is important. For any ultrasound examination, the patient should be fasted to decrease the artefacts caused by gas, which will reduce the size of the usable windows and hinder visibility of the relevant structures. The haemostatic status of the patient should be assessed, in particular when core biopsies are considered or whenever risk of significant haemorrhage is suspected (cavitated lesions for example).

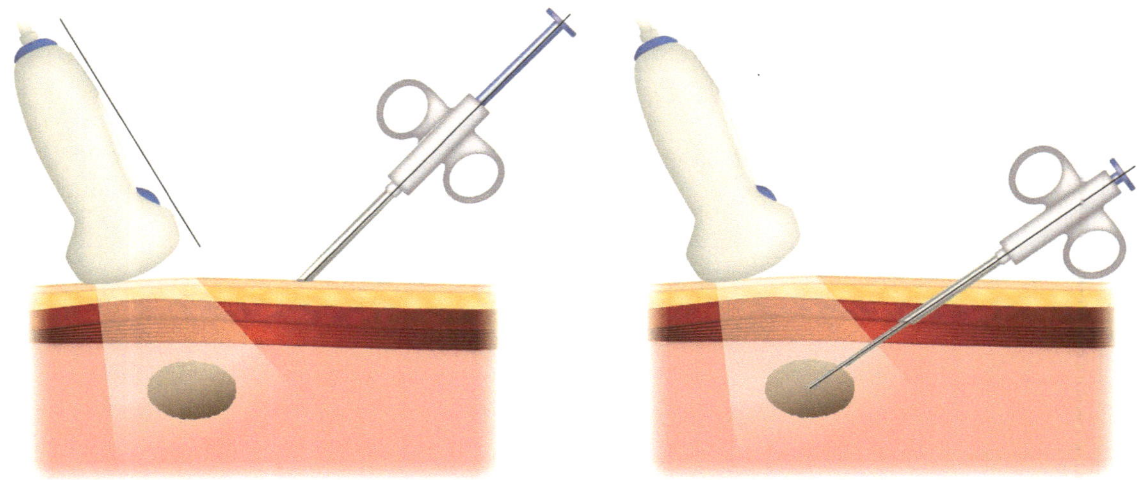

Figure 23. Sampling diagram by means of ultrasound-guided biopsy.

The safest path from the skin to the lesion to be biopsied should be identified. This is most commonly the shortest path, although presence of another organ between the skin and the targeted lesion/organ in the path may guide towards a longer route. The needle should not pass through more than one body cavity and should be changed for every lesion sampled. The skin should be cleaned aseptically over a wide area to allow positioning of both the probe and the sampling device.

Several devices exist that are attached to the ultrasound probe to allow the needle to slide at a precise angle along a predetermined path that can be visualised on the screen. These devices are often voluminous and cumbersome to use. Freehand technique is preferred by experienced sonographers allowing more flexibility in choosing the safest path to the lesion for each individual patient. Continuous visualisation of the needle path and tip is achieved by perfect alignment of the needle shaft with the ultrasound beam. The needle bevel should be orientated toward the ultrasound probe to allow a better visualisation of the needle tip with precise monitoring of the area sampled. Bevelled tip injection needles, spinal needles, or Tru-Cut® biopsy needles are most commonly used, depending on the purpose of the sampling:

- **bevelled tip injection** needles are mainly used for tapping fluid and obtaining cells for cytological examination;
- **spinal needles** are used when the lesion to be sampled is located deep within normal tissue to avoid collecting material on the way to the lesion; and
- **Tru-Cut® biopsy needles are** preferred for histological samples.

Once the needle is in position, small back and forth movements, aspiration of material or Tru-Cut® biopsy can be performed. For Tru-Cut® biopsies, it is essential to keep in mind, and also in the field of view, the final length to which the needle will extend once triggered to avoid complications. These complications will depend on the experience of the operator, the size of the needle and the nature of the lesion being sampled. Haemorrhage is the most common complication, although pneumothorax is also common for thoracic procedures.

Computed Tomography: Principles and Interpretation of Clinical Cases

Computed tomography uses X-rays like radiography, but the images obtained are cross sectional, i.e. slices through the body region under assessment. The X-rays are produced by a tube rotating around the body, and the X-rays are received on the other side by electronic sensors rotating in synchrony. The information received is transformed into a cross sectional picture of the body by a software system and the images obtained are displayed on a high resolution computer screen. Although the images are only obtained in a transverse plane, volumetric reconstructions can be processed in all planes, allowing for dorsal and sagittal reconstructions. This provides three dimensional information that could not be gained with conventional radiography. Maximum intensity projection and volume rendered reconstructions can also be obtained providing useful support for treatment planning.

CT is the imaging modality of choice for planning radiotherapy treatment. It allows the most accurate assessment of the tumour volume and tumour margins with regard to surrounding organs at risk.

The principles of CT interpretation are similar to conventional radiography, relying on the differential attenuation of the X-rays by the body structures. The image obtained can be reconstructed with different algorithms and visualised in different windows to allow better assessment of bones, lungs, and soft tissues. To optimise the resolution of the images, multiple factors are to be considered and therefore it is paramount to have adequate protocols set up for the different areas under investigation. **A strong point of CT is the ability to assess several areas of the body with a single imaging modality under a single anaesthesia**, allowing assessment of a primary lesion in one area of the body, as well as staging the rest of the body during the same procedure.

Patient preparation and patient restraint are also important, as any movement during image acquisition will lead to blurring of the images. Therefore, general anaesthesia is usually favoured. If the patient's condition allows for it, hyperventilation of the patient is used to induce apnoea to avoid undesirable respiratory movement artefacts. **Severely dyspnoeic patients may not be good candidates for CT examination.** Recognition of common artefacts is essential for accurate image acquisition and interpretation.

In CT angiography, use of iodinated contrast agents does not only allow assessment of the vascularity of a lesion, but also allows assessment of lesions in arterial and venous phases. Image acquisition can be triggered by the presence of contrast density in a predefined area (aorta for arterial phase), providing mapping of the arterial supply to the lesion, then acquisition is repeated after a period of time providing mapping of the venous drainage of the lesion. This is called "bolus tracking" and requires the use of a power injector pump. Recent development of interventional vascular treatment techniques such as intra-arterial chemotherapies or embolisation rely on accurate mapping of arterial supply to a tumoural lesion.

Skeletal Structures

Principles of interpretation are similar to radiography; most primary bone tumours present with a degree of bone lysis and poorly organised periosteal reaction. **The length of the transition zone between the centre of the lesion to normal bone structure is better appreciated with CT than conventional radiography** and is usually long. CT provides excellent definition of the architecture of the medullary bone and better delineation of the bone cortices. It is **extremely sensitive for detecting areas of early bone lysis**, and these can be seen much earlier than with radiography. It also detects more subtle new bone formation such as early periosteal reactions. Hence, precise assessment of the extent of long bone lesions can be made. Reconstructions along the long axis of the bone are very helpful and accurate measurements can be obtained for salvage procedures such as limb sparing surgery (Figure 24). Regional lymph nodes and staging for pulmonary metastatic lesions can be obtained during the same procedure.

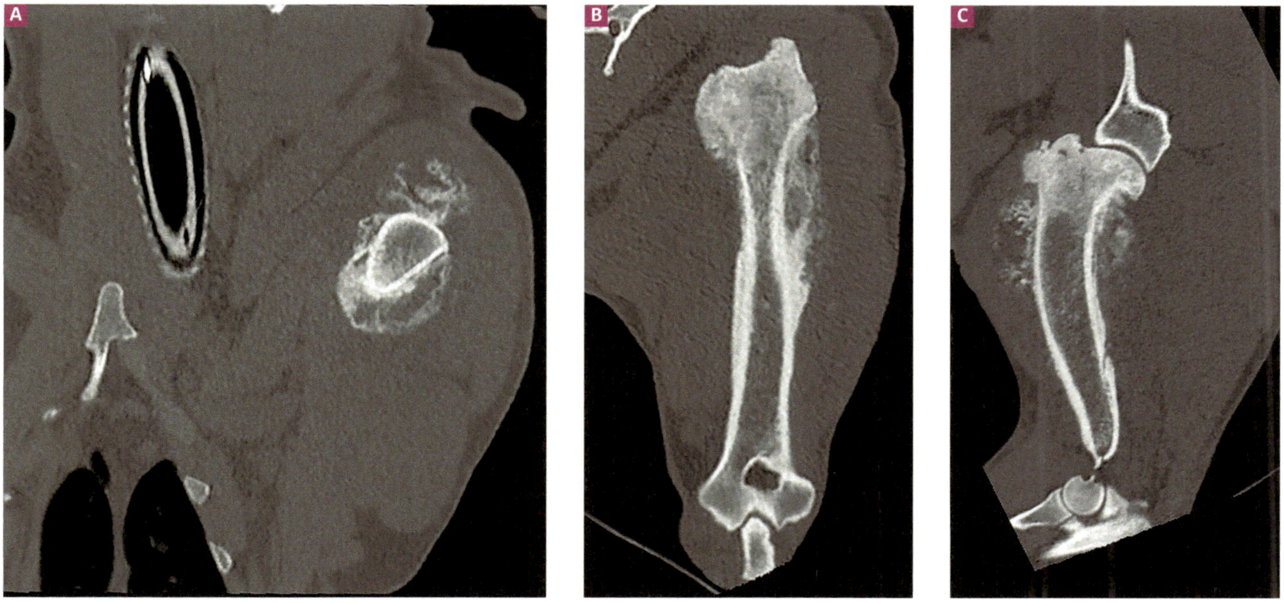

Figure 24. CT images in a bone window of a primary osteosarcoma of the proximal humerus in transverse (**A**), dorsal (**B**) and sagittal (**C**) reconstruction planes. Note the classical features associated with malignancy.

Primary vertebral tumours are common. They affect the thoracic spine more frequently, although all segments can be affected. They tend to affect a solitary vertebra and tend to be more lytic than osteoproliferative. Differential diagnoses include osteosarcoma, chondrosarcoma, fibrosarcoma and haemangiosarcoma. Occasionally they may lead to pathological fracture of the vertebra. Diffuse tumours such as multiple myeloma tend to be polyostotic and present as numerous focal punctuated lytic lesions mainly affecting sternebrae, ribs and vertebrae.

Head and Neck

The **head is one of the most challenging areas to image** due to the concomitant presence of multiple soft tissue structures, numerous bones of various sizes, and nervous structures.

Although positioning is less crucial than for conventional radiography, **achieving a symmetrical image remains important** to compare the anatomical structures from one side to the other. Opening the mouth with a plastic object such as a syringe, and even removing the endotracheal tube are little tips that will aid obtaining good quality studies and help visualisation of lesion extent, particularly for oral, pharyngeal, and laryngeal tumours. Good knowledge of species variations is important particularly when it comes to nasal chambers and sinuses.

Interpretation principles rely on **identifying an organomegaly or a space occupying lesion**, displacing adjacent soft tissue structures and/or distorting or eroding adjacent bones. Subtle erosion of fine bony structures such as nasal turbinates or the cribriform plate can be identified at an early stage with CT (Figure 25). Infiltrative tumours can be more difficult to identify and should be suspected when diffuse changes are present, in particular when they are unilateral. Fluid accumulation can be differentiated from vascularised soft tissue by comparing precontrast and postcontrast studies.

Ultimately **biopsy will be necessary to reach a final diagnosis**. Although CT-guided biopsies can be performed, obtaining

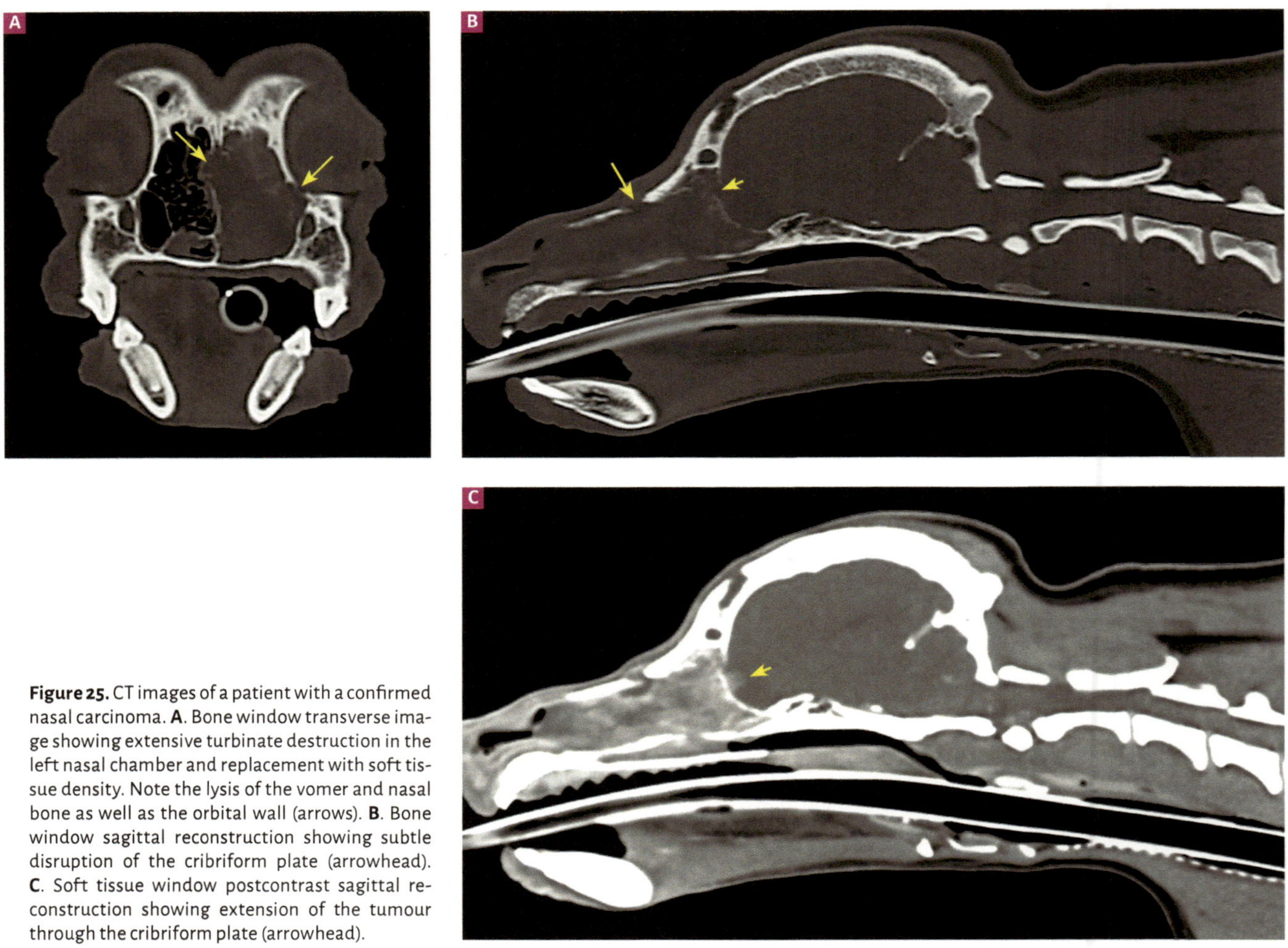

Figure 25. CT images of a patient with a confirmed nasal carcinoma. **A**. Bone window transverse image showing extensive turbinate destruction in the left nasal chamber and replacement with soft tissue density. Note the lysis of the vomer and nasal bone as well as the orbital wall (arrows). **B**. Bone window sagittal reconstruction showing subtle disruption of the cribriform plate (arrowhead). **C**. Soft tissue window postcontrast sagittal reconstruction showing extension of the tumour through the cribriform plate (arrowhead).

either ultrasound-guided or endoscopy-guided biopsies are preferred, depending on the location.

In the **neck**, like for the head, comparison between both sides is extremely helpful to identify a mass lesion. In cases of thyroid carcinoma, CT is particularly useful to assess the margins of the lesions, as well as early dystrophic mineralisations that are reported in some carcinomas.

Thoracic Structures

With its high inherent contrast between the bony structures and the air filled lungs, **CT is the best imaging technique to assess the thorax** as a whole. To minimise artefacts associated to breathing movements, manually induced apnoea or ventilators may be used.

Thoracic structures include the mediastinum (including the oesophagus, lymph nodes, the heart, and vessels), the trachea, the lungs, the bronchi, the pleura, and the thoracic wall. Images should be viewed in all windows – mediastinal, lung and bone – to assess all structures and all possible aspects of a lesion. **Precontrast and postcontrast** images should be obtained whenever a neoplastic condition is suspected. Positioning in sternal recumbency is usually best, although images should be acquired as soon as possible to avoid development of settling pulmonary atelectasis. Images should be obtained from the caudal thorax to the thoracic inlet.

Primary lung tumours are described most commonly as a solitary large mass lesion with more or less bronchograms visible within the lesion. The bronchi are narrowed or obstructed by the tumour, eventually causing the clinical signs. They present mild or moderate contrast enhancement and some intralesional dystrophic mineralisations can be present. Once they reach a large volume, they may eventually cavitate (Figure 26). Regional lymphadenopathy may or may not be present but is commonly associated with histiocytic sarcoma. Diffuse multicentric neoplasia such as lymphoma are reported although they are much less common. They usually present as a diffuse interstitial infiltrate.

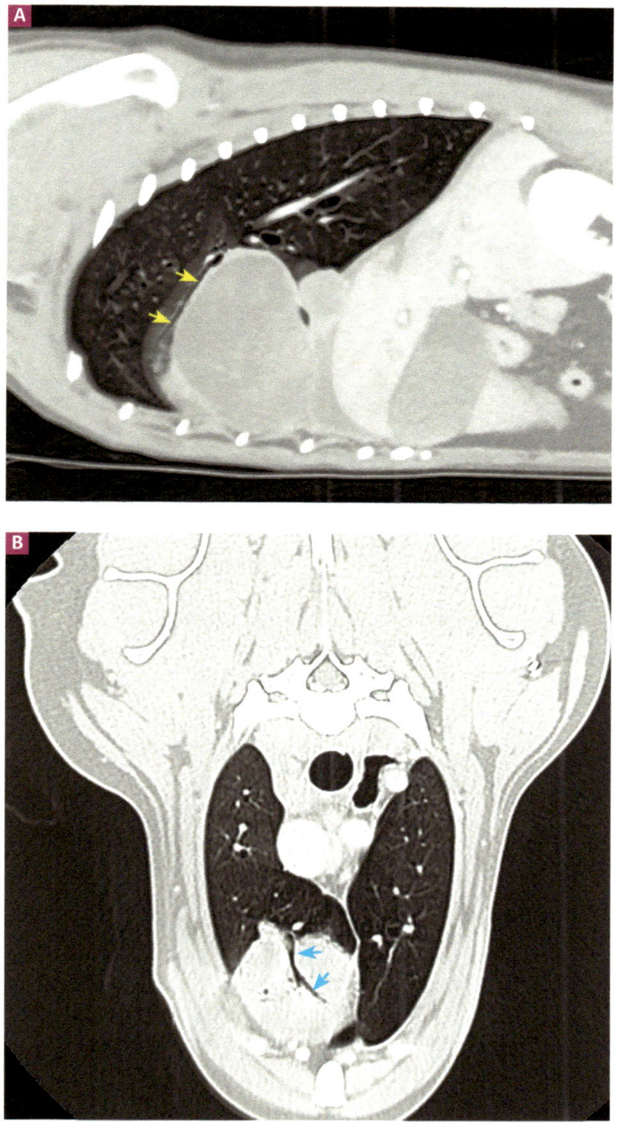

Figure 26. CT images in lung windows of patients with pulmonary neoplasia. **A**. Sagittal reconstruction of a pulmonary carcinoma, showing compression of the adjacent main bronchus (arrowheads). **B**. Transverse image of a histiocytic sarcoma showing nodular consolidation and the air bronchogram running through its centre (arrowheads).

Mediastinal tumours will present invariably in the presence of a mediastinal mass, associated with a mass effect, as per Table 3. CT allows a more accurate identification of the organ of origin of the tumour. The lesions present as a homogeneous mass presenting a variable contrast uptake depending on their vascularisation. Central necrosis can be observed as a poorly enhancing core in the lesion.

In the **cranial mediastinum**, lymphoma, lymphosarcoma and thymoma are the most common tumours. The first is more likely to present as lymphadenopathy of variable size, but affecting several lymph nodes, while the latter two are more likely to present a large solitary mass displacing the trachea dorsally and the heart caudally (Figure 27). Megaoesophagus may be present in case of thymoma as a secondary finding.

Heart-based tumours will be identified in the perihilar region. These will cause displacement of the carina and/or a filling defect in the iodinated contrast material present in the adjacent cardiac chamber, most commonly the right atrium or ventricle.

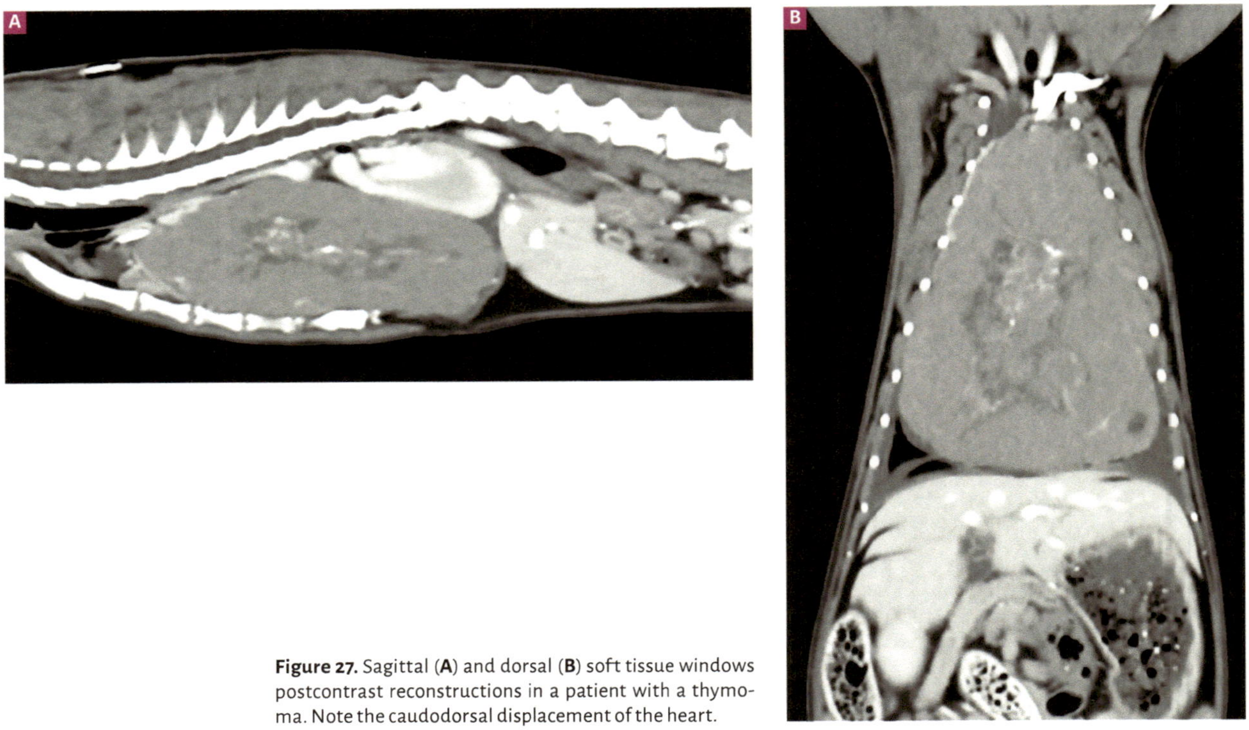

Figure 27. Sagittal (**A**) and dorsal (**B**) soft tissue windows postcontrast reconstructions in a patient with a thymoma. Note the caudodorsal displacement of the heart.

They may be poorly defined due to infiltration of the myocardium or pericardium. Secondary pericardial effusion may be present.

Neoplasia of the pleura, mesothelioma, are particularly difficult to identify as they often present as an irregular, or less commonly, nodular thickening of the pleura. Contrast uptake is helpful in identification of the affected area of the pleura. Pleural and/or pericardial effusion may be the only significant changes.

The thoracic wall contains a variety of structures including ribs, sternum and vertebrae, and their related soft tissue structures including muscles, fat, and skin. Finally, the diaphragm delineates the caudal thoracic boundary. All these structures can be affected by neoplastic conditions.

Primary rib tumours are uncommon, osteosarcoma and chondrosarcoma being the most common. They are associated with various degrees of osteolysis and irregular periosteal reactions. They usually affect the distal half of a solitary rib (Figure 28). The associated soft tissue swelling often displaces the adjacent ribs and extends intrathoracically. **Tumours of the sternum** are very uncommon and usually associated with multiple myeloma, as described above in the skeletal structures section.

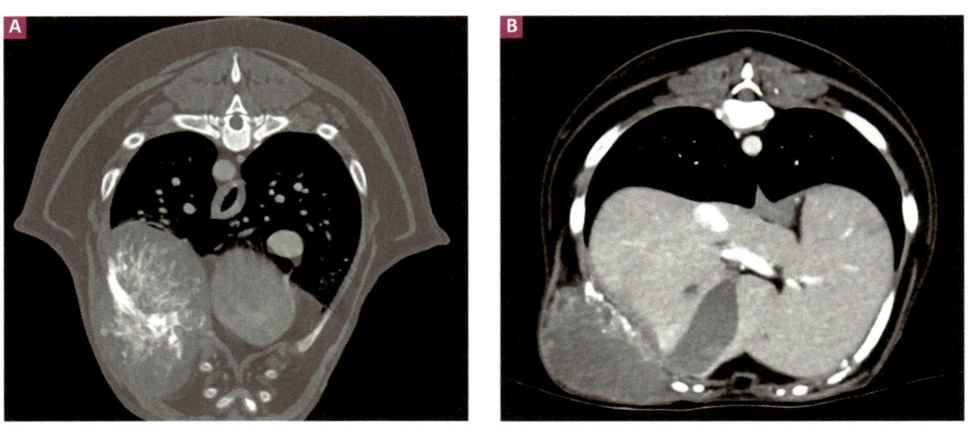

Figure 28. CT images of chondrosarcomas affecting the thoracic wall. **A.** Transverse CT image in bone window of a large chondrosarcoma affecting rib 7, left side in a canine patient. **B.** Transverse CT image in soft tissue window postcontrast of an osteosarcoma in a canine patient. Depending on the rib affected, note that the mass effect may be observed in the abdominal cavity rather than in the thorax.

Soft-tissue tumours, fibrosarcoma, and haemangiosarcoma are more likely to present as a large mass extending both inward and/or outward from the thoracic wall, invading the soft tissue, and be more or less cavitated depending on their size, possibly involving several ribs leading to lysis and periosteal reaction and eventually leading to pathological fractures.

Lipomas are common, often presenting with a capsule delineating them from the surrounding subcutaneous fat. They usually show almost no contrast uptake. Unlike simple lipomas, infiltrative lipomas and liposarcomas are locally invasive, infiltrating the muscles and the fibrous tissue and may present soft tissue components and contrast uptake.

Abdominal Structures

CT provides a useful way to assess all the abdominal organs during the same exam, in particular regarding their vascularisation. The patient is positioned in sternal recumbency. IV contrast injection should be performed for all studies, and a dual phase CT angiography is preferred, one acquisition is obtained during the arterial phase (Figure 29 A), and a second acquisition during the venous phase. Ideally an injector pump should be used to achieve a good arterial phase.

Primary hepatic and splenic tumours tend to be large in size with an irregular shape. They may have cystic/necrotic areas and haemangioma/sarcoma are often poorly vascularised (Figure 29 B).

Pancreatic tumours are difficult to identify but CT is certainly very helpful. Pancreatic carcinomas tend to be large mass lesions, poorly enhanced compared to the normal adjacent pancreatic tissue. To the contrary insulinoma, gastrinoma or other endocrine tumours are often small and usually present a strong contrast enhancement in the arterial phase. Regional lymphadenopathy is often present at the time of diagnosis representing early metastatic disease.

CT features of **gastrointestinal tumours** are poorly reported, although occasionally CT can provide information on the degree of the extent of a lesion (Figure 30 A). CT gastrography has been described and will outline mass lesions in the stomach and the proximal segments of the small intestinal tract. The excellent results obtained with ultrasound and endoscopy have pushed CT into a second place.

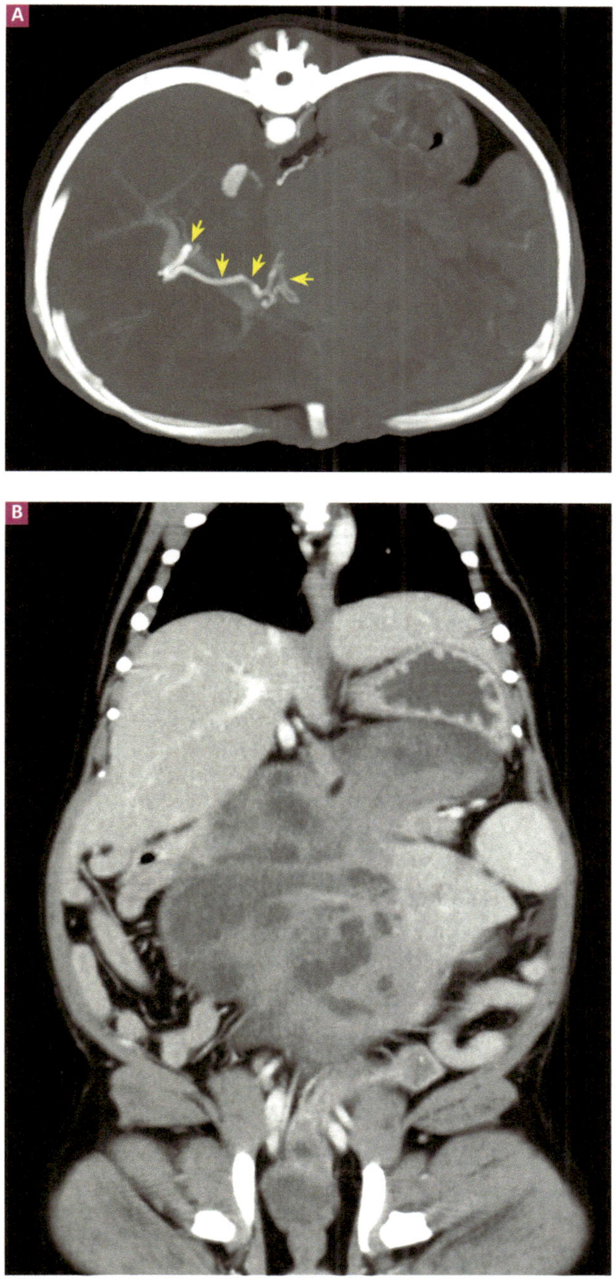

Figure 29. A. Maximum intensity projection CT image (MIP-CT) demonstrating the arterial supply (arrowheads) to a hepatic carcinoma. **B.** Sagittal soft tissue postcontrast reconstruction showing a large splenic haemangiosarcoma. Note the heterogeneous contrast uptake suggestive of intralesional cavitation.

Adrenal tumours present as adrenomegaly of variable size, shape, and density. The larger and more irregular the outline, the more likely a malignant process. Dystrophic mineralisations are also suggestive of a malignant process. As mentioned in the ultrasound section, assessment for vascular invasion is a key element both for prognosis and treatment purposes. Therefore, CT angiography is essential. Invasion of the vessels will show as a hypodense filling defect occupying a variable degree of the vessel lumen (Figure 30 B). Also, if the material represents neoplastic tissue, it will show some degree of contrast uptake whilst a thrombus will not enhance.

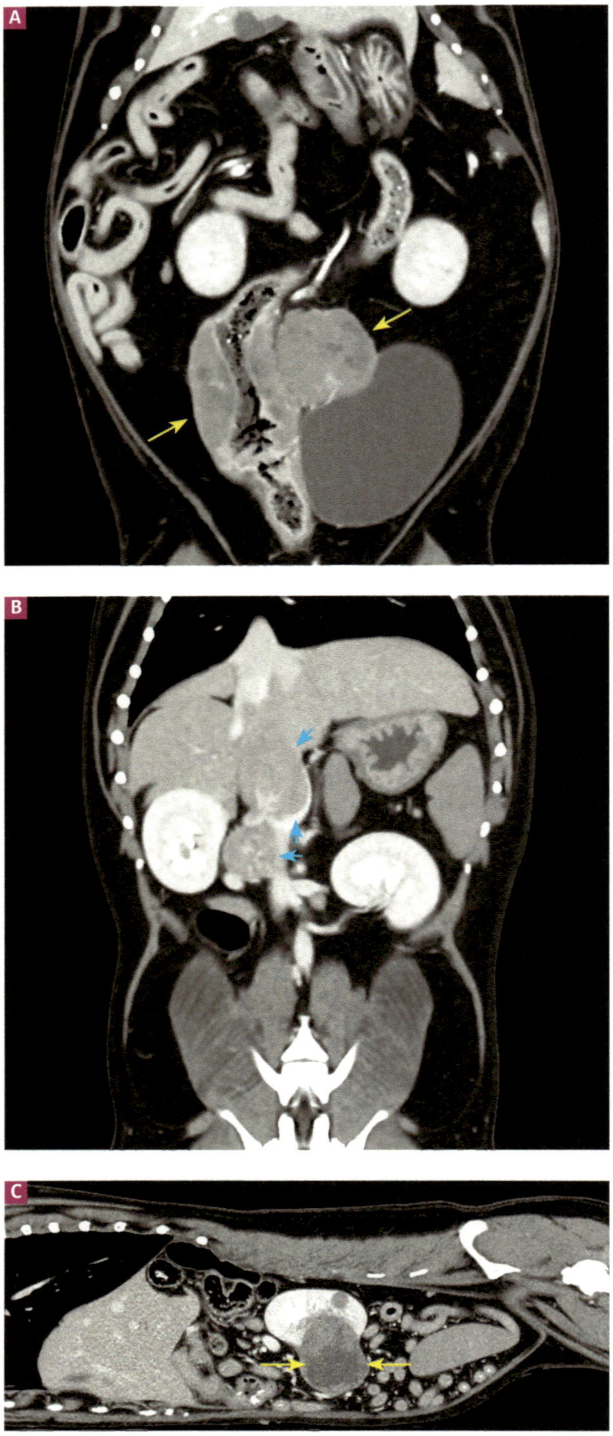

Figure 30. A. Dorsal reconstruction CT soft tissue window postcontrast of a canine patient with a colic carcinoma (arrows). The extent can be more precisely assessed in view of surgical planning. **B**. Dorsal reconstruction CT soft tissue window postcontrast venous phase, showing a large pheochromocytoma on the right side, invading the cranial vena cava (arrowheads). This is the same patient as in Figure 17. **C.** Sagittal reconstruction soft tissue window postcontrast in a canine patient with a renal carcinoma (arrows). This patient also presented metastatic lesions in the primarily affected kidney and the lungs.

CT is a valuable tool for investigation of the **urinary system, in particular the kidneys and the ureters**. The patient should be positioned in sternal recumbency with the pelvis elevated. Postcontrast sequences should be obtained for the parenchymal phase immediately after contrast injection, and for the excretory phase two to four minutes postinjection. Care should be taken when using iodinated contrast agents if the patient already has a compromised renal function and good studies can often be achieved with only half the normal dose of contrast agent. **Renal tumours** usually present as masses of variable sizes and variable contrast enhancement, replacing the normal parenchymal structure (Figure 30 C). The lesions show a variable contrast uptake, and some will present a cystic or cavitated component best appreciated on postcontrast sequences. They may cause ureteral obstruction and secondary pyelectasia. **Bladder tumours** can be identified on CT, but they are better assessed with ultrasound. A thickening of the wall or a mass formation will be outlined with excreted iodinated contrast.

Unlike with ultrasound, the **genital system** can be fully assessed with CT. Ovaries, uterine horns, cervix, and vagina can all be visualised. **Ovarian tumours** are often large heterogeneous soft tissue lesions, with moderate contrast enhancement. As mentioned in the ultrasound section they are often displaced ventrally and commonly found in the mid abdomen. Retrograde vaginography helps identification of mass lesions affecting the distal segments (**vagina and vestibule**). A neoplastic lesion causing a nodule or mass will cause a defect in the contrast filling. Intravenous contrast uptake helps to define the extent of lesion.

CT is more useful to identify and characterise **neoplastic retained testicles** than nonretained ones, which are very amenable to ultrasonographic examination. Retained neoplastic testicles are often large masses identified in the mid-abdomen, with a heterogeneous soft tissue density, showing moderate contrast uptake. Dystrophic mineralisations may also be identified. CT findings of **prostatic tumours** include various degrees of prostatomegaly. The lobes may become asymmetrical although a generalised tumour may cause a diffuse symmetrical enlargement of the gland. Postcontrast enhancement is present although cystic areas may appear as poorly enhancing intralesional areas. Dystrophic mineralisations are often a feature of carcinoma.

Nervous System

CT imaging of the brain necessitates a good knowledge of anatomy. A narrow window width should be used in order to distinguish between cerebrospinal fluid, white and grey matter. Postcontrast sequences should be obtained, as the uptake in the pituitary gland, choroid plexus and vessels will help the interpretation of the images. Although the differential diagnoses for brain tumours are varied, they will usually present as a mass lesion with a variable contrast uptake. Displacement of the *falx cerebri*, loss of symmetry/compression of the ventricles, and herniation of the brain parenchyma are clues to the **presence of a mass effect**. Location of the mass effect helps organise the differential diagnoses in order of likelihood.

Meningiomas are extra-axial broad-based masses contacting the adjacent bone, they are most commonly solitary, iso or hyperdense to the parenchyma and present a strong enhancement. A triangular area of contrast uptake can sometimes be seen at the periphery of the mass called a "dural tail". Occasionally in cats, the adjacent bone can become significantly thickened, a feature called hyperostosis.

Gliomas are intra-axial tumours presenting as solitary masses of varying size, shape, and definition (Figure 31 A). They have variable density and contrast enhancement. When isodense to the brain parenchyma and poorly enhancing, secondary signs of mass effects may be the only indication of the presence of a mass. **Choroid plexus tumours** arise within the ventricular system, mainly the third and fourth ventricles. They present as significantly enhancing mass lesions in the affected ventricle and may cause secondary hydrocephalus.

Peripheral nerve sheath tumours usually present as well-defined oval mass lesions in the path of the affected nerve. If reaching a sufficiently large volume, they will displace the adjacent muscle and cause muscle atrophy of the dependant area. They often present an intense contrast enhancement.

Although the pituitary gland is not clearly part of the nervous system, pituitary gland tumours of sufficient size may cause, as well as endocrinological symptoms, central nervous symptoms due to their location inside the skull and the mass effect this induces on the brain. Pituitary adenoma is more common than pituitary carcinoma. They present as a suprasellar mass of variable size causing a variable degree of mass effect on the adjacent brain. Reasonable contrast uptake is usually present (Figures 31 B and C).

Cranial nerve tumours are difficult to diagnose on CT as this relies on accurate identification of the skull foramina, allowing appreciation of the widening of a foramen compared to its contralateral pair. The easiest malignant peripheral nerve sheath tumour to identify is one affecting the trigeminal nerve, causing widening of the rostral alar foramen and ipsilateral secondary atrophy of the temporal muscle. Occasionally the tumour is large enough to become visible following intravenous contrast injection.

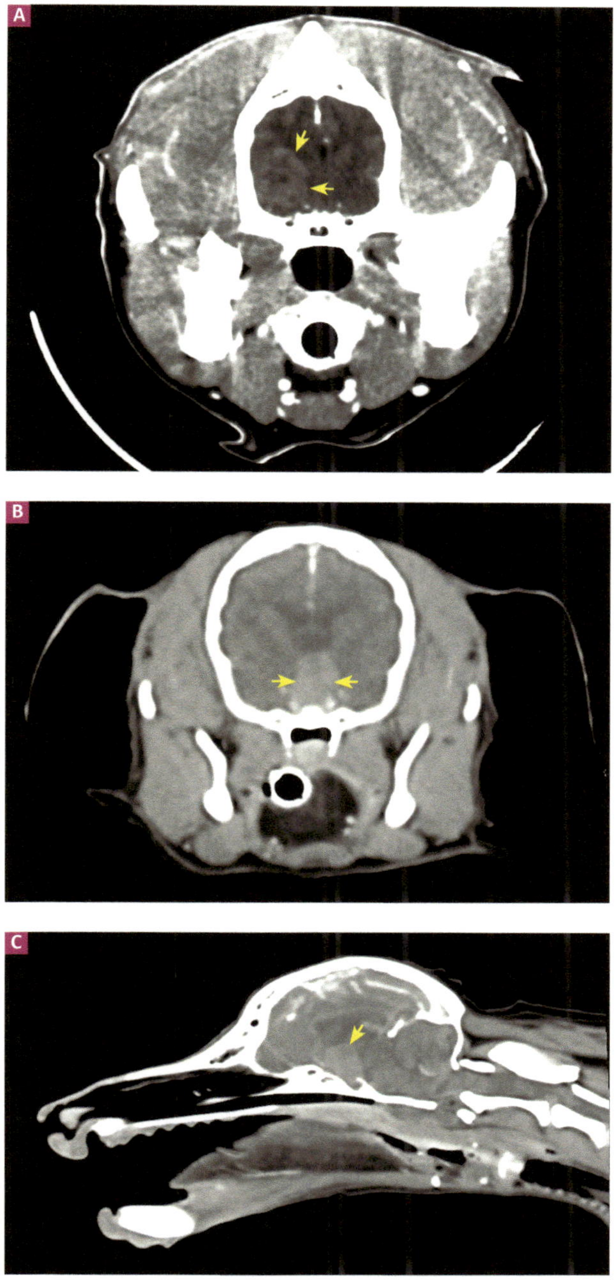

Figure 31. A. Transverse CT brain window postcontrast of a patient with a suspected large glioma (arrowheads). **B**. Transverse CT soft tissue window postcontrast of a patient with a suspected large pituitary adenoma (arrowheads). **C**. Sagittal CT soft tissue window postcontrast in the same patient.

Spine Tumours

To obtain good quality CT images of the spine, the patient should be positioned in dorsal recumbency and the head should be maintained extended with tape. If the main region of interest is the cervical spine, the limbs should be pulled caudally; and for the thoracic and lumbar spine, the limbs should be pulled cranially. Intravenous contrast injection should be performed if a neoplastic condition is suspected, as contrast enhancement of the vertebral venous sinuses and vessels may be useful for interpretation of images. Myelography can also be considered to assess spinal cord compression, as well as helping accurate localisation of the lesion (extradural vs intradural vs intramedullary).

The most common tumours affecting the spinal cord are extramedullary, arising from the vertebrae and causing secondary compression. They are covered in the skeletal section above. **Intradural extramedullary tumours** include meningioma, neurofibrosarcoma, lymphosarcoma, nerve root tumours and nephroblastoma. Myelography is necessary to identify these tumours. The contrast outlines the tumour causing a split in the contrast column at the level of the mass effect called a "golf tee" sign. It can be very difficult to differentiate these from intramedullary lesions. With nerve root tumours, the mass effect may cause a widening of the intervertebral foramen. They may also have an intramedullary component.

The **other intramedullary type of tumours** are gliomas – mainly in dogs – and lymphosarcoma in cats. CT myelography shows a focal swelling of the spinal cord surrounded by a thinning to disappearing myelogram. Occasionally intravenous sequences may show a focal enhancement of the spinal cord itself.

Metastatic Disease

Lungs are a predilection site for metastatic neoplasia in dogs and cats. Most metastatic lesions present as small size interstitial nodular lesions, representing a population which is homogeneous in size and shape (Figure 32 A). The advantage of CT compared to radiography is the detection of smaller lesions, but also of lesions in a difficult location, between

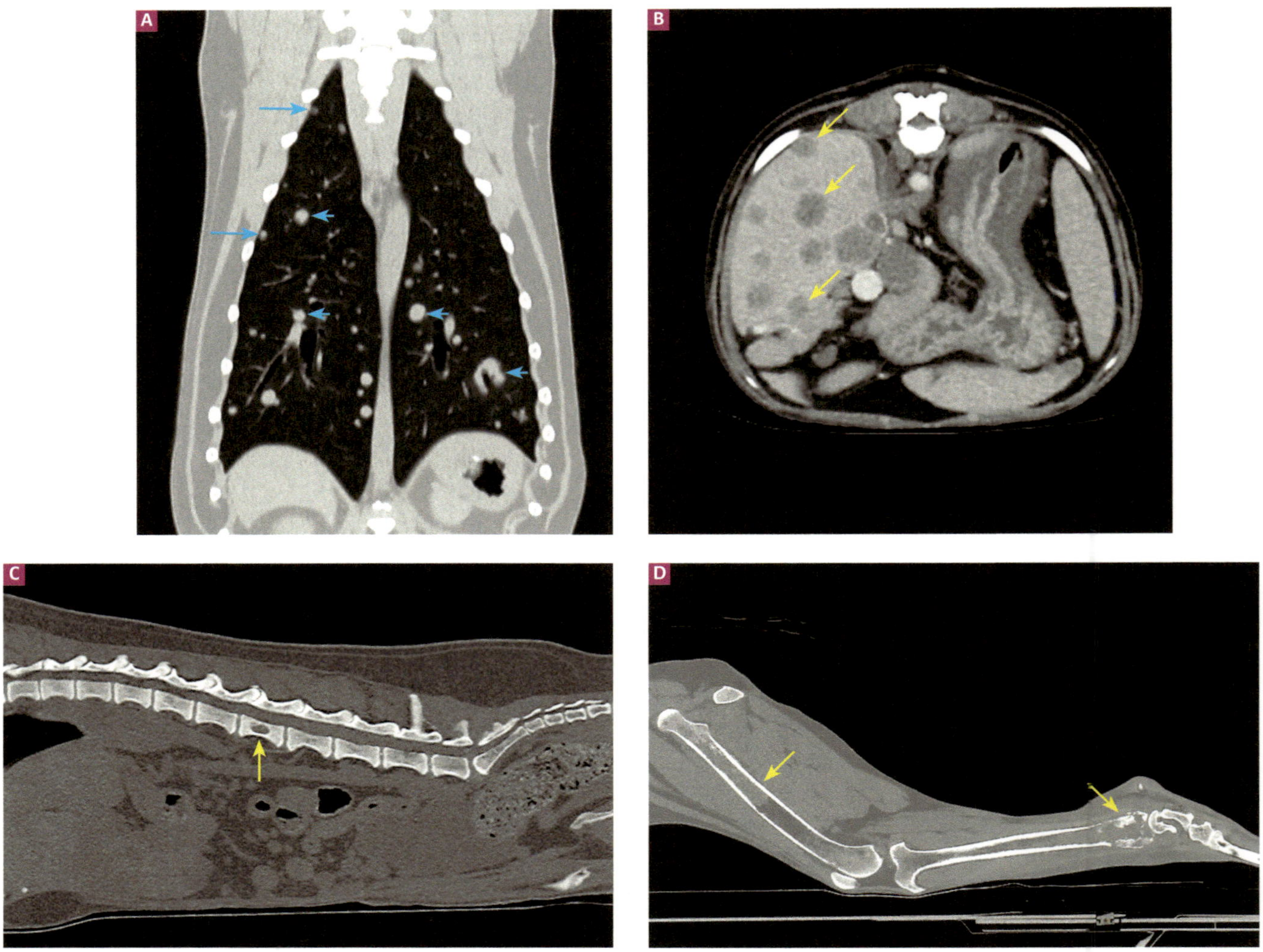

Figure 32. Examples of metastatic lesions. **A**. Dorsal reconstruction lung window of pulmonary metastatic lesions (arrows and arrowheads). Note that the smaller peripheral lesions would be unlikely to appear on thoracic radiographs (arrows). **B**. Transverse soft tissue postcontrast image of metastatic lesions affecting the liver (arrows). **C**. Sagittal reconstruction bone window of metastatic lesion affecting the third lumbar vertebral body (arrow). **D**. Sagittal reconstruction bone window of metastatic lesions affecting the femur and the distal tibia (arrows).

the heart and the diaphragm or along the pleura for example. Unlike the primary lesions, they rarely mineralise. If only a solitary lesion is present, a repeat CT should be considered after 4 to 6 weeks to assess the rate of progression. Metastatic spread to the pleura, pleural carcinomatosis, can be identified as thickening of the pleura and is often associated with a variable volume of pleural effusion.

CT is a very useful imaging tool to screen the entire body. It allows identification of widespread lesions in the parenchymal organs (Figure 32 B), but also in the bones, including the spine and long bones. Metastatic bone lesions are often, but not always, polyostotic, usually affecting the diaphysis of long bones, the proximal half of the ribs, or the vertebral bodies (Figure 32 C and D). They produce less periosteal/new bone than primary bone tumours, and are generally mainly lytic focal or multifocal lesions. The exceptions to this are metastatic lesions from prostatic tumours, which produce a florid periosteal reaction along the vertebral bodies and/or along the pelvic bones.

CT lymphography has recently been described as a complementary technique for lymph node staging. The technique consists of injecting iodinated contrast in the four quadrants surrounding the primary site of the tumour and assessing the progression of the contrast into the sentinel lymph nodes. These can then be assessed by sampling for cytology or removed for histopathology (Figure 33).

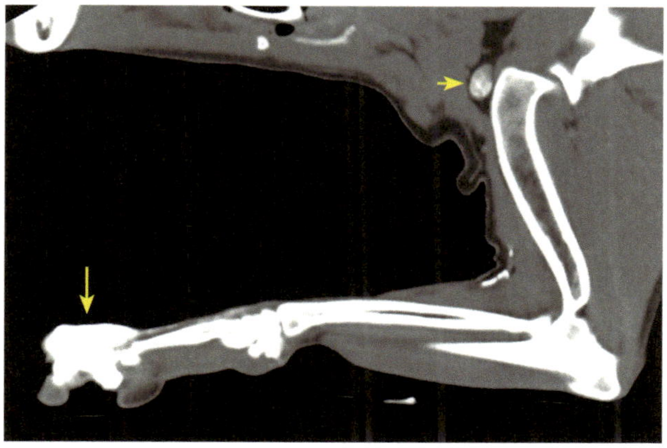

Figure 33. Sagittal reconstruction soft tissue window postlymphography. The primary lesion, a mast cell tumour, is located on the dorsal aspect of the metacarpi/digits where contrast has been injected (arrow). Contrast uptake in the prescapular lymph node identifies it as a sentinel lymph node (arrowhead) and was therefore sampled for staging purposes.

Other Advanced Imaging Techniques: Scintigraphy, PET-CT, MRI, and DCE-MRI

Several other imaging modalities are being used to image cancer patients. **Scintigraphy** is based on the metabolisation of a radiopharmaceutical in an organ of interest. Concentration of gamma emission is measured with a gamma camera. Two dimensional images are obtained mapping the areas of high concentration of the injected pharmaceutical (Figure 34). **Positron emission tomography (PET)** is a type of nuclear imaging producing three dimensional images. Scintigraphy and PET provide images of poor anatomical resolution and can now be superimposed onto CT images to provide a combination of good resolution images and precise localisation of the radioisotope concentration. These two modalities can be reunited in a single gantry and are then called **PET-CT**. In human medicine, this imaging modality is currently in use, and it is likely that its use will progress in veterinary oncology. Its main application is whole body staging, looking for distant metastatic lesions, in particular skeletal lesions.

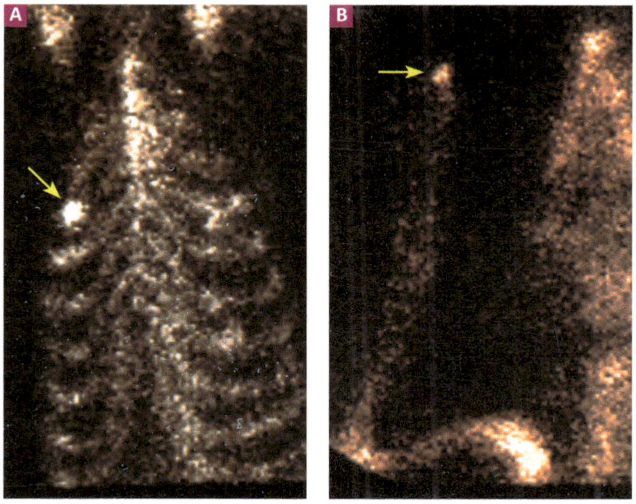

Figure 34. Images from a full body scintigraphy study for staging purposes in a canine patient with a palatine osteosarcoma; an injection of Technetium 99mHDP has been applied. **A**. The thorax is showing accumulation of radionuclide in one rib (arrow). **B**. In the right forelimb, the accumulation of radionuclide can be appreciated in a digit (arrow).

MRI (magnetic resonance imaging) is a tomographic imaging modality that relies on the return to alignment of hydrogen atoms of the different tissues, when placed in a large magnetic field. In the magnetic field, the hydrogen atoms align along the line of the magnetic flux. These hydrogen atoms are taken out of alignment when submitted to a radiofrequency. If the signal stops, they return to their alignment emitting a radiofrequency "listened to" by the receiver.

The time taken by the hydrogen atoms of each type of tissue back to the receiver is different and the software maps these times to create the image. Depending on the radiofrequency, the time taken to realign for each type of tissue varies from one type of series to another; comparison between series allows the type of tissue image to be determined. The software provides grey scale images and images can be acquired directly in all three planes: transverse, dorsal and sagittal. Acquisition of a single series takes a few minutes; several series should be performed to obtain a complete study. Studies are acquired in all three planes and do not rely on reconstructions like CT. Contrast agents for MRI are based on the presence of gadolinium instead of iodine, and are less nephrotoxic, although anaphylactic reactions have been reported.

MRI interpretation is complex and necessitates good familiarity with the images and knowledge of anatomy. MRI studies are significantly more time consuming than CT, requiring longer sessions of general anaesthesia. **MRI** provides superior imaging of soft tissue structures and is considered **the gold standard to assess the central nervous system**, due to its excellent differentiation between white and grey matter (Figure 35 A). Its superior soft tissue discrimination allows very precise assessment of soft tissue tumour margins (Figure 35 B and C) as well as early identification of tumour regrowth. As a downside, imaging of bony structures is not as good as with CT, due to the specifics of hydrogen protons in mineralised structures, although infiltrative neoplastic conditions of the skeleton are well assessed with MRI (Figure 35 D). MRI is extremely susceptible to movement artefacts and as a result, imaging of the thoracic structures can be challenging due to a combination of respiratory movement and cardiac contractions.

Dynamic contrast enhanced MRI (**DCE-MRI**) is used to assess perfusion of tissues, including for soft-tissue sarcoma and CNS tumours. These advanced imaging techniques are only in their early stages in veterinary medicine but will undoubtedly progress in parallel to oncology advances.

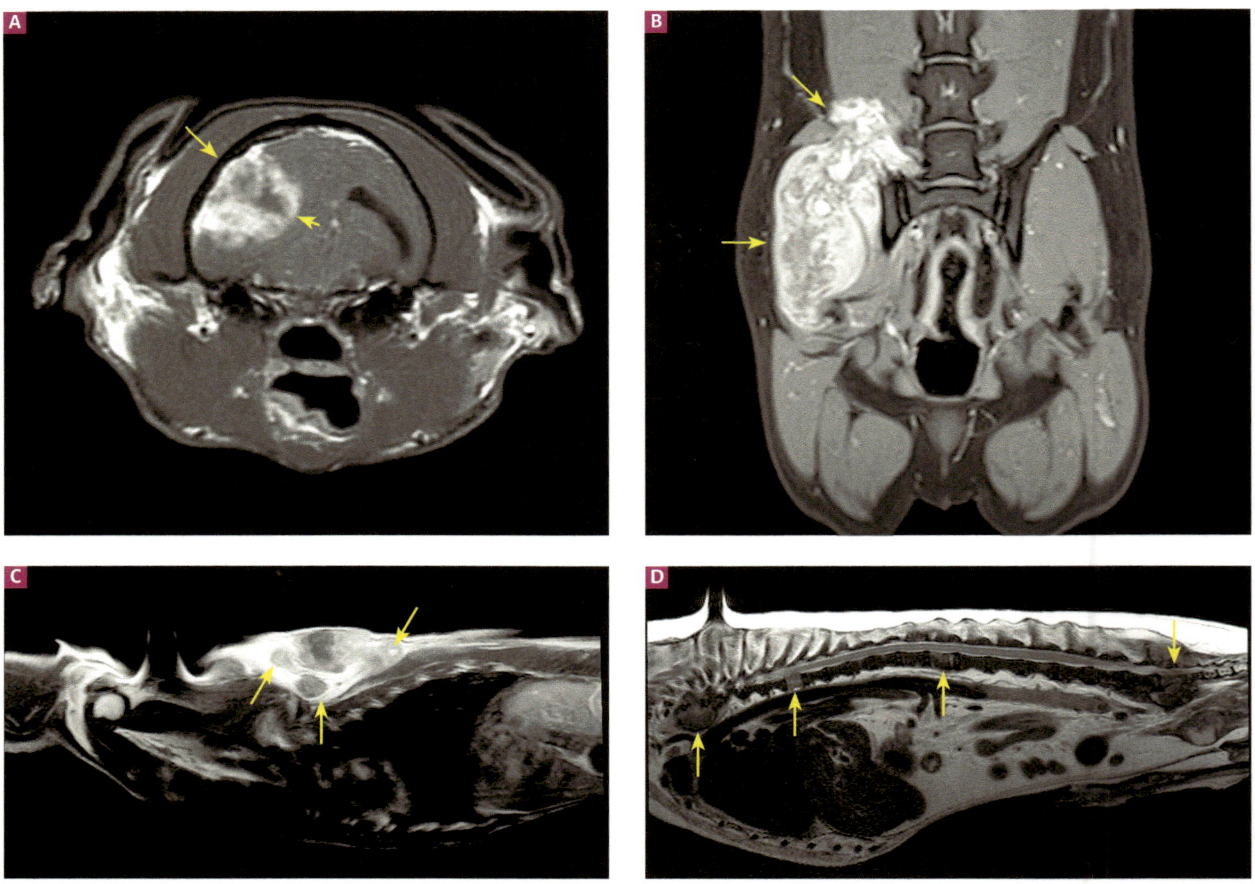

Figure 35. Examples of MRI studies in cancer patients. **A**. Transverse FSE (fat spin echo) T1 postcontrast image of a feline patient with a meningioma (arrowhead). Note the mass effect as well as the thickening of the adjacent calvarium (arrow). **B**. Dorsal FS (fat suppression) T1 postcontrast image of a canine patient with a sciatic nerve tumour (arrows). **C**. Sagittal T1 postcontrast image of a feline patient with an injection site sarcoma with its satellite nodular extensions (arrows). **D**. Sagittal T2 image of a patient with prostatic carcinoma with metastatic lesions in several vertebral bodies (arrows).

Bibliography

- Armbrust, L.J., Biller, D.S., Bamford, A. et al. (2012) Comparison of three-view thoracic radiography and computed tomography for detection of pulmonary nodules in dogs with neoplasia. *J Am Vet Med Assoc*, 240:1088–94.
- Barr, F., Gaschen. L. eds. (2011) *BSAVA Manual of Canine and Feline Ultrasonography*. 1st ed. Gloucester: British Small Animal Veterinary Association.
- Beer, P., Pozzi, A., Rohrer Bley, C. et al. (2018) The role of sentinel lymph node mapping in small animal veterinary medicine: a comparison with current approaches in human medicine. *Vet Comp Oncol*, 16:178–87.
- Bigio Marcello A., Gieger, T.L., Jiménez, D.A. et al. (2015) Detection of comorbidities and synchronous primary tumours via thoracic radiography and abdominal ultrasonography and their influence on treatment outcome in dogs with soft tissue sarcomas, primary brain tumours and intranasal tumours. *Vet Comp Oncol*, 13:433–42.
- Cuccovillo, A., Lamb, C.R. (2002) Cellular features of sonographic target lesions of the liver and spleen in 21 dogs and a cat. *Vet Radiol Ultrasound*, 43(4):275–278.
- Dennis, R., Kirberger, R.M., Barr, F., Wrigley, R.H. eds. (2010) *Handbook of Small Animal Radiology and Ultrasound: Techniques and Differential Diagnoses*. 2nd ed. Edinburgh: Churchill Livingstone Elsevier.
- De Swarte, M., Alexander, K., Rannou, B. et al. (2011) Comparison of sonographic features of benign and neoplastic deep lymph nodes in dogs. *Vet Radiol Ultrasound*, 52(4):451–456.
- Flemming, K., Nemanic, S., Löhr, C.V. et al. (2019) CT angiography and MRI imaging features do not predict the tumour type and grade of feline injection site sarcoma. *Vet Radiol Ultrasound*, 60(6): 668–679.
- Forrest, L.J. Computed tomography imaging in oncology (2016) *Vet Clin North Am Small Anim Pract*, 46:499–513.
- Gendler, A., Lewis, J.R., Reetz, J.A. et al. (2010) Computed tomographic features of oral squamous cell carcinoma in cats: 18 cases (2002-2008). *J Am Vet Med Assoc*, 236:319–25.
- Grimes, J.A., Secrest, S.A., Northrup, N.C. et al. (2017) Indirect computed tomography lymphangiography with aqueous contrast for evaluation of sentinel lymph nodes in dogs with tumors of the head. *Vet Radiol Ultrasound*, 58:559–64.
- Hanson, J.A., Pappageorges, M., Girard, E. et al. (2001) Ultrasonographic appearance of splenic disease in 101 cats. *Vet Radiol Ultrasound*, 42(5):441–445.
- Hecht, S., Penninck, D., Keating, J.H. (2007) Imaging findings in pancreatic neoplasia and nodular hyperplasia in 19 cats. *Vet Radiol Ultrasound*, 48(1):45–50.
- Kafka, U.C., Carstens, A., Steenkamp, G. et al. (2004) Diagnostic value of magnetic resonance imaging and computed tomography for oral masses in dogs. *J S Afr Vet Assoc*, 75:163–8.
- Karnik, K.S., Samii, V.F., Weisbrode, S.E. et al. (2012) Accuracy of computed tomography in determining lesion size in canine appendicular osteosarcoma. *Vet Radiol Ultrasound*, 53:273–9.
- Lang, J., Wortman, J.A., Glickman, L.T. et al. (1986) Sensitivity of radiographic detection of lung metastases in the dog. *Vet Radiol Ultrasound*, 27:74–8.
- Langenbach, A., McManus, P.M., Hendrick, M.J. et al. (2001) Sensitivity and specificity of methods of assessing the regional lymph nodes for evidence of metastasis in dogs and cats with solid tumors. *J Am Vet Med Assoc*, 218:1424–8.
- Laurenson, M.P., Skorupski, K.A., Moore, P.F. et al. (2011) Ultrasonography of intestinal mast cell tumours in the cat. *Vet Radiol Ultrasound*, 52(3):330–334.
- Magestro, L.M., Gieger, T.L. (2017) Detection of synchronous primary tumours and previously undetected metastases in 736 dogs with neoplasia undergoing CT scans for diagnostic, staging and/or radiation treatment planning purposes. *Vet Comp Oncol*, 15:576–81.
- Mai, W. (2018) *Diagnostic MRI in dogs and cats*. CRC Press.
- Majeski, S.A., Steffey, M.A., Fuller, M. et al. (2017) Indirect Computed Tomographic lymphography for iliosacral lymphatic mapping in a cohort of dogs with anal sac gland adenocarcinoma: technique description. *Vet Radiol Ultrasound*, 58(3):295–303.
- Mattoon, J.S., Bryan, J.N. (2013) The future of imaging in veterinary oncology: learning from human medicine. *Vet J*, 197:541–52.
- Nemanic, S., London, C.A., Wisner, E.R. (2006) Comparison of thoracic radiographs and single breath-hold helical CT for detection of pulmonary nodules in dogs with metastatic neoplasia. *J Vet Intern Med*, 20:508–15.
- Ober, C.P., Barber, D. (2006) Comparison of two- vs. three-view thoracic radiographic studies on conspicuity of structured interstitial patterns in dogs. *Vet Radiol Ultrasound*, 47:542–5.
- Palladino, S., Keyerleber, M.A., King, R.G. et al. (2016) Utility of computed tomography versus abdominal ultrasound examination to identify iliosacral lymphadenomegaly in dogs with apocrine gland adenocarcinoma of the anal sac. *J Vet Internal Med*, 30:1858–63.
- Paoloni, M.C., Penninck, D.G., Moore, A.S. (2002) Ultrasonographic and clinicopathologic findings in 21 dogs with intestinal adenocarcinoma. *Vet Radiol Ultrasound*, 43(6):562–567.
- Penninck, D., d'Anjou, M.A., eds. (2008) *Atlas of Small Animal Ultrasonography*. 1st ed. Oxford, UK: Blackwell Publishing.
- Petite, A. and Dennis, R. (2006) Comparison of radiography and magnetic resonnance imaging for evaluating the extent of nasal neoplasia in dogs. *J Small Anim Pract*, 47:529–536.
- Prieto, S., Gomez-Ochoa, P., De Blas, I. et al. (2009) Pathologic correlation of resistive and pulsatility indices in canine abdominal lymph nodes. *Vet Radiol Ultrasound*, 50(5):525–529.
- Rebhun, R.B., Thamm, D.H. (2010) Multiple distinct malignancies in dogs: 53 cases. *J Am Anim Hosp Assoc*, 46:20–30.
- Rossi, F., Körner, M., Suárez, J. et al. (2018) Computed tomographic-lymphography as a complementary technique for lymph node staging in dogs with malignant tumors of various sites. *Vet Radiol Ultrasound*, 59:155–62.

■ Schwarz, T. and Saunders, J. (2011) *Veterinary Computed Tomography.* Wiley-Blackell.
■ Skinner, O.T., Boston, S.E., Giglio, R.F. et al. (2018) Diagnostic accuracy of contrast-enhanced computed tomography for assessment of mandibular and medial retropharyngeal lymph node metastasis in dogs with oral and nasal cancer. *Vet Comp Oncol,* 16:562–70.
■ Taeymans, O., Penninck, D.G., Peters, R.M. (2013) Comparison between clinical, ultrasound, CT, MRI, and pathology findings in dogs presented for suspected thyroid carcinoma. *Vet Radiol Ultrasound,* 54:61–70.
■ Talbott, J.L., Boston, S.E., Milner, R.J. et al. (2017) Retrospective evaluation of whole body computed tomography for tumour staging in dogs with primary appendicular osteosarcoma. *Vet Surg,* 46:75–80.
■ Vignoli, M., Terragni, R., Rossi, F. et al. (2013) Whole body computed tomographic characteristics of skeletal and cardiac muscular metastatic neoplasia in dogs and cats. *Vet Radiol Ultrasound,* 54:223–30.
■ Williams, L.E., Packer, R.A. (2003) Association between lymph node size and metastasis in dogs with oral malignant melanoma: 100 cases (1987-2001). *J Am Vet Med Assoc,* 222:1234–6.

Test

Answers on Page 86

1. **The objective of diagnostic imaging in the oncology patient is:**
    a. To help identify the origin of the tumour and its effects on adjacent structures.
    b. Establish a prioritised list of differential diagnoses and, subsequently, a definitive diagnosis through biopsies.
    c. Answers a) and b) are correct.
    d. None of the above are correct.

2. **Which is the correct answer?**
    a. It does not take much experience to carry out MRI diagnoses, interpretation of the technique is simple.
    b. Complete assessment of an oncology patient usually requires more than one diagnostic imaging technique.
    c. Diagnostic techniques using radiography, ultrasound and CT are based on X-rays.
    d. Digital radiography is the technique of choice for assessing head injuries.

3. **When examining the lymphatic system, which of the following should be taken into account?**
    a. Each lymph node drains a single area of the body, so it is easy to link a lymph node metastasis to its origin.
    b. The presternal lymph node drains the lungs, bronchi, trachea, oesophagus, aorta, heart, and diaphragm.
    c. The hepatic lymph node drains the liver, stomach, duodenum, pancreas, and spleen.
    d. The axillary lymph node drains superficial structures of the dorsal thoracic area, posterior aspect of the forelimb, thoracic mammary glands, and cranial abdominal muscles.

4. **Regarding radiography as a diagnostic method, which answer is incorrect?**
    a. The main drawback of radiography is that the organs included in the projection overlap.
    b. This technique is mainly used as a screening modality.
    c. Bone loss needs to reach 50% of the mineralised matrix to be detected on radiography.
    d. Changes in the surrounding soft tissue may also be assessed radiographically, e.g. muscle loss, soft tissue inflammation, and/or joint effusion.

5. **Which is the correct answer?**
    a. In the head, the use of radiography is limited to assessing bone tumours.
    b. The radiographic protocol for the detection of pulmonary masses should not include dorsoventral projections.
    c. The thoracic wall is the first structure to be evaluated radiographically in case of neoplasia.
    d. If on radiography an increase in size of the cranial mediastinal space is seen, this suggests the presence of a diaphragmatic tumour.

6. **Which answer is incorrect?**
    a. Round cell tumours have a nodular or mass lesion appearance when assessed with ultrasound.
    b. The lungs are one of the most frequent locations of metastatic disease.
    c. Lymphadenopathies may be more or less visible on radiographs depending on the location of the draining lymph nodes.
    d. Ultrasound is the first choice of technique for observation and evaluation of abdominal organs.

7. **What additional information does Doppler ultrasound provide?**
    a. None, in practice it is used because coloured ultrasound scans have a greater effect on the patient's owner.
    b. If it shows an increase in peripheral arterial vascularisation of the tumour this may be indicative of a malignant lesion.
    c. Colours are used to differentiate the different densities of tissue, which facilitates diagnosis.
    d. None of the above.

8. **When performing an ultrasound assessment of the structures of the head and neck, which of the following is correct?**
    a. Ultrasound is a good technique for evaluation of bone neoplasms of the structures of the head and neck.
    b. The parathyroid gland is seen especially clearly on ultrasound, as hyperechogenic nodular structures.
    c. It allows evaluation of the deep structures of the eye even if an opaque barrier such as cataracts are found.
    d. The parathyroid gland can measure up to 5 mm and this is normal.

9. Which of the following is incorrect?

a. A radiograph cannot provide reliable information about whether a tumour is present in an abdominal organ or what the extent of the tumour is.

b. Colour Doppler allows the vascular invasion of the vessels adjacent to a tumour to be assessed and detection of the presence of thrombi.

c. Hepatic or biliary cystadenoma has a cystic component with an anechoic appearance.

d. Ultrasound assessment of diffuse round cell tumours always shows a modification of the ultrasound structure of the organ where they are present.

10. Regarding ultrasound-guided biopsies, which answer is correct?

a. The ability to perform ultrasound-guided sampling is one of the key features of ultrasound.

b. Fine needle aspiration is the correct technique for diagnosing sarcomas, which tend to exfoliate more easily than round cell tumours.

c. The safest route to the lesion is always the shortest route.

d. The bevel of the needle should be oriented towards the opposite side of the ultrasound probe, to allow better visualisation of its tip.

11. Why is CT the technique of choice for planning treatment with radiation therapy?

a. It is a simple and fast diagnostic method, so patients with respiratory failure do not need to be sedated.

b. It allows irradiation of large areas to be planned, so that treatment is much more effective.

c. It provides real time evidence of blood flow surrounding the tumour without injecting contrast media into the patient.

d. It allows both the size of the tumour and its margins to be assessed very accurately.

12. Using CT to assess the skeletal system has its advantages. Which of the following is not one of them?

a. It allows detection of the amplitude of the transition zone between the centre of the lesion and the normal structure of the bone better than conventional radiography.

b. It shows evidence of bone lysis long before it is evident on radiographs.

c. It enables a precise assessment of the extension of the lesion in long bones.

d. It allows the type of tumour (osteosarcoma, chondrosarcoma, fibrosarcoma etc.) to be determined without the need for biopsy.

13. Regarding the use of CT to assess thoracic structures, what is the correct answer?

a. CT is the best imaging technique for assessing the thorax as a whole.

b. Although it is very useful for assessing certain thoracic structures, ultrasound is much more effective.

c. The recommended positioning of the patient is in right lateral recumbency, so as not to compress the heart in prolonged scans.

d. The most common tumour detected in the pleura by CT is lymphoma.

14. Regarding the use of CT to assess abdominal structures, what is the correct answer?

a. CT is very useful for diagnosing pancreatic tumours.

b. CT is not very effective for assessing abdominal structures due to the overlap of the organs.

c. CT is far superior to radiography or ultrasound for the diagnosis of gastrointestinal tumours.

d. The urinary system, mainly kidneys and ureters, are not well visualised by CT, ultrasound is preferable.

15. Regarding the evaluation of nervous system structures and the spine by CT, which answer is incorrect?

a. To evaluate brain tumours, a narrow window should be used that allows differentiation of the cerebrospinal fluid, grey matter, and white matter.

b. Meningioma usually presents as an extra-axial mass, with a wide base implantation that is in contact with the adjacent bone.

c. Gliomas present as multiple intra-axial masses of varying size, shape, and definition.

d. Tumours of the choroid plexus occur in the ventricular system, primarily in the third and fourth ventricles.

16. Which of the following is correct?

a. Scintigraphy allows creation of 3D images based on the metabolisation of a radiopharmaceutical in a certain organ of interest.

b. Positron emission tomography (PET) scans produce images with poor anatomical resolution.

c. MRI is based on the same principles as radiography and CT; therefore, the images are three dimensional.

d. Digital magnetic resonance imaging is the best technique for assessing bone structures.

Notes

Correct Answers:

1. c
2. b
3. d
4. c
5. a
6. a
7. b
8. c
9. d
10. a
11. d
12. d
13. a
14. a
15. c
16. b

Notes

Practical Chemotherapy for Dogs and Cats

Ana Lara García

Chemotherapy, although a word that simply means medical treatment through the use of chemicals, is commonly associated with the use of cytotoxic drugs for the treatment of cancer. It is estimated that **25% of dogs and cats will develop cancer throughout their lives** and that this is the **cause of death in half of pets over 10 years of age**. The development of veterinary oncology has made it possible for more and more pets with cancer to be treated just like with any other chronic disease.

In recent years, the development of veterinary specialisation in this area, the increase in continuous professional development and the greater number of studies and publications in veterinary oncology, added to a growing number of owners who demand therapeutic options for their pets diagnosed with cancer, have provided greater knowledge, and contributed to the change of mentality on the part of veterinarians towards the treatment of cancer in small animals. This has made it possible for veterinary clinics to offer chemotherapy treatments and for veterinary referral centres to begin offering cancer surgery and radiotherapy as additional treatment modalities.

Chemotherapy as a single modality of cancer treatment is a palliative therapy, which rarely cures the patient, as is the case with the symptomatic treatment of other chronic diseases (chronic kidney failure, congestive heart disease, diabetes mellitus, hyperadrenocorticism, inflammatory bowel disease, etc.) that are treated on a daily basis in practice.

The main goal of chemotherapy treatment for pets with cancer is to **treat the disease while maintaining or improving quality of life for as long as possible**. It is the veterinarian's responsibility to set realistic expectations and maintain a high degree of communication with the owners of these pets to ensure that they understand the patient's prognosis and the goal of treatment.

It is important to make it very clear what the possible adverse effects are, explain what is acceptable and what is not tolerable and establish a symptomatic action plan with the support of the owner to minimise the impact on the patient if these complications appear.

The relationship between owner and veterinarian is extremely important to achieve the objectives mentioned above.

Tumour Biology and Mechanism of Action of Chemotherapeutic Agents

To understand the mechanism of action and effects, on the tumour and on normal tissues, understanding cell and tumour kinetics is necessary. In general, normal cells and tumour cells follow a similar **cell cycle** that includes four phases (Figure 1).

- **G1 phase**, where the enzymes necessary for DNA synthesis are produced.
- **S phase**, synthesis, where DNA is synthesised.
- **G2 phase**, where proteins are synthesised.
- **M phase**, where mitosis occurs.

After mitosis, the cell can start the cycle again reaching a new division or entering a **resting phase (G0)**. The mitotic index indicates the percentage of dividing cells in a tissue (normal or tumour) and because chemotherapy mainly affects dividing cells, tissues with a high mitotic index will be more sensitive to chemotherapy.

In general, the types of neoplasia with a high mitotic index may be more sensitive to cytotoxic drugs while tumour types with a low mitotic index often do not respond to this treatment or do so very slowly. On the other hand, the adverse effects of cytotoxic drugs appear in healthy tissues with a high mitotic or proliferation index. In general, only the epithelium of the intestinal villi and bone marrow has a high mitotic index in normal tissues, which explains the sensitivity of these tissues to cytotoxic drugs.

Tumour Growth

Tumour growth is considered Gompertzian, which is where there is a rapid initial growth followed by a plateau in growth (Figure 2). During the rapid growth phase, the growth fraction is high, and chemotherapy is more effective, as cells are more susceptible to chemical damage (and radiation) when they are dividing. At a later stage, a smaller proportion of cells are dividing, and growth reaches a plateau phase (for example, when the blood supply becomes insufficient for tumour volume). Unfortunately, tumours are often only found clinically relatively late, towards the end of the initial growth phase.

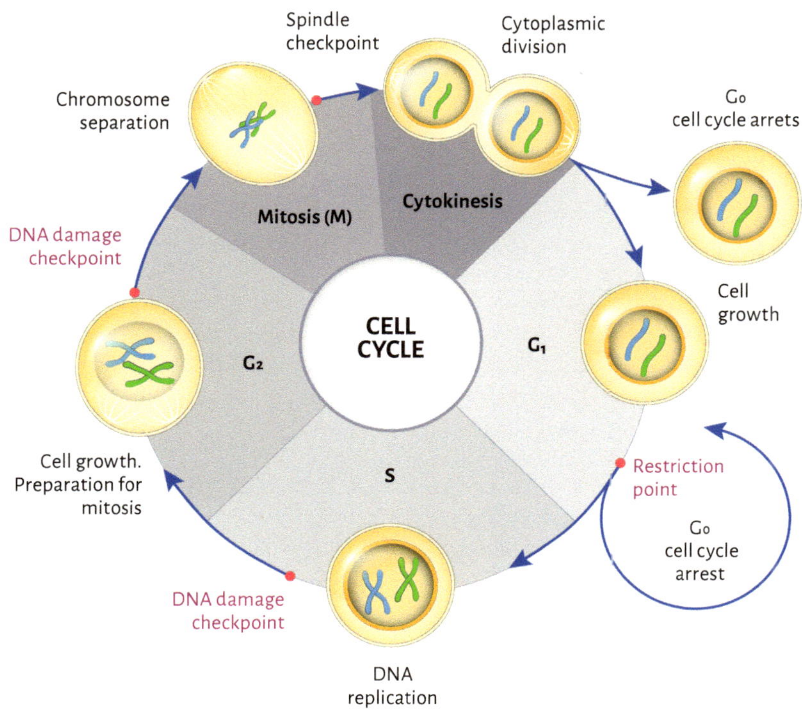

Figure 1. The cell cycle.

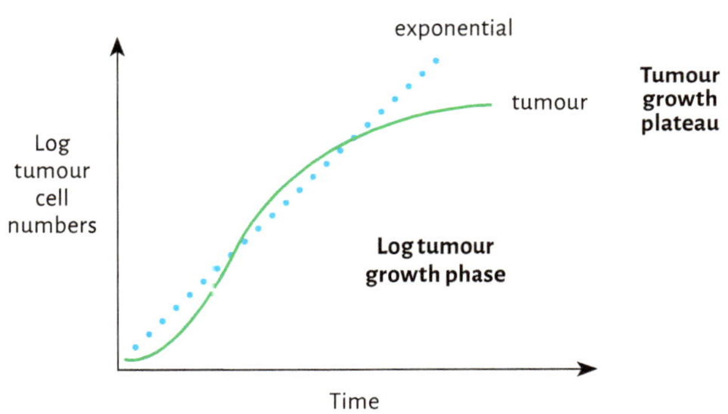

Figure 2. Gompertzian tumour growth curve.

The fraction of cells in the resting phase (G_0) in the tumour population will dictate the outcome of chemotherapy.

When referring to malignant neoplasms with a high replication rate, they show their highest mitotic index when they are smaller in size than when they can be detected by imaging or physical examination. However, this index decreases when the tumour increases in size and presents more areas of necrosis and has a more limited vascular supply. For this reason, better responses to chemotherapy are given in these types of tumours when microscopic disease is present (for example, micrometastasis or residual tumour after surgery with incomplete margins).

The effects of chemotherapy follow logarithmic kinetics. That is, they kill a percentage of tumour cells, not a constant number of them. Doses are usually given at regular intervals, determined by the time it takes for normal tissue (gastrointestinal and bone marrow) to recover, but tumour cells that survive each dose will proliferate between each treatment session. In neoplasms with a high replication rate, reducing the dose decreases the effectiveness of the treatment against the tumour, as well as the side effects, and the same occurs if the timing between each dose is increased. On the other hand, the individual idiosyncrasy of each patient must be taken into account in terms of risk of toxicity with cytotoxic treatments: minimising this risk is more important than the rules on efficacy associated with dose and frequency of treatment, and it is important to remember that the goal is to treat cancer in pets, while maintaining quality of life. Furthermore, in patients who suffer more adverse effects a more pronounced antitumour effect of chemotherapy is often seen.

Tumour Response to Chemotherapy

Different types of neoplasms have different sensitivities to chemotherapy, so some types are insensitive to the cytotoxic drugs used in veterinary oncology.

The most important factors that determine the response of a certain type of cancer to cytotoxic drugs are:

- the growth fraction or **mitotic index** of the cancer to be treated
- development of **resistance mechanisms** to cytotoxic drugs.

It must be taken into account that although some types of neoplasms have a very high mitotic index, they may be inherently resistant to conventional cytotoxic drugs, as is the case with malignant oral melanoma and many types of carcinomas.

In any case, it should be borne in mind that the doses of cytotoxic drugs administered in veterinary oncology are minuscule compared to those in humans, despite the fact that tumour biology is similar in both species. For this reason, responses to chemotherapy in some types of pet cancer are often more limited or non-existent compared to human oncology, even when similar drugs are used. The most satisfactory responses to the doses used in veterinary oncology are seen in high-grade neoplasms that are also chemosensitive.

Considerations Regarding the Choice and Dose of Cytotoxic Drugs

In general, drug combinations have been shown to be more effective than the use of one drug alone (exceptions to this are vincristine in transmissible venereal tumour (TVT) or doxorubicin or carboplatin in osteosarcoma).

These combinations must follow some basic rules.

- Each individual drug must have demonstrated **efficacy against the tumour**.
- They should have **different mechanisms of action**.
- They should not have overlapping **toxicities**.

Dose Intensity

There is ample evidence in human and veterinary oncology that optimal dose intensity improves chemotherapy outcome.

Dose intensity is defined as the amount of drug administered per unit of time (mg/m²/week). Therefore, the dose intensity can be increased by increasing the dose of any of the drugs in the chemotherapy protocol or by shortening the time interval between consecutive administrations. As a general rule, the dose intensity should be the maximum tolerated by the patient with minimal toxicity. It is very important to think that this theory, at the doses that are used in veterinary medicine, will be effective for neoplasms sensitive to chemotherapy and, among these, those that have a high proliferation rate. In other words, in neoplasms resistant to cytotoxic chemotherapy such as, for example, malignant oral melanoma, mammary or pulmonary carcinomas or neoplasms with a low proliferation rate such as low-grade lymphoma, intensification of cytotoxic therapy will not provide greater effectiveness, but it will put the patient at risk of further toxicity. Likewise, it is very important to know the mechanisms of action of the drugs used and their possible interactions when combining different cytotoxic substances.

Chemotherapy Dose Calculation

Dosage recommendations for cytotoxic drugs in small animals are largely based on body surface area (BSA, m^2). Conversion tables for kg to m^2 to calculate the body surface area in cats and dogs are used. In general, the following formula can also be used:

$$S = K \times \text{weight (kg)}^{0.66}/10^4$$

Where K = 10.1 in dogs and 10 in cats

Using this formula, smaller dogs would receive a higher dose in proportion to body weight than larger dogs, thus compensating, in theory, for the faster distribution, metabolism and excretion of the drugs in small animals. If this is correct, the exposure to the drug and therefore its efficacy and toxicity should be uniform for different species. In reality, this is not the case and **for veterinary use this body surface-based system is not perfect**. For some cytotoxic drugs, small dogs and cats require lower doses. For example, reducing the dose of doxorubicin in dogs less than 15 kg or in cats to 1 mg/kg instead of 30 mg/m² is recommended.

Problems with the body surface calculation formula have been evaluated in different studies. In the formula, as it was designed, the constant K would supposedly be associated with a constant body shape for the same species, but in reality, the phenotype of different breeds of dogs can be very variable and there should probably be different constants for different breeds. Even in cats, various studies have shown that the K constant is not accurate despite the relative uniformity of body shape in different feline breeds. This constant does not correlate with the concentration of haematopoietic progenitor cells by species or breed, liver, or kidney function, and it does not include other factors such as age, breed, and type of disease, all of which affect drug distribution, metabolism, and excretion. Despite all these limitations, for now this system is the only one available. The veterinarian should use a body surface conversion table and be informed of which drugs require dose reduction for small animals.

Estimation of body surface area can also lead to overdose in obese animals. In obese dogs, the normal weight should be estimated, and the body surface calculated based on that estimate. It should also be remembered that different species may present different metabolisation or elimination of drugs and, therefore, not only are the doses of chemotherapy drugs in dogs and cats often different, but also the toxicities for the same drug.

Effects of Body Systems on Cytotoxic Drugs (Pharmacokinetics and Pharmacodynamics)

There are four important factors that affect the dosing of cytotoxic drugs in dogs and cats. These factors must be evaluated in each patient individually. As many cancer patients are also geriatric, it must be taken into account that in older animals, sometimes the most important body systems may have reduced function, and this can affect the toxicity or effectiveness of the substances used.

- **Absorption**. For example, animals with malabsorption syndrome may have decreased digestive absorption when receiving oral cytotoxic drugs such as cyclophosphamide or methotrexate and, therefore, the activity of these drugs could be lower than expected.
- **Distribution**. In cases of hypoproteinaemia, when drugs are administered that require binding to plasma proteins, such as the vinca alkaloids, mitoxantrone or cisplatin, a higher proportion than expected may remain pharmacologically active or may be eliminated more quickly.
- **Excretion**. The concentration of drug in the blood over time is a function of the elimination rate of all the elimination or metabolism systems. When the glomerular filtration rate is decreased, it affects drugs that depend on the urinary system for elimination, such as carboplatin. In fact, in humans, cats, and dogs, the dose that most reliably predicts carboplatin toxicity is that calculated from measurements of renal creatinine clearance. This is particularly useful in patients with kidney dysfunction. Disruptions in bile flow can reduce the elimination of drugs that require this pathway for metabolism, such as vincristine or doxorubicin (asparaginase can increase the toxicity of vincristine when both are administered simultaneously by delaying hepatic metabolism of vincristine). In patients with decreased renal filtration or decreased hepatic metabolism, it should be taken into account that if they receive drugs eliminated by these routes, they could suffer toxicities (haematological and gastrointestinal) to a greater degree, as well as being more prolonged since the elimination of the active compound is delayed. In these cases, consideration should be given to whether a temporary dose reduction is appropriate.
- **Metabolism**. Liver dysfunction can reduce the metabolism of doxorubicin, increasing its toxicity. Cyclophosphamide, lomustine, and dacarbazine require hepatic activation, so reduced hepatic metabolism may reduce the efficacy of these drugs.

Chemotherapy Strategies in Veterinary Medicine

Neoplasms grow faster when they are smaller. As explained previously, when they increase in size, the growth rate decreases due to a decrease in the proportion of cells in active phases of the cell cycle and an increase in cell death due to reduced blood supply, leading to poor nutrition and hypoxia. Poor tumour vascular support can lead to chemotherapy not reaching the neoplastic tissue in adequate concentrations to exert its effect. Furthermore, resistance to chemotherapy can occur through spontaneous mutations in the tumour cell. The possibility of these mutations occurring is directly proportional to the number of cell divisions that have occurred in a tumour, so acquired resistance to cytotoxic drugs is more common in larger tumours.

In general, cytotoxic chemotherapy is most effective against small tumours, either after detection or after a cytoreductive process such as surgery or radiation. It is rare for chemotherapy to be effective against large or extensive tumours, unless these are extremely chemosensitive, such as high-grade lymphoma and transmissible venereal tumour.

Chemotherapy Resistance

The first studies for the treatment of lymphoma using single agents such as vincristine or cyclophosphamide obtained dramatic responses in cats and dogs, but with a short duration, but continued use of the same drug produced no response after relapse. In other words, these animals developed resistance. Tumour resistance is common, especially in high-grade neoplasms with a high or very high proliferation rate, sometimes even before treatment has started (intrinsic resistance), and rapidly dividing tumour cells acquire resistance to drugs quickly after exposure due to high mutation rates.

The mathematical model called the "Goldie-Coldman hypothesis" was developed to predict the possibility of cellular neoplastic mutations that would lead to resistance to chemotherapy. This theory proposes that spontaneous mutations occur every 10 000 to 1 000 000 cell divisions. The hypothesis predicts that as the number of neoplastic cells grows, the probability of resistance increases, such that:

- treatment should start **as soon as possible** when the tumour population is small;
- **multidrug** regimens minimise the possibility of development of resistant cell clones; and
- the drugs should be administered with the **highest possible intensity**, specifically in high-grade neoplasms.

Another problem is the development of cross-resistance between multiple different drugs. This happens with substances that are eliminated cellularly by means of the transmembrane excretion pump called P-glycoprotein, present in several normal tissues and also in some tumours at high levels. Their presence in tumour cells reduces the intracellular concentration of these drugs. The prevalence and amount of P-glycoprotein has been seen to increase with continued exposure to chemotherapeutic drugs. This MDR (multiple drug resistance) phenomenon affects drugs from the anthracycline family (such as doxorubicin), vinca alkaloids (vincristine), corticosteroids, and other substances such as actinomycin, paclitaxel, and etoposide.

In practical terms, a patient who is resistant, for example, to vincristine and prednisone could be resistant to other drugs from the same families and also other active substances whose elimination is carried out through P-glycoprotein, such as doxorubicin. In practice, the only way to know is to administer the new drug and see if there is a response or not. On the other hand, using subtherapeutic doses should be avoided as much as possible to minimise the risk of resistance and, whenever possible, solid protocols established for the prevention of adverse effects that avoid reductions in chemotherapeutic drugs. On the other hand, it must be remembered that, in principle, the drugs from the alkylating family do not usually present cross-resistance.

Combinations of Chemotherapeutic Drugs

The combination of chemotherapeutic agents with different mechanisms of action can reduce the risk of developing tumour resistance, since cells that are resistant to a certain drug can be eliminated by another included in the treatment combination, through a mechanism of action for which the cell has not developed resistance. A combination of active ingredients can increase the risk of toxicity, so the toxicity patterns of the different drugs to be combined should be studied in such a way that improves the elimination of tumour cells without increasing toxicity. For example, non-immunosuppressive substances, such as asparaginase, or slightly immunosuppressive, such as vincristine, can be administered one week after an agent that is more immunosuppressive such as doxorubicin or high-dose cyclophosphamide (as is done in CHOP or VAC protocols).

Guidelines for Chemotherapy

Chemotherapy is indicated as the main therapy in animals with systemic neoplasms (lymphoma, multiple myeloma, leukaemia) or in local neoplasms with a high metastatic potential after resection, to delay their recurrence, or when there are metastases.

Sometimes it can be used in inoperable tumours sensitive to chemotherapy or refractory to other therapeutic modalities, such as radiation.

Adjuvant Chemotherapy

This is the name given to the use of cytotoxic drugs after resection of a type of primary tumour that has a high rate of metastasis and/or recurrence after incomplete resection. The most typical example would be the administration of carboplatin or doxorubicin after amputation of a canine appendicular osteosarcoma. The effectiveness of adjuvant chemotherapy is greater the smaller the volume of neoplasia in the patient: for example, in the case that there are only microscopic foci of metastatic disease, since the number of cells is low, these are less likely to be resistant and, in addition, the growth fraction is high and in principle sensitive to cytotoxic drugs.

The decision to administer adjuvant chemotherapy should be based on a definitive diagnosis and knowledge of the biological behaviour of the excised neoplasm. It is indicated as adjuvant therapy after surgery in tumours with a high rate of metastasis (osteosarcomas, haemangiosarcomas, grade II mast cell tumours–Patnaik classification–with mitotic index >5 or grade III).

Neoplasms with a low rate of metastasis have a high percentage of cure if excision is complete and they do not require adjuvant chemotherapy. If the removal has been incomplete, chemotherapy is not an appropriate treatment to prevent recurrence: a second surgery to obtain larger margins or radiotherapy is more appropriate. A low-grade tumour with incomplete resection (for example, a soft-tissue sarcoma), is not very likely to respond to cytotoxic therapy as it has a low proliferation rate, as demonstrated by the long time to recurrence in the low percentage of cases where this occurs. In high-grade sarcomas, cytotoxic therapy could help delay recurrence, but is highly unlikely to prevent it.

Neoadjuvant Chemotherapy

This use of chemotherapy before surgery is neoadjuvant chemotherapy. It is applied in neoplasms very sensitive to chemotherapy (high-grade mast cell tumours, subcutaneous haemangiosarcomas). The goal of neoadjuvant chemotherapy is to reduce tumour volume after several cycles of chemotherapy to a point that allows surgical removal. Chemotherapy can also be used in animals with inoperable tumours or in which surgery with curative intentions is not possible (it is not possible to achieve the appropriate margins or the degree of reconstructive surgery after "en bloc" removal of the tumour is not feasible), such as for example, to reduce the possible effects of degranulation before starting radiation therapy in inoperable high-grade mast cell tumours.

As a general rule, chemotherapy should not be used as a replacement therapy for surgery or radiation when these treatment modalities are indicated as the treatment of choice and can be carried out. It should also not be administered in patients with severe multiorgan failure (or should be administered with caution, modifying the doses) because the risk of systemic toxicity is increased.

Things to Consider

Although the general indications for chemotherapy have already been mentioned, a number of factors must be taken into account when choosing a chemotherapy regimen for a given patient.

- **Factors related to the patient**. The general evaluation of the patient, age, presence or absence of systemic diseases, functional abnormalities, etc. directly influence the choice of treatment for a given tumour. For example, while amputation – plus chemotherapy – is the treatment of choice in dogs with osteosarcoma, it may not be an option in animals with severe osteoarthritis or significant neurological deficits in other limbs.
- **Owner-related factors**. Treatment predisposition, tolerance to side effects, availability for necessary visits to the practice, and cost of treatments should be discussed with owners and taken into account when choosing a chemotherapy protocol.
- **Disease related factors**. The main objective is to cure the disease, but when using chemotherapy (without surgery) this can rarely be achieved. If the chances of cure are low, the goal of treatment is to maintain a good quality of life and try to achieve tumour remission. Different clinical stages of the same tumour (for example, presence of metastatic disease or not) require different approaches to treatment, but in general, early diagnosis and treatment increase the chances of cure when they exist or, at least, of achieving control of the disease for longer periods.

What are Cytotoxic Drugs and How do they Work?

Many pharmacologically different drugs have been identified for their anticancer activity (Table 1). These agents can be divided into groups by their mode of action, antitumour activity, and toxicity.

- **Alkylating agents**, which substitute alkyl groups for an H^+ ion in DNA, cause crosslinking and breakdown of DNA molecules. This interferes with DNA replication and RNA transcription. They are not drugs with an action associated with specific phases of the cell cycle.
- **Antimetabolites**, which replace normal substrates necessary for DNA or RNA synthesis and cause enzymatic inhibition or lead to the synthesis of non-functional molecules. These act in the S phase of the cell cycle.
- **Anti-tumour antibiotics**, which use various mechanisms to inhibit DNA and RNA synthesis, including DNA strand breaks, DNA base pair cross-linkage, inhibition of topoisomerase II (an enzyme important in the unwinding of DNA strands) and the production of free radicals. The action of these drugs is not associated with specific phases of the cell cycle.
- **Vinca alkaloids** are antimitotic and act specifically on the mitotic spindle, binding to tubulin and causing a metaphase cell cycle arrest (they act in the M phase of the cell cycle).
- **Platinum complexes**, which produce crosslinking between the same DNA chain or between adjacent chains, interfering with its replication and RNA synthesis. The action of these drugs is not associated with specific phases of the cell cycle.
- **Hydroxyurea** inhibits ribonucleoside diphosphate reductase and prevents the conversion of ribonucleotides to deoxyribonucleotides (acts in the S phase of the cell cycle).

All these agents exert their action in phases of cell growth and division, for this reason cytotoxic drugs are more effective against cells in active phases of growth or division (Figure 3). The high rate of cell division in certain normal body tissues, such as bone marrow and gastrointestinal tissue, makes them susceptible to the effect of cytotoxic drugs, causing what is known as toxicity or adverse effects.

Table 1. Most widely used cytotoxic agents in veterinary oncology and possible side effects.

Drugs		Side effects	
		Immune suppression	Gastrointestinal toxicity
Alkylating agents	Cyclophos-phamide	High (high dose)	Low
	Melphalan	Low	Low
	Chlorambucil	Low	Low
	Lomustine	Very high	Low
	Procarbazine	Low	Low-moderate
	Dacarbazine	Very high	High-very high
Antimetabolites	Cytarabine	Moderate (with infusion), low (SC)	Low
	5-fluorouracil	Low-moderate	Low
	Methotrexate	Low	Moderate
	Gemcitabine	Moderate	Low-moderate
Antitumour antibiotics	Doxorubicin	High	High
	Epirubicin	High	High
	Mitoxantrone	High	High
	Actinomycin D	High-very high	High-very high
Vinca alkaloids	Vincristine	Moderate	Low-moderate
	Vinblastine	Moderate-high	Low-moderate
	Vinorelbine	Moderate-high	Low-moderate
Platinum complexes	Carboplatin	High-very high	Low
	Hydroxyurea	Low	Low

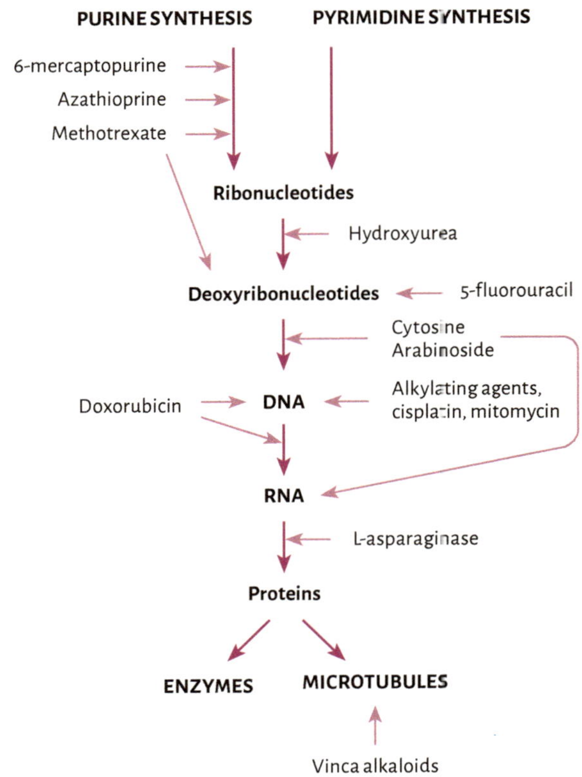

Figure 3. Point of cellular action of cytotoxic drugs.

Other Agents Used in Cancer Treatment

L-asparaginase

An enzyme that breaks down the amino acid asparagine to form aspartic acid, preventing it from being used in protein synthesis. It is used in the treatment of lymphoma and acute lymphoblastic leukaemia. Neoplastic lymphoid cells cannot synthesise asparagine and depend on an external source. In the presence of L-asparaginase, asparagine is depleted and, as neoplastic lymphoid cells are unable to synthesise protein, this leads to their cell death.

Corticosteroids

Corticosteroids, such as prednisolone, dexamethasone, etc., cause apoptosis of tumour cells that present a membrane receptor for glucocorticoids, such as lymphoid cells and cells of other round cell tumours such as mast cell tumours and plasma cell tumours. In addition, they reduce the inflammation associated with neoplastic infiltration in healthy tissues. Corticosteroids have no anticancer effect in carcinomas or sarcomas.

Nonsteroidal Anti-inflammatories (NSAIDs)

The mechanism of antitumour action of NSAIDs is not fully understood, but they are thought to be associated with inhibition of COX-2 receptors. NSAIDs inhibit angiogenesis, promote apoptosis, and are anti-inflammatory and analgesic. They are part of the treatment of transitional cell carcinoma of the bladder/urethra and of metronomic therapy protocols.

Routes of Cytotoxic Drug Administration

Intravenous Administration of Chemotherapy

The most commonly used route for the administration of chemotherapeutic drugs is the **intravenous route**. Most of these drugs, if they are extravasated, produce effects ranging from local irritation to severe tissue necrosis, and for this reason it is essential to ensure intravenous administration through the use of small diameter catheters and to be extremely careful regarding their correct fixation. On the other hand, drugs such as L-asparaginase, cytosine arabinoside, bleomycin or gemcitabine can be administered **subcutaneously** since they do not cause tissue damage.

As a general rule, venous access should be achieved on the first attempt to minimise possible vascular damage and, thus, the potential for extravasation. If the attempt is unsuccessful, using a different peripheral vein or a portion proximal to where the first attempt was initially made is recommended. The correct positioning of the catheter, before and after drug administration, must be confirmed by infusion of saline, preferably not heparinised, since some chemotherapeutic agents can precipitate on contact with heparin.

Box 1. Additional recommendations for the administration of intravenous chemotherapeutics

- **The jugular veins should be used to take blood for complete blood counts or any other blood tests in patients undergoing chemotherapy treatment. This avoids repeated damaged to peripheral veins for procedures which do not involve the administration of chemotherapy.**
- **Different veins should be alternated between for chemotherapy administration, to allow possible phlebitis caused by previous treatments to resolve.**
- **Sedation prior to administration should be considered in patients which become stressed in the hospital or have an aggressive character.**
- **In extremely aggressive patients treated with long duration protocols (such as the Madison-Wisconsin protocol for lymphoma), as well as curative radiation protocols which require numerous anaesthetics the placement of permanent catheters for vascular access can be considered or the chosen chemotherapy protocol reconsidered. Permanent access catheters can remain in place in the patient for up to three years and allow blood samples to be obtained as well as administration of intravenous medications via an access placed in the subcutaneous tissue connected to a silicone catheter commonly implanted in the femoral vein.**

What to do in Case of Chemotherapy Extravasation

Before proceeding with intravenous administration of vesicant drugs, owners must be **informed of the possible risks** if extravasation occurs. When extravasation of vesicant chemotherapy occurs, the degree of subsequent tissue damage will depend on the type and amount of extravasated drug, ranging from pruritus, erythema, and dermatitis to severe tissue necrosis. These symptoms usually appear in the days after extravasation, although in the case of doxorubicin they can take a week or more. Once these signs have appeared, only symptomatic treatment with anti-inflammatories, local antibiotics, bandages, use of a buster collar to prevent self-mutilation and surgical debridement in the case of severe tissue necrosis can be performed. For these reasons, the measures taken to prevent extravasation are extremely important as they will prevent it from occurring and, if it does occur, will minimise the amount of drug extravasated and, therefore, the consequences for the patient (Box 1).

In the event of extravasation, immediate action should be taken, and drugs that are known to prevent the adverse effects of extravasation should be used. In veterinary practices where chemotherapy is administered routinely, an action plan must be established for cases of extravasation and the drugs required in this situation must be kept in stock.

To follow are some recommendations that can be applied immediately after extravasation of vesicant cytotoxic drugs in order to reduce the degree of subsequent tissue damage.

- If extravasation of chemotherapy with a strict intravenous route occurs, or if there are simply doubts during the administration of the correct positioning of the intravenous route, the **administration should be stopped immediately** and the syringe with the drug in question should be disconnected.
- **Effectiveness of venous access should be checked** first by exerting negative pressure to visualise blood flowing into the syringe. If this does not happen, the infusion of a set volume of saline solution should be attempted.
- If the catheter is out of the vein or a certain extravascular volume has been administered, **the catheter should not be removed and attempts should be made to aspirate** with negative pressure into an empty syringe or saline solution.
- **Injectable corticosteroids should be administered** (dexamethasone 0.15 mg/kg IV or SC) and the instructions below followed depending on the type of drug extravasated.

Box 2. Useful considerations in neutropaenic patients

- **For neutrophil counts less than 1 000/µl** there is a significant risk of sepsis, especially in patients with parallel clinical signs compatible with damage to the gastrointestinal barrier and the possibility of bacterial translocation.
- **If the neutrophil count is 500–1000/µl (grade III neutropaenia)** chemotherapy treatment should be delayed for 2–4 days. If the patient does not present clinical signs (gastrointestinal or pyrexia), administration of broad-spectrum oral antibiotic therapy for a few days and monitoring until the next complete blood count is usually sufficient. The neutrophil nadir rarely persists for more than a few days.
- **For patients with neutrophil counts less than 500/µl (grade IV neutropaenia)**, administration of intravenous antibiotics for 24 hours and monitoring is recommended. If they also present with pyrexia or gastrointestinal symptoms, hospitalisation is necessary and intravenous fluids, antibiotics and symptomatic treatments should be administered.

Although the neutrophil count returns to normal quickly (2 to 4 days), when **nadirs with a number of neutrophils** ≤500/µl are detected, a reduction in the dose should be considered of around 15 to 20% for the next administration or an improved plan for prevention of side effects. If the dose is reduced, a complete blood count should be performed again at the nadir to determine if the new dose has the desired effect. The myelosuppressive effect of each drug included in the chemotherapy protocol should be assessed separately.

For neutrophil counts of 1000–3000/µl (grade I–II neutropaenia), if the patient is well, the treatment can be administered. If highly immunosuppressive drugs (doxorubicin or lomustine, for example) should be administered and the patient has a count of 1000–1500/µl, it can be delayed 48–72 hours if the disease is under control. As an alternative, if administering treatment is a priority, antibiotics which reach high concentrations in the digestive tract can be used preventively, such as sulfa-trimethoprim, until the nadir.

If the patient is not clinically well (for example, has anorexia, diarrhoea, vomiting...) or has a temperature, regardless of the neutrophil count (even if the count is normal), treatment should not be administered and symptomatic treatment should be administered.

In addition, consideration should be given to the need for additional clinical testing to differentiate whether clinical signs are due to treatment or disease (e.g., gastrointestinal signs as a result of intestinal lymphoma progression or secondary to chemotherapy).

In certain breeds, especially **sighthounds** (Greyhound, Podenco, Afghan Hounds, etc.) a neutrophil count below 3000/µl is normal.

When deciding whether to treat or not, it is important to take into consideration, together with the number of neutrophils and the patient's clinical status, the type of neoplasia the patient presents (degree of malignancy) and the clinical stage of the neoplasia (in remission, out of remission, existence of metastasis).

Vincristine/Vinblastine Extravasation

- Infiltrate the area with a total of 1500 subcutaneous hyaluronidase units, covering the extravasated area with various injections.
- Apply warm compresses.
- Apply anti-inflammatory ointment.
- Continue over the following days with oral and topical anti-inflammatories.

Doxorubicin/Epirubicin/Actinomycin/Mitoxantrone Extravasation

- Apply cold compresses to induce vasoconstriction and minimise drug distribution.
- Doxorubicin: administer IV dexrazoxane at a dose of 10 times the amount of doxorubicin administered within 3 hours of extravasation. If feasible, repeat this procedure at 24 and 48 hours. This treatment has been described in isolated cases, showing complete avoidance or, at least, significant reduction of tissue damage after doxorubicin extravasation.
- Apply topical dimethyl sulfoxide (DMSO) every 2–4 hours.
- Apply anti-inflammatory ointment and administer oral anti-inflammatories over subsequent days.

Oral Administration of Chemotherapy

When using oral chemotherapy drugs, it can be difficult to administer the exact dose, especially in small dogs or cats, due to a limited availability of different milligram presentations of the drugs. In these cases, it can be extremely helpful to find chemists or laboratories with availability to reformulate these drugs into capsules containing fewer milligrams.

This is especially useful for the use of lomustine in cats or cyclophosphamide in metronomic therapy. It should be remembered that tablets or capsules should never be split or opened **because these practices can result in improper dosing and exposure to cytotoxic substances**. It is also important to instruct owners to wear gloves for the administration of these drugs.

Intracavitary Administration of Chemotherapy

Chemotherapy can also be administered intracavitarily in dogs and cats with malignant pleural or abdominal effusions (mesotheliomas disseminated carcinomatosis). For this, the use of thoracic catheters or permanently implanted pleural catheters (Pleuroport®, Norfolk Veterinary products, Illinois, United States) is recommended. Drugs such as cisplatin, carboplatin, mitoxantrone, and fluorouracil have been shown to be effective in reducing malignant effusions in dogs over long periods.

Adverse Effects of Chemotherapy, Monitoring and Medical Management

The toxicity of chemotherapeutic agents is normally related to the dose, although other factors must always be remembered, such as insufficiencies in the organ systems responsible for the metabolisation and elimination of these drugs (hepatic and urinary system). Because cytotoxic drugs are effective in the active phases of the cell cycle, tissues with high rates of cell replication are the most commonly affected. Dogs of breeds with increased frequency of mutations of the MDR (multi drug resistance) gene, which cause exacerbated toxicity of drugs that are substrates of P-glycoprotein, should be tested before receiving these drugs (more information at http://vcpl.vetmed.wsu.edu/affected-breeds).

In patients with decreased renal filtration or decreased hepatic metabolism, it should be borne in mind that if they receive drugs that are eliminated by these routes, they could suffer higher and longer lasting toxicities (haematological and gastrointestinal), as the elimination of the active compound is delayed.

Haematological Toxicity

Myelosuppression is a general term applied to the toxic effects of chemotherapy on the bone marrow. The limiting factor for myelosuppression is usually neutropaenia (Table 2).

In general, the prognosis for animals with uncomplicated neutropaenia is good: most patients have no clinical signs and the neutrophil count returns to normal within a few days. The **nadir for peripheral blood neutrophils** (lowest point in the number of neutrophils after chemotherapy administration) occurs between 5 and 10 days after treatment for most drugs used in veterinary oncology, except for carboplatin (nadir 10 to 14 days). This is why administration is usually every one or two weeks, except for lomustine or carboplatin, which require longer intervals as they cause greater myelosuppression.

A complete blood count including platelet count should be performed one week after chemotherapy administration, when the nadir for neutrophils is being assessed. For carboplatin, a complete blood count at 10 and another at 14 days after administration should be evaluated, at least after the first treatment, to find out exactly when the nadir produced by this drug occurs and to see if it is of clinical significance or not. In high intensity protocols, the next dose of chemotherapy will often be given at the time of the nadir (as in high-grade lymphoma protocols).

It must be taken into account that after the administration of cytotoxic drugs, a **platelet nadir** will also occur, which is usually a little later than that for neutrophils and rarely causes clinically significant thrombocytopaenia. Sometimes, in patients who are quite sensitive to the substances used, a platelet count below normal at the time of neutrophil nadir can be seen. After the platelet nadir, as after the neutrophil nadir, the counts return to normal within a few days (usually 2–4 days). It should be taken into account that the Greyhound and Cavalier King Charles have lower physiological platelet counts than normal.

It is important to remember that some drugs can cause cumulative thrombocytopaenia after long periods of treatment (usually months). This is the case with melphalan and sometimes lomustine. In patients who have been treated with numerous cytotoxic drugs for a prolonged period, an exacerbation of haematological toxicity and a slower recovery of cell counts is sometimes seen. A "depletion" and slowing down of the bone marrow response can also be observed.

There are some specific cases in which it is not absolutely necessary to carry out a continuous complete blood count in the nadir period, for example, in dogs receiving carboplatin or doxorubicin as adjunctive treatment for osteosarcoma. After the first or second cycle, after determining that the patient has an acceptable number of neutrophils at nadir and instructing the owner to monitor the patient in the period in which the greatest immunosuppression is expected, blood counts can then be performed only on the day the patient is to receive treatment.

Gastrointestinal Toxicity

Gastrointestinal toxicity is **one of the factors with the greatest impact on the quality of life** of pets treated with chemotherapy and it is not acceptable. Therefore, the development of measures for its prevention are almost more important than the treatment of this toxicity. It is the responsibility of the veterinarian to assess the patient's risk of developing gastrointestinal toxicity, taking into account the prevalence of this adverse effect with each drug included in the chosen chemotherapy protocol, as well as individual factors such as the patient's breed, individual sensitivity (for example, previous history of frequent gastroenteritis with any change in diet) or if the neoplasm to be treated affects the gastrointestinal tract (for example, gastrointestinal lymphoma).

It is imperative to inform owners of the clinical signs to expect when this toxicity occurs, when they are expected to occur, and what they should do in case of their occurrence. The most common clinical signs of gastrointestinal toxicity are loss of appetite, anorexia, nausea, vomiting, small or large intestinal diarrhoea, abdominal pain, and constipation.

Sometimes, especially when a drug with a high prevalence of gastrointestinal toxicity is to be administered for the first time, prescribing symptomatic treatments (antiemetics, antidiarrhoeals) that owners can use immediately if toxicity appears is indicated. Likewise, instructing the owners to contact the clinician if this happens is important, so the severity of the symptoms can be assessed, and a decision made as to whether it is necessary for them to come to the practice or whether the plan for symptomatic treatment and monitoring is sufficient.

It must be taken into account that patients with gastrointestinal toxicity, which have a damaged intestinal epithelial barrier, are at greater risk of developing sepsis due to bacterial translocation if they subsequently develop neutropaenia at the nadir. In addition, as gastrointestinal symptoms are secondary to damage and inflammation of the gastrointestinal mucosa (inflammation composed of neutrophils, among other cells), these patients are also more likely to have lower neutrophil counts at nadir due to additional consumption in the process of gastroenteritis. Therefore, efforts towards the prevention or early detection and treatment of gastrointestinal toxicity should be maximised. Dose reductions or changes in the chemotherapy protocol should be considered when this toxicity is unacceptable or cannot be avoided with preventive measures.

When it occurs, diarrhoea usually appears three to five days after chemotherapy administration. In addition to proper dietary management for patients with diarrhoea, drugs such as sulfasalazine, metronidazole, loperamide, and probiotics are useful. Doxorubicin tends to cause colitis more frequently than small intestinal diarrhoea and metronidazole at anti-inflammatory doses is quite useful in managing this adverse effect.

Other causes of diarrhoea such as dietary indiscretion should be ruled out, especially when animals with poor appetites are fed products they are not used to, or parasites. Some patients may have inadequate bacterial overgrowth or, less frequently, diarrhoea from organisms such as *Campylobacter* or *Cryptosporidium* after prolonged immunosuppression. Faecal analysis is useful in diarrhoea that does not respond to symptomatic therapy and in non-dewormed patients.

Methotrexate, used in maintenance protocols for lymphoma, can cause anorexia, vomiting, or diarrhoea after a long period of treatment. If this occurs, its administration should be discontinued.

Vincristine often produces neurotoxicity in the myenteric plexus, especially at high doses and more frequently in cats. This toxicity can vary in its clinical manifestations and does not always cause a clear paralytic ileus, although it is present. Pronounced loss of appetite, anorexia, abdominal pain, or constipation (sometimes only loss of appetite) may be observed. It is usually self-limiting, but sometimes the clinical signs take weeks to disappear. If this toxicity is suspected, the dose should be reduced, vincristine replaced by vinblastine, or discontinued. Prokinetic drugs such as metoclopramide or cisapride can help in the management of this toxicity.

Loss of appetite or anorexia can sometimes be the only manifestation of nausea secondary to chemotherapy. There are chemotherapeutic drugs that are highly emetogenic, such as actinomycin or cisplatin, and antiemetic prophylaxis should be administered before administration. In the case of patients treated with doxorubicin, antiemetic prophylaxis should be administered during the first three or four days of treatment, including the day of chemotherapy administration, especially if nausea or vomiting has been observed after a previous administration of this drug. Antiemetic prophylaxis may also be indicated with other active ingredients before the first treatment, if the clinician suspects an increased risk for the patient based on their individual characteristics.

Serotonin antagonists have dramatically reduced gastrointestinal toxicity in pets treated with different chemotherapy drugs. Maropitant (1 mg/kg SC or 2 mg/kg PO), an antiemetic for veterinary use that antagonises neurokinin, has shown good results in preventing vomiting secondary to the administration of doxorubicin. Ondansetron (0.2–0.5 mg/kg IV, SC, or PO) administered 20–30 minutes before treatment markedly reduces the prevalence of chemotherapy-associated nausea. It can be given up to twice a day for two to three days, if necessary. It is usually an effective choice, especially in patients who do not respond to other antiemetics. In injectable forms it used to be expensive, but more recently the availability of generics, especially in the oral form, has contributed to its increase in use. The effect of metoclopramide is usually inferior as an antiemetic in chemotherapy.

Anorexia is the most common clinical sign of gastrointestinal toxicity in cats and is quite common after administration of cyclophosphamide. Sometimes, it can be a manifestation of the development of nausea or paralytic ileus after administration of doxorubicin or vincristine, respectively. In the case of paralytic ileus, the use of antiemetics, prokinetics or the possibility of changes in dosage are indicated, in addition to offering appetite stimulants. Cyproheptadine (0.35–1 mg/kg PO every 12–24 hours in cats and 0.3–2 mg/kg PO every 12 hours in dogs) may be effective.

It must be taken into account that, in cats, high doses of cyproheptadine can cause behavioural changes and hyperactivity. Mirtazapine also exerts an appetite-stimulating effect (0.6 mg/kg PO q 24 h or 3–3.75 mg/cat PO q 48 h).

Cardiotoxicity

Doxorubicin can cause cardiotoxicity with cumulative doses (>180 mg/m²) in the dog as well as in humans. In the cat, cardiomyocyte damage and echocardiographic changes have been shown at cumulative doses greater than 170 mg/m², but no clinical evidence of heart disease has been documented. This drug, in addition to inducing cell death by inhibiting topoisomerase II, also causes oxidative cellular damage by producing free radicals. Myocardial cells are especially sensitive to this type of cell damage. Although induction of cardiac arrhythmias has been reported during administration, they rarely have any clinical significance, especially when slow administration is performed for at least 20–30 minutes. Cumulative cardiac toxicity is directly proportional to the peak concentration of doxorubicin reached in the blood, which is why slow intravenous infusion is obligatory. Damage to myocardial cells is reflected in a progressive decrease in cardiac contractility that, if allowed to progress, can lead to the development of dilated cardiomyopathy.

In dogs with normal contractility before starting doxorubicin treatment, only cumulative levels would be reached from which some change in cardiac contractility could begin to be observed with total doses of more than 180 mg/m² that is, after the administration of at least about six doses of doxorubicin at standard doses (30 mg/m²). If cardiac contractility is decreased before starting treatment or if subclinical myocardial disease is present (possible in breeds predisposed to dilated cardiomyopathy) cardiotoxicity may develop at a lower cumulative dose. In general, since most protocols that include doxorubicin only include administration of 4–5 doses, performing an echocardiogram on the patient before the first dose is sufficient. This can be repeated at the end of the protocol or if considering giving more than 4–5 doses of doxorubicin.

In breeds predisposed to dilated cardiomyopathy (such as the Dobermann and others) or dogs with suboptimal cardiac contractility, the use of doxorubicin is not recommended if there is another feasible alternative for the patient's neoplastic disease (for example, carboplatin instead of doxorubicin as adjunctive therapy for appendicular osteosarcoma). If a clinically significant decrease in cardiac contractility is detected during treatment with doxorubicin, discontinuation is recommended.

If the patient needs to continue with chemotherapy treatment, it can be replaced by another drug from the same family such as mitoxantrone, actinomycin or epirubicin. It should be considered that these substances may be less effective for the treatment of some neoplasms and produce more adverse effects with a high impact on the immediate quality of life (gastrointestinal toxicity). Epirubicin can also be cardiotoxic. Likewise, it must be considered that some diseases such as canine visceral haemangiosarcoma or osteosarcoma have relatively short survival periods, which means that the impact of a possible adverse effect in the medium-long-term future must be put into context.

Another alternative is the administration of doxorubicin together with dexrazoxane, a chelator that prevents cardiotoxicity if given before doxorubicin. The dose in dogs is 10 times the dose of doxorubicin and it is administered intravenously as a slow infusion over 10 minutes. The biggest drawback of this drug is its cost. Along the same lines, the β-blocker carvedilol has significant antioxidant properties and in experimental studies protects myocardial cells from damage induced by doxorubicin. It appears that it may have a similar effect in the dog, although there are no clinical studies on this at the moment.

Urinary System Toxicity

Sterile haemorrhagic cystitis is a side effect of **cyclophosphamide** administration and is due to the effect on the cells of the urinary mucosa of one of its metabolites, acrolein. The approximate prevalence is believed to be around 15% in dogs treated with this drug. This toxicity is not seen in the cat. It appears that high intravenous doses or prolonged treatment at low oral doses (several months of treatment) increase the risk, but it also depends on individual sensitivity.

An attempt can be made to minimise this risk by ensuring that the patient has access to water and periods for urination during the hours after administration, as well as by dividing the dose over several days when given as a high dose of 200–300 mg/m² PO (for example, over 48 hours, morning and evening) or simultaneously administering a low dose of furosemide (0.5 mg/kg/day PO). In the case of metronomic therapy with cyclophosphamide, the prevalence of this toxicity is 30% for which the continued use of daily furosemide is recommended. Once this side effect appears, it may take several weeks or months for clinical signs to disappear. Sometimes they can be irreversible, especially in cases in which the administration of this drug has been continued despite the development of clinical signs of cystitis.

The treatment of this complication consists of discontinuing the use of this drug for the rest of the patient's life and establishing symptomatic therapy. Urinalysis and urine culture are recommended to differentiate the condition from a urinary infection. Sometimes, in patients with cystitis there may be a secondary urinary infection as they are more immunosuppressed and present significant damage to the mucosa of the urinary bladder. The administration of nonsteroidal or sometimes steroidal anti-inflammatory drugs, which increase water intake and therefore the emptying of the bladder with greater volumes of urine, has shown relief of the clinical signs. Other drugs such as oxybutynin hydrochloride (0.2–0.3 mg/kg PO 2–3 times a day) can help improve clinical symptoms. Urinary bladder instillation of DMSO diluted in 25% saline for 30–60 minutes once a week has also been described as potentially effective in very severe cases.

Cisplatin is highly nephrotoxic in dogs (in cats it is fatal, causing death). The alternative is to use carboplatin, since it does not present this toxicity at the recommended doses and has a similar range of effectiveness. The use of cisplatin is questionable not only because of its toxicity but also because of the high risk of exposure to this drug by veterinary personnel when the recommended diuresis protocols are carried out to avoid its nephrotoxicity.

Hepatotoxicity

Lomustine can cause hepatotoxicity in the dog, which can be irreversible, although it is rare: it has only been documented in 7% of dogs treated with this active ingredient. On the other hand, it is much more frequent for it to cause an increase in liver enzymes, generally reversible with discontinuation of the drug, whose long-term relevance is not very clear. Monitoring serum liver enzymes (alanine aminotransferase, ALT) before each lomustine administration is recommended. In general, about 50% of dogs treated with lomustine experience increases in ALT that can reach values 4 or 5 times above the maximum normal limit for this enzyme, or even more in some cases. When these extreme values are recorded, increasing the interval between administrations is recommended. If with this precaution in place a return to normality is observed, a decision should be taken whether to discontinue treatment depending on the magnitude of the increase in ALT. Cases without excessive elevations of ALT during treatment have been seen to develop long-term irreversible liver disease if they have a long survival time.

For this reason, when lomustine is used as adjuvant chemotherapy (for example, in young or middle-aged dogs with mast cell tumours after incomplete surgical resection or to reduce the risk of metastasis) it is advisable to use the lowest dose within the therapeutic range (60 mg/m²) and for a limited time (four to six months). One publication described that the use of S-adenosylmethionine can minimise the magnitude of the increase in liver enzymes in dogs receiving lomustine, although it does not prevent the increase itself. The publication does not provide information on the impact of this practice on late hepatocellular tissue damage in patients with long survival times. In general, in dogs where lomustine is usually indicated (high-grade T-cell lymphoma, malignant histiocytosis, or high-grade mast cell tumours) fatal hepatotoxicity is not usually seen, probably due to their limited survival time.

Hypersensitivity

L-asparaginase can cause hypersensitivity reactions in dogs with repeated administrations, although this does not occur frequently if subcutaneous or intramuscular routes are used. It manifests with skin reactions, facial oedema, hyperthermia or dyspnoea. To reduce the risk, the use of intramuscular antihistamines half an hour before drug administration (such as diphenhydramine 2 mg/kg IM) is recommended.

Doxorubicin, if administered rapidly, can cause mast cell degranulation and rapid histamine release, which, although not a true hypersensitivity reaction, can present the same clinical symptoms. This adverse effect is extremely rare if the recommended protocol for slow intravenous infusion over 20–30 minutes is followed. Either way, if desired, an antihistamine can be administered prior to the administration of doxorubicin. Due to the low frequency of this adverse effect, the practice of administering corticosteroids before doxorubicin is not necessary, thus minimising the risk of gastrointestinal toxicity in patients who are usually already receiving corticosteroids or NSAIDs.

Specific Toxicities in Cats

Cisplatin should never be administered systemically to felines, as it causes acute pulmonary oedema leading to death. Similarly, **fluorouracil** should not be used in cats as it causes fatal neurotoxicity.

Doxorubicin and **lomustine** can cause nephrotoxicity in cats. Monitoring kidney parameters and specific urinary gravity are indicated before starting treatment with these substances and these should be re-evaluated at least after every two treatments. The risk of developing this type of toxicity is much higher if the feline patient has suboptimal kidney function. The development of pulmonary fibrosis has been described in cats after long-term continuous therapy with lomustine.

Herding Dog Breeds and Sensitivity to Chemotherapeutic Agents

Some herding breeds such as Collies, Shetland Sheepdogs, Australian Shepherds, and Border Collies, among others, have shown high toxicity after the administration of chemotherapy drugs such as **vincristine** or **doxorubicin** due to a mutation in their MDR1 gene that leads to a decrease in the P-glycoprotein cell membrane pump, which is normally responsible for removing drugs from the cell cytoplasm. Dogs carrying this mutation will show toxicity with all substances that are substrates of P-glycoprotein. Blood and saliva PCR tests exist for the detection of this mutation (available from the University of Giessen, Germany, or Laboklin, Manchester, UK, among other laboratories).

While awaiting results, chemotherapy drugs such as cyclophosphamide and prednisolone (e.g. for the treatment of lymphoma) can be safely used in these dogs. If the dog is homozygous for the mutation, it is best not to treat it with drugs that are eliminated by P-glycoprotein, such as vincristine or doxorubicin. If it is heterozygous, it is also better to avoid this type of drug, but if absolutely necessary, treatment with reduced doses of cytotoxic agents can be attempted.

A reduction in the vincristine dose of at least 25% has been proposed along with a comprehensive plan for prevention and detection of adverse effects. For doxorubicin, there is no proposed dose reduction and even with a 25% reduction the degree of toxicity expected in a given individual is unpredictable (limited published data available).

Management Guidelines for Cytotoxic Chemotherapy Drugs

Cytotoxic drugs have very narrow therapeutic indices, **resulting in toxic effects even at standard therapeutic doses**. Effects that personnel administering these drugs may suffer have also been described in the literature: side effects caused by this exposure include headache, nausea, liver disease, and impaired reproductive function. A safe level of exposure has not been identified, but all necessary precautions should be taken to limit the exposure of personnel to cytotoxic drugs during their preparation and administration. Recently, a consensus by the American College of Internal Medicine on the safe use of cytotoxic drugs in Veterinary Medicine (ACVIM small animal consensus statement on safe use of cytotoxic chemotherapeutics in veterinary practice, 2018), freely accessible online, has been published.

Reconstitution of cytotoxic drugs should be performed in a class II vertical laminar flow chamber. Although the cost of this equipment is not excessive for large hospitals (6000–9000 €), its frequency of use does not usually justify this outlay, especially in small veterinary clinics. There are several closed systems for chemotherapy preparation and administration (Phaseal™ or Equashield™ are some examples) that are practical, relatively inexpensive, and reduce operator and environmental exposure to virtually zero levels of cytotoxic drugs. If these devices are not available, drugs should be prepared and/or reconstituted in a hospital or human pharmacy, to minimise the risk of exposure to the operator and hospital environment.

It is necessary to take into account the half-life of reconstituted drugs, which should be administered as soon as possible. Each dose should be calculated and double checked by a second person if possible. The use of a specific chemotherapy dose calculation sheet is recommended for each patient that can be used as a written record that allows the dates of administration, total dose administered and weight that was used to calculate the dose which can be checked retrospectively if necessary. This record becomes a safety document in the event of any unpredictable adverse effects after a treatment. Drugs should be distributed from the place of preparation to the place of administration in sealed plastic bags.

The syringes must be clearly labelled with which drug they contain, the amount in mg and concentration, and the name of the patient for whom they have been prepared. Cytotoxic drug vials used for multiple doses should have the date on which they were opened or reconstituted and should be stored at the temperature required by their manufacturer. The prospectus for each medication used and the preparation and storage instructions must be followed. In case of doubts regarding the management and administration of cytotoxic drugs, contacting a veterinary oncologist is recommended.

Personnel preparing, handling, and administering cytotoxic drugs should have a minimum of training in this area and have adequate protective equipment. In human medicine, proper protective equipment has been shown to limit the exposure of auxiliary personnel to cytotoxic drugs when combined with conservative and safe handling practices. All personnel present during the administration of chemotherapy (veterinarians, assistants, and other personnel) must wear thick latex gloves specific for chemotherapy or two pairs of latex gloves commonly used for examinations.

From a protection point of view, the thickness of the glove is more important than its composition. Ideally, personnel should also have disposable waterproof gowns, as well as eye protection and masks that filter particles when there is a risk of aerosolisation or spillage, that is, when subcutaneous injections of cytotoxic drugs are administered or when they are reconstituted outside of a laminar flow chamber.

The chemotherapy administration area should be an area of the hospital with minimal traffic of personnel and animals; isolation areas minimise staff exposure to drugs. When chemotherapy is given orally, the pills must be prepared in advance and moved to the area where patients can receive chemotherapy. If oral cytotoxic medication is provided to owners to administer at home, verbal and written instructions should be provided on safe administration and storage precautions for the product.

To reduce environmental contamination, all infusion sets should be flushed before adding drugs to the fluids when administering drugs by drip; in addition, all potentially contaminated material such as gown, gloves, fluid bottles or infusion sets should be placed in bags or containers for biohazard material. Disposal of material potentially contaminated with cytotoxic drugs can be handled through a human hospital or can be carried out by companies approved by the Environmental Protection Agency.

The materials used in the preparation and administration of chemotherapy cannot be reused. Patient waste (urine, faeces) must be eliminated with the precautions mentioned during the first 24–48 hours after administration and the personnel attending the hospitalisation of these patients must wear the protective equipment recommended above (disposable gown and gloves) when cleaning any type of excretions from the patient or from the hospitalisation cage. Pregnant women should not prepare or administer chemotherapy or participate in the management of these patients while they are hospitalised. Once the patient has received chemotherapy, their cage should be clearly identified, and staff should have information on the precautions to take when caring for these patients and their waste.

Summary of Guidelines for the Administration of Chemotherapy

To finish this section, a summary of the guidelines for administration of available chemotherapy drugs in dogs and cats is shown in Table 2.

Metronomic Therapy in Veterinary Oncology

Metronomic therapy (MT) offers a new concept in cancer treatment, from a different viewpoint to conventional cytotoxic therapy. Traditional chemotherapy regimens are based on the administration of drugs at maximum doses to kill as many tumour cells as possible. These treatments are associated with toxicity and require a rest period to allow recovery of healthy tissues with a high rate of cell proliferation. In contrast, the metronomic administration of cytotoxic drugs implies a **continuous administration without pause for a long period of time at doses much lower than those used conventionally, which minimises the risk of toxicity**.

This therapy was developed as a new strategy to treat cases that are refractory to conventional chemotherapeutic regimens with the idea of using tumour vasculature or angiogenesis as a therapeutic target instead of directly attacking neoplastic cells. Recent research proposes that metronomic therapy may also be related to the restoration of the antitumour immune response that is often diminished in humans and animals with cancer.

In the last decade, several clinical studies in medicine have established the efficacy and low toxicity of MT using different cytotoxic drugs (Tables 3 and 4).

Low-dose cyclophosphamide has probably been the most widely used active ingredient as part of MT regimens and, probably, also the most widely studied in preclinical and clinical MT models in terms of its mechanism of action. Nonsteroidal anti-inflammatory drugs (NSAIDs) are frequently included in MT regimens, which appear to share part of the mechanism of action attributed to low-dose cytotoxic drugs. The **combined use of MT with conventional chemotherapy, radiation or even molecular targeted therapy** is emerging as a new treatment strategy against cancer. In veterinary medicine, MT has been described in studies published since 2007 with promising results, especially for neoplasms with a limited response to cytotoxic chemotherapy regimens. It represents a very attractive therapy for the treatment of pets with cancer due to its low cost, need for infrequent monitoring, and low prevalence of adverse effects (Table 5)

Mechanism of Action

Antiangiogenic Effects of Metronomic Therapy

In relation to the mechanism of action of metronomic therapy, its inhibitory effect on the tumour angiogenesis process

Table 2. Summary of guidelines for administration of chemotherapy in dogs and cats (from chapters about specific neoplasms from: Withrow SJ, Vail DM, Page RL (eds) (2012) *Withrow and MacEwen's Small Animal Clinical Oncology*, 5th Edition. St Louis: Saunders-Elsevier).

Neoplasm	VId (cm)	SIVd (cm)
Lymphoma	· Vincristine · Cyclophosphamide · Doxorubicin · Prednisolone · Methotrexate · L-asparaginase · Lomustine · Procarbazine	· First line treatment with combined drug protocols. Disease-free interval (DFI) ~250 days with Madison-Wisconsin protocol in dogs with B-cell lymphoma · Dogs with T-cell lymphoma have a longer median survival time (MST) with protocols which include alkylating agents such as lomustine and procarbazine
Multiple myeloma	· Melphalan and prednisolone	· MST ~18 months in dogs, less in cats
Chronic lymphocytic leukaemia and low-grade canine/feline lymphoma	· Chlorambucil + prednisolone (±vincristine)	· MST ~1–2 years
Osteosarcoma	· Carboplatin or doxorubicin	· Adjuvant chemotherapy increases survival time after amputation from a few months with just surgery to 8–11 months; ST at one year is 40%
Haemangiosarcoma and high-grade sarcoma	· Doxorubicin combined with cyclophosphamide · (AC) ± vincristine (VAC)	· Adjuvant chemotherapy increases survival time after amputation from 2 months with just surgery to 6–9 months for visceral HAS and 1–1.5 years for subcutaneous HSA
Feline injection site sarcoma	· Doxorubicin/carboplatin	· Adjuvant chemotherapy increases time in remission after surgery and radiotherapy, especially in high-grade sarcoma
Mast cell tumours (high-grade or metastatic)	· Vinblastine/lomustine + prednisolone · Vinblastine + prednisolone · Lomustine + prednisolone · Chlorambucil + prednisolone · Masitinib/toceranib	· Adjuvant chemotherapy is used after surgery for grade II mast cell tumours with a mitotic index >5 or for grade III (Patnaik) or Tier 2 (Kiupel); it is also used as sole therapy in patients with inoperable mast cell tumours or systemic metastases
Transitional cell carcinoma of the urinary bladder	· Vinblastine + NSAID · Chlorambucil + NSAID · Mitoxantrone + piroxicam · Carboplatin + NSAID	· RR: 86%, with 21% partial or complete; MST: 147 days as second line treatment · RR: 70%, con 3% partial or complete; MST: 221 days as second line treatment · RR: 81%, con 35% partial or complete; MST: 291 days · RR: 83%, con 38% partial or complete; MST: 161 days
Anal sac carcinoma	· Carboplatin · Melphalan · Toceranib · Metronomic therapy · Mitoxantrone	· Can be used as adjuvant therapy after surgery +/- radiation, but their contribution is controversial, especially with cytotoxic drugs. New treatments have shown efficacy against metastasis
Mammary gland carcinoma (cats)	· Doxorubicin/carboplatin	· Evidence of limited effectivity
Thyroid carcinoma (dogs)	· Doxorubicin	· Evidence of limited effectivity compared to local therapy
Polycythaemia vera	· Hydroxyurea	· MST >1 year
Malignant histiocytosis	· Lomustine	· As sole therapy in systemic disease or adjuvant therapy after surgery; response rate of 40% in inoperable disease

MST: median survival time; RR: response rate; ST: survival time; HAS: haemangiosarcoma.

has been the most studied part to date. There may certainly be several contributing mechanisms, but the antiangiogenic aspects of this therapy are believed to be the result of three main factors.

- **Chemotherapy affects endothelial cells** in a much more direct and selective way compared to other cells and tissue types.
- **Progenitor endothelial cells derived from bone marrow** appear to be direct targets of metronomic chemotherapeutic action.
- Chemotherapy modulates the levels of angiogenic growth factors and inhibitors in favour of the latter and thus **indirectly influences the angiogenic balance**.

Table 3. Results of clinical trials using metronomic therapy in women with breast cancer (extracted from: Pasquier E, Kavallaris M, André N. (2010) Metronomic chemotherapy: new rationale for new directions. *Nat Rev Clin Oncol*; 7(8):455–65).

Patients	Metronomic therapy protocol	RR and CB (%)	Best responses
Metastasis in patients previously treated with conventional chemotherapy	· Cyclophosphamide PO daily · Methotrexate PO twice a week	· RR: 19 · CB: 32	· CR: 2/63 · PR: 10/63 · SD: 8/63 (all *)
Untreated senior patients	· Letrozole PO daily	· RR: 72	· CR: 23/57 · PR: 18/57
	· Letrozole PO daily · Cyclophosphamide PO daily	· RR: 88	· CR: 25/57 · PR: 25/57
Patients not treated or previously treated with conventional chemotherapy	· Cyclophosphamide PO daily · Methotrexate PO twice a week	· RR: 21 · CB: 41.5	· CR: 3/86 · PR: 15/86 · SD: 18/86 (all *)
	· Cyclophosphamide PO daily · Methotrexate PO twice a week · Thalidomide PO daily	· RR: 12 · CB: 41.5	· CR: 3/85 · PR: 7/85 · SD: 25/85 (all *)
HER2 positive metastasis previously treated with trastuzumab and conventional chemotherapy	· Cyclophosphamide PO daily · Methotrexate PO twice a week · Trastuzumab every three weeks	· RR: 18 · CB: 45	· CR: 0/22 · PR: 4/22 · SD: 10/22 (6*)
Previously treated with conventional chemotherapy	· Capecitabine PO TID · Cyclophosphamide PO daily · Bevacizumab every two weeks	· RR: 48 · CB: 68	· CR: 1/46 · PR: 21/46 · SD: 19/46 (8*)
Patients with metastases refractory to anthracycline and taxane	· Cyclophosphamide PO daily · Methotrexate PO twice a week · Bevacizumab every two weeks	· RR: 32 · CB: 64	· CR: 0/22 · PR: 7/22 · SD: 7/22 (all *)
Metastases previously treated or not treated with conventional chemotherapy	· Cyclophosphamide PO daily · Dalteparin SC daily · Methotrexate PO twice a week · Prednisone PO daily	· RR: 17 · CB: 24	· CR: 1/41 · PR: 6/41 · SD: 3/41 (all *)
	· Cyclophosphamide PO daily · Prednisone PO every other day · Epirubicin IV weekly · 5-fluoracil IV weekly · Vincristine IV weekly	· RR: 59 · CB: 93	· CR: 12/63 · PR: 25/63 · SD: 22/63

RR: response rate; CB: clinical benefit; CR: complete response; PR: partial response; SD: stable disease; *for more than six months.PO: *per os* (orally).

Table 5. Summary of some clinical studies with metronomic therapy performed in veterinary oncology.

Tumour type	Protocol	Number of animals	Results
Soft-tissue sarcomas with incomplete resection	· Cyclophosphamide 10 mg/m² · Piroxicam 0.3 mg/kg PO daily or on alternate days	30 dogs treated and 55 control	· Disease-free period 410 days vs 211 days without treatment
Transitional cell carcinoma of the urinary bladder	· Chlorambucil 4 mg/m² PO daily ± NSAIDs	30 dogs	· 70% clinical benefit · MST 271 days
Different types of advanced stage neoplasms	· Chlorambucil 4 mg/m² PO daily	36 dogs	· 58% partial response or stable
Splenic stage II haemangiosarcoma	· Cyclophosphamide 12.5–25 mg/m² PO daily or on alternate days · Etoposide 50 mg/m² PO daily · Piroxicam 0.3 mg/kg PO daily	9 dogs treated and 24 control	· MST 178 days
Different types of tumours	· Lomustine average dose 2.82 mg/m² (NSAIDs allowed)	64 dogs	· 36% clinical benefit. Some dogs received other treatments simultaneously
	· Satraplatin 5 mg/m² daily oral	24 dogs	· 70% clinical benefit that includes 6 dogs with microscopic disease
	· Cyclophosphamide	24 cats	· Low-grade toxicity assessment (GI and renal only)

Clinical benefit (complete response + partial response + stable disease). PO: *per os* (orally).

Table 4. Results of clinical studies with metronomic therapy in patients with different types of cancer (extracted from: Pasquier E, Kavallaris M, André N (2010) Metronomic chemotherapy: new rationale for new directions. *Nat Rev Clin Oncol*; 7 (8): 455–65).

Patients	Metronomic therapy protocol	RR and CB (%)	Best responses
Recurrent ovarian cancer previously treated with metronomic therapy	· Cyclophosphamide PO daily · Bevacizumab every two weeks	· RR: 44 · CB: 67	· CR: 2/9 · PR: 2/9 · SD: 2/9
	· Cyclophosphamide PO daily · Bevacizumab every two weeks	· RR: 24 · CB: 56	· CR: 0/70 · PR: 17/70 · SD: 44/70 (22*)
Hormonal prostate cancer previously treated with androgen deprivation	· Cyclophosphamide PO daily · Dexamethasone PO daily	· RR: 64 · CB: 70	· CR: 22/34 · SD: 2/34
	· Cyclophosphamide PO daily	· RR: 45	· OR: 26/58
	· Dexamethasone PO daily · Celecoxib PO BID	· RR: 32	· OR: 9/28
Recurrent or refractory aggressive non-Hodgkin's lymphoma	· Cyclophosphamide PO daily · Celecoxib VO BID	· RR: 37.5 · CB: 59	· CR: 2/32 · PR: 10/32 · SD: 7/32
Progressive multiple myeloma previously treated with conventional chemotherapy	· Cyclophosphamide PO daily · Prednisone PO daily	· RR: 69	· OR: 29/42
Recurrent glioblastoma and malignant glioma previously treated with radiotherapy and/or conventional chemotherapy	· Temozolomide PO daily	· RR: 16 · CB: 58	· CR: 0/12 · PR: 2/12 · SD: 5/12
	· Temozolomide PO daily	· RR: 14 · CB: 59	· CR: 0/49 · PR: 7/49 · SD: 22/49
	· Etoposide PO daily for three weeks · Bevacizumab every two weeks	· RR: 22 · CB: 90	· CR: 3/59 · PR: 10/59 · SD: 40/59
	· Etoposide PO daily for three weeks alternated with cyclophosphamide PO daily for three weeks · Thalidomide PO daily · Celecoxib PO BID	· RR: 10	· CR: 0/47 · PR: 1/47 · MR: 4/47 · SD: 26/47
Progressive, locally advanced, or metastatic renal cell carcinoma	· Cyclophosphamide PO daily · Celecoxib PO BID	· RR: 3 · CB: 12.5	· CR: 0/32 · PR: 1/32 · SD: 3/32 (all *)
	· Capecitabine PO BID · Gemoltabine IV weekly · Sorafenib PO BID	· RR: 24 · CB: 93	· PR: 20/40 · SD: 17/40
Locally advanced or metastatic neuroendocrine carcinoma	· 5-fluoroacil IV daily · Long-acting octreotide once a month	· RR: 24 · CB: 93	· CR: 0/29 · PR: 7/29 · SD: 20/29
Metastatic melanoma previously treated with conventional chemotherapy	· Paolitaxel IV for three days, repeat weekly · Celecoxib PO BID	· RR: 5 · CB: 35	· CR: 0/20 · PR: 1/20 · SD: 7/20 (3*)
Advanced solid tumours of various types previously treated with conventional chemotherapy	· Cyclophosphamide PO daily · Rofecoxib PO BID · Vinblastine IV weekly ± minocycline	· RR: 13 · CB: 30	· CR: 2/47 · PR: 4/47 · SD: 8/47 (all *)
	· Capecitabine PO BID	· CB: 34	· SD: 11/35 (all *)
	· Celecoxib PO BID · Vinorelbine PO three times a week	· RR: 13 · CB: 45	· OR: 8/62 · SD: 20/62 (all *)

RR: response rate; CB: clinical benefit; CR: complete response; PR: partial response; SD: stable disease; *for more than six months; OR: objective response; MR: minor response. PO: *per os* (orally); BID: twice a day.

Selective Cytotoxicity towards Endothelial Cells

Many traditional chemotherapy drugs act as antiangiogenic drugs simply because the endothelial cells that supply blood for tumour growth are highly proliferative, while most normal blood vessels remain quiescent.

In vitro laboratory experiments designed to compare the cytotoxicity of chemotherapeutic drugs on various cell types demonstrate the inhibition of endothelial cell proliferation and migration at picomolar concentrations of the drug. However, the concentrations of drugs such as cyclophosphamide, methotrexate, vinblastine, and paclitaxel required to produce similar effects in non-endothelial cell lines, such as tumour cells, epithelial cells, lymphocytes, and fibroblasts, are 10 to 100 000 times higher. These effects demonstrate an **intrinsic sensitivity of endothelial cells to ultra-low doses of chemotherapy** and explain why healthy tissues may be relatively protected during metronomic chemotherapy protocols, while new tumour blood vessels are selectively inhibited.

Circulating Progenitor Endothelial Cells

Endothelial progenitor cells (EPCs) derived from bone marrow are now known to be vital in the process of tumour angiogenesis. These cells can be mobilised from the bone marrow, enter the peripheral circulation, settle in areas where angiogenesis occurs, join the lumen of a growing ramification, and differentiate into endothelial cells.

EPC mobilisation occurs in response to several proangiogenic molecules (for example, vascular endothelial growth factor – VEGF) and, therefore, they are considered a target for antiangiogenic treatment strategies that neutralise these growth factors. On the other hand, PECs are also direct targets of chemotherapy, regardless of the use of high or metronomic doses.

EPC levels decline markedly and suddenly when high-dose chemotherapy is given, only to reappear during the rest period between doses. In contrast, with MT, this regrowth and its consequent contribution to angiogenesis can be avoided. This has been demonstrated using cyclophosphamide metronomically in pre-clinical murine lymphoma models. The continuous suppression of these cells could represent a major component of the antiangiogenic mechanisms of metronomic chemotherapy. EPCs can be measured and quantified in the bloodstream with flow cytometry, allowing their monitoring to be used as a non-invasive marker of angiogenesis that is currently being used in human clinical trials with MT. A canine EPC detection method has been described that could be incorporated as a possible biomarker in veterinary metronomic chemotherapy trials.

Modulation of Growth Factors in Metronomic Therapy

Two independent studies have shown that elevation of the endogenous angiogenesis inhibitor TSP-1 (thrombospondin) may be a factor associated with metronomic chemotherapy dosing. Results from a clinical trial in human medicine using metronomic cyclophosphamide and etoposide in paediatric cancer patients showed that elevated TSP-1 levels were associated with a prolonged response. It is not known whether these levels were induced by therapy or whether patients had increased endogenous levels unrelated to treatment. In any case, a possible implication supported by preclinical studies is that **metronomic chemotherapy potentiates the antiangiogenic effects of TSP-1**. Several studies have also monitored blood VEGF levels during MT as a possible marker of response to therapy, but the results have been contradictory.

Tumour Immunology

The other postulated mechanism of action for MT is based on the ability of some low-dose cytotoxic drugs, especially cyclophosphamide, to exert an **immunomodulatory effect on immune cells present in the tumour microenvironment**. Tumour cell destruction can be mediated by lymphocytic responses by cytotoxic T and T-helper cells and also by natural killer type cells.

These immune responses are influenced by another group of lymphocytes called regulatory T-cells that normally play a major role in autoimmune disease processes and tumour self-tolerance. In humans and dogs with cancer, especially with solid neoplasms (carcinomas, melanomas, sarcomas), a higher level of regulatory T-cells has been demonstrated than in healthy individuals and this seems to be associated with greater tumour tolerance.

Low dose cyclophosphamide causes a reduction in the number of regulatory T-cells and is believed to thereby contribute to the restoration of the antitumour immune mechanism. In women with advanced breast cancer receiving metronomic therapy with cyclophosphamide, a decrease in the percentages of regulatory T-cells and an increase in reactive T-lymphocytes in tumour tissue have been associated with an objective response to treatment and a better prognosis.

Recently, in dogs with sarcomas also treated with low doses of cyclophosphamide it was found that only when the drug was administered daily and at a dose of 15 mg/m² (compared to alternate day regimens and lower doses of cyclophosphamide) could depletion of the percentages of regulatory cells be observed, as well as a decrease in the tumour microvascular density, documenting an antiangiogenic and immunomodulatory activity of this treatment regimen.

The effect of metronomic chemotherapy on the immune system is in the early stages of research, but current evidence supports its role in stimulating the antitumour immune response.

Results of Clinical Trials in Humans

The clinical trial that sparked the greatest interest in a more comprehensive evaluation of metronomic combination chemotherapy was a study looking at the effect of low daily dose cyclophosphamide and twice weekly methotrexate in 64 women with advanced, progressive, refractory breast cancer. The overall response rate in this heavily pre-treated population was 32% including two complete responses, 10 partial responses, and 12 patients who had stable disease for 6 months or more. In addition, favourable results for MT have been reported in people with cancers of particular relevance to veterinary oncology, including non-Hodgkin's lymphoma, haemangiosarcoma, melanoma, soft-tissue sarcoma, and prostate cancer.

Currently, several phase II clinical trials are investigating metronomic combinations against malignant glioma, non-small cell lung cancer, ovarian carcinoma, squamous cell carcinoma of the head and neck, renal carcinoma, hepatocellular carcinoma and pancreatic carcinoma and this list is getting longer and longer (Table 4). Most of these trials combine oral cyclophosphamide with a commercially available anti-angiogenic molecular therapy (e.g. bevacizumab) or a nonsteroidal anti-inflammatory drug (such as celecoxib) on a daily basis. Other alkylating agents, such as trophosphamide or temozolomide, or other antiangiogens such as thalidomide and the oral hypoglycaemic agent pioglitazone, have also been popular choices in published clinical studies thus far.

As in treatment with tyrosine kinase inhibitors, with MT the concept of clinical benefit is considered as a measure of response to therapy; clinical benefit (CB) includes the total percentage of cases not only with partial response and complete response, but also with stable disease, which is often the type of response expected with this therapy due to the mechanism of action explained above.

Results of Clinical Trials in Veterinary Oncology

The metronomic therapy protocols in veterinary oncology described so far generally **use chlorambucil or cyclophosphamide, often in combination with a nonsteroidal anti-inflammatory drug (NSAID)**, due to the antiangiogenic and immunomodulatory effects of NSAIDs.

There are few published studies evaluating MT in veterinary oncology: to date it has been evaluated in dogs with incomplete resection of soft-tissue sarcomas, splenic haemangiosarcoma, transitional cell carcinoma of the urinary bladder, and a variety of other tumours refractory to conventional therapies which presented an advanced tumour stage (Table 5).

There is a study published on the tolerability of MT in cats with cancer. These studies offer a good starting point but are limited due to the low number of patients, the lack of uniformity of the selected cases, the lack of control groups and the evaluation of biomarkers of response to treatment and, often, their retrospective nature. It is useful to note that, in general, a percentage of positive responses has been described in all the studies that, although not very high, is comparable in some cases to the responses historically obtained with conventional cytotoxic regimens, which are probably not very effective either.

Metronomic cyclophosphamide administered together with piroxicam appears to delay the time to recurrence in incompletely resected soft-tissue sarcomas and is considered a viable option when surgery to obtain complete margins or postoperative adjuvant radiotherapy is not possible. Although, on the other hand, it must be taken into account that only 35% of grade I and II soft-tissue sarcomas will recur after incomplete resection. No significant differences were found between MT with cyclophosphamide, etoposide and piroxicam when compared with doxorubicin as a single agent in the treatment of patients with stage II splenic haemangiosarcoma (without metastasis).

The number of dogs included in this study was particularly low (9 dogs treated with MT and 25 dogs with doxorubicin) so it is difficult to draw conclusions, but the idea that MT could be therapeutically equivalent to doxorubicin used as a single agent is a very interesting idea in the treatment of this disease. On the other hand, more recent studies are contradictory in the use of MT in canine haemangiosarcoma after splenectomy: while some propose a greater effectiveness of the use of MT after treatment with doxorubicin, others have not found any difference in mean survival times. Neither has a difference in survival times been seen for canine osteosarcoma when metronomic therapy has been combined with carboplatin or with carboplatin and doxorubicin or has been administered after completion of carboplatin chemotherapy treatment.

On the other hand, another study proposes that the use of MT in lung carcinomas that are not candidates for surgery or where metastases were present provided longer median survival times than when cytotoxic drugs are administered which, although traditionally have been used against non-operable or metastatic, have not shown significant therapeutic effects on this type of neoplasm.

The use of metronomic chlorambucil (with or without concomitant treatment with NSAIDs) was associated with a 70%

clinical benefit rate in dogs with transitional cell carcinoma of the urinary bladder. In another study, the clinical benefit of MT with chlorambucil in dogs with a wide variety of advanced tumours (13.8% with regional metastases and 50% with distant metastases) in which conventional therapy had failed was 58% (47% showed disease stabilisation and 11% partial or complete response) with a mean survival time of 153 days.

The use of MT with such low doses of cyclophosphamide in dogs or cats often implies the need to reformulate the drugs used in lower dose capsules. It should be kept in mind that with reformulations there may be some variability in the exact amount of drug per capsule. Chlorambucil and low-dose cyclophosphamide are well tolerated in MT protocols with a low prevalence of toxicity at 4 mg/m² PO daily; regimens of 6–8 mg/m² showed greater toxicity and no increase in therapeutic effectiveness. Low-dose cyclophosphamide can induce sterile hemorrhagic cystitis (SHC) in far fewer patients (approximately 22% of the total) than when used at a dose of 25 mg/m². Studies in which doses of 10–15 mg/m² were used have presented a prevalence of cystitis between 10–30% and there is a clear association between this prevalence and the amount of time over which MT is administered.

Recently, the use of low-dose furosemide (0.5–1 mg/kg) in combination with metronomic cyclophosphamide has been shown to reduce the prevalence of SHC by 10%. Although the percentage of dogs that develop SHC is low, it is an adverse effect that must be avoided, since it has a high impact on the quality of life and the time until resolution is unpredictable. For this reason, it is necessary to seriously consider in which cases a decision is taken to use MT based on the type of neoplasia, presence of macroscopic disease or not, life expectancy, evidence of effectiveness or not and, also, for how long this therapy is used.

There are other drugs that have been used as part of MT, but their use has been limited. A study evaluated the toxicity of reformulated lomustine for administration in a metronomic regimen in dogs with a wide variety of primary and metastatic tumours (some heavily pre-treated), showing a low to moderate toxicity profile (higher prevalence of toxicity than with cyclophosphamide or chlorambucil). Although the aim of the study was to assess toxicity, the response to lomustine was also assessed with a response rate of 36% (although some dogs received additional adjuvant treatment). Another phase I clinical trial has been published using a metronomic regimen with satraplatin: of the 24 dogs evaluated, 17 had stable disease and, in general, the drug was well tolerated. Although the risk of toxicity is low with MT, the accumulated doses of these drugs can cause late onset toxicity and permanent monitoring of complete blood count parameters, biochemistry and urinalysis is recommended during treatment (generally, every 4 to 8 weeks depending on the protocol).

When evaluating the above results, it is important to bear in mind that several of the studies using MT have included patients with advanced disease stages (inoperable masses, presence of local and distant metastases). This is common when evaluating the toxicity of new therapies in phase I studies. On the other hand, it should be kept in mind that this study population itself has a worse prognosis and this may influence the results obtained in terms of the effectiveness of the treatment, so it is likely that the results of MT were more effective in patients with a lower disease volume or in less advanced stages. In addition, adjusting expectations when evaluating the clinical results of MT is necessary, since, like other antiangiogenic therapies, objective results take time to appear. Therefore, if disease stabilisation is seen, especially in patients with advanced stage neoplasms, this can be considered a significant success for the treatment as long as it is associated with a good quality of life. Thus, it could be considered that the objective of MT could be to turn the patient's disease into a chronic maintained disease, in which treatment is aimed at prolonging a good quality of life instead of hoping for a cure.

Tyrosine Kinase Inhibitors in Veterinary Oncology

Cancer is a disease characterised by uncontrolled cell growth, decreased apoptosis, and stimulation of cell migration, invasion, and angiogenic processes. The molecular mechanisms responsible for this biological behaviour are diverse and complex, but one of the families of molecules that has received great attention, especially due to their potential as a target for new cancer therapies, is the receptor tyrosine kinase family (RTK). These molecules are receptors for extracellular growth factors that facilitate the communication of extracellular signals within the cell, mediating growth, survival, invasion, and angiogenesis functions. Almost all tumour cells express a range of different RTKs, which play different and important roles in neoplastic pathogenesis.

Most RTKs are formed as monomers that are homodimerised or heterodimerised at the moment in which the union with the corresponding growth factor occurs, which induces a change in the conformation of the molecule that allows the phosphorylation of tyrosine residues in the intracellular domain of the receptor. This phosphorylation triggers a chain of intracellular signals that induce cell proliferation and culminate in a cell with abnormal gene expression and, frequently, in a tumour cell phenotype with additional malignant characteristics (Figure 4).

There are several drugs in medicine that act by inhibiting the signalling cascade that is triggered after the activation of one

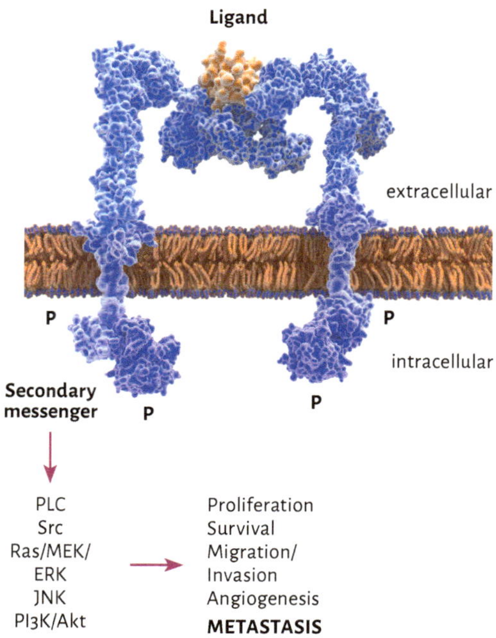

Figure 4. Diagram of receptor tyrosine kinase.

or more RTKs and that are currently available on the market or are in the final stages of clinical study. These substances could have a potential use in veterinary medicine, but, on the other hand, there are also RTK inhibitors (RTKIs) marketed especially for veterinary patients. As veterinary oncology continues to advance, an understanding of RTKs, their inhibitors, and their therapeutic potential is critical.

Activation of Tyrosine Kinase Receptors

Under normal circumstances, RTKs are only activated when extracellular growth factor binds to the receptor. But there can also be **inappropriate activation** by a series of mechanisms.

- **Autocrine stimulation**: tumour cells themselves produce growth factor.
- **RTK overexpression** leading to spontaneous receptor dimerisation.
- **RTKs mutations** that lead to a morphological change in the receptor, in which there is constant activation in the absence of the growth factor or ligand.

Any of these alterations can lead to inappropriate intracellular signalling, which, in turn, results in a neoplastic phenotype.

Inhibition of Receptor Tyrosine Kinase as Antitumour Therapy

One of the first tyrosine kinase-like proteins that was shown to be involved in the human tumour genesis process was the Bcr-Abl fusion protein, which was present and functional in many cases of chronic myeloid leukaemia (CML). This abnormal protein is produced as a result of a translocation between chromosomes 9 and 22 (called the Philadelphia translocation or chromosome), resulting in a protein that fuses the activation domain of Bcr to the kinase-like domain of the Abl protein. This leads to an active protein capable of constantly sending signals to the nucleus, providing an endless stimulus for cell proliferation and protection against apoptosis.

Malignant cells in CML depend on this fusion protein for their proliferation and survival, so a drug capable of specifically inhibiting the intracellular signalling cascade caused by the Bcr-Abl protein was designed. As a consequence, the molecule that was first called ST571 was developed, and which was later known as **imatinib** or Gleevec®. The effects of this molecule resulted in decreased proliferation and increased apoptosis of CML cells, which resulted in excellent antitumour activity for this disease. This drug is currently being tested as a treatment for CML.

Imatinib's success in treating CML was a revolution in human oncology: it meant the start of a new era in cancer treatment, representing a completely new type of anticancer therapy. Since then, great efforts have been made by researchers and pharmaceutical companies to design many other active compounds of this type that could be beneficial in the fight against a greater variety of neoplasms. Several of these drugs have been approved for use in human oncology (Table 6).

Tyrosine Kinase Receptors in Veterinary Medicine

Mast Cell Tumours and the Receptor Tyrosine Kinase KIT

Although in general the expression patterns of RTK in veterinary oncology have not been studied as much as in humans, there are several examples where its presence, activation and function are well documented and RTK blocking therapies have been developed with success. The best example is the **stem cell factor receptor, also called KIT**. This receptor is present in all mast cells and in most canine mast cells. Furthermore, in about a third of mast cell tumours, the gene that encodes the structure of KIT has a mutation that causes this receptor to be constantly constitutively activated.

Table 6. RTK inhibitors approved for human use.

Name	Class	Molecular target	Use
Imatinib (Gleevec®)	Small molecule	Bcr-Abl, KIT, PDGFR	Chronic myeloid leukaemia (CML), gastrointestinal stromal tumour (GIST)
Trastuzumab (Herceptin®)	Monoclonal antibody	HER2 (erbb2)	Breast cancer
Gefitinib (Iressa®), Erlotinib (Tarceva®)	Small molecule	EGFR	Lung cancer
Cetuximab (Erbitux®)	Monoclonal antibody	EGFR	Colon cancer
Monoclonal Antibody	Monoclonal antibody	$VEGFR_2$	Colon cancer
Sorafenib (Nexavar®)	Small molecule	KIT, FLT3, VEGFR2/3, PDGFR	Renal carcinoma (RC)
Sunitinib (Sutent®)	Small molecule	KIT, FLT3, VEGFR1-3, PDGFR, CSF-1R, RET	RC, GIST
Dasatinib (Sprycel®)	Small molecule	Bcr-Abl, Src, KIT, EPHA2, PDGFR	CML, acute lymphoblastic leukaemia
Nilotinib (Tasigna®)	Small molecule	Bcr-Abl, KIT, PDGFR	CML
Lapatinib (Tykerb®)	Small molecule	EGFR, HER2	Breast cancer
Panitumumab (Vectibix®)	Monoclonal antibody	EGFR	Colon cancer

An association has been found between the presence of the mutation and more aggressive biological behaviour (high-grade mast cell tumours).

Currently, two small molecules are available on the market, toceranib (Palladia®) and masitinib (Masivet®), which inhibit KIT and, consequently, have the potential to stop the growth of mast cell tumours, especially those that carry the mentioned mutation, as demonstrated in recent clinical studies.

Recent research has shown the presence of RTK in other common neoplasms in pets. Most injection-induced sarcomas in cats express PDGFR, which is the receptor for platelet-derived growth factor (PDGF). PDGFR and other RTKs such as HER2 (one of the epidermal growth factor receptors), IGF-1R (insulin-like growth factor receptor) and MET (hepatocyte growth receptor) have also been identified in canine osteosarcoma). Table 7 provides a more comprehensive list of RTKs identified in veterinary oncology and some information on their potential utility as molecular therapy targets.

Receptor Tyrosine Kinase Inhibitors (RTKIs) Marketed in Veterinary Medicine

To follow, the information available on the use in veterinary oncology of the two RTKIs specifically designed for use in small animals that are currently on the market is summarised. Firstly, dosages and management of adverse effects will be discussed, then therapeutic effectiveness against mast cell tumours and in the final section the information available on their use and effectiveness in other types of neoplasms wi l be covered.

Toceranib

Palladia (toceranib) was approved in 2009 by the FDA (Food and Drug Administration) for use in the United States and a year later its commercialisation was extended to Europe. **Toceranib is a molecule that blocks several types of RTK in addition to KIT such as VEGFR, PDGFR, CSF-1, Flt-3 and probably Ret**.

Although this drug was marketed for use in inoperable grade II and III mast cell tumours due to its action on the KIT receptor, it is evident that it has a much broader potential for antitumour activity due to the greater spectrum of RTK that it can block and, above all, given its action on VEGFR and PDGFR, it also has significant antiangiogenic activity.

Toceranib Dosage

The dose listed on the label of toceranib is 3.25 mg/kg every other day, a dose that can be reduced in fractions to a minimum of 2.2 mg/kg if adverse effects appear in the patient.

It is important to know that, in the phase I clinical study with Palladia, of the dogs treated with 2.5 mg/kg, 68% presented

Table 7. RTK expression, function, and inhibition in canine and feline neoplasms.

RTK	Ligand	Tumour type	Level of evidence
KIT	Stem cell factor	Canine mast cell tumour (MCT) and haemangiosarcoma (HSA)	Expressed in the majority of MCTs and HSAs: ~30% of MCTs have a functional activation mutation. Small molecules capable of inhibiting the signalling and antitumour effects have been identified in vitro and in patients
		Feline mast cell tumour	Expressed in the majority of MCTs. No functional mutations have been identified
MET	Hepatocyte growth factor (scatter factor)	Multiple canine tumours, including osteosarcoma (OSA), melanoma, histiocytic sarcoma, and mast cell tumour	Expressed in the majority of the tumours of the histotypes examined. Constitutive activation detected in OSA. Functional receptor and signalling can be inhibited in vitro with small molecules
IGF-1R	Insulin-like growth factor type 1	Canine OSA, melanoma	Expressed in the majority of the tumours of the histotypes examined. Functional receptor and signalling can be inhibited in vitro with small molecules
EGFR	Epidemic growth factor, transforming growth factor α, others	Mammary, lung, transitional cell, and nasal carcinomas in the dog. Oral squamous cell carcinoma in cats	Documented expression of most of the tumours of the histotypes examined. The receptor is functional in canine mammary carcinoma and signalling can be inhibited in vitro with small molecules
HER2	Epidemic growth factor, transforming growth factor α, others	Canine and feline mammary carcinoma. Canine OSA	Expressed in a large minority of canine and feline mammary tumours, it appears overexpressed in some canine OSAs. The coreceptor for EGFR may contribute to the biological effects of EGF in mammary carcinoma
PDGFR	Platelet-derived growth factor	OSA and canine HSA. Injection site associated sarcoma in cats	Expressed in canine OSA. Expressed, functional and can be inhibited with small molecules in vitro and in murine models of injection site-associated sarcoma
VEGFR2	Vascular endothelial growth factor	HSA melanoma, nasal carcinoma and vascular tumour in dogs	Expressed in some melanomas and nasal carcinomas and most of the HSA evaluated. Some evidence of functionality in canine HSA cells. Increased concentrations of ligand detected in the serum of patients with HSA
FGFR1 and 2	Basic fibroblast growth factor	Canine HSA. Vascular tumour	Expressed in the majority of the HSAs evaluated. Evidence of functionality in canine HSA cells. Increased ligand concentrations in the urine of patients with HSA
TrkA	Nervous growth factor	Canine OSA	Expressed in the majority of OSA. TrkA blockade induces apoptosis
Panitumumab (Vectibix®)	Monoclonal antibody	EGFR	Colon cancer

a biological response (sum of patients with complete response, partial response and stable disease) compared with a 60% response at a dose of 3.25 mg/kg. Based on these data, it is reasonable to assume that for many dogs, doses lower than those proposed on the label of 3.25 mg/kg may be therapeutically effective, especially when considering that at lower doses this drug may present less toxicity that would allow a more continuous treatment, without the need for discontinuation periods, and would lead to owners committing to prescribed treatment guidelines more easily.

Administration three days a week (for example, Monday, Wednesday, Friday) is tolerated quite well, has shown therapeutic effectiveness and allows Palladia to be easily combined with other drugs such as NSAIDs or cyclophosphamide (metronomic therapy).

A multi-institutional clinical study is currently underway in the United States using Palladia at doses lower than 3.25 mg/kg three days per week to provide more information on its therapeutic effect at low doses.

Masitinib

Masitinib is an RTKI has been marketed as Masivet® in Europe since late 2008 for use in recurrent or inoperable grade II/III MCTs and in the United States since 2011. This molecule has been specifically designed to optimise its **selectivity for RTK KIT, PDGF, Lyn, Fyn and Lck**. This high specificity allows its administration at higher doses while maintaining a good level of tolerance as it has a safer toxicity profile than other RTKIs that block a broader spectrum of RTKs.

This molecule was designed to block mast cells and hence, apart from its efficacy against canine mast cells, it also offers potential benefit in diseases such as feline asthma and canine atopic dermatitis. Likewise, it is postulated that it could be used against other types of neoplasms due to its antiangiogenic potential, by blocking PDGF, and by inhibiting the protumoural action that inflammatory tumour infiltrates can cause in solid neoplasms, which often contain mast cells.

Masitinib Dosage

The recommended dose in dogs is 12.5 mg/kg daily. So far, there are no studies documenting the therapeutic activity of this drug at lower doses or in a regimen other than daily administration. Some oncologists mention activity at lower doses or administered every other day in isolated cases.

Management of RTKI Toxicity in Veterinary Oncology

RTKIs can present adverse effects like any other anticancer treatment, mostly associated with the inhibition of RTKs present in normal cells. The most common effects are **gastrointestinal disturbances** (anorexia, loss of appetite, weight loss, nausea, vomiting, intestinal bleeding, diarrhoea) with a prevalence of between 40–50% for toceranib and masitinib in clinical studies performed in dogs with mast cell tumours. The appearance of these symptoms can be highly variable, from a few days after starting treatment to after several weeks. Other less frequently described adverse effects are neutropaenia, thrombocytopaenia, vasculitis, pulmonary thromboembolism, muscle pain, lameness, liver toxicity, nephrotic syndrome, etc.

It is very important to recognise the existence of adverse effects to RTKIs as early as possible, since, due to their mechanism of action, although in principle they are mild, they tend to worsen over time if they are not treated, both in severity and frequency of appearance. They may not disappear within a few days after initiation of symptomatic therapy and discontinuation of RTKI; unlike toxicity secondary to cytotoxic chemotherapy, resolution can sometimes take weeks. On the other hand, given the limited experience of clinicians in the use of these drugs due to their short commercialisation period, the real prevalence, severity, and degree of reversibility of each of these adverse effects is still being discovered.

As a general rule to promote early detection of adverse effects, monitoring of the patient with history, physical examination, blood count, biochemistry, urinalysis and blood pressure is recommended at the beginning of treatment, at two weeks and, thereafter, every four weeks if possible.

Pets with cancer can present a variety of problems that can predispose to the development of toxicity with the use of toceranib, which is especially true for patients with mast cell tumours, which can present with subclinical (or clinical) intestinal bleeding secondary to degranulation of mast cell tumours, which would make them more susceptible to the development of vomiting, diarrhoea, and additional intestinal bleeding with the use of RTKIs. To minimise the risk of these adverse effects, these patients should be pre-treated with symptomatic therapy (starting a few days before the start of RTKI therapy may offer advantages). When gastrointestinal adverse effects appear during treatment, if they are mild to moderate, the use of symptomatic therapy is recommended on the days the RTKI is administered. If there is no response or if they are moderate to severe effects, then a period of rest and use of symptomatic therapy is recommended until these adverse effects cease, with subsequent reinitiation of RTKIs at a reduced dose.

The use of antacids (famotidine, omeprazole), antihistamines (diphenhydramine or chlorphenamine) and sucralfate is recommended in dogs that are positive for faecal occult blood. The use of maropitant, metoclopramide or ondansetron is usually effective in patients who present inappetence or vomiting. In relation to the control of diarrhoea, the use of metronidazole or loperamide can also be effective when administered on the same days that toceranib is administered.

The use of NSAIDs together with toceranib can exacerbate gastrointestinal toxicity, so administration on the same day is not recommended when using combination therapies, as well as the preventative use of gastrointestinal protectors. In a recent study combining toceranib and piroxicam, no increased toxicity was observed using this alternating regimen. The combination with cyclophosphamide (metronomic therapy) every other day does not appear to increase the gastrointestinal or myelosuppressive toxicity of this drug. It should be taken into account that, in general, dogs with mast cell tumours tend to show a higher prevalence of gastrointestinal toxicity than dogs with other types of neoplasia.

Evidence of Effectiveness against Mast Cell Tumours

Toceranib

Toceranib was marketed for use in canine mast cell tumours based on the results obtained in a randomised double-blind clinical study in patients with inoperable grade II and III mast cell tumours. During the blind phase, the response rate was 37.2% with 7 complete responses (CR) and 25 partial responses (PR) in the group that received toceranib (n = 86) compared with a response of 7.9% in the placebo group (n = 63).

Given the evidence of progressive disease, 58 more dogs that initially received placebo were subsequently treated with toceranib, with a response rate of 41.4% (8 CR, 16 PR). The response rate of all Palladia-treated dogs in the study (n = 145) was 42.3% (21 CR, 41 PR). Dogs with KIT mutation-positive mast cell tumours had a higher response rate than those without the mutation (82% versus 55%). This shows that, although part of toceranib's activity against mast cell tumours lies in the blockage of KIT receptors, another part of the drug's activity is probably based on its antiangiogenic nature, as a result of blocking VEGFR and PDGR.

A more recent study in 88 dogs compared the effect of prednisone plus toceranib or vinblastine in inoperable mast cell tumours, all either grade II or III and 43% with the presence of metastases. The response to treatment was 46% and 30% respectively, and there were no significant differences in time to progression or survival between the two groups, nor when the presence or absence of mutation in c-KIT was analysed.

Masitinib

The results of a randomised double-blind phase II clinical study (Table 8), which included 202 dogs with inoperable grade II/III mast cell tumours and no evidence of metastasis, did not demonstrate a higher response rate between the placebo group and the group that received masitinib at 6 weeks of treatment (15% versus 16%), but they did show a significant difference in the time to disease progression, with a more pronoun-ced effect when masitinib was used as the first line of therapy, regardless of the presence of the KIT mutation. A higher survival rate at 12 and 24 months was also seen in the masitinib group. When the response was evaluated after 6 months of treatment, a significant difference was found between both groups, with a 29% response for the placebo group and 50% for the RTKI group. Tumour control at 6 months had a high predictive value for survival at 24 months with specificity and sensitivity of 88% and 76% respectively.

Table 8. Summary of the results of the phase II clinical study with masitinib.

Results	Masitinib	Placebo
Response rate at 6 months	50%	29%
Mean time to disease progression (DPT)	173 days	75 days
DPT (cases without KIT mutation)	140 days	75 days
DPT (with KIT mutation)	241 days	83 days
12-month survival rate	62%	36%
24-month survival rate	40%	15%
Median survival time (using masitinib as first line of therapy)	803 days	322 days

A more recent study that included inoperable and metastatic grade II and III mast cell tumours treated with masitinib had a response rate of 50% with 27% complete responses, 15% partial responses, and 42% with stable disease. Response to masitinib was a significant prognostic factor in terms of survival and not tumour grade, stage, or location. In 2016, another clinical study described a response of 82% in dogs with gross mast cell tumours (mostly high-grade), 38.5% of dogs had a complete response and 43.6% a partial response. The mean time to progression was 79 days (14–667 days).

Apparently, KI67, KIT cytoplasmic pattern and presence or absence of mutation in c-KIT exon 11 do not appear to be predictive of the response to masitinib in high-risk mast cell tumours. The initial clinical response seems to be the safest prognostic factor for predicting survival in these cases for now.

Use of RTKI in Combination with Cytotoxic Drugs in the Treatment of Mast Cell Tumours

The first study combining RTKI with cytotoxic therapy for mast cell tumours has been performed combining toceranib with vinblastine. The objective response to this therapy in dogs with gross disease was 71% despite the fact that the maximum tolerated dose of vinblastine was only 1.6 mg/m² due to the pronounced immunosuppression caused by this regimen (toceranib was administered at 3.25 mg/kg every other day).

More studies are needed to explore the efficacy of traditional cytotoxic drug combinations in combination with RTKIs, although based on the response observed in this study the strategy appears promising, especially for the treatment of high-grade mast cell tumours with a high rate of metastasis. When toceranib is used at a dose of 2.75 mg/kg, in combination with weekly vinblastine at 2 mg/m², immunosuppression is less than in the study mentioned and the combination is satisfactory with mild adverse effects. Currently, the efficacy of the use of toceranib and vinblastine as adjunctive therapy after complete resection of high-grade mast cell tumours is being investigated, but standardised studies with homogeneous cases in terms of mast cell characteristics and staging are needed.

The combination of lomustine and toceranib has been described in inoperable mast cell tumours with response rates of 50% but the rate of occurrence of adverse effects is considered unacceptable: 3 out of 10 dogs died from the adverse effects.

Use of RTKI in Combination with Radiation in the Treatment of Mast Cell Tumours

A prospective study using toceranib in combination with radiation (hypofractionated) in dogs with inoperable mast cell tumours has recently been started, with the goal of obtaining information on the efficacy, tolerability, and adverse effects of this combination. Preliminary results in 17 dogs indicate an objective response of 78% (53% CR, 24% PR) and an additional 12% had stable disease (SD), with a total clinical benefit (CR + PR + SE) of 90%. The protocol was well tolerated. All dogs received prednisone, omeprazole, and diphenhydramine 72 hours before starting toceranib administration (which was dosed at 2.75 mg/kg on Monday, Wednesday, and Friday one week before the first radiation session). The most frequently observed adverse effect was grade I gastrointestinal toxicity.

Use of RTKIs for the Treatment of Feline Mast Cell Tumours

In general, feline skin mast cell tumours are benign and surgery is usually curative. However, some show aggressive behaviour, as with feline visceral mast cell tumours and antineoplastic therapy would be indicated in all cases.

There are no specific studies on the activity of masitinib or toceranib against feline mast cell tumours. In a study using the human RTKI, imatinib, a complete response was documented in 2 of 9 cases and a partial response in 6 of 9 cases positive for the c-KIT mutation. In a recent study (2017) on toceranib toxicity in cats with cancer, it was documented that of seven cats with mast cell tumours treated, two had a complete response and five a partial response and that the treatment was well tolerated, although the effectiveness study was not the primary goal of this publication.

Biological Activity of RTKI in Dogs and Cats with Neoplasms other than Mast Cell Tumours

There is little information regarding the use, efficacy, or tolerability of toceranib or masitinib in neoplasms other than mast cell tumours or their combination with other antitumour drugs for the treatment of these diseases. Following initial publications, where toceranib was administered to groups of dogs with different types of neoplasms (Table 9), multi-institutional clinical studies with toceranib have been conducted in the United States. One of them has shown that treatment with toceranib as a single agent in 22 dogs with metastatic osteosarcoma provided limited survival times (LST) of 89 days (7–574 days) and another parallel study only demonstrated a clinical benefit in 10% of the cases with a mean time to progression of 36 days and comparable survival.

Similarly, the use of toceranib as maintenance therapy after amputation and conventional chemotherapy in canine osteosarcoma did not increase the survival percentage at one year compared to adjuvant chemotherapy alone. Similarly, postoperative use of toceranib in stage I or II canine splenic haemangiosarcoma had no impact on survival times compared to doxorubicin monotherapy.

Meanwhile, more information on the use of toceranib or masitinib in neoplasms continues to be collected through the OncoListserve shared by oncologists certified by the American College of Veterinary Internal Medicine (ACVIM) and from international veterinary oncology congresses. The majority of patients with solid neoplasms treated with RTKI are refractory to conventional therapies and often present advanced stages (inoperable masses and/or local/distant metastases). In this situation, finding a therapy that allows for a good quality of life and is capable of stabilising disease or even providing a partial response for several months is certainly of great value.

There are several studies documenting a synergistic antitumour effect in the addition of masitinib to the treatment of canine tumour cell cultures with cytotoxic drugs. However, the in vivo results of these combinations can be very different. There are also preliminary results of the joint therapy of masitinib in combination with carboplatin or doxorubicin in dogs, which showed good tolerability and low toxicity. The maximum tolerated dose of carboplatin was 200 mg/m² when used in combination with toceranib (2.75 mg/kg every other day) in a pilot study with ten dogs. On the other hand, no clinical benefit was demonstrated when adding toceranib to vinblastine therapy in the treatment of transitional cell carcinoma of the bladder compared to vinblastine therapy and COX-2 inhibitors. Likewise, the use in inflammatory mammary carcinomas has shown a low response rate of 21% when toceranib was used in combination with piroxicam and thalidomide (Table 9).

In relation to efficacy in the treatment of haematopoietic neoplasms, there is information describing the treatment of a dog with cutaneous lymphoma and two dogs with multicentric T-cell lymphoma in which the disease was controlled for a period of three to eight months. More recently, the results of the use of masitinib in the treatment of ten dogs with cutaneous epitheliotropic lymphoma have been published: two dogs showed complete remission and five partial remission, with a mean duration of response of 60.5 days.

The use of tyrosine kinase inhibitors in cats has been limited and most studies have provided data only on toxicity, which is usually mild to moderate with myelosuppression and gastrointestinal toxicity as the most common adverse effects, and some cases of severe hepatotoxicity. In feline squamous cell carcinoma, survival time with NSAIDs and toceranib was 123 days in 23 cats with a clinical benefit of 56.5% mostly with stable disease, and 45 days in another 23 cats treated only with NSAIDs. Its use in 18 cats with inoperable injection site sarcomas did not demonstrate evidence of clinical response.

Table 9. Clinical efficacy of toceranib in canine and feline neoplasms.

Tumour type	Patients	Toceranib dosage	Response
Thyroid carcinoma (n = 15)	· Treated with surgery (n = 5), radiation (n = 3), or chemotherapy (n = 7) · Primary tumour present (n = 13) · Metastasis (n = 10, 1 = liver/spleen, 9 = pulmonary)	· Average dose 2.75 mg/kg (2.47–3.25) · 9/15 MWF	· PR: 4 · SD: 8 · CB: 80% · Duration of treatment (for n = 12): 24.5 weeks (11–50)
Head and neck carcinomas (n = 8; nasal plane SCC, n = 3; oral SCC, n = 4; carcinoma of ceruminous glands, n = 1)	· Treated with radiotherapy or surgery (n = 3) · Metastasis (n = 3, 2 = LN, 1 = pulmonary)	· Average dose 2.87 mg/kg (2.5–3.2) · 4/8 MWF	· CR: 1 · PR: 5 · CB: 75% · Duration of treatment (for n = 6) 19.5 weeks (19–48)
Osteosarcoma with pulmonary metastasis (n = 23, n = 20)	· Treated with surgery and chemotherapy (n = 21)	· Average dose 2.7 mg/kg (2.3–3.25) · 13/23 MWF	· PR: 1 · SD: 10 · CB: 47.8% · Duration of treatment (for n = 11) 24 weeks (10–42) · CB: 10% · Average time to progression: 36 days · MST: 90 days
Nasal carcinoma (n = 7)	· Previous radiation therapy (n = 4) · Metastasis (n = 3)	· Average dose 2.67 mg/kg (2.4–3.2) · 5/7 MWF	· CR: 1 · SD: 1 · Improvement of clinical signs, but CT scan not performed: 3 · CB: 71.4% · Duration of treatment (for n = 6) 18 weeks (12–20)
Anal sac carcinoma (n = 32)	· Previous therapy (n = 25) · Metastasis (n = 28, 25 = sublumbar LN, 9 = pulmonary, 2 = liver, 11 = others)	· Average dose 2.81 mg/kg (2.2–3.25) · 22/32 MWF	· PR: 8 (25%) · Duration of treatment 22 weeks (10–40) · SD: 20 (62.5%) · Duration of treatment 30.5 weeks (10–47) · CB: 87.5% · Duration of treatment (for n = 32) 25 weeks (0–47)
Inflammatory mammary carcinoma (n = 14) in combination with piroxicam and thalidomide	· Response rate: 21% · Clinical benefit: 64%		· Average time to progression: 28 days · MST: 59 days
Treatment with toceranib in cats with different neoplasms (n = 41)	· SCC: 13 · OR: 8% · CB: 54% · ISS: 8 · OR: 42.9% · CB: 71% (3 PR and 2 SD) · MCT: 6 · OR: 33% · CB: 100%	· Average dose 2.8 mg/kg (1.67–4) · 3–4 times per week	· Adverse effects: anorexia/weight loss (n = 6), vomiting (n = 5), tumour necrosis (n = 2), elevated liver enzymes (n = 1), lameness (n = 1), fever (n = 1), diarrhoea (n = 1)
Treatment with toceranib and NSAIDs in cats with oral SCC (n = 23)			· CR: 1 · PR: 2 · SD: 10 · PD: 10 · CB: 56.5% · MST: 123 days

SCC: squamous cell carcinoma; ISS: injection site sarcoma; MCT: mast cell tumour; OR: objective response (CR + PR); CR: complete response, PR: partial response; SD: stable disease; PD: progressive disease; CB: clinical benefit (CR + PR + SD); MWF: therapy administered on Monday, Wednesday and Friday; LN: lymph nodes; MST: median survival time.

Annex: Chemotherapy Protocols

Lymphoma

Remission induction

- **Canine COAP/feline COP**
  - **Duration**: 8 weeks in dogs; 6 weeks in cats.
  - **Cyclophosphamide**: 50 mg/m² PO every 48 hours in dogs. In cats 200–250 mg/m² PO in week 1 and week 4 (about 2–3 days after vincristine so that the immunosuppression caused by both drugs does not overlap).
  - **Vincristine**: 0.5–0.7 mg/m² IV one day per week.
  - **Cytarabine**: 300 mg/m² on the first day only, SC or as an IV drip for 4–24 hours in dogs. In cats, administer this drug if there is renal or CNS extension. In this case, start with vincristine followed by cytarabine infusion at 250 mg/m² IV over 4–12 hours.
  - **Prednisone**: 40 mg/m² PO every 24 hours for one week and then 20 mg/m² PO every 48 hours.

  This protocol is continued with the LMP or LMPV maintenance protocol in dogs and with LP in cats.

  For complicated presentations or with neutropaenia secondary to the disease, the protocol with L-asparaginase can be started.
- **Madison-Wisconsin 25 (does not use maintenance chemotherapy)**
  - **Week 1**. Vincristine: 0.5–0.7 mg/m² IV. L-asparaginase: 400 IU/kg IM or SC (optional). Prednisone: 2 mg/kg PO every 24 hours.
  - **Week 2**. Cyclophosphamide: 200–250 mg/m² PO. Prednisone: 1.5 mg/kg PO every 24 hours.
  - **Week 3**. Vincristine: 0.5 mg/m² IV. Prednisone: 1 mg/kg PO every 24 hours.
  - **Week 4**. Doxorubicin: 30 mg/m² IV (or 1 mg/kg if <15 kg or in cats) IV.
    - Prednisone: 0.5 mg/kg PO every 24 hours.
  - **Week 6**. Vincristine: 0.5 mg/m² IV.
  - **Week 7**. Cyclophosphamide: 200–250 mg/m² PO.
  - **Week 8**. Vincristine: 0.5 mg/m² IV.
  - **Week 9**. Doxorubicin: 30 mg/m² IV (or 1 mg/kg if <15 kg or in cats) IV.
  - **Week 11**. Vincristine: 0.5 mg/m² IV.
  - **Week 13**. Cyclophosphamide: 200–250 mg/m² PO.
  - **Week 15**. Vincristine: 0.5 mg/m² IV.
  - **Week 17**. Doxorubicin: 30 mg/m² IV (or 1 mg/kg if <15 kg or in cats) IV.
  - **Week 19**. Vincristine: 0.5 mg/m² IV.
  - **Week 21**. Cyclophosphamide: 200–250 mg/m² PO.
  - **Week 23**. Vincristine: 0.5 mg/m² IV.
  - **Week 25**. Doxorubicin: 30 mg/m² IV (or 1 mg/kg if <15 kg or in cats) IV.

  For complicated cases, the protocol can be started with L-asparaginase.
- **LOPP for dogs with T lymphoma**
  - **Day 1**. Vincristine: 0.5 mg/m² IV.
  - **Day 7**. Lomustine: 50–60 mg/m² PO. Prednisone: 40 mg/m² PO every 24 hours for one week and then 20 mg/m² PO every 48 hours.
  - **Day 1–14**. Procarbazine: 50 mg/m² PO BID for 14 days. Dogs <0.4 m² use 50 mg every other day.

  Duration: 6 months, the duration of each cycle is 3 weeks.

  This protocol is continued with the LMP or LMPV maintenance protocol.

  If procarbazine is not available, it can be eliminated or replaced with cyclophosphamide 50 mg/m² PO every other day for 14 days.

Maintenance

- **LMP**
  - Chlorambucil: 20 mg/m² PO every 2 weeks.
  - Methotrexate: 2.5 mg/m² PO two or three times a week.
  - Prednisone: 20 mg/m² PO every 48 hours.

  Duration: indefinite, until remission.
- **LMPV**
  - Vincristine: 0.5 mg/m² IV every 2 weeks.
  - Chlorambucil: 20 mg/m² PO every 2 weeks (alternate week to vincristine).
  - Methotrexate: 2.5 mg/m² PO two or three times a week.
  - Prednisone: 20 mg/m² PO every 48 hours.

  Duration: indefinite, until remission.
- **LP**
  - Chlorambucil: 20 mg/m² PO every 2 weeks.
  - Prednisone: 20 mg/m² PO every 48 hours.

  Duration: indefinite, until remission.

Rescue

- **DMAC (for dogs)**
  - **Day 1**. Actinomycin D: 0.5–0.7 mg/m². Cytarabine: 300 mg/m² SC or IV infused over 4–6 hours.
  - **Day 8**. Melphalan: 20 mg/m² PO on day 8. Substitute with chlorambucil after 3 months, at the same dose. Dexamethasone: 1 mg/kg PO or SC on days 1 and 8.

  Duration: indefinite, until remission or maximum 6 months. Each cycle is 2 weeks.

Canine Mast Cell Tumour

- **LVP**
  - **Day 1**. Lomustine: 50–60 mg/m² PO.
  - **Day 10 or 14**. Vinblastine: 2 mg/m² IV. Prednisone: 40 mg/m² PO every 24 hours for one week and then 20 mg/m² PO every 48 hours.

Duration: 4–6 months when used as adjuvant therapy and indefinite in dogs with gross disease (unresectable or visceral lymph node metastases). The duration of each cycle is 3 or 4 weeks, depending on the stage of the disease.

- **LP**
  - Lomustine: 50–60 mg/m² PO every 3 or 4 weeks.
  - Prednisone: 40 mg/m² PO every 24 hours for one week and then 20 mg/m² PO every 48 hours.

  Duration: 4–6 months when used as adjuvant therapy and indefinite in dogs with metastatic or visceral mastocytosis.
- **VP**
  - Vinblastine: 2 mg/m² IV, once a week for 4 weeks, then once every 2 weeks for another 4 doses (in total 8 doses as adjunctive therapy after resection of high-grade mast cell tumours without evidence of metastatic disease). Prednisone: 40 mg/m² PO every 24 hours for one week and then 20 mg/m² PO every 48 hours.

  Duration: indefinite in dogs with metastatic or visceral mastocytosis.

Canine Metronomic Therapy

Indicated as adjunctive therapy in splenic haemangiosarcomas and soft-tissue sarcomas where resection was incomplete. Also in carcinomas, although there are no publications on its effectiveness in this type of neoplasia.

- **Cyclophosphamide**: 15 mg/m² PO BID.
- **Nonsteroidal anti-inflammatory**: (piroxicam or cox-type NSAIDs) PO BID.

If the treatment is effective and is continued for more than 2–3 months, using furosemide 0.5 mg/kg BID is recommended to minimise the possibility of developing sterile hemorrhagic cystitis.

Carcinomas in Dogs

- **Carboplatin**: 300 mg/m² IV every 3 weeks.

  Duration: each cycle is 21 days. At least 4–6 cycles when used as adjunctive therapy.
- **Gemcitabine**: 675 mg/m² IV infused over 20 minutes every 2 weeks.

  Duration: each cycle is 14 days. At least 6 cycles when used as adjunctive therapy.
- **Mitoxantrone/piroxicam**: mitoxantrone 5 mg/m² IV infused over 10 minutes every 3 weeks. **Piroxicam**: 0.3 mg/m² PO every other day.

Duration: indefinite if there is evidence of disease until evidence of progression is seen.

- **FAC**
  - **Day 1**. Doxorubicin: 30 mg/m² (or 1 mg/kg if <15 kg) IV.
  - **Day 8**. 5-fluorouracil: 150 mg/m² IV.
  - **Day 10**. Cyclophosphamide: 200–300 mg/m² PO.
  - **Day 15**. 5-fluorouracil: 150 mg/m² IV. Sulpha-trimethoprim: 15 mg/kg/12 hours PO.

  Duration: each cycle is 21 days. At least 4–6 cycles when used as adjunctive therapy.

Feline Carcinomas and Fibrosarcomas

- **AC protocol**
  - **Day 1**. Doxorubicin: 1 mg/kg IV.
  - **Day 10**. Cyclophosphamide: 200–250 mg/m² PO.

  Duration: each cycle is 21 days. At least 4–6 cycles when used as adjunctive therapy.
- **Carboplatin**: 200–250 mg/m² IV every 3–4 weeks.

  Duration: each cycle is 3–4 weeks. At least 4–6 cycles when used as adjunctive therapy.

Canine Soft-tissue Sarcomas and Haemangiosarcomas

- **Modified VAC protocol**
  - **Day 1**. Doxorubicin: 30 mg/m² (or 1 mg/kg if <15 kg) IV.
  - **Day 8**. Cyclophosphamide: 200–250 mg/m² PO.
  - **Day 15**. Vincristine: 0.5–0.75 mg/m² IV.

    Duration: each cycle is 21 days. At least 4–6 cycles and 6 cycles are recommended when used as adjunctive therapy to treat haemangiosarcoma.
- **AC protocol**
  - **Day 1**. Doxorubicin: 30 mg/m² (or 1 mg/kg if <15 kg) IV.
  - **Day 10**. Cyclophosphamide: 200–250 mg/m² PO.

  Duration: each cycle is 21 days. At least 4–6 cycles and 6 cycles are recommended when used as adjunctive therapy to treat haemangiosarcoma.

Osteosarcomas in Dogs

- **Doxorubicin**: 30 mg/m² (or 1 mg/kg if <15 kg) IV.

  Duration: each cycle is 14 days. 6 cycles are recommended.
- **Carboplatin**: 300 mg/m² IV every 3 weeks.

  Duration: each cycle is 21 days. 6 cycles are recommended.

Bibliography

- Bavcar, S., de Vos, J., Kessler, M., et al. (2017) Combination toceranib and lomustine shows frequent high-grade toxicities when used for treatment of non-resectable or recurrent mast cell tumours in dogs: A European multicentre study. *Vet J*, 224:1–6.
- Biller, B.J., Elmslie, R.E., Burnett, R.C. et al. (2007) Use of FoxP3 expression to identify regulatory T cells in healthy dogs and dogs with cancer. *Vet Immunol Immunopathol*, 116(1–2):69–78. Epub 2006 Dec 16.
- Burton, J.H., Mitchell, L., Thamm, D.H. et at. (2011) Low-dose cyclophosphamide selectively decreases regulatory T cells and inhibits angiogenesis in dogs with soft tissue sarcoma. *J Vet Intern Med*, 25(4):920–6. doi:10.1111/j.1939–1676.2011.0753.x.
- Cadot, P., Hensel, P., Bensignor, E. et al. (2011) Masitinib decreases signs of canine atopic dermatitis: a multicentre, randomized, double-blind, placebo-controlled phase 3 trial. *Vet Dermatol*, 22(6):554–64.
- Carlsten. K.S., London, C.A., Haney, S. et al. (2012) Multicenter prospective trial of hypofractionated radiation treatment, toceranib, and prednisone for measurable canine mast cell tumors. *J Vet Intern Med*, 26(1):135–41.
- Chon, E., McCartan, L., Kubicek, L.N. et al. (2011) Safety evaluation of combination toceranib phosphate (Palladia®) and piroxicam in tumour-bearing dogs (excluding mast cell tumours): a phase I dose-finding study. *Vet Comp Oncol*. doi: 10.1111/j.1476–5829.2011.00265.x.
- ECVIM-CA (2007) *Guidelines - Preventing occupational and environmental exposure to cytotoxic drugs in veterinary medicine*, 2nd version (http://www.ecvim-ca.org/guide_lines.htm)
- Elmslie, R.E., Glawe, P., Dow, S.W. (2008) Metronomic therapy with cyclophosphamide and piroxicam effectively delays tumor recurrence in dogs with incompletely resected soft tissue sarcomas. *J Vet Intern Med*, 22(6):1373–9. Epub 2008 Oct 3.
- Gardner, H.L., London, C.A., Portela, R.A. (2015) *Maintenance therapy with toceranib following doxorubicin-based chemotherapy for canine splenic hemangiosarcoma. BMC Vet Res*,11:131.
- Gustafson, D., Page, R.L. (2012) *Cancer chemotherapy*. In: Withrow, S.J., Vail, D.M., Page, R.L. (eds): Withrow and MacEwen's Small Animal Clinical Oncology, 5th Edition. St Louis: Saunders-Elsevier, 157–179.
- Hahn, K.A., Legendre, A.M., Shaw, N.G. et al. (2010) Evaluation of 12- and 24-month survival rates after treatment with masitinib in dogs with nonresectable mast cell tumors. *Am J Vet Res*, 71(11):1354–61. Erratum in: Am J Vet Res. 2011 Feb;72(2):247.
- Hahn, K.A., Ogilvie, G., Rusk, T. et al. (2008) Masitinib is safe and effective for the treatment of canine mast cell tumors. *J Vet Intern Med*, 22(6):1301–9.
- Harper, A., Blackwood, L. (2017) Toxicity and response in cats with neoplasia treated with toceranib phosphate. *J Feline Med Surg*, 19(6):619–623.
- Hayes, A. (2005) Safe use of anticancer chemotherapy in small animal practice. *In Practice*, 27, 118–127.
- Holtermann, N., Kiupel, M., Hirschberger, J. (2017) The tyrosine kinase inhibitor toceranib in feline injection site sarcoma: efficacy and side effects. *Vet Comp Oncol*, 15(2):632–640.
- Horiuchi, Y., Tominaga, M., Ichikawa, M. et al. (2009) Increase of regulatory T cells in the peripheral blood of dogs with metastatic tumors. *Microbiol Immunol*, 53(8):468–74.
- Horiuchi, Y., Tominaga, M., Ichikawa, M. et al. (2010) Relationship between regulatory and type 1 T cells in dogs with oral malignant melanoma. *Microbiol Immunol*, 54(3):152–9.
- Horta, R.D.S., Giuliano, A., Lavalle, G.E. et al. (2018) Clinical, histological, immunohistochemical and genetic factors associated with measurable response of high-risk canine mast cell tumours to tyrosine kinase inhibitors. *Oncol Lett*, 15(1):129–136.
- Kim, C., Matsuyama, A., Mutsaers, A.J. et al (2017) Retrospective evaluation of toceranib (Palladia) treatment for canine metastatic appendicular osteosarcoma. *Can Vet J*, 58(10):1059–1064.
- Klahn, S. (2014) Chemotherapy safety in clinical veterinary oncology. *Vet Clin North Am Small Anim Pract*, 44(5):941–63.
- Knobloch, A., Mohring, S.A., Eberle, N. et al. (2010) Cytotoxic drug residues in urine of dogs receiving anticancer chemotherapy. *J Vet Intern Med*, 24(2):384–90.
- Knobloch, A., Mohring, S.A., Eberle, N. et al. (2010) Drug residues in serum of dogs receiving anticancer chemotherapy. *J Vet Intern Med*, 24(2):379–83.
- Lana, S., U'ren, L., Plaza, S. et al. (2007) Continuous low-dose oral chemotherapy for adjuvant therapy of splenic hemangiosarcoma in dogs. *J Vet Intern Med*, 21(4):764–9.
- Laver, T., London, C.A., Vail, D.M. et al. (2017) Prospective evaluation of toceranib phosphate in metastatic canine osteosarcoma. *Vet Comp Oncol*.
- Lawrence, J., Saba, C., Gogal, R. et al (2012) Masitinib demonstrates anti-proliferative and pro-apoptotic activity in primary and metastatic feline injection-site sarcoma cells. *Vet Comp Oncol*. doi: 10.1111/j.1476–5829.2011.00291.x.
- Leach, T.N., Childress, M.O., Greene, S.N. et al (2011) Prospective trial of metronomic chlorambucil chemotherapy in dogs with naturally occurring cancer. *Vet Comp Oncol*. doi:10.1111/j.1476–5829.2011.00280.x.
- Leo, C., Stell, A., Borrego, J. et al. (2014) Evaluation of low-dose metronomic (LDM) cyclophosphamide toxicity in cats with malignant neoplasia. *J Feline Med Surg*, 16:671–678.
- London, C., Mathie, T., Stingle, N. et al. (2011) Preliminary evidence for biologic activity of toceranib phosphate (Palladia®) in solid tumours. *Vet Comp Oncol*. doi: 10.1111/j.1476–5829.2011.00275.x.
- London, C.A., Gardner, H.L., Mathie, T., et al. (2015) Impact of Toceranib/Piroxicam/Cyclophosphamide Maintenance Therapy on Outcome of Dogs with Appendicular Osteosarcoma following Amputation and Carboplatin Chemotherapy: A Multi-Institutional Study. *PLoS One*, 10(4):e0124889.

■ London, C.A., Malpas, P.B., Wood-Follis, S.L. et al. (2009) Multi-center, placebo-controlled, double-blind, randomized study of oral toceranib phosphate (SU11654), a receptor tyrosine kinase inhibitor, for the treatment of dogs with recurrent (either local or distant) mast cell tumor following surgical excision. *Clin Cancer Res*, 15(11):3856–65.

■ London, C.A. (2009) Tyrosine kinase inhibitors in veterinary medicine. *Top Companion Anim Med*, 24(3):106–12. Review.

■ Martinez de Merlo, E., Ruano, R., Arconada, L., et al. (2013) Treatment of canine cutaneous epitheliotrophic lymphoma of T cell origin with masitinib. *Proceedings of the 2013 South European Veterinary Conference*. Barcelona, Spain, pp 87.

■ Matsuyama, A., Poirier, V.J., Mantovani, F. et al. (2017) Adjuvant Doxorubicin with or without Metronomic Cyclophosphamide for Canine Splenic Hemangiosarcoma. *J Am Anim Hosp Assoc.*, 53(6):304–312.

■ Matsuyama, A., Schott, C.R., Wood, G.A. et al (2018) Evaluation of metronomic cyclophosphamide chemotherapy as maintenance treatment for dogs with appendicular osteosarcoma following limb amputation and carboplatin chemotherapy. *J Am Vet Med Assoc*, 252(11):1377–1383.

■ Mealey, K.L., Fidel, J., Gay, J.M. et al. (2008) ABCB1-1 Delta polymorphism can predict hematologic toxicity in dogs treated with vincristine. *J Vet Intern Med*, 22(4):996–1000.

■ Mealey, K.L. (2006) Adverse drug reactions in herding-breed dog: the role of p-glycoprotein. *Compendium of continuing education for the practising veterinarian*, 28:23–33.

■ Merrick, C.H., Pierro, J., Schleis, S.E. et al. (2017) Retrospective evaluation of toceranib phosphate (Palladia®) toxicity in cats. *Vet Comp Oncol*, 15(3):710–717.

■ Moore, A.S., Frimberger, A. (2008) Anticancer drugs and protocols: Traditional drugs. En: Bonagura, J.D., Twedt, D.C. (eds): *Kirk's Current Veterinary Therapy XIV*. Section 4: Hematology, oncology and immunology, 14th Edition. St Louis: Saunders-Elsevier, 305–331.

■ Mutsaers, A.J. (2009) Metronomic chemotherapy. *Top Companion Anim Med*, 24(3):137–43. Review.

■ Olmsted, G.A., Farrelly, J., Post, G.S. et al. (2017) Tolerability of toceranib phosphate (Palladia) when used in conjunction with other therapies in 35 cats with feline oral squamous cell carcinoma: 2009-2013. *J Feline Med Surg*, 19(6):568–575.

■ Olsen, J.A., Thomson, M., O'Connell, K. (2018) Combination vinblastine, prednisolone and toceranib phosphate for treatment of grade II and III mast cell tumours in dogs. *Vet Med Sci*. doi: 10.1002/vms3.106.

■ O'Neill, K., Guth, A., Biller, B. et al (2009) Changes in regulatory T cells in dogs with cancer and associations with tumor type. *J Vet Intern Med*, 23(4):875–81.

■ Pasquier, E., Kavallaris, M., André, N. (2010) Metronomic chemotherapy: new rationale for new directions. *Nat Rev Clin Oncol*, 7(8):455–65.

■ Polton, G., Finotello, R., Sabattini, S. et al (2018) Survival analysis of dogs with advanced primary lung carcinoma treated by metronomic cyclophosphamide, piroxicam and thalidomide. *Vet Comp Oncol*. doi: 10.1111/vco.12393.

■ Rippy, S.B., Gardner, H.L., Nguyen, S.M. et al (2016) A pilot study of toceranib/vinblastine therapy for canine transitional cell carcinoma. *BMC Vet Res*, 12(1):257.

■ Rissetto, K.C., Rindt, H., Selting, K.A. et al. (2010) Cloning and expression of canine CD25 for validation of an anti-human CD25 antibody to compare T regulatory lymphocytes in healthy dogs and dogs with osteosarcoma. *Vet Immunol Immunopathol*, 135(1–2):137–45.

■ Robat, C., London, C., Bunting, L. et al. (2011) Safety evaluation of combination vinblastine and toceranib phosphate (Palladia®) in dogs: a phase I dose-finding study. *Vet Comp Oncol*. 2011. doi: 10.1111/j.1476–5829.2011.00261.x.

■ Rossi, F., Sabattini, S., Vascellari, M. et al. (2018) The impact of toceranib, piroxicam and thalidomide with or without hypofractionated radiation therapy on clinical outcome in dogs with inflammatory mammary carcinoma. *Vet Comp Oncol*. doi: 10.1111/vco.12407.

■ Schrempp, D.R., Childress, M.O., Stewart, J.C. et al. (2013) Metronomic administration of chlorambucil for treatment of dogs with urinary bladder transitional cell carcinoma. *J Am Vet Med Assoc*, 242(11):1534–8.

■ Selting, K., Henry, C., Axiak, S. (2010) Tolerability of Metronomic Satraplatin in Dogs with Spontaneously Occurring Tumors. *VCS Proceedings*, San Diego. p 116.

■ Setyo, L., Ma, M., Bunn, T. et al. (2017) Furosemide for prevention of cyclophosphamide-associated sterile haemorrhagic cystitis in dogs receiving metronomic low-dose oral cyclophosphamide. *Vet Comp Oncol*, 15(4):1468–1478.

■ Smith, A.N., Klahn, S., Phillips, B. et al. (2018) ACVIM small animal consensus statement on safe use of cytotoxic chemotherapeutics in veterinary practice. *J Vet Intern Med*. doi.org/10.111/jvim.15077.

■ Smrkovski, O.A., Essick, L., Rohrbach, B.W. et al. (2013) Masitinib mesylate for metastatic and non-resectable canine cutaneous mast cell tumours. *Vet Comp Oncol*. doi: 10.1111/vco.12053.

■ Thamm, D.H., Rose, B., Know, K. et al. (2012) Masitinib as a chemosensitizer of canine tumor cell lines: A proof of concept study. *Vet J*, 191(1):131–4.

■ Tripp, C.D., Fidel, J., Anderson, C.L. et al. (2011) Tolerability of Metronomic Administration of Lomustine in Dogs with Cancer. *J Vet Int Med*, 25:278–284.

■ Weishaar, K.M., Ehrhart, E.J., Avery, A.C. et al. (2018) c-KIT Mutation and Localization Status as Response Predictors in Mast Cell Tumors in Dogs Treated with Prednisone and Toceranib or Vinblastine. *J Vet Intern Med*, 32(1):394–405.

■ Wiles, V., Hohenhaus, A., Lamb, K. et al. (2017) Retrospective evaluation of toceranib phosphate (Palladia) in cats with oral squamous cell carcinoma. *J Feline Med Surg*, 19(2):185–193.

■ Wouda, R.M., Hocker, S.E., Higginbotham, M.L. (2018) Safety evaluation of combination carboplatin and toceranib phosphate (Palladia) in tumour-bearing dogs: A phase I dose finding study. *Vet Comp Oncol*, 16(1):E52-E60.

Test

Answers on Page 124

1. **Regarding gastrointestinal toxicity associated with the administration of cytotoxic drugs, which of the following statements is false?**
    a. With those with a high prevalence of gastrointestinal toxicity, prophylactic treatment is recommended since gastrointestinal toxicity has a high impact on the quality of life of the animal.
    b. Gastrointestinal toxicity is very common with alkylating agents such as chlorambucil.
    c. Gastrointestinal toxicity can exacerbate neutropaenia at the leucocyte nadir by increasing the consumption of neutrophils at sites of gastrointestinal inflammation.
    d. Loss of appetite or anorexia may be manifestations of nausea or intestinal paralytic ileus.

2. **Regarding extravasation of cytotoxic drugs, which of the following statements is false?**
    a. Doxorubicin causes severe tissue damage if it extravasated, but tissue damage is usually only apparent days or weeks after administration.
    b. Dilution of doxorubicin and close monitoring during administration minimise complications that could occur in the event of extravasation.
    c. Hyaluronidase infiltrations can minimise tissue damage secondary to vincristine extravasation.
    d. Administration of dexrazosan can completely reverse tissue damage, even if several days have elapsed after doxorubicin extravasation.

3. **After exposing tumour cells to a vinca alkaloid, in what phase of the cell cycle should maximum lethal toxicity to cells be expected?**
    a. G_0.
    b. G_1.
    c. G_2.
    d. M.

4. **Regarding tyrosine kinase inhibitors and their relationship with cancer in pets, which of the following statements is false?**
    a. A large part of the receptor tyrosine kinase (RTK) family are receptors for extracellular growth factors.
    b. Inappropriate inactivation of RTK can occur when there are mutations in these receptors that lead to constant activation.
    c. The expression of a RTK in a given neoplasm guarantees the successful anticancer activity of tyrosine kinase inhibitors for that tumour.
    d. One third of canine mast cell tumours have mutations in the RTK c-KIT.

5. **P-glycoprotein is a transmembrane cell pump; it has the ability to actively eliminate certain drugs from the cell cytoplasm including chemotherapeutic agents in both normal and tumour cells. The following drugs have been shown to act as substrates for P-glycoprotein with its consequent cellular excretion, except:**
    a. Doxorubicin.
    b. Carboplatin.
    c. Vincristine.
    d. Actinomycin-D.

6. **Regarding haematologic toxicity after administration of cytotoxic drugs, which of the following statements is correct?**
    a. For all cytotoxic drugs, if the neutrophil and platelet count on the blood count are normal 10 days after the drug administration, the next dose of chemotherapy can be administered.
    b. If a patient has a fever, but there is no neutropaenia on the blood count, the next dose of chemotherapy can be administered.
    c. Neutrophil counts less than 2000/µL require hospitalisation and administration of intravenous antibiotics.
    d. Patients with neutrophil counts of 1200/µl can be treated with cytotoxic drugs if they are clinically well, especially if the drug to be received is moderately immunosuppressive.

7. **Which of the following statements regarding cyclophosphamide is false?**
    a. Cyclophosphamide is inactive in vitro and must be metabolised by P450 enzymes in the liver to their active species.
    b. Concomitant use of furosemide may be protective against sterile haemorrhagic cystitis in dogs treated with standard doses of cyclophosphamide.
    c. Acrolein is the metabolite largely responsible for sterile haemorrhagic cystitis.
    d. Hepatotoxicity is the limiting toxicity of cyclophosphamide.

8. **Regarding metronomic therapy, which of the following statements is false?**
    a. In veterinary medicine, it usually consists of a combination of a low dose cytotoxic drug with an NSAID.
    b. One of its mechanisms of action is direct toxicity to tumour cells.
    c. One of its mechanisms of action is based on the inhibition of endothelial cell replication.
    d. In veterinary medicine, low-dose regimens of chlorambucil or cyclophosphamide have shown some degree of effectiveness against tumour proliferation.

9. **Which of the following answers is correct?**
    a. Cytarabine is an alkylating drug.
    b. 50% of carboplatin is excreted via the urinary tract.
    c. Actinomycin D belongs to the family of antitumour antibiotics.
    d. Vinorelbine belongs to the family of antimetabolite drugs.

10. **Which of the following statements regarding adverse effects is correct?**
    a. Lomustine can cause increased liver enzymes in 90% of patients and tissue hepatotoxicity in 30%.
    b. Cisplatin produces cutaneous oedema in felines, which causes death in 50% of treated cats.
    c. Asparaginase can cause anaphylactic reactions when first administered.
    d. Doxorubicin can produce cumulative cardiotoxicity in dogs when the patient receives total doses greater than 180 mg/m².

Clinical Case

Signalment

Neutered 11-year-old, male Podenco, diagnosed with osteosarcoma. The decision was made to treat him with 6 doses of doxorubicin, one every two weeks. The first dose was administered a week ago.

Reason for consult

The check-up was scheduled to evaluate a complete blood count at the point where the white blood cell nadir should occur. The owner comments that the dog has been lethargic for the past three days, with decreased appetite and vomiting. He has also suffered from several episodes of colitis with tenesmus and haematochezia.

Physical examination

The physical examination is not remarkable except for a depressed attitude and a temperature of 40.1 °C (normal up to 38.9 °C at rest).

Complete blood count

The neutrophil count is 300/µl (normal range: 2060–10 600/µl).

Questions:

1. **Based on the information provided, what should the immediate plan be?**
    a. Send the patient home and repeat the complete blood count in a week's time.
    b. Prescribe oral antibiotics, send home with symptomatic therapy, and repeat complete blood count after 3–7 days.
    c. Hospitalise the patient for supportive therapy including intravenous antibiotics until fever subsides and delay the next doxorubicin treatment.
    d. Hospitalise, administer intravenous antibiotics. Make a prophylactic plan and consider dose reduction before the next administration of doxorubicin.

2. **What is the most likely cause of the observed neutropaenia and clinical signs?**
    a. Immunosuppression caused by doxorubicin.
    b. The effect of doxorubicin on the gastrointestinal tract.
    c. The poor immune status of the patient while suffering from cancer.
    d. The combination of the effect on the gastrointestinal tract (inflammation and consumption of neutrophils) and effect on the bone marrow of doxorubicin.

3. What antibiotics should be administered in this situation?

a. Amoxicillin-clavulanate.
b. Imipenem.
c. Marbofloxacin.
d. Sulfonamides-trimethoprim.

4. And if the dog had the same symptoms, but without pyrexia, which of the following treatment plans should have been followed?

a. Send the patient home and repeat the complete blood count in a week's time.
b. Prescribe oral antibiotics, send home with symptomatic therapy, and repeat the complete blood count in 3–7 days.
c. Hospitalise the patient for supportive therapy including intravenous antibiotics until fever subsides and delay the next doxorubicin treatment.
d. Hospitalise, administer intravenous antibiotics. Make a prophylactic plan and consider dose reduction before the next administration of doxorubicin.

5. What would an appropriate prophylactic plan be before giving the next dose of doxorubicin (including suggested dose reduction)?

a. 15–20% reduction with prophylactic administration of antiemetics and metronidazole.
b. Reduction by 50%.
c. The dose cannot be reduced.
d. 15–20% reduction with prophylactic administration of antiemetics.

6. If the owner does not want to continue with doxorubicin due to the adverse effects and impact on the quality of life of the dog, what other effective alternatives are available to treat osteosarcoma, with a lower possibility of adverse effects?

a. Vincristine.
b. Lomustine.
c. Carboplatin.
d. Cisplatin.

Notes

Correct answers:

Test

1. b
2. d
3. d
4. c
5. b
6. d
7. d
8. b
9. c
10. d

Clinical Case

1. d
2. d
3. a
4. b
5. a
6. c

Notes

Diagnosis and Treatment of Lymphoma and Leukaemia in Dogs and Cats

Ana Lara García

Diagnosis of Lymphoma in Dogs and Cats

Lymphoma encompasses a **diverse group of diseases with a common origin in the lymphoreticular organs**. It is characterised by uncontrolled clonal proliferation of lymphoreticular cells and usually has its origin in lymphoid tissues such as lymph nodes, spleen, and bone marrow, although it can originate in any tissue in the body. Given that lymphoma is a systemic disease that, although it can present locally, in most cases usually affects more than one organ or body system, when evaluating patients where this disease is suspected focus should not only be on obtaining cytological or histological evidence of the disease, but also on forming a diagnostic plan that establishes how many organs the disease is present in, or, determining the clinical stage, which amounts to the same thing.

Physical Examination

Suspicions of lymphoma usually begin with findings during the physical examination. This should be detailed, regardless of the clinical history, and special attention should be paid to the examination of anatomical locations in which the patient presents clinical signs. In multicentric lymphoma, the peripheral lymph nodes, which are often involved, can be palpated. In patients affected by the disease, various clinical signs and lesions can be observed such as abdominal organomegaly, thickening of the intestinal loops, enlarged pelvic lymph nodes on rectal palpation, skin or mucosal lesions, increased size of the tonsils, abnormal thoracic auscultation as well as signs of the possible presence of mediastinal lymphadenopathy or ocular lesions.

Non-invasive Diagnostic Tests

The findings of the physical examination can sometimes be highly indicative of lymphoma and on other occasions they can be more non-specific, and a list of possible differential diagnoses should be established, whilst also continuing with a diagnostic plan that helps to rule out or confirm the different possibilities.

Non-invasive tests that can help and that will be necessary anyway to provide a minimum amount of information if the diagnosis is lymphoma include:

- **complete blood count**
- **biochemistry**
- **urinalysis**
- **total T4 levels, cobalamin, and folate in FeLV/FIV cats**.

Complete Blood Count

The information it provides is **not usually relevant for diagnosis, although it is essential to rule out other pathologies** (such as systemic infectious diseases) **and assess the general condition of the patient**.

The most common abnormalities are non-regenerative anaemia, resulting from the chronicity of the condition and/or a variable degree of bleeding in the case of gastrointestinal involvement or if there is thrombocytopaenia due to bone marrow involvement. In the latter, other cytopaenias and even malignant cells in circulation may be observed.

Malignant lymphoid cells are seen in the blood smear in 30% of canine lymphoma cases and in 15–80% of cats with large granular cell lymphoma.

Studies have been published that confer a prognostic value to thrombocytopaenia, absolute neutrophil values, and different leucocyte indices at the time of diagnosis of canine multicentric lymphoma.

Blood Biochemistry

In some cases **biochemistry tests can be completely normal**.

Elevations in liver or kidney parameters may indicate neoplastic infiltration of these organs or simply concomitant disease in these patients, who are frequently geriatric. On the other hand, when these parameters are normal, the involvement of these organs cannot be completely ruled out.

The presence of hypoalbuminaemia is frequent in cases of gastrointestinal involvement since the loss of albumin through the intestinal lumen exceeds the hepatic production capacity. In feline gastrointestinal lymphoma, cobalamin is usually reduced in 80% of cases. Detecting these abnormal levels and supplementing with vitamin B_{12} when appropriate cause an improvement in digestive symptoms.

The presence of hypercalcaemia is usually associated with T-cell lymphomas in the dog and can have an impact on the clinical course in the short and medium term, since if it is not treated quickly azotaemia and irreversible kidney damage can occur that complicate the clinical picture. Therefore, the finding of this paraneoplastic sign has significant relevance.

Urinalysis

Malignant lymphoid cells can sometimes be seen in renal lymphoma by analysing the urine sediment. It is also important to rule out urinary tract infections before starting immunosuppressive therapies and as baseline information to get an idea of renal function along with renal biochemical parameters in geriatric patients.

Diagnostic Imaging Tests

Diagnostic imaging tests **allow the extent of the disease to be determined and, with it, the clinical stage**, but they rarely provide information that leads to changes in the treatment plan.

In cases where the animal is ill, they normally provide useful information. In fact, they are extremely useful in patients with lymphoma who do not have external evidence of the disease: for example with gastrointestinal, mediastinal, hepatosplenic, renal lymphoma, etc.

Thoracic or abdominal radiographs may be helpful in determining the presence of mediastinal masses or hepato-/splenomegaly.

Ultrasound allows visualisation of the different abdominal organs and mediastinal masses, if they exist, in great detail and their size can be documented by taking measurements. In addition, this technique can be used to facilitate obtaining ultrasound-guided samples of organs where there are obvious lesions or, for example, of the spleen and liver if a complete staging is being performed.

CT may also be useful to determine if there is intrathoracic or intra-abdominal lymphadenopathy, as well as other extranodal lesions produced by lymphoma.

Histological and Immunophenotypic Classification and Biological Behaviour

One of the reasons for the differences observed in the percentage of response and remission when treating lymphoma is that the **biology of the disease is highly variable**. Malignant transformation of B, T, or NK lymphocytes can occur at different points in their maturation and as a result of different cell mutations. Although common behavioural patterns can be observed, each malignant transformation is unique, which explains why lymphoma in different patients can show different biological behaviour even with the same immunophenotype.

Although high-grade lymphomas which are the most common, are easily diagnosed by cytology since the neoplastic population is quite different from normal lymphocytes, with evident characteristics of malignancy, in veterinary oncology the cytological diagnosis of lymphoma does not provide enough information to choose an appropriate treatment and gain a good understanding of the prognosis. Knowing the immunophenotype and an estimate of the grade is necessary.

It has been widely demonstrated that the histological grade is related to the biological behaviour of the disease and the response to treatment. This can be determined easily with a peripheral lymph node biopsy in most cases.

Although there are several histological classifications of lymphoma (Kiel system and the working formulation), in 2002 the World Health Organization (WHO) published a classification system to define the different categories of haematopoietic and lymphoid tumours in domestic animals that incorporated anatomical, histological and immunophenotypic criteria, in order to allow a more precise and reproducible diagnosis of this disease. Several studies assess the application of this classification system and show the percentages of each subtype. In that of Valli et al. (2011) the concordance between a group of pathologists when applying this classification system was also evaluated. They examined 300 cases and the agreement reached among the 17 pathologists was 83% which amounts to 87% in the most frequent subtypes: diffuse large B-cell lymphoma (40%), marginal zone lymphoma (3.7%), peripheral T-cell lymphoma (15%), T-zone lymphoma (12.7%), lymphoblastic T-cell lymphoma (4%), and follicular hyperplasia (3.7%). Because these six categories include about 80% of all canine lymphomas, the application of this system is practical for most pathologists and a high degree of efficacy can be achieved in the diagnosis of canine lymphoma according to the WHO classification.

In 2013, Valli et al. published the results obtained by correlating histological classification, subtype, mitotic index, clinical stage and treatment with respect to survival in 992 dogs with lymphoma diagnosed by histopathology. Due to the numerous types of type B and T lymphomas, they grouped the cases into seven diagnostic categories. Based on the mitotic index, they also established three categories: low, intermediate, and high-grade lymphomas.

Intermediate or high-grade lymphomas have a high mitotic rate, rapid progression, and are most commonly type B-cells. This type of lymphoma, especially high-grade types, are characterised by a rapid progression that leads to the death of the patient if effective therapy is not implemented promptly. They tend to respond fairly quickly to chemotherapy, and remission is frequently achieved. The biggest problem with high-grade lymphomas is that they can also develop resistance relatively easily, given the high potential for developing mutations that favour the survival of cells with a high mitotic index. For this reason, implementing chemotherapeutic protocols that include several drugs with different mechanisms of action is indicated.

In dogs with this type of lymphoma, although short induction protocols followed by a maintenance protocol can be effective, sometimes the remission period is longer with more aggressive protocols with a longer induction duration. In recent years, several publications have presented evidence that high-grade T-cell lymphomas (peripheral T-cell lymphoma) may have longer survival times when alkylating agents such as lomustine, procarbazine, or mechlorethamine are included (LOP-like protocols) in induction chemotherapy protocols. High-grade B-cell lymphomas (diffuse large B-cell lymphoma) have shorter survival times than was thought previously and respond well to COP or CHOP protocols. The COP protocol includes the drugs cyclophosphamide, vincristine sulfate (Oncovin®) and prednisolone; and the CHOP protocol includes the drugs cyclophosphamide, doxorubicin hydrochloride (hydroxydaunorubicin), vincristine sulfate (Oncovin®), and prednisone.

On the other hand, **low-grade lymphomas** are less common (5–29%), have a lower mitotic rate, and are more frequently T-cell types. These lymphomas do not respond to chemotherapy quickly nor with less or more aggressive protocols. Sometimes it takes several weeks to reach a state of remission, or it is never fully reached, although, on the other hand, dogs with this type of lymphoma show a slow disease progression and can have a long survival time with non-aggressive chemotherapy protocols (such as COAP followed by LMP). There are low-grade and immunophenotype T-cell lymphomas that behave indolently (T-zone lymphoma) that are only treated if there are associated symptoms and with oral protocols.

For all of the above, it is important to determine the phenotype when making a diagnosis of lymphoma. The techniques that can be used to reach a diagnosis are described below.

Which Tests Can be Performed to Classify and Identify the Immunophenotype of the Lymphoma?

Apart from the anatomical classification described above, lymphoma can be classified **morphologically**, for which a biopsy of the affected lymph node or tissue is required for histopathological study, and by its **immunophenotype**, by performing molecular diagnostic techniques such as immunohistochemistry (IHC), flow cytometry (FC) and clonality tests (PARR). These techniques can help to make a definitive diagnosis by showing that the cell population of interest is of a single type (type B or T-cells) rather than a mixed population as occurs in most inflammatory processes and, at the same time, provide the immunophenotype of the lymphoma. In addition to better characterising the type of lymphoma, they are also used to diagnose it in cases that represent a diagnostic challenge (in which neither cytology nor histopathology can differentiate between reactive lymphocytosis and lymphoma, as frequently occurs in cases of low-grade lymphoma).

Removal of an entire lymph node, including the capsule, is recommended for effective histopathologic evaluation. Although biopsy may be sufficient, it is important to avoid crush artefacts or inadequately sized samples. Most pathologists prefer to receive the entire lymph node, as it provides maximum information by allowing the architecture of the organ to be properly examined.

An experienced cytologist can try to estimate the lymphoma subtype of greatest prognostic significance, or at least the grade, based on cell/nuclear size, chromatin pattern, and the number, size, and location of nucleoli in combination with the immunophenotype obtained by FC, IHC and, least preferably, PARR. For this to be possible, samples of excellent quality are required, in which the cytological criteria are very evident. Molecular diagnostic techniques can be performed on tissues and cells from peripheral blood, lymph nodes, non-lymphoid tissues, and effusions. To diagnose large granular cell lymphoma, special stains such as IHC with granzyme-B are required.

FC and IHC determine the immunophenotype by assessing the expression of plasma membrane proteins (CDs – cluster of differentiation) of lymphocytes and other immune system cells. For the detection of these antigens, the use of specific monoclonal antibodies is necessary. Development to detect specific markers in canine lymphocytes has allowed the immunophenotyping of tumours in dogs and cats on a routine basis. These techniques can be performed on formalin-fixed tissue, paraffin samples, cytological samples obtained by puncture or, in the case of FC, on cell suspensions obtained from neoplastic tissue (such as a lymph node or other organ aspirate), blood and effusions. These cell suspensions are stained with specific fluorochromes and passed through a FC chamber where they are analysed using a laser.

FC is very useful for the immunophenotyping of lymphomas and leukaemia (it identifies the cell line involved), as well as for determining the difference between lymphoma and acute lymphoblastic leukaemia and reactive lymphocytosis. It can also provide information on other parameters of prognostic importance, such as proliferation factors (Ki67) or expression of the major histocompatibility complex (MHC).

The most important antigens in canine and feline lymphoma from a diagnostic point of view are CD3 (expressed by T lymphocytes) and CD79 (expressed by B lymphocytes). However, a larger panel is usually tested to obtain more information and better typing of the lymphoma (Table 1). With this technique, different subtypes of lymphoma can be identified, although results must be correlated with cytological or histological studies. The main drawback is that the sample must be processed quickly (ideally within 48 hours), since the cells are only viable for a short time.

PCR for Antigen Receptor Rearrangement (PARR)

The polymerase chain reaction (PCR) technique can be used to **distinguish lymphoma or leukaemia from reactive processes**, using samples from aspirates, blood (in the case of leukaemia), or appropriately formalin-fixed tissue or blood.

This technique is based on the fact that lymphocytes contain regions of DNA that are unique in length and sequence. PARR amplifies the DNA gene that encodes the clonally rearranged antigen receptor (in the variable region of the lymphocyte membrane receptor; TCR or BCR), which allows the diagnosis to be confirmed by demonstrating that the population considered neoplastic consists only of type T or type B lymphocytes (monoclonal population), rather than a mixture of the two that is typical of inflammatory diseases (polyclonal population indicative of a reactive process). In the dog, this test identifies approximately 91% of lymphomas. In addition, by means of this method it is also possible to obtain the immunophenotype of lymphoid neoplasms, although its precision is lower than that of FC (Table 2).

It should be taken into account that some cases of infectious diseases, as in the case of ehrlichiosis, can cause a monoclonal expansion of lymphocytes, generating false positive results for a malignant lymphoproliferative disease. The term PARR is used to distinguish this test from other types of PCR analysis and from other methods to determine clonality. PARR is useful in cases in which, even after biopsy and immunohistochemistry have been performed, it is difficult to differentiate between lymphoma and lymphoid hyperplasia or other lymphoproliferative inflammatory diseases, a problem that is often seen with low-grade lymphomas. The sensitivity of PARR to detect T-cell lymphoma in cats is 78–90%.

The choice of one or another test within the diagnostic protocol depends on the clinical state of the patient, the objective to be achieved (Table 3) and its diagnostic efficacy (Table 2).

Table 1. Tested markers using flow cytometry for immunophenotyping of canine and feline lymphoma (extracted from: Martínez de Merlo, E.M., Royón Mayordomo, E. Diagnóstico del linfoma canino y clasificación en subtipos de importancia pronóstica. *Canis et felis*. Junio 2018; 152:6-15).

Marker	Cellular distribution
CD34	Precursor cell
CD45	Leucocyte (all)
CD21*	Mature B lymphocyte
CD79*	B lymphocyte in transformation into plasma cell
CMH II	Mature B lymphocyte; prognostic marker: low expression, high mortality
CD3*	T lymphocyte
CD5*	T lymphocyte
CD4*	Helper T lymphocyte
CD8*	Cytotoxic T lymphocyte
CD14*	Monocyte/neutrophil
Ki67	Cell proliferation marker: <20% greater survival

*Markers used in feline species.

Table 2. Comparison of diagnostic efficiency between FC and PARR (extracted from: Martínez de Merlo, E.M., Royón Mayordomo, E. Diagnóstico del linfoma canino y clasificación en subtipos de importancia pronóstica. *Canis et felis*. Junio 2018; 152:6–15).

		FC (%)	PARR (%)
Sensitivity	B lymphoma	91	67
	T lymphoma	100	75
Positive predictive value	B lymphoma	100	100
	T lymphoma	94	92
Negative predictive value	B lymphoma	80	52
	T lymphoma	100	100
Concordance with IHC		94	70

Table 3. In which cases is the use of PARR, IHC or FC recommended to reach a diagnosis? (Extracted from: Martínez de Merlo, E.M., Royón Mayordomo, E. Diagnóstico del linfoma canino y clasificación en subtipos de importancia pronóstica. *Canis et felis.* Junio 2018; 152:6–15).

Cases	IHC	FC	PARR
Diagnosed lymphoma awaiting phenotyping	+	+	
Suspected lymphoma (homogenous population of lymphocytes)	+	+	
Suspected lymphoma (heterogenous population of lymphocytes)			+
Difficulty containing a simple with high cellularity due to anatomical location			+
Mediastinal mass (lymphoma/thymoma)		+	
Peripheral blood – lymphocytosis		+	
Peripheral blood – suspicious cells without lymphocytosis			+
Bone marrow – neoplastic lymphocytes		+	
Bone marrow – no evidence of neoplastic lymphocytes			+
Cerebrospinal fluid with lymphocytosis			+

Practical Considerations of Multicentric and Non-multicentric Canine Lymphoma

Lymphoma (LSA) is the **most common type of canine cancer** diagnosed in clinical veterinary practice and the most common malignant haematopoietic neoplasm in the dog, representing between 7% and 24% of all canine neoplasms. The incidence of lymphoma in dogs is 24 cases/100 000 dogs/year. Chromosomal aberrations and genetic predisposition have also been identified in dogs with lymphoma, as well as differences in the prevalence of certain immunophenotypes between different breeds. For example, the Spitz-type breeds (Akita, Basenji, Siberian Husky, Alaskan Malamute), Shih Tzu, Lhasa Apso, and Boxer tend to be more likely to develop T-cell lymphoma.

In most cases, this disease has a multicentric presentation that affects lymph nodes and other haematopoietic organs in a generalised way, and is considered a systemic condition, although recently some types of lymphoma that affect a specific anatomical area have been revealed, in which a different approach that uses localised therapy as the primary form of treatment will be covered.

Is It Worth Investing in Lymphoma Diagnosis?

Sometimes clients are on a limited budget. It is useful to adapt the planned tests based on the prognostic information or the relevance to treatment decisions that they can provide. This approach makes it **possible to optimise the financial resources available, obtain the best possible prognostic information and invest in the best treatment** for the specific type of LSA affecting the canine patient.

As mentioned above, recent research has shown the prognostic importance of gathering as much information as possible on morphological classification (classification according to the parameters of the World Health Organization), grade, and immunophenotype.

If the diagnosis is made on a lymph node biopsy, the pathologist can provide a morphological classification and an immunophenotype with immunohistochemistry should be obtained. In practice, the diagnosis is often based on a cytological specimen as it is cheaper, and the results are more readily available. Important prognostic information can be provided with an interpretation of the cytological characteristics of the neoplastic lymphoid cells together with the immunophenotype obtained with flow cytometry or PARR.

Multicentric Lymphoma: Immunophenotype, Grade, Chemotherapy Treatment and Prognosis

On a practical level, most multicentric lymphomas in the dog will be as follows.

- **High-intermediate or high-grade** lymphomas.
- They are characterised by a **high mitotic rate and rapid progression**.
- They will be of the **most common immunophenotype: B-cell**.

High-grade LSA progresses rapidly without treatment and responds rapidly to chemotherapy. Likewise, it can develop resistance relatively easily as a result of their high potential for the development of mutations that favour the survival of cells with a high mitotic index. Therefore, it is advisable to use chemotherapy protocols that include several drugs with different mechanisms of action.

The most common type of multicentric LSA is diffuse large B-cell lymphoma (DLBCL), which can be immunoblastic or centroblastic. A recent study has described a mean remission period of 252 days when CHOP is used as induction and 147 days with COP-type protocols. Increased age, globulin concentration, neutrophil count, neutrophil/lymphocyte ratio, or presence of anaemia or thrombocytopaenia were associated with shorter periods of remission.

Median survival in DLBCL is independent of the induction protocol received, as long as rescue therapy is instituted after relapse, and it includes doxorubicin. The survival rate at one year is 39–44% and 10% at two years. On the other hand, the median survival time (MST) for DLBCL (322 days; 402 if rescue therapy is received) appears to have a better prognosis compared to high-grade B-cell lymphoblastic lymphoma (MST 160 days).

Peripheral T-cell and lymphoblastic LSA are high-grade lymphomas with an aggressive clinical course. With flow cytometry they can be shown to be $CD4^+$, $CD45^+$ and class II MHC, with a MST of 159 days. Multicentric high-grade T-cell LSAs are often inherently resistant to doxorubicin, which would explain the low response rate (50%) to this drug and the short periods of median remission described (over 104 days when treated with CHOP-type protocols). However, the mean remission periods are longer (175–200 days) when treated with MOPP, LOPP or VELCAP-TSC protocols, which include alkylating agents such as lomustine, procarbazine or mechlorethamine. Reported MST varies between 237–323 days, compared to 235 days with CHOP.

Low-grade or intermediate-grade lymphomas are less common (5–29%), have a low mitotic rate, and are more commonly of T-cell origin, although they can also be of B-cell origin. These lymphomas will not respond quickly to chemotherapy, regardless of whether aggressive protocols are used or not. It can take several weeks to reach a state of remission, and sometimes it is never fully achieved.

This is the case for T-zone LSAs, the most common type of low-grade T-cell lymphoma. They usually have a multicentric presentation and show the biological behaviour of indolent lymphoma, with a favourable prognosis and mean survival of 21.2–33.5 months, without the need for therapy or with very mild oral protocols such as the combination of chlorambucil and prednisolone. They are often accompanied by lymphocytosis as an accidental finding, which in principle is of no prognostic relevance.

Golden Retrievers are overrepresented among breeds affected by this type of indolent lymphoma. They can be diagnosed by histology based on their morphological classification or by cytology and flow cytometry due to their distinctive profile ($CD45^-$ MHC class 2^+ and a high percentage is $CD21^+$).

What are the Chemotherapy Protocols of Choice for Treating Canine Lymphoma with a Tight Budget?

Protocols that include multiple cytotoxic drugs will always have a better and longer-lasting response and are the treatment of choice to induce remission in intermediate to high-grade multicentric lymphomas. If the owner is on a tight budget, **COP-type protocols** (combination of cyclophosphamide, vincristine, and prednisolone) with a short induction of 8 weeks are, in general, affordable and effective in cases of both multicentric B and T-cell lymphoma. The prevalence of adverse effects and the monitoring requirements are, in general, lower than for the CHOP or LOPP protocols. Oral maintenance therapy (LMP) with chlorambucil, methotrexate, and prednisolone is a reasonable option once this short induction is over.

Protocols with a single cytotoxic drug in combination with corticosteroids can achieve a high response rate, but the duration of remission is shorter than with multi-agent protocols due to the rapid development of resistance. In principle, there are no specific studies providing this information for T or B-cell lymphoma. Doxorubicin given every 3 weeks provides response rates of 60–75% and remission periods of 4–5 months, so it may be an appropriate option for DLBCL. As a single agent, prednisolone induces remissions of 1–3 months in about 50% of patients.

Other drugs with proven efficacy as single agents in the treatment of canine LSA include cyclophosphamide, L-asparaginase, epirubicin, mitoxantrone, actinomycin D, and lomustine. In dogs with lymphoma, lomustine as a single agent has a response rate of 52% and MST of 3.5 months. This response can be higher by combining lomustine with L-asparaginase, a combination that could be appropriate for high-grade lymphomas and T-cells in a scenario where there are economic limitations.

Options after Relapse: Reinduction Protocols

Most dogs with lymphoma will come out of remission at some point. When this occurs, reinduction with chemotherapy should be considered. As a general rule, **the remission rate after a first relapse is lower and the second remission period is shorter** than after initial treatment, but about 70–80% of dogs will still present a response; this is especially evident for DLBCL cases.

In general, if the patient relapses when on maintenance treatment or when not undergoing any treatment, it is advisable to revert to the initial induction protocol. When CHOP is used as a rescue, response rates of 78% and duration of about 5.5 months are described. When the original induction protocol fails, a rescue protocol can be used.

On a tight budget, all of the individual agents mentioned above can be used as rescue protocols, but the most popular in this setting are oral lomustine after a single dose of L-asparaginase or doxorubicin as a single agent, with response rates around 70% and mean remission times of 2–3 months. DMAC is a frequently used rescue protocol (dexamethasone, actinomycin D, cytarabine and melphalan), which has presented remission rates of up to 74% in reinduction with a mean duration of 2–3 months in high-grade B and T-cell lymphoma. Other protocols or reinduction agents are MOPP (mechlorethamine, procarbazine, vincristine, prednisolone) and L-asparaginase followed by lomustine as a single agent.

The use of carboplatin, melphalan or vinblastine as sole rescue agents has recently been described, as well as combinations of bleomycin and cytarabine, lomustine and procarbazine, temozolomide and doxorubicin. All these protocols have response rates of 30 to 60% and remission times between 15 days and 3.5 months.

Radiotherapy

In recent years, several studies have evaluated the role of radiotherapy in the treatment of canine lymphoma. **Lymphoma is very sensitive to radiation therapy**. Currently, the most common indication is the treatment of dogs with lymphoma located in a particular anatomical region, such as the nasal cavity, CNS, skin, etc., in combination with systemic chemotherapy. In emergency situations, lymphomas confined to a single anatomical region associated with severe clinical symptoms (anterior mediastinal lymphoma or CNS lymphomas) can be effectively treated and vital functions quickly restored.

Another possible scenario is the use of radiation in terminal situations, to treat chemotherapy-resistant lymphoma. Radiation alone usually produces short remission periods, but the patient may benefit in the short term. There are also studies that have evaluated whole-body radiation, divided into sequentially irradiated body halves and in combination with chemotherapy. The usefulness of this technique as an additional treatment to chemotherapy is still being researched. In addition, it must be remembered that whole-body radiation therapy can present subsequent haematological toxicity due to radiation received by the bone marrow.

Non-multicentric Anatomical Forms and Prognosis

Certain specific anatomical presentations of canine LSA may have very different therapies and prognoses compared to multicentric LSA.

Mediastinal lymphoma is the second most common presentation. It is usually associated with hypercalcaemia and with the T phenotype, for which historically it is also associated with shorter survival times. However, as previously discussed, certain protocols seem to produce better results for dogs with this phenotype. In this presentation, the clinical signs may be respiratory or related to high serum calcium levels (polyuria, polydipsia, lethargy).

Marginal zone or mantle cell splenic LSAs are both indolent forms of B-cell LSAs that primarily affect the spleen, often without further spread to other organs. Diagnosis requires histopathology and immunophenotyping. Associated lymphocytosis is often seen, and haemoabdomen may also develop. The survival rate after splenectomy one year after diagnosis is 75% without reaching the MST since most of the affected animals do not die from this disease. After surgery, chemotherapy treatment has no impact on prognosis as it is not recommended.

In splenic marginal zone lymphoma, the MST with splenectomy is 383 days; for asymptomatic dogs it is 1153 days. In a recent study, it was observed that metastases to lymph nodes, haemoabdomen, postoperative adjuvant chemotherapy, anaemia, and the presence of another tumour did not affect survival times.

Cutaneous epitheliotropic LSA is usually low-grade and of T-cell origin. It presents diffuse skin involvement, sometimes with peripheral lymphadenopathy. The highest responses with chemotherapy, of 80% have been described with oral lomustine and prednisolone instead of the traditional protocols with injectable drugs, but their mean duration is about 90 days with an MST of 130 days. The use of retinoids is also an option for this presentation and recent evidence supports treatment with the oral tyrosine kinase inhibitor masitinib when there is relapse, with responses of 40–70% and a duration between 2–3 months. It is interesting to know that when there are only isolated lesions, surgery or radiotherapy can be sufficient to control of the disease. For example, dogs with only oral mucocutaneous involvement without lymph node involvement have a MST of 770 days with radiotherapy. The MST of dogs with solitary lesions in the mucosa or mucocutaneous areas is 491 days with surgery or radiation and medical treatment. A small percentage of these cases can progress to circulating malignant cells in the blood, which is called Sézary syndrome.

Canine **alimentary lymphoma** has traditionally been associated with a poor prognosis. It usually presents with predominantly diffuse involvement of the gastrointestinal tract and treatment with CHOP-type chemotherapy is unsuccessful, with a MST of 77 days. On the other hand, 62% of responses have been described with the use of oral lomustine and survival times of 120 days and 354 days for dogs with a partial or complete response respectively to this treatment. Recently, a more favourable prognosis has been described for canine T-type low-grade alimentary lymphoma treated with alkylating agents and corticosteroids, with a MST of 628 days. On the other hand, if the LSA is limited to the large intestine (colon, rectum, or both), the prognosis with chemotherapy is excellent, with mean remission periods of 1318 days and a MST of 1845 days, with no differences in prognosis between the use of the COP or CHOP protocol. This makes the use of COP more attractive, since it is cheaper and produces fewer adverse effects.

Nasal lymphoma is very common in cats, but quite rare in dogs. If a case is diagnosed, it is important to know that, as in cats, they respond to combinations of radiotherapy and chemotherapy with a MST of 455 days. The response is associated with the grade of the lymphoma: thus, low-grade LSAs present a MST of 823 days.

When treating **primary central nervous system lymphoma or multicentric lymphoma with nervous or ocular system involvement**, it must be taken into account that it is extremely important to use drugs that cross the blood-brain barrier: cytarabine, lomustine, procarbazine, and temozolomide, in addition to corticosteroids. It should be taken into account that, with localised lesions, such as spinal lymphoma, radiotherapy can be very useful, as in combination with chemotherapy a rapid response can be achieved and provides median survival times of 179 days.

Staging: Does it Really Help with the Decision-making Process Regarding Treatment?

The economic factor can be a limiting factor for clinical staging of canine LSA. This is especially important when the cost of these tests could affect the owner's subsequent financial ability to perform the treatment. To this end, it is useful to be aware of in which situations staging would have an impact on the therapeutic approach and prognosis and in which situations this is unlikely.

Staging consists of **documenting the extent of the lymphoma in the patient and determining the corresponding stage** (Box 1).

Box 1. Classification of clinical staging for lymphoma in small animals according to the World Health Organization

- **Anatomical location**

A. multicentric
B. alimentary
C. thymic
D. cutaneous
E. leukaemia (only blood and bone marrow affected)
F. others (including renal).

- **Stage** (applicable to multicentric lymphoma)

I. Involvement of a single lymph node.
II. Involvement of several lymph nodes on one side of the diaphragm.
III. Generalised lymphadenopathy.
IV. Liver or spleen involvement (± stage III).
V. Presence in peripheral blood and bone marrow and/or other organs (± stage I–IV).

Each stage is subclassified in turn into:
a. no clinical signs
b. with clinical signs.

The minimum tests required before initiating therapy for canine LSA are a complete blood count with blood smear evaluation, blood chemistry, and urinalysis. Complete staging consists of imaging of the thorax and/or abdomen with or without fine needle aspirates of internal organs (liver and spleen). Most dogs with multicentric, non-diseased (substage-a) LSA, with a complete blood count and blood chemistry without clinically relevant abnormalities, are likely to be classified as stage III or IV, in which case their prognosis and treatment would be similar. Staging is particularly useful in cases of non-multicentric LSA, when all evidence of disease is in internal cavities.

One third to 50% of dogs with multicentric LSA will have bone marrow infiltration (stage V) at the time of diagnosis, but malignant circulating cells are not always seen in peripheral blood. Stage V correlates with a shorter MST when treated with chemotherapy protocols. Bone marrow infiltration can be determined when circulating malignant cells are seen in the blood smear. Performing PARR or flow cytometry in peripheral blood can confirm that these circulating cells are neoplastic and similar to those in peripheral ganglia, avoiding the need for bone marrow aspirates and therefore saving money.

When there are cytopaenias in peripheral blood, it may be due to infiltration of the bone marrow or to an immune-mediated cytopaenia secondary to LSA in the bone marrow, although the latter is uncommon. Bone marrow aspiration is helpful in these cases.

On a practical level, if the patient has clinically irrelevant cytopaenias, they are unlikely to have any impact on the treatment plan. If the dog presents severe neutropaenia, treatment with broad-spectrum antibiotics and non-immunosuppressive chemotherapy with L-asparaginase should be started, followed by the chosen protocol once the neutrophil count has returned to an appropriate level. Adequate production of platelets, white and red blood cells will not be restored until treatment decreases or eliminates a large percentage of malignant cells in the bone marrow. Some studies advocate the benefit of the use of continuous intravenous infusions (12–24 hours) of cytarabine as part of induction protocols for cases of LSA with bone marrow involvement.

Dogs with substage-b (with clinical symptoms at the time of diagnosis) have a worse prognosis, probably due to a more advanced form or critical involvement of vital body systems. Establishing the extent of the disease with imaging tests and internal organ sampling can help with modification of induction therapy, at least initially, to avoid more adverse effects or further deterioration.

Thoracic imaging tests are very useful when there are respiratory signs secondary to mediastinal masses or pleural effusion. In addition to visualising the disease, they allow samples to be obtained which can be used to reach a diagnosis if there is no external manifestation of the disease. Drugs that have a rapid effect, such as L-asparaginase and dexamethasone, can be used to initiate induction in these cases and achieve a rapid reduction in the size of the mediastinal mass, which can reduce or eliminate the pleural effusion rapidly.

When there are gastrointestinal signs, it is important to determine whether high-grade focal LSA in the form of intestinal or gastric masses is present using abdominal ultrasound. In this scenario, there may be a serious risk of ulceration or perforation when commencing chemotherapy treatment: the gastrointestinal mucosa will already be altered by the infiltration of neoplastic cells and when treatment begins, a large number of tumour cells infiltrating the intestine or stomach will be rapidly destroyed. Subsequently, there may be damage associated with the impact of chemotherapy on the gastrointestinal tract, which when healthy is a tissue with a high replication rate.

This means there is a higher risk of toxicity in this type of case. If known in advance, steps can be taken to avoid a higher rate of adverse effects, so initiating symptomatic gastrointestinal therapy before starting chemotherapy is helpful. Avoiding fast-acting medications (such as L-asparaginase) will also help, as well as considering the use of medications with a lower prevalence of gastrointestinal toxicity or decreasing drug doses, at least initially, until the patient shows a response to treatment.

In dogs with multicentric LSA that present with symptoms of liver dysfunction such as elevated ALT or clinically relevant bile acid levels, abdominal ultrasound examination and fine needle aspiration of the liver are helpful to determine if there is malignant liver involvement or concomitant liver disease.

Many medications used to treat LSA require liver activation (especially alkylating agents such as cyclophosphamide or lomustine) and often require liver inactivation as well (e.g. vinca alkaloids, alkylating agents, or tumour antibiotics such as doxorubicin). This could lead to reduced efficacy of the cytotoxic drug or increased adverse effects if hepatic metabolism is decreased. When starting treatment in these patients, the type of drugs which can be used is limited. Using reduced doses to avoid greater adverse effects should be considered, especially in cases of primary hepatic lymphoma.

Considerations in the Treatment of Specific Breeds

Some breeds, such as Collies, Shetland Sheepdogs, Australian Shepherds, etc., have a higher prevalence of mutations in the MDR (multidrug resistance) gene, which produces a decrease in cellular P-glycoprotein (GpP) and an increased risk of adverse effects after the administration of certain chemotherapeutic drugs. The test for the mutation can be performed on peripheral blood or saliva, depending on the laboratory. Drugs that are a known substrate for GpP should not be used in these patients until results are available. Once they are, if the patient is heterozygous or homozygous for the mutation, dose reductions of 25% are recommended before administering these substances and extreme precautions to prevent gastrointestinal toxicity are recommended.

Canine Lymphoid Leukaemia

Lymphoid leukaemia is the most relevant in the dog in terms of prevalence and knowledge of treatment and prognosis. It is defined as the proliferation of neoplastic cells in the bone marrow, although it can sometimes originate in the spleen. Most of the time, these cells are found circulating in the bloodstream, although in rare cases they may not be detected in the blood.

The diagnosis of leukaemia in general has been greatly optimised in recent years, with the use of flow cytometry and molecular techniques. On the other hand, there is very little information on the treatment and prognosis of leukaemia with the exception of chronic lymphocytic leukaemia (CLL). The distinction between true leukaemia and stage V lymphoma can be difficult and arbitrary and is often based on the absence of pronounced lymphadenopathy, the degree of bone marrow and peripheral blood involvement, and immunophenotypic features.

Incidence, Risk Factors, and Aetiology

Lymphoid leukaemia is more common than acute myeloid leukaemia and myeloproliferative disorders, although the actual incidence is unknown. Lymphoid leukaemia occurs most often in middle to old aged dogs (7–10 years). The aetiology of this disease is unknown, although it is probably associated with genetic factors. Retroviruses have been shown to be involved in the development of leukaemia in felines, bovines, fish, snakes, birds, rodents, non-human primates, and humans, but not in dogs. In people, acute lymphoblastic leukaemia (ALL) has been associated with several genetic factors, radiation, exposure to benzenes, phenylbutazone, and antineoplastic agents. Given the large difference in the immunophenotypic profile between canine and human leukaemia, an extrapolation of predisposing factors does not appear to be appropriate.

Pathology and Classification

Lymphoid leukaemia can be divided based on **cell size, degree of maturation, genetic aberrations, microRNA expression, and immunophenotype**. The simplest classification divides leukaemia into two groups: **chronic** (small cells with a mature cytological phenotype) and **acute** (large cells with an immature cytological phenotype). The immunophenotype is usually determined using flow cytometry.

There are three primary types of CLL described in the dog based on immunophenotype.

- **T-CLL**, which is the most common form. In most cases, the cells are large granular $CD8^+$ lymphocytes.
- **B-CLL**, which is the second most common type.
- **Atypical CLL**, representing a combination of immunophenotypes.

In humans, this disease is primarily type B lymphoid cells. In CLL, neoplastic cells are often morphologically indistinguishable from normal small lymphocytes and have a low proliferation rate. Hence the increase in circulating numbers, largely due to the long-life expectancy of these cells than because of the speed with which they proliferate.

The immunophenotype of ALL is most commonly of B origin ($CD21^+$, $CD3^-$, $CD4^-$, $CD8^-$), although there is a small percentage (<10%) that originate from T cells ($CD3^+$, $CD4^-$, $CD8^-$, $CD21^-$). In general, these cells are medium to large in size, with moderate amounts of basophilic cytoplasm.

Perhaps the most notable feature of lymphoblasts is the nuclear chromatin pattern, which is more condensed than chromatin in myeloblasts. The difficulty lies in the fact that, most of the time, immature ALL cells cannot be distinguished morphologically from immature cells from other haematopoietic lines, which is why a correct diagnosis usually requires the help of specific markers using immunocytochemistry or flow cytometry. If the cells express CD34, this stem cell marker implies the diagnosis of acute leukaemia, but the use of lymphoid (B or T) or myeloid (myeloperoxidase) markers to know the exact origin are necessary.

History and Clinical Signs

Dogs **affected by CLL are often asymptomatic**, but some owners describe lethargy and decreased appetite. Mild lymphadenopathy and splenomegaly may be seen, although in advanced stages splenomegaly may be marked. The white cell blood count is usually greater than 30 000 cells/µl but can range from a normal count up to more than 100 000 cells/µl. Lymphocytosis is persistent, and granulocytes are usually found in normal counts. In dogs with neoplastic lymphoid cell counts above 30 000 cells/µl, no other significant findings are usually found on the blood count. Sometimes CLL is accidentally diagnosed when the animal goes to the vet for an unrelated problem.

Mild anaemia, neutropaenia, and thrombocytopaenia may occur, which are more common and marked when the disease is advanced, and the patient has lymphocyte counts greater than 30 000 cells/µl. Although neoplastic cells are very similar to normal lymphocytes, they function abnormally. CLL-associated paraneoplastic syndromes such as monoclonal gammopathy, immune-mediated haemolytic anaemia, red blood cell aplasia, and rarely hypercalcaemia have been reported.

Dogs with ALL often present with clinical signs such as anorexia, weight loss, and lethargy. Splenomegaly is typical, and other findings may include bleeding, lymphadenopathy, and hepatomegaly. Infiltration of the bone marrow by neoplastic lymphoid cells can be extensive and result in a significant decrease in the components of other haematopoietic lines or myelophthisis. Anaemia, neutropaenia and thrombocytopaenia are much more serious than in CLL and often become a cause of mortality. Infiltration of extramedullary sites such as the CNS, bone, and gastrointestinal tract can occur, resulting in neuropathies, bone pain, and gastrointestinal symptoms.

Diagnosis and Clinical Staging

To make an accurate diagnosis, it is essential to jointly consider the characteristics of the patient, clinical history, findings on the physical examination and morphological appearance of the neoplastic cells, as well as the immunophenotype. When there are atypical lymphoid cells in circulation or if the immunophenotype of the circulating lymphocytes is homogeneous, in addition to being increased in number or if the clonality of the lymphocytes has been documented (for example, with PARR) lymphoid leukaemia should be suspected. Other differential diagnoses for lymphocytosis are infectious diseases such as chronic ehrlichiosis, postvaccine reactions in young dogs, administration of IL-2, epinephrine-induced or transient physiological lymphocytosis. Sometimes it is difficult to distinguish reactive lymphocytes from neoplastic ones, especially when the counts are only slightly outside the normal range.

Expansion and infiltration into the bone marrow is the hallmark of ALL and, in most cases, also of CLL. In cases with marked lymphocytosis with atypical cells, peripheral blood can be used to establish phenotypic analysis or clonality, without the need for bone marrow examination. Peripheral blood evaluation with smear evaluation and flow cytometry is important, since in most cases it can provide a definitive diagnosis. When performing a bone marrow aspirate, it is important that it be evaluated by an experienced cytopathologist to establish a diagnosis. Bone marrow biopsies are only useful when an adequate bone marrow aspirate has not been possible. In ALL, lymphoblasts predominate in the bone marrow and are also present in peripheral blood, with a decreased presence of other cell lines. In CLL, an expansion in the bone marrow of small mature lymphocytes (>30% of all nucleated cells) will be observed. In the case of T-CLL, eosinophilic granules can be seen within the neoplastic lymphocytes.

Although according to the WHO staging system all dogs with leukaemia are classified as stage V, this system has limited utility for this disease since, despite the fact that in most cases the leukaemia affects the bone marrow, the prognosis is very different depending on the type of leukaemia.

Treatment of CLL

The decision to treat CLL is **usually based on the patient's clinical signs and laboratory findings**. When CLL is diagnosed incidentally and there are no significant clinical signs or significant haematological abnormalities, most oncologists recommend monitoring with physical examination and a complete blood count without treatment. Treatment is usually started if the animal is anaemic or thrombocytopaenic, has significant lymphadenomegaly or hepatosplenomegaly, or has a high lymphocyte count (>60 000 cells/µl). It should be recognised that the term "high lymphocyte count" is arbitrary and there is no medically standard count established for starting treatment. The author prefers to make treatment decisions based on the presence of relevant clinical signs and/or blood cytopaenias.

Treatment consists of chlorambucil (2 mg/m² PO every other day or 20 mg/m² PO every 20 weeks) and prednisolone (20 mg/m² PO every other day). The dose and regimen of chlorambucil should be adjusted according to the response and tolerance of the bone marrow. When CLL is refractory to this treatment, the use of cyclophosphamide or lomustine may be considered instead of chlorambucil. CLL treatment is palliative with rare complete remissions due to the somewhat indolent nature of the disease, however, this explains why survival periods are between one and three years with a good quality of life. The rare possibility of CLL that evolves into an acute phase with the development of a fast-growing type of lymphoma, with rapid progression, characterised by the presence of immunoblasts in the bloodstream, has been described; in people this is called Richter syndrome. The prognosis for treatment in this phase is poor.

Treatment of ALL

Most of the clinical signs in dogs with ALL derive from invasion and spread into the bone marrow, with the development of severe cytopaenias that can often result in death. Neutropaenia, thrombocytopaenia, and anaemia can be quite serious in these patients, requiring intensive supportive therapy with blood transfusions, broad-spectrum antibiotics, fluid therapy, and nutritional support. Monitoring for the possible development of sepsis, haemorrhage, and DIC is important.

The treatment of ALL requires aggressive chemotherapy to reduce the volume of neoplastic cells in the bone marrow and stabilise the patient, although on the other hand there are no protocols that have been consistently effective in veterinary medicine. The same protocols are used as for multicentric lymphoma, often including asparaginase or cytarabine infusions. Usually the biggest problem is that, although there is usually a response to treatment, the duration of this response is generally short-lived. In affected people, the standard treatment of acute leukaemia includes bone marrow transplants, which are not usually available in veterinary oncology.

Prognosis

CLL is a slow, progressive disease, and some animals do not require therapy for some time, even years. For cases in which treatment is administered, the normalisation of the lymphocyte count occurs in 70% of cases. The mean survival time described is 930 days for T-CLL, 480 days for B-CLL and 22 days for atypical CLL. Young age and anaemia were considered negative prognostic factors. In another study that included immunophenotyping results, it was found that dogs with CD8⁺ CLL and <30 000 cells/µl had median survival times of 1098 days.

The **prognosis for ALL is generally poor**. In a study with 21 dogs treated with vincristine and prednisone, 30% achieved a complete or partial response and the median survival time was 120 days This is very similar to 129 days regardless of the treatment protocol used in a study of dogs with B-cell ALL. In another study that used CHOP as a treatment, the survival time range ranged from 3 to 128 days with a mean of 16 days. A more recent study in dogs with acute leukaemia found that in 36 dogs that received cytotoxic therapy, 23 went into complete or partial remission for a mean of 56 days (range 3–218 days). Median survival time for treated dogs was 55 days (range 1–300 days), with most animals rapidly developing resistance to it. Dogs that were not treated or that received only palliative treatment had a mean survival time of 7.5 days.

Plasma Cell Tumours and Multiple Myeloma

Plasma cell tumours **arise when precursors to B lymphocytes or plasma cells undergo malignant transformation**. There are several clinical entities within this group, among which **multiple myeloma (MM)**, **solitary bone plasmacytoma** or **extramedullary plasmacytoma stand out**.

Multiple Myeloma

MM is a **relatively rare** lymphoproliferative disease, accounting for less than 8% of haematopoietic tumours. There does not appear to be any breed or sex predisposition and geriatric dogs are more frequently affected. In the case of cats, it is less frequent, with an average age of occurrence of 12 to 14 years.

The causes of the disease are largely unknown, although it is believed that cellular control mechanisms such as overexpression of the cell cycle control component (cyclin D1) and dysregulations in tyrosine kinase receptors may be involved in the development of these tumours. It should also be noted that isolated cases of progression from solitary plasma cell tumours to MM, as well as progression from B-cell lymphoma to MM, have been described, but this occurs rarely.

Pathology

MM is a tumour characterised by the infiltration and growth of clonal plasma cells at different points in the bone marrow (BM). In the case of cats, on many occasions the classic presentation of MM that is seen in dogs does not occur, in which the bone marrow is mainly affected, but there is abundant involvement of the abdominal organs without involvement of BM. This makes the disease more difficult to diagnose in cats if only BM samples are taken.

Being a clonal expansion of neoplastic cells, these plasma cells produce the same type of immunoglobulin called paraprotein, monoclonal protein or, M component. This paraprotein can be detected in conventional laboratory protein electrophoresis as a monoclonal peak and can be represented by the heavy or light (Bence Jones protein) immunoglobulin chains. IgA and IgG gammopathies are the most common in dogs and cats; IgM (Waldenström's macroglobulinaemia) is quite rare. In dogs, the ratio of IgG to IgA is similar, but IgG is much more common in cats (4:1).

It is important to remember that there are other pathologies in dogs and cats that can cause a monoclonal gammopathy: MGUS (monoclonal gammopathy of undetermined significance), chronic infection (FIP, ehrlichiosis, pyoderma, leishmaniasis) and other lymphoid-type tumours (B-cell lymphoma, chronic and acute lymphoid leukaemia). The pathological findings associated with MM are the result of high levels of paraprotein in the blood, infiltration of organs with neoplastic cells, or both at the same time. Possible clinical signs are bone disease, bleeding diathesis, hyperviscosity syndrome, kidney disease, hypercalcaemia, immunodeficiency, cytopaenia secondary to myelophthisis, and heart failure.

Hyperviscosity syndrome is due to increased blood viscosity due to the high concentration of circulating paraprotein, manifesting as neurological signs, retinopathy, and cardiomyopathy. IgA and IgM are the most frequently associated with this presentation because they form dimers (IgA) and pentamers (IgM). Heart failure can occur due to increased cardiac load and cardiac hypoxia caused by hyperviscosity. In studies in cats, it has been seen that up to 2/3 of them had cardiomegaly on radiographs, and half of them had heart murmurs.

Osteolytic lesions associated with MM include the typical areas of malignant osteolysis with a "punched out" appearance or, less frequently, generalised osteopaenia. They are mainly located in flat bones and are frequent in vertebral bodies and spinous processes, but also in the pelvis and ribs. These injuries can be associated with bone pain, spinal cord compression, pathologic fractures, and hypercalcaemia. Only 50% of dogs affected by MM present radiographic evidence of bone disease, the incidence in cats is not clear. An attempt can be made to increase the probability of detection by performing radiological studies of both the thorax and abdomen. CT is more sensitive, although serial radiological studies are still preferred in human medicine.

When **bleeding diathesis** is observed, it is the consequence of different factors, such as thrombocytopathies and the interaction of paraprotein with coagulation factors. Approximately 1/3 of dogs and cats show signs of bleeding (epistaxis, intraocular bleeding or bleeding of the gums among others). Clotting times are frequently increased and thrombocytopaenia is present in up to 50% of cases.

Regarding **haematological abnormalities**, one of the most frequent findings on the complete blood count is a non-regenerative normochromic normocytic anaemia, which can be caused by multiple mechanisms such as coagulopathies, chronic disease, myelophthisis or destruction of red blood cells. Pancytopaenia may be seen in cases where the bone marrow is severely affected, although this occurs very rarely at diagnosis.

Hypercalcaemia may be the consequence of osseous resorption (mediated by tumour necrosis factor alpha (TNF–α) and interleukins 1, 2 and 6 secreted by plasma cells), and be associated with malignancy (PTHrp secreted by plasma cells) or be caused by hyperglobulinaemia. Hyperglobulinaemia can cause calcium to bind to paraprotein while maintaining normal ionised calcium, so it is vital to assess ionised calcium in these cases.

MM-associated **kidney disease** occurs only in 1/3 of cases. The two most common mechanisms are hypercalcaemia and circulating immunoglobulin light chains that damage tubules and cause inflammation. Despite the abundance of antibodies in the blood, they are usually not functional, and this can predispose animals with MM to bacterial infections. In addition, if the bone marrow is affected (myelophthisis) with an increased production of malignant plasma cells, the rest of leucocyte components may be reduced and, as a consequence, the predisposition to develop infections increases.

Clinical Signs

The duration of clinical signs before diagnosis is highly variable, but the average duration is usually at least one month. The most common clinical signs in order of frequency include lethargy and weakness, lameness, bleeding diathesis, abnormalities on fundus examination, polyuria/polydipsia, and neurologic deficits.

Diagnosis and Staging

The diagnosis of MM is usually based on the presence of plasmacytosis in the bone marrow, the presence of lytic lesions, and the detection of M component. A minimum database should be obtained at diagnosis with complete blood count and biochemical profile, as well as urinalysis, to establish if there are any of the most frequent findings described above (azotaemia, anaemia, hypercalcaemia, hyperglobulinaemia, etc.).

A urine culture should be submitted from these patients to rule out a subclinical urinary infection, given their predisposition to developing infections. Both blood and urine samples can be sent for a proteinogram. A blood proteinogram usually reveals a monoclonal gammopathy with a peak in the beta or gamma zone or, less frequently, a biclonal gammopathy. Urine can also be tested for small chain proteins using the Bence Jones precipitation method or immunoelectrophoresis. Urine test strips are not useful, since the proteinuria that is detected is mainly albumin. If only Bence Jones proteinuria is detected in urine without a monoclonal peak in blood, it is diagnostic for light chain MM. Abdominal radiographs or ultrasound are used to evaluate possible spleen and liver involvement. Splenic involvement is common in feline MM (85%) and can also be seen in dogs. In addition, they can facilitate the detection of lytic bone lesions.

Normally, to reach a diagnosis of MM at least two of the criteria described in Box 2 should be present in the patient, although a definitive diagnosis can be made simply if it is shown that there is an excess of plasma cells in the bone marrow and/or in the spleen.

Box 2. Criteria for diagnosing MM (at least two must be met)

- **Monoclonal gammopathy.**
- **Radiographic evidence of osteolytic bone lesions.**
- **>5% neoplastic cells or >10–20% plasma cells in the bone marrow.**
- **Light chain proteinuria (Bence Jones).**
- **Infiltration of visceral organs (spleen) with >5% neoplastic cells or >10–20% plasma cells.**

Treatment

Treatment of patients with MM is aimed at **killing tumour cells, but also treating the systemic symptoms** that patients present. That is why patients usually need aggressive fluid therapy in cases in which it is required to control azotaemia, hypercalcaemia or preexisting dehydration in some cases.

Antibiotics are also necessary in cases with clinical or subclinical infections secondary to MM-induced immunosuppression. The use of analgesics such as gabapentin or paracetamol-codeine is usually necessary in patients who present lytic lesions since, although there are no visible signs of associated pain, these lesions are usually quite painful. Radiation is very effective in treating large osteolytic foci in the case of plasma cell neoplasia, albeit palliatively. It is more effective than medical treatment in alleviating the pain and discomfort associated with these injuries.

In cases of hyperviscosity syndrome, it usually resolves after a few months of commencing cytotoxic drug therapy. In cases in which there is a serious clinical sign that requires rapid medical action, plasmapheresis can be useful, which consists of extracting blood from the patient and separating the different components, and then removing the plasma and reintroducing it, however, this technique has limited availability in veterinary practices.

Chemotherapy

Most dogs with this disease respond very well to treatment. In the case of cats half respond to cytotoxic therapy and there are few long-term survivors. The median survival time in dogs is 540 days, with a treatment based on alkylating agents, such as **melphalan, combined with prednisolone** (1.5 mg/kg PO BID for 1–2 weeks and then every other day).

The most frequently used dose of melphalan is 6–8 mg PO/m²/24 h for 5 consecutive days, repeating an administration cycle every 3 weeks. Control blood counts can be done every 3 weeks for the first 2–3 months and every 2 cycles thereafter is considered reasonable. Immunoglobulin levels will be monitored and should gradually decrease to or approach near normal levels, although melphalan therapy at these doses and the proposed regimen is not very immunosuppressive and neutropaenias are rarely seen. On the other hand, the platelet count should be evaluated since the chronic use of melphalan can cause cumulative thrombocytopaenia, usually after months of therapy. If this is the case, the medication should be discontinued until platelet levels return to normal.

The other published dosing schedule is 0.1 mg/kg for 10 days and then 0.05 mg/kg once daily. It is more intense than the one previously described, which is why it is often used only if the former does not achieve complete remission. It should be borne in mind that the normalisation of neoplastic immunoglobulin production does not occur rapidly in most cases, but rather after months of therapy, given that MM is usually a well-differentiated neoplasm with a low proliferation rate.

In the treatment of MM in dogs in situations of resistance to initial treatment with melphalan, other alkylating agents such as **cyclophosphamide or lomustine** are used. The VAD protocol (vincristine, doxorubicin, and dexamethasone) has also been described, but with few results.

New agents such as **thalidomide and toceranib** may offer therapeutic benefits in this disease. In the case of thalidomide, it is one of the most widely used drugs in humans and Palladia® has been shown to have biological activity in at least one dog. In sick patients in whom a much faster response is required, a single dose of IV cyclophosphamide can be given at the same time as melphalan for a faster response (200 mg/m²).

In cats, melphalan has a fair immunosuppressive effect and severe myelosuppression is often seen with this treatment. Therefore, **chlorambucil** is often used at a dose of 20 mg/m² every 2 weeks or 2 mg total dose per cat every other day, combined with prednisolone (1.5 mg/kg PO BID for 1–2 weeks and then every two days). When melphalan is used in cats, the dose is 0.1 mg/kg (or 0.5 mg total dose) for 10–14 days and then every other day until the animal improves or cytopaenias occur.

Response Monitoring

The improvement in clinical signs and laboratory tests usually occurs in the first 4–8 weeks of treatment. A complete remission is considered present when serum immunoglobulin levels return to normal values, while a partial remission is classified where there is a 50% reduction.

If there are visible lesions on physical examination or imaging tests, they should also be monitored to see if there is resolution or a partial response.

Prognosis

The response rate in dogs is close to 92% with 43% achieving a complete response and 48% a partial response, with a median survival time of 540 days. In comparison, cases that are only treated with prednisolone have a median survival time of 220 days. Some of the negative prognostic factors in dogs include hypercalcaemia, light chain proteinuria, and extensive osteolytic lesions.

The response to and the duration of therapy appears much more variable in the case of cats. In this species, negative prognostic factors are pathological fractures associated with lytic bone lesions, anaemia, light chain proteinuria, azotaemia, and poor response to treatment.

Solitary or Extramedullary Plasma Cell Tumours

These are plasma cell neoplasms that can originate in soft tissue (**extramedullary plasmacytoma, EMP**) or bone (**osseus extramedullary plasmacytoma, OEP**).

The most common location of EMP is cutaneous (86%) or in the oral and lip mucosa (9%), although it can also appear in other portions of the gastrointestinal tract such as the rectum or colon (4%) or, more rarely, the oesophagus, stomach, or small intestine. Cutaneous EMPs are generally benign, and the treatment of choice is local therapy with surgery, although they may also respond to radiotherapy. EMPs that are not cutaneous or oral may show more aggressive behaviour, with metastases to regional nodes. Colorectal EMPs tend to show less aggressive behaviour, and most do not recur after resection, with median survival times of 15 months.

The treatment of OEP, which can be located in the appendicular skeleton, ribs or skull, consists of aggressive surgery with margins clear of tumour cells; a percentage of these cases will progress to MM after months or years, for which they are treated with chemotherapy after resection. Protocols based on prednisolone and melphalan can be used, as well as for those with recurring EMP or metastasis.

On the other hand, the recurrence rate after incomplete resection in cutaneous and oral mucocutaneous EMPs is only 5% with only 2% developing metastases.

Canine Cutaneous Plasmacytosis

Canine cutaneous plasmacytosis is a recently described syndrome with **multiple cutaneous plasmacytomas and absence of MM**.

The most commonly affected breeds are the Golden Retriever and Labrador Retriever. Most of the cases described have more than 10 lesions, with some presenting more than 100. The lesions are round, raised, pink or reddish, variably alopecic, and sometimes ulcerated.

The response to prednisolone and melphalan is 73.7% and the response to lomustine is 71.4%. The mean time to disease progression is 153 days and the mean survival time is 542 days.

Bibliography

■ Álvarez, F.J., Kisseberth, W.C., Gallant, S.L. et al. (2006) Dexamethasone, melphalan, actinomycin D, cytosine arabinoside (DMAC) protocol for dogs with relapsed lymphoma. *J Vet Intern Med*, 20(5):1178–83.

■ Avery, P.R., Burton, J., Bromberek, J.L. et al. (2014) Flow cytometric characterization and clinical outcome of CD4+ T-cell lymphoma in dogs: 67 cases. *J Vet Intern Med*, 28(2):538–46.

■ Batschinski, K., Dervisis, N., Kitchell, B. et al. (2018) Combination of Bleomycin and Cytosine Arabinoside Chemotherapy for Relapsed Canine Lymphoma. *J Am Anim Hosp Assoc.* doi: 10.5326/JAAHA-MS-6617.

■ Beaver, L.M., Strottner, G., Klein, M.K. (2010) Response rate after administration of a single dose of doxorubicin in dogs with B-cell or T-cell lymphoma: 41 cases (2006–2008). *J Am Vet Med Assoc*, 237(9):1052–5.

■ Bennett AL, Williams LE, Ferguson MW, et al. (2017) Canine acute leukaemia: 50 cases (1989-2014). *Vet Comp Oncol*, 15(3):1101–1114.

■ Berlato, D., Schrempp, D., Van Den Steen, N. et al. (2012) Radiotherapy in the management of localized mucocutaneous oral lymphoma in dogs: 14 cases. *Vet Comp Oncol*, 10(1):16–23.

■ Boostrom, B.O., Moore, A.S., DeRegis, C.J. et al. (2017) Canine Cutaneous Plasmacytosis: 21 Cases (2005–2015). *J Vet Intern Med*, 31(4):1074–1080.

■ Brodsky, E.M., Maudlin, G.N., Lachowicz, J.L. et al. (2009) Asparaginase and MOPP Treatment of Dogs with Lymphoma. *J Vet Intern Med*, 23(3): 578–584.

■ Brown, P.M., Tzannes, S., Nguyen, S. et al. (2018) LOPP chemotherapy as a first-line treatment for dogs with T-cell lymphoma. *Vet Comp Oncol*, 16(1):108–113.

■ Couto, K.M., Moore, P.F., Zwingenberger, A.L. et al. (2018) Clinical characteristics and outcome in dogs with small cell T-cell intestinal lymphoma. *Vet Comp Oncol.* doi: 10.1111/vco.12384.

■ Comazzi, S., Martini, V., Riondato, F. et al. (2017) Chronic lymphocytic leukemia transformation into high-grade lymphoma: a description of Richter's syndrome in eight dogs. *Vet Comp Oncol*, 15(2):366–373.

■ Comazzi, S., Gelain, M.E., Martini, V. et al. (2011) Immunophenotype predicts survival time in dogs with chronic lymphocytic leukemia. *J Vet Intern Med*, 25(1):100–6.

■ Davies, O., Szladovits, B., Polton, G. et al. (2017) Prognostic significance of clinical presentation, induction and rescue treatment in 42 cases of canine centroblastic diffuse large B-cell multicentric lymphoma in the United Kingdom. *Vet Comp Oncol.* doi: 10.1111/vco.12378.

■ Desmas, I., Burton, J.H., Post, G. et al. (2017) A. Clinical presentation, treatment and outcome in 31 dogs with presumed primary colorectal lymphoma (2001–2013). *Vet Comp Oncol*, 15(2):504–517.

■ Childress, M.O., Ramos-Vara, J.A., Ruple, A. (2018) Retrospective analysis of factors affecting clinical outcome following CHOP-based chemotherapy in dogs with primary nodal diffuse large B-cell lymphoma. *Vet Comp Oncol*, 16(1):E159–E168.

■ Flory, A.B., Rassnick, K.M., Erb, H.N. et al. (2011) Evaluation of factors associated with second remisión in dogs with lymphoma undergoing retreatment with a cyclophosphamide, doxorubicin, vincristine, and prednisone chemotherapy protocol: 95 cases (2000–2007). *J Am Vet Med Assoc*, 238(4):501–6.

■ Gillem, J., Giuffrida, M., Krick, E. (2017) Efficacy and toxicity of carboplatin and cytarabine chemotherapy for dogs with relapsed or refractory lymphoma (2000–2013). *Vet Comp Oncol*, 15(2):400–410.

■ George, R., Smith, A., Schleis, S. et al. (2016) Outcome of dogs with intranasal lymphoma treated with various radiation and chemotherapy protocols: 24 cases. *Vet Radiol Ultrasound*, 57(3):306–312.

■ Goodman, I.H., Moore, A.S., Frimberger, A.E. (2016) Treatment of canine non-indolent T cell lymphoma using the VELCAP-TSC protocol: A retrospective evaluation of 70 dogs (2003–2013). Vet J, 211:39–44.

■ Holtermann, N., Kiupel, M., Kessler, M. et al (2016) Masitinib monotherapy in canine epitheliotropic lymphoma. *Vet Comp Oncol*, 14 Suppl1:127–35.

■ Hosoya, K., Kisseberth, W.C., Lord, L.K. et al. (2007) Comparison of COAP and UW-19 protocols for dogs with multicentric lymphoma. *J Vet Intern Med*, 21(6):1355–63.

■ Lana, S.E., Jackson, T.L., Burnett, R.C. et al. (2006) Utility of polymerase chain reaction for analysis of antigen receptor rearrangement in staging and predicting prognosis in dogs with lymphoma. *J Vet Intern Med*, 20(2):329–34.

■ Lenz, J.A., Robat, C.S., Stein, T.J. (2016) Vinblastine as a second rescue for the treatment of canine multicentric lymphoma in 39 cases (2005 to 2014). *J Small Anim Pract*, 57(8):429–434.

■ Marconato, L., Bonfanti, U., Stefanello, D. et al. (2008) Cytosine arabinoside in addition to VCAA-based protocols for the treatment of canine lymphoma with bone marrow involvement: does it make the difference? *Vet Comp Oncol*, 6(2):80–9.

■ Martinez de Merlo, E.M., Royón Mayordomo, E. (2018) Diagnóstico del linfoma canino y clasificación en subtipos de importancia pronóstica. *Canis y felis*, 152:6–15.

■ Mastromauro, M.L., Suter, S.E., Hauck, M.L., Hess, P.R. (2018) Oral melphalan for the treatment of relapsed canine lymphoma. *Vet Comp Oncol*, 16(1):E123–E129.

■ Mealey, K.L., Meurs, K.M. (2008) Breed distribution of the ABCB1-1Delta (multidrug sensitivity) polymorphism among dogs undergoing ABCB1 genotyping. *J Am Vet Med Assoc*, 233(6):921–4.

■ Modiano, J.F., Breen. M., Burnett, R.C. et al. (2005) Distinct B-cell and T-cell lymphoproliferative disease prevalence among dog breeds indicates heritable risk. *Cancer Res*, 65(13):5654–61.

■ O'Brien, D., Moore, P.F., Vernau, W., et al. (2013) Clinical characteristics and outcome in dogs with splenic marginal zone lymphoma. *J Vet Intern Med*, 27(4):949–54.

■ Ponce, F., Magnol, J.P., Ledieu, D. et al. (2004) Prognostic significance of morphological subtypes in canine malignant lymphomas during chemotherapy. *Vet J*, 167(2):158–66.

■ Ponce, F., Marchal, T., Magnol, J.P. et al. (2010) A morphological study of 608 cases of canine malignant lymphoma in France with a focus on comparative similarities between canine and human lymphoma morphology. *Vet Pathol*, 47(3):414–33.

■ Rassnick, K.M., Moore, A.S., Collister, K.E. et al. (2009) Efficacy of combination chemotherapy for treatment of gastrointestinal lymphoma in dogs. *J Vet Intern Med*, 23(2):317–22.

■ Rebhun, R.B., Kent, M.S., Borrofka, S.A. et al (2011) CHOP chemotherapy for the treatment of canine multicentric T-cell lymphoma. *Vet Comp Oncol*, 9(1):38–44.

■ Risbon, R.E., de Lorimier, L.P., Skorupski, K. et al. (2006) Response of canine cutaneous epitheliotropic lymphoma to lomustine (CCNU): a retrospective study of 46 cases (1999–2004). *J Vet Intern Med*, 20(6):1389–97.

■ Rout, E.D., Avery, P.R. (2017) Lymphoid Neoplasia: Correlations Between Morphology and Flow Cytometry. *Vet Clin North Am Small Anim Pract*, 47(1):53–70.

■ Saba, C.F., Hafeman, S.D., Vail, D.M. et al. (2009) Combination chemotherapy with continuous L-asparaginase, lomustine, and prednisone for relapsed canine lymphoma. *J Vet Intern Med*, 23(5):1058–1063.

■ Seelig, D.M., Avery, P., Webb, T. et al. (2014) Canine T-zone lymphoma: unique immunophenotypic features, outcome, and population characteristics. *J Vet Intern Med*, 28(3):878–86.

■ Simon, D., Moreno, S.N., Hirschberger, J. (2008) Efficacy of a continuous, multiagent chemotherapeutic protocol versus a short-term single-agent protocol in dogs with lymphoma. *J Am Vet Med Assoc*, 232(6):879–85.

■ Treggiari, E., Elliott, J.W., Baines, S.J. et al. (2017) Temozolomide alone or in combination with doxorubicin as a rescue agent in 37 cases of canine multicentric lymphoma. *Vet Comp Oncol*. doi: 10.1111/vco.12335.

■ Vail, D.M, Young, K.M. (2013) *Hematopoyetic tumors, Section A, Canine Lymphoma and Lymphoid leukemia.* In: Withrow, S.J., Vail, D.M. (eds): Withrow and MacEwen's Small Animal Clinical Oncology, 5th Ed, St Louis, Saunder-Elsevier, pp. 608–638.

■ Valli, V.E., Vernau, W., de Lorimier, L.P. (2006) Canine indolent nodular lymphoma. *Vet Pathol*, 43(3):241–56.

■ Valli, V.E., Kass, P.H., San Myint, M. (2013) Canine lymphomas: association of classification type, disease stage, tumor subtype, mitotic rate, and treatment with survival. *Vet Pathol*, 50(5):738–48.

■ van Stee, L.L., Boston, S.E., Singh, A. et al. (2015) Outcome and Prognostic Factors for Canine Splenic Lymphoma Treated by Splenectomy (1995–2011). *Vet Surg*, 44(8):976–82.

■ Wilkerson, M.J., Dolce, K., Koopman, T. (2005) Lineage differentiation of canine lymphoma/leukemias and aberrant expression of CD molecules. *Vet Immunol Immunopathol*, 106(3–4):179–96.

TEST

ANSWERS ON PAGE 146

1. **Which of the following techniques could be used to differentiate if the following image corresponds to lymphoid hyperplasia or lymphoma on a lymph node cytology?**
   a. Flow cytometry.
   b. PARR.
   c. Immunohistochemistry.
   d. Immunocytochemistry.

2. **Which of the following types of canine multicentric lymphoma has an indolent course?**
   a. Diffuse large B-cell lymphoma (DLBCL).
   b. Peripheral T-cell lymphoma.
   c. T-zone lymphoma.
   d. Epitheliotropic T-cell lymphoma.

3. **Regarding the treatment of canine multicentric lymphoma, which of the following statements is correct?**
   a. Diffuse type B large cell lymphoma (DLBCL) presents mean remission periods of 252 days when treated with CHOP-type protocols (Madison-Wisconsin).
   b. Peripheral T-cell lymphoma (PTCL) has response rates of 90% to Madison-Wisconsin-type protocols.
   c. COP-like protocols provide the longest median remission times for PTCL, at 252 days.
   d. LOPP-like protocols are associated with remission times of 175–200 days in dogs with DLBCL.

4. **Regarding the different anatomical forms of canine lymphoma, which of the following statements is correct?**
   a. Mediastinal lymphoma is usually associated with immunophenotype B.
   b. Colorectal lymphoma shows short, brief responses to chemotherapy.
   c. The most common cutaneous lymphoma is immunophenotype B non-epitheliotropic lymphoma.
   d. Lymphoma involving the central nervous system requires the use of drugs that cross the blood-brain barrier.

5. **Among the prognostic factors for feline alimentary lymphoma, the most important positive prognostic factor is:**
   a. Presence of anaemia.
   b. Immunophenotype B.
   c. That the lymphoma is large granular cell lymphoma.
   d. Existence of response to treatment.

6. **Which of the following statements regarding the treatment of feline digestive lymphoma is correct?**
   a. Large granular cell lymphoma has remission times of 7–10 months with CHOP protocols.
   b. Low-grade lymphoma responds to treatment with chlorambucil and corticosteroids with survival times of more than 2 years.
   c. High/intermediate-grade lymphoma responds to CHOP-type protocols with survivals of more than 2 years.
   d. Low-grade lymphoma responds to COP protocols with remission times of 7–10 months.

7. **What is the most common primary type of chronic lymphoid leukaemia?**
   a. T-CLL $CD4^+$.
   b. T-CLL $CD8^+$.
   c. Atypical T-CLL.
   d. B-CLL.

8. **Regarding the treatment and prognosis of lymphoid leukaemia, which of the following statements is true?**
   a. CLL is always treated with chemotherapy, usually with COP protocols.
   b. Treatment of ALL with protocols such as COP or CHOP achieves survival times of about 3 months.
   c. Median survival for CLL is less than a year.
   d. ALL only requires treatment if the dog shows any clinical signs.

9. **Which of the following clinical signs is not one of the criteria used for the diagnosis of multiple myeloma?**
   a. Monoclonal gammopathy.
   b. Radiographic evidence of osteolytic bone lesions.
   c. >5% neoplastic cells or >10–20% plasma cells in the bone marrow.
   d. Hypercalcaemia.

10. **The first line of treatment for canine multiple myeloma is:**
   a. The VAD protocol.
   b. Cyclophosphamide and vincristine.
   c. Prednisone and melphalan.
   d. Protocols that include doxorubicin.

Clinical Case

An 11-year-old neutered male Border Collie arrives for a consultation. He has presented with severe generalised lymphadenopathy and splenomegaly on abdominal palpation for 10 days, as well as polyuria and polydipsia for the last 4 days. Vital signs are normal, including body temperature.

1. **The primary differential diagnosis is lymphoma. Which of the tests presented below would allow a diagnosis to be reached and to establish the immunophenotype of this lymphoma?**
   a. Histopathology.
   b. Cytology.
   c. Cytology plus histopathology.
   d. Cytology plus flow cytometry.

2. **Fine needle aspiration and corresponding cytology of several peripheral nodes is performed with results that are compatible with high-grade lymphoma (Figure A). Which of the following statements is true for high-grade lymphomas?**
   a. The most common are type B and progress slowly.
   b. The most common are type T and progress rapidly.
   c. The most common are type B and progress rapidly.
   d. They are usually indolent in nature and progress slowly.

3. **Based on the findings of the physical examination, what stage of lymphoma would this dog present and what impact would it have on the prognosis?**
   a. Stage 2 with a better prognosis than higher stages.
   b. Stage 3 with a better prognosis than higher stages.
   c. Stage 4 with a better prognosis than higher stages.
   d. Stage 5 with a worse prognosis than lower stages.

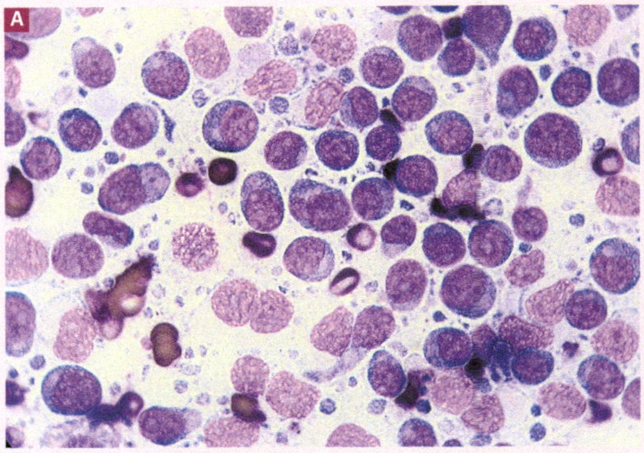

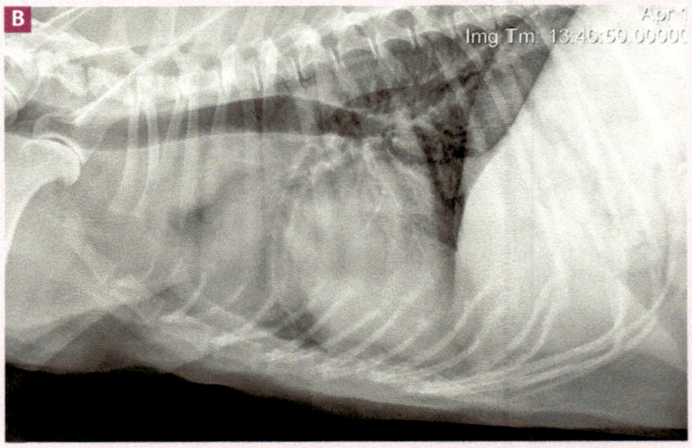

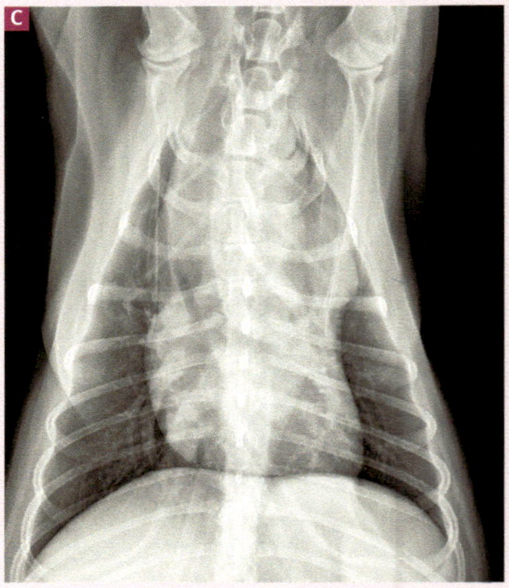

4. Blood count and biochemistry are performed, as well as staging with thoracic radiographs (Figures B and C) and abdominal ultrasound. What effects on the diagnosis could the information obtained have?

a. It is still stage 4, so the prognosis does not change.
b. Hypercalcaemia is more likely in T-cell lymphomas.
c. Thoracic findings are more common with B-cell lymphoma.
d. Anaemia and thrombocytopaenia are typical of T-cell lymphoma.

5. This dog is a Border Collie. What should be taken into consideration before starting chemotherapy treatment?

a. Test for MDR mutation.
b. No special considerations.
c. This breed is more prone to type B lymphoma.
d. This breed is more prone to type T lymphoma.

6. What type of chemotherapy protocol would be an appropriate choice for this patient if only considering the grade of the lymphoma, the most probable immunophenotype, and the clinical stage?

a. A Madison-Wisconsin protocol, since the immunophenotype does not affect the response and the combination of cytotoxic drugs is more effective in high-grade lymphomas, as they have a high replication rate.
b. A LOPP protocol, since the immunophenotype does affect the response and the combination of cytotoxic drugs is more effective in high-grade lymphomas, as they have a high replication rate.
c. A protocol with only doxorubicin, since the immunophenotype does not affect the response and the combination of cytotoxic drugs is less effective in high-grade lymphomas, as they have a low replication rate.
d. A protocol with only chlorambucil, since the immunophenotype does not affect the response and the combination of cytotoxic drugs is less effective in low-grade lymphomas, as they have a low replication rate.

Correct answers:

Test

1. b
2. c
3. a
4. d
5. d
6. b
7. a
8. b
9. d
10. c

Clinical Case

1. d
2. c
3. c
4. b
5. a
6. b

Notes

Mast Cell Tumours, Skin Neoplasms, Soft-tissue Sarcomas, and Feline Injection Site Sarcoma

Mónica Clemente

Canine Mast Cell Tumours

Mast cells come from the bone marrow and migrate to peripheral tissues where, under the influence of local cytokines, they differentiate into mature mast cells. Mast cells are present in almost all normal animal tissues. They are occasionally found in the bone marrow, but never in the systemic circulation, under normal circumstances. Mast cell tumours (MCTs) are neoplastic proliferations of mast cells. Cutaneous mast cell tumours arise from tissue mast cells in the dermis and subcutaneous tissue.

Incidence and Predisposition

MCTs are the most common skin tumour in dogs: 16–21% of all skin tumours and their appearance is extremely varied. They are usually solitary tumours, although some dogs can present with multiple. The mean age of onset is 9 years of age, but they have been described in dogs from 3 weeks to 19 years old. There is no sex predisposition.

Some breeds are at higher risk: Boxer, Bulldog, Pug, Boston Terrier (and terriers in general), Labrador, and Golden Retriever and Shar Pei. In one study, Boxers and Boston Terriers accounted for more than 50% of dogs with MCT. Shar Pei's often have highly malignant MCTs, which often appear in young dogs. Pugs, Boston Terriers, and Boxers can develop multiple MCTs during their life, but most of then tend to develop low-grade MCTs.

Aetiology

The aetiology of mast cell tumours is unknown and is **probably multifactorial**. It has been documented that there is a genetic predisposition in some breeds, which indicates that there is a genetic factor associated with this fact. Chronic skin irritation can contribute to the formation of MCTs. Mutations in c-kit have been detected in some tumours; mutations in this proto-oncogene can predispose dogs to MCT. SCF (stem cell factor) is an essential growth factor for normal mast cells, KIT is the surface receptor with tyrosine kinase activity for SCF and is encoded for it by the proto-oncogene c-kit. KIT-SCF interactions are necessary for mast cell differentiation, survival, and function. Mutations in c-kit leading to activation of KIT receptors in the absence of SCF binding have been described in 30–40% of dogs with MCT.

The molecular aetiology for most of these tumours remains unknown, although characterisation of genomic alterations in canine MCTs could identify genomic regions responsible for development and progression. In a recent publication, a DNA study of 109 canine MCTs in different breeds (Boxer, Labrador, Pug, other breeds, and mongrels) was conducted and showed that there is a greater number of copy number aberrations as the tumour grade increases. KIT sequencing showed that mutations in these receptors were less frequent in MCTs in Pugs and that they were also associated with histological grade.

Behaviour

Mast cells originate in the bone marrow and are normally found in places such as the lung, liver, skin, and the gastrointestinal tract, where they participate in allergic reactions and inflammatory processes.

IgE binds to the surface of mast cells and causes the release of **granules** inside mast cells, which contain histamine, heparin, and prostaglandins. The **release of granules** is called **degranulation** and can lead to some paraneoplastic syndromes or complications.

- **Gastrointestinal ulceration**. Histamine stimulates gastric acid secretion by parietal cells. Clinical signs secondary to ulceration include vomiting, gastrointestinal bleeding, anorexia, and abdominal pain. Anaemia secondary to a lack of iron or peritonitis may occur as a consequence of digestive tract perforation. Necropsy studies have shown gastrointestinal ulceration in 35–83% of cases.
- **Hypotension** during surgery or vigorous palpation of the tumour due to histamine, prostaglandin, and other vasoactive amines released from the granules.
- **Coagulopathies** due to heparin released from the granules.
- **Delayed healing after surgery** possibly due to proteolytic enzymes present in the granules that inhibit normal fibroblast proliferation.

- Rarely, a sudden, massive release of histamine from neoplastic cells can occur causing an **acute anaphylactic reaction and collapse episode**. Animals with extensive disease are at higher risk.
- **Darier's sign**. Mechanical manipulation of the tumour can cause the release of histamine, heparin, etc.; degranulation with erythema and wheal formation may occur in surrounding tissues.

They can develop anywhere on the body, but MCTs in dogs are generally found in the dermis and subcutaneous tissue. They rarely occur in extra-cutaneous locations such as the oral and nasal cavities or the gastrointestinal tract. Recently, two cases of pulmonary MCT and seven cases of intramuscular MCT have been described. 60% of MCTs appear on the trunk and it is also common to observe them on the extremities (25–40%), although they can appear anywhere (for example, 10% of cases appear on the head and neck).

The gross appearance is highly varied and can resemble any other skin tumour and other non-neoplastic skin conditions; some subcutaneous MCTs may look and feel like lipomas. Therefore, **MCT should always be on the differential diagnosis list for any skin nodule**. The gross appearance correlates in some way with the histological grade.

- **Well-differentiated cutaneous tumours**. Low-grade tumours tend to be solitary, alopecic, slow growing, 1–4 cm in diameter, and generally present for about 6 months before diagnosis (Figure 1).
- **Poorly-differentiated tumours**. Fast-growing, with a tendency to ulcerate and show pruritic lesions, and there may be evidence of local lymphadenopathy or organomegaly on abdominal palpation (Figure 2).

Between 10 and 40% of patients have multiple cutaneous MCTs at the time of diagnosis or will develop new MCTs after treatment. It is **very important** to always explain to clients

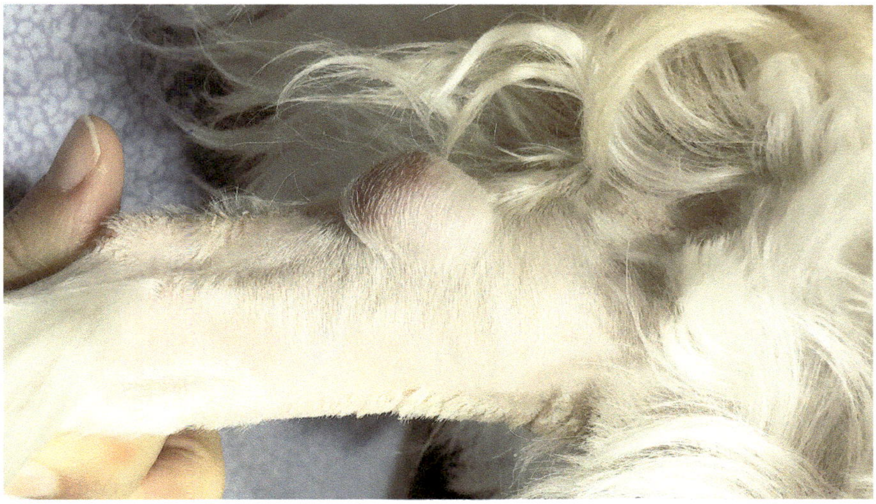

Figure 1. Low-grade, well-differentiated mast cell tumour on the forelimb of a dog. The tumour is well defined and not ulcerated or attached to deep planes.

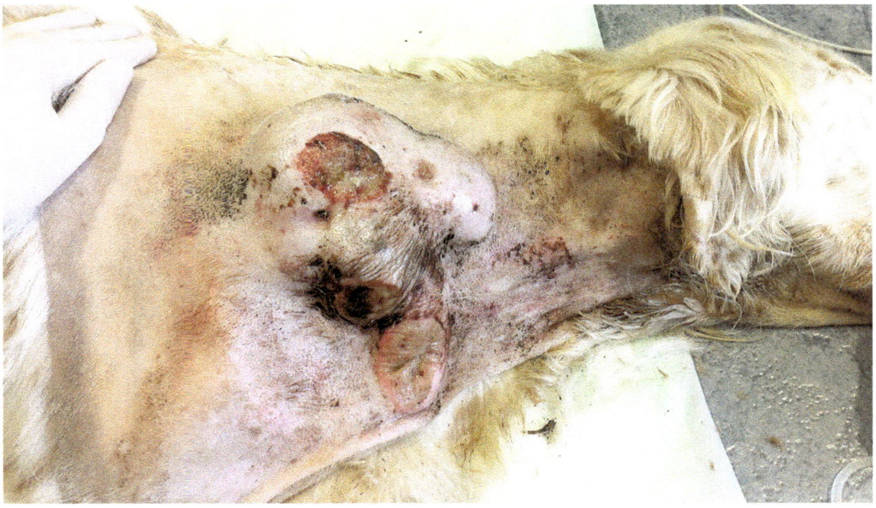

Figure 2. High-grade, poorly differentiated mast cell tumour affecting all of the right side of the neck of a dog. The mass is large, ulcerated, poorly defined, and attached to deep tissue planes.

that dogs with a history of mast cell tumours should be **examined as soon as possible** for any lumps/bumps/protuberances. In the case of **primary visceral MCT**, it can present with or without evidence of cutaneous MCT.

Diagnosis

The clinical history of a mass that **changes in size**, increasing or decreasing in size, is suggestive of a mast cell tumour (linked to intermittent degranulation). However, since MCTs can resemble any skin lesion, fine needle aspiration is recommended.

Cytology

A cytological diagnosis of MCT can practically always be made (92–96% of cases). Mast cells exfoliate very well. Mast cell tumours are round cell tumours that contain characteristic metachromatic granules (purple, red, or blue granule staining) (Figure 3).

In poorly differentiated tumours, the granules may not be detected microscopically and special stains for mast cell granules (toluidine blue, Wright-Giemsa) must be performed to reach a diagnosis; alternatively, a positive staining for c-kit receptors can be used to diagnose MCT. Very poorly differentiated MCTs tend to lose granules.

Cytologic analysis does not accurately report tumour grade (i.e. you cannot tell whether a tumour is well differentiated based solely on cytologic analysis), but rather a histopathologic analysis is required. Although it is true that a few studies have been published that describe cytological characteristics that could help determine the grade of the tumour. According to one study, MCTs can be classified as high or low-grade based on:

- loss of granules
- presence of mitotic figures
- bi- or multinucleated cells
- presence of nuclear pleomorphism
- anisokaryosis of more than 50%.

According to another study in which the characteristics of the **Kiupel 2-tier histopathology grade system** are used, they are classified as high if they present any of the characteristics indicated in Table 1 (Figure 4).

These studies show that cytology has a sensitivity of 86–88% and a specificity of 94–97% to correctly diagnose high- or

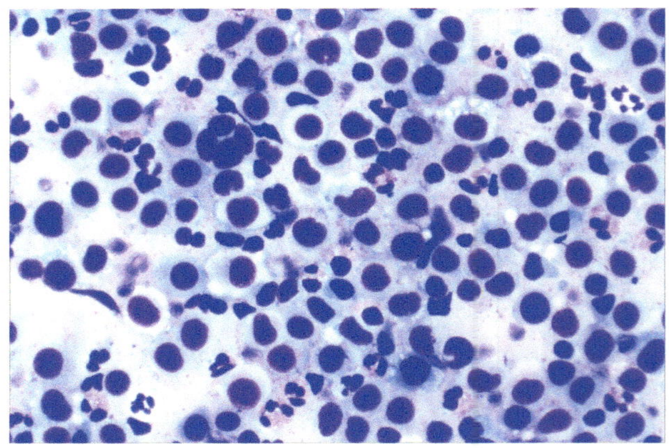

Figure 4. Cytology of a high-grade canine mast cell tumour where a population of round cells can be seen where the "typical" granules seen in mast cells can barely be seen and different characteristics of malignancy can be seen. To help with the diagnosis of a mast cell tumour, the presence of abundant eosinophils should be noted.

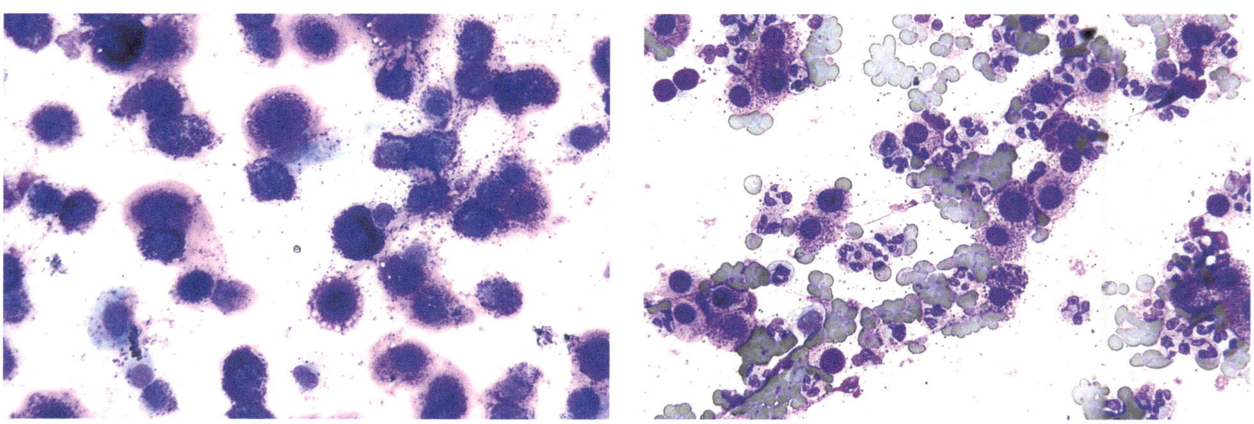

Figure 3. Cytological images of a well-differentiated mast cell tumour. The diagnosis of a mast cell tumour is simple in these cases, as the presence of granules in the mast cells is obvious.

low-grade mast cell tumours. However, approximately 33% of those diagnosed as high-grade by cytology are false positives when compared to histologic grade, and 13% of tumours were diagnosed as low-grade by cytology but reclassified as high-grade by histopathology. Therefore, the application of the histological grade in cytology is useful initially, but the **evaluation of the grade should be based primarily on the histological study**

Biopsy

The histological appearance of MCTs is highly varied. Tumours are classified by grades according to their histological appearance. Traditionally, the Patnaik classification was used (Table 1), but currently there is an additional classification for mast cell tumours, which is the Kiupel classification (Box 1).

Table 1. Patnaik grading system.

Grade	Patnaik grade	Microscopic description	Rate of metastasis
High-grade (anaplastic, poorly differentiated)	III	· Irregular size and shaped nuclei · Frequent mitosis · Few cytoplasmic granules	>55%
Intermediate-grade	II	· Infrequent mitotic figures · More granules than in the anaplastic type · Nucleus/cytoplasmic ratio lower than in the anaplastic type	10–20%
Low-grade (well differentiated)	I	· Spherical or ovoid nuclei · Mitotic figures uncommon or absent · Large well stained cytoplasmic granules	<10%

The **Kiupel grade classification system seems to better predict the biological behaviour of the tumour**, that is, it better predicts the possibility that dogs will die from this disease than Patnaik's classification.

In a study which evaluated whether the Patnaik or Kiupel systems were more accurate, it determined that the Kiupel 2-tier method had a higher prognostic value and was better at predicting the negative behaviours of some Patnaik grade II tumours. However, it also confirmed that the histological grade system is not always sufficient by itself to determine the prognosis and the tumour's biological behaviour and that all the characteristics of the animal and the tumour must be considered. In addition, it may be necessary to supplement this information with molecular techniques.

Box 1. Kiupel 2-tier grade classification system

- **According to this classification system, mast cell tumours are divided into two grades:**
  - **high-grade**
  - **low-grade.**

- **Classification is based on some histopathological characteristics. They are high-grade if at least one of the following criteria is present:**
  - **≥7 mitotic figures/10 high power field (HPF)**
  - **≥3 multinucleated cells/10 HPF**
  - **≥3 atypical nuclei/10 HPF**
  - **karyomegaly (more than 10% of neoplastic cells with a nucleus diameter more than twice the normal size).**

- **According to this system, the associated survival is:**
  - **4 months for high-grade**
  - **2 years for low-grade.**

Poorly Differentiated MCTs (Anaplastic)

They may show little or no granulation and can be difficult to diagnose by routine light microscopy. Biopsies of these tumours can be interpreted as "undifferentiated round cell tumour" or even "undifferentiated sarcoma".

If a mast cell tumour is suspected based on the clinical signs of the tumour (peritumoural oedema, other signs of degranulation), the pathologist should be contacted.

Toluidine blue staining can be helpful in identifying mast cell granules. c-kit (CD117) can be used to diagnose agranular MCTs and electron microscopy (to visualise granules) is useful in some cases.

Metastasis

Histological grade is the most predictive factor of biological behaviour.

MCTs almost always spread to local lymph nodes first, which may be followed by spread to the spleen, liver, bone marrow, and other skin areas. In cases of widespread metastasis, mast cells often appear in the peripheral blood.

Although recently described, cases of pulmonary mast cell tumours are scant and metastases from mast cell tumours rarely affect the thorax, but a pleural effusion can occur, especially in cases with numerous abdominal tumours and peritoneal effusion.

Prognostic Factors for Canine Mast Cell Tumours

The behaviour and progression of MCTs is highly variable. However, **histological grade is the most important individual prognostic factor** and the one most closely related to tumour behaviour and clinical outcome.

Histopathology (Histological Grade)

Poorly differentiated tumours (Patnaik grade III or high-grade 2-tier) have shorter survival times and more metastases, compared to other grades. Lymph node metastases are directly related to tumour grade.

In general, most dogs with well-differentiated tumours have long-term survival times after complete surgical removal. The metastatic rate for high-grade MCTs is elevated (55–96%), and most of the patients die of their disease within 1 year.

Lymph Node Involvement

Lymph node cytology is crucial in clinical staging since the **presence or absence of metastases in the regional lymph node is directly related to survival**. The problem is that the interpretation of lymph node involvement is complicated.

Dogs with regional lymph node metastases (not distant or extended metastases) may have a longer survival time if the metastatic lymph node is treated with surgery or radiation therapy.

Location

Historically, MCTs which develop in mucocutaneous, muzzle, perioral, oral, and inguinal areas have been considered highly malignant, regardless of the histological grade.

- **Mucocutaneous localisation**: in general, MCTs of the ocular conjunctiva are usually associated with a better prognosis, provided they are treated locally in an appropriate manner. However, in other mucocutaneous areas, they are associated with a worse prognosis.
- **Muzzle/perioral/oral**: approximately 50–60% of dogs with MCT located on the muzzle, oral or perioral area, present with metastasis in the regional node at the time of diagnosis (compared to the 10% of metastases described for other cutaneous MCT). Survival is much higher if there is no regional lymph node involvement, or if the lymph node is also treated/removed at the time of the local treatment of the primary MCT. Estimated survival is approximately 14 months for cases with lymph node metastases, whereas these same MCT sites without regional node metastases are associated with a 52-month survival time.
- **Inguinal**: historically, the caudal half of the dog has always been considered to have a worse prognosis (for those that affect the inguinal area, prepuce, and scrotum). Although there are contradictory studies, from a clinical point of view tumours in or between the toes and the scrotal and preputial areas are still considered to tend to metastasise at an early stage of the pathological process and present with an aggressive local behaviour (Figure 5).
- **Subcutaneous**: according to the Patnaik classification, the fact that they are subcutaneous classifies them as grade II. A 2011 study determined that subcutaneous MCTs have a good prognosis, and in general, they show a more benign type of behaviour. They recur 8% of the time

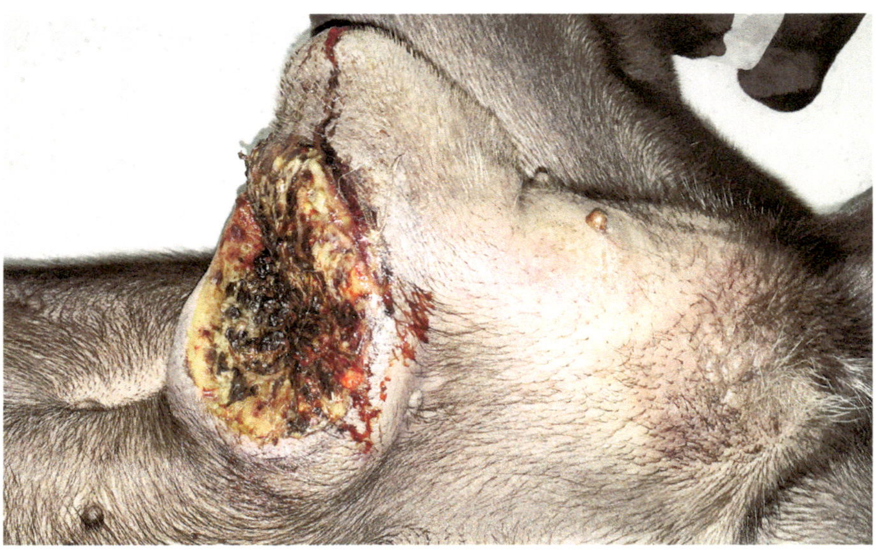

Figure 5. High-grade mast cell tumour in the inguinal region, around the prepuce, with oedema, erythema, and ulceration

(12% if the margin is incomplete, compared to 23–33% for grade II; in the case of a complete margin, 2% versus 11% for grade II), metastasise in 4% of cases and associated mortality is only 9% (compared to 18% of grade II in general). Although a priori subcutaneous mast cell tumours can be considered to have better prognosis than grade II mast cell tumours; recently new studies have shown that not all the subcutaneous mast cell tumours behave as a low grade tumours and careful attention must be taken to the prognostic factors associated to this tumour. The factors associated with a worse prognosis in subcutaneous MCT are:

- mitotic index greater than 4
- multinucleation or infiltration
- Ki67, Ki67+ + AgNOR and KIT cell localisation.

The prognostic factor with the strongest correlation is the **mitotic index**. The rest of the markers are not usually requested.

- **Visceral**: dogs with primary intestinal MCTs without a history of cutaneous MCTs. In one study that included 10 cases, all dogs died from the tumour within 8 weeks of diagnosis.

In general, **tumours located on the trunk** have a worse prognosis than those in the extremities, except in the case of digital MCTs (Figure 6).

Growth Rate and Size

The growth rate of the tumour is a **significant prognostic factor** for its behaviour.

- Tumours that grow slowly and that are localised for long periods of time (months or years) are usually well differentiated.
- Tumours that have not changed in more than 7 months: 83% live at least 30 weeks.
- Tumours that grow in less than 7 months: 25% live 30 weeks.
- Larger tumours have a worse prognosis after surgery or radiotherapy.

Clinical Signs

Local or generalised clinical signs such as anorexia, vomiting, generalised erythema, oedema, ulceration or itching, gastrointestinal ulceration, etc. in dogs are usually associated with poorly differentiated tumours.

Recurrence or Failure of Treatment

Recurrent tumours after surgical removal are often highly malignant and have a worse prognosis.

Breed

There is a **relationship between breed and the histopathological grade** of mast cell tumours, which indicates the presence of genetic factors associated with aggressive behaviour of high-grade MCTs. Some breeds are more predisposed to develop malignant tumours and others benign ones.

- **Shar Pei** often develop highly malignant MCTs that are common in young dogs (mean age 4 years).
- **Pugs, Boston Terriers, Boxers**, and **other breeds** are more prone to develop low-grade MCTs. For example, one study showed that 56% of Pugs will have multiple MCTs in their lifetime and that 98% will be low-grade.

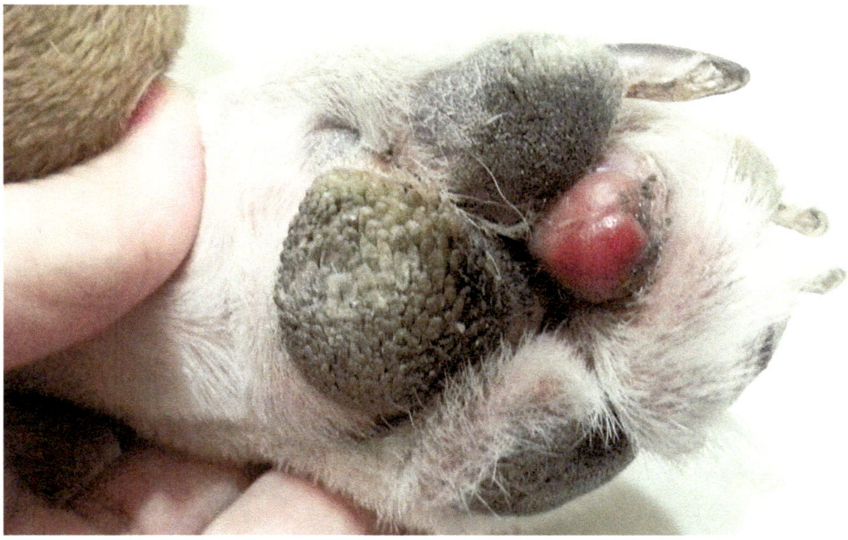

Figure 6. Digital high-grade mast cell tumour associated with the third toe. An erythematous lesion which is about to become ulcerated can be seen.

Clinical Stage

At present, **many studies question the usefulness of the WHO clinical staging system** (Table 2), especially regarding stage III since the fact that an animal has multiple MCTs is not always associated with a worse prognosis. The histological grade is much more predictive of behaviour and outcome.

The presence of distant metastases is indicative of a poor prognosis. Some dogs with multiple cutaneous MCTs can have a long survival time; brachycephalic dogs frequently have multiple low-grade MCTs.

Table 2. WHO clinical staging for canine MCT.

Clinical stage	Description
-1	Single tumour removed with clean margins and negative lymph node
0	Skin tumour incompletely removed and positive or negative lymph node
1	Tumour confined to the dermis with negative lymph node
2	Tumour confined to the dermis with positive local or regional lymph node
3	Multiple dermal tumours or large infiltrating tumour with positive or negative lymph node
4	Any tumour with distant metastasis

Table 3. Relationship between mitotic index and growth markers with grade of survival in dogs with mast cell tumours.

Parameter	Significance	Prognostic value
Mitotic index	· >5: low survival rate, independent of grade · >7: predictive of recurrence	Useful test which should be requested in all histopathology reports
Ki-67	· High: associated with an increase in mortality, recurrence rate, appearance of metastasis. Helps to determine aggressiveness of grade II (cut off point: 1.8)	Useful if available, factor independent from grade
AgNOR	· High: associated with increase in death, recurrence, and metastasis	Not a prognostic factor independent of grade, but can be helpful in grade II
PCNA	· High: associated with an increase in mortality	Not a prognostic factor independent of grade

Systemic Mastocytosis

Systemic mastocytosis is very rare and there is little information regarding prognosis. In a 2018 study, dogs with lymph node metastases lived longer than those with mastocytosis, and those with metastases in more than two different sites had a worse prognosis than those with metastases in a single location. Furthermore, in these cases, the animals that received lomustine, vinblastine, and prednisone showed better responses than those that received prednisone or Palladia® (toceranib phosphate). In general, patients with systemic mastocytosis have a very poor prognosis.

Mitotic Index

Mitotic index is directly related to the grade of the tumour and is an **important factor in predicting survival**, the problem is that there are different studies that establish a different cut-off mitotic index. For subcutaneous MCTs, it was established (2011) that a mitotic index greater than 4 is associated with a lower survival and disease-free time, as well as a higher risk of metastasis and local recurrence. According to the most recent classification system (Kiupel 2011), MCTs will be classified as high-grade if the MI is 7 or higher than 7.

In general, a mitotic index below or above 5 is considered very significant. A 2007 study, determined that the survival times of dogs, regardless of tumour grade, were:

- MI <5: 70 months
- MI >5: 2 months.

Proliferation Markers

Proliferation markers (AgNOR, Ki-67 and PCNA) (Table 3): the higher Ki-67, PCNA and AgNOR, the higher the tumour grade. Furthermore, the mitotic index, Ki-67, the combination of Ki-67 and AgNOR, and the cellular localisation of KIT have been associated with local recurrence and metastasis for subcutaneous MCTs.

C-kit Mutation

The KIT ligand is a stem cell factor. The expression of KIT has been demonstrated with immunohistochemistry in normal and tumour mast cells. However, the expression is much higher in neoplastic mast cells, with a higher expression the less differentiated the mast cells are.

The proto-oncogene c-kit, whose product is c-kit (which is a receptor tyrosine kinase), is expressed in mast cells and is critical for their differentiation, proliferation, survival, and activation. Mutations have been detected in c-kit that correlate with a more aggressive MCT phenotype.

The c-kit mutation is associated with:

- higher grade
- increased risk of metastasis
- greater local recurrence
- higher rate of tumour proliferation.

Staging

Once a diagnosis of MCT is made, a **complete staging** that defines the extent of the disease should be performed. Frequent metastatic sites include the local lymph nodes, skin, spleen, liver and bone marrow. The thorax is rarely affected by metastatic disease.

Most dogs will have tumours that are unlikely to metastasise, and not all patients need full staging. However, if extensive/aggressive or expensive treatment is being planned or a poorly differentiated tumour has been identified, full staging is recommended.

In a recent study, the usefulness of different staging methods was evaluated, considering the prevalence of metastasis. At presentation, 31% of the dogs had lymph node metastases and 7% had distant metastases. No dog had or developed distant metastases without regional lymph node metastases and no dog had evidence of pulmonary metastasis.

Low-grade Appearance

If the cytological diagnosis of MCT is made in an **area where surgical removal can be performed and in the absence of negative prognostic indicators** (e.g. peritumoural oedema/haematoma/ulceration, signs of gastrointestinal ulceration):

- **the regional lymph node should be aspirated** so that it can be removed simultaneously with surgery (if there is already or is the possibility of lymph node metastasis exists);
- **blood tests** before surgery (complete blood count, biochemical analysis, urinalysis if indicated);
- ideally, an **abdominal ultrasound** should be included in every patient with MCT, before surgery is performed. However, if there is a high suspicion of a low-grade tumour, it could be done after surgery if the report is indicating higher grade;
- as a general rule, a wide **surgical resection** is performed (objective: a layer of fascia below, 2 cm laterally); and
- tissue should be sent for **evaluation of histologic grade and margins**.

Postoperatively, if the margins are incomplete or the tumour is poorly differentiated (Patnaik grade III) or high-grade, further staging tests are needed and treatment should be continued.

High-grade Appearance

If there are **negative prognostic indicators** (i.e. peritumoural oedema/haematoma/ulceration, signs of gastrointestinal ulceration) or if there are lymph node metastases at the time of diagnosis, **additional tests should be performed before applying definitive treatments, which are detailed below.**

Complete Blood Count

To determine the presence of:

- **mastocytosis**: rare in dogs, more common in cats;
- **eosinophilia**: quite common in dogs with MCT, since mast cells contain the eosinophil chemotactic factor;
- **basophilia**;
- **regenerative or non-regenerative anaemia**: can be seen when there is gastrointestinal ulceration or bleeding from the tumour; and
- **mature neutrophilia or left shift**: if gastrointestinal perforation has occurred (rare).

Serum Biochemistry and Urinalysis

Serum biochemistry and urinalysis tests are used to assess for signs of concurrent disease.

Abdominal Ultrasound with Spleen and Liver Aspirates

There are different studies on the aspiration of the liver and spleen in normal ultrasonographic organs. In general, aspiration of the liver and spleen is always recommended because they are highly indicative of prognosis and ultrasound is not sufficiently sensitive.

One study states that a splenic aspirate should be performed, even if it appears normal, because in 43% of spleens and 0% of the livers in this study of dogs with metastasis produced a normal ultrasound image. 36% of cases with grade II or III MCT have infiltration of the liver and/or spleen. In practice, and accordance with oncologists, aspirations are only performed if there are abnormalities on ultrasound or suspicion of high-grade tumours. In addition, during ultrasound, it should be determined whether there is mesenteric lymphadenopathy, organ infiltration, peritoneal effusion, etc.

Thoracic Radiographs

Thoracic radiographs are generally **not useful** in cases of MCTs because these tumours rarely metastasise to the lungs. In fact, thoracic radiographs can be useful to evaluate the sternal lymph node if the mass is in the ventral abdomen, but to evaluate metastases to the lung they are generally unnecessary.

Tumour Biopsy

If a MCT is large and inoperable, a small punch biopsy should be performed to determine tumour grade and mitotic index (MI).

If an incisional biopsy is performed, only opting for a punch biopsy (versus a large and open biopsy or surgical debulking of the tumour) is recommended to try to avoid the risk of degranulation, among other problems, such as healing issues. Only small tumour samples are needed to determine histological grade and MI.

Bone Marrow Aspirate

Normal bone marrow contains one mast cell for every 1000 nucleated cells; a higher number is indicative of metastasis. In one study, only 2% of dogs with cutaneous MCT (at diagnosis) had bone marrow metastases, so this test is not routinely performed. However, it has been determined that 19% may have bone marrow involvement in cases of recurrence or progressive disease.

The clinical signs associated with bone marrow invasion are non-specific (lethargy, weakness, weight loss...). If the bone marrow is affected, the estimated survival time is 43 days.

Lymph Node Evaluation

Cytologic evaluation of the regional node is very important, even if the node feels normal when palpated. There are numerous studies which describe that palpation is not sufficient since an affected node is not always enlarged.

Normal lymph nodes contain a small number of mast cells. It can be difficult to determine if the mast cells in the lymph node are mast cells drained from the tumour or true metastases: if there are aggregates of mast cells or if the mast cells are less differentiated than the mast cells from the primary tumour, it is very likely that it is a true metastasis.

Node excisional biopsy may be more effective than cytology in identifying metastasis. In general, if a lymph node is suspected of having MCT metastases based on cytologic analysis, it should be removed during removal of the primary tumour.

In the case of dogs with MCT, **lymph node metastasis is not necessarily a poor prognostic indicator**, as long-term survival is possible if the lymph nodes are properly treated.

There are different indications for identifying whether a lymph node has metastasis from an MCT or whether it is the normal mast cell population of the node. A study was published in 2016 that is based on the histological criteria used by the 2-tier grading system for MCTs. The system developed had 88% sensitivity and 94% specificity relative to histological grade. Dogs with high histological and cytological grades were at 39 and 25 times, higher risk of dying within a 2-year period respectively than dogs with low-grades. Furthermore, high-grade was associated with a higher rate of recurrence or development of new tumours.

Special consideration must be taken regarding the lymph node status because the regional lymph node (the closest to

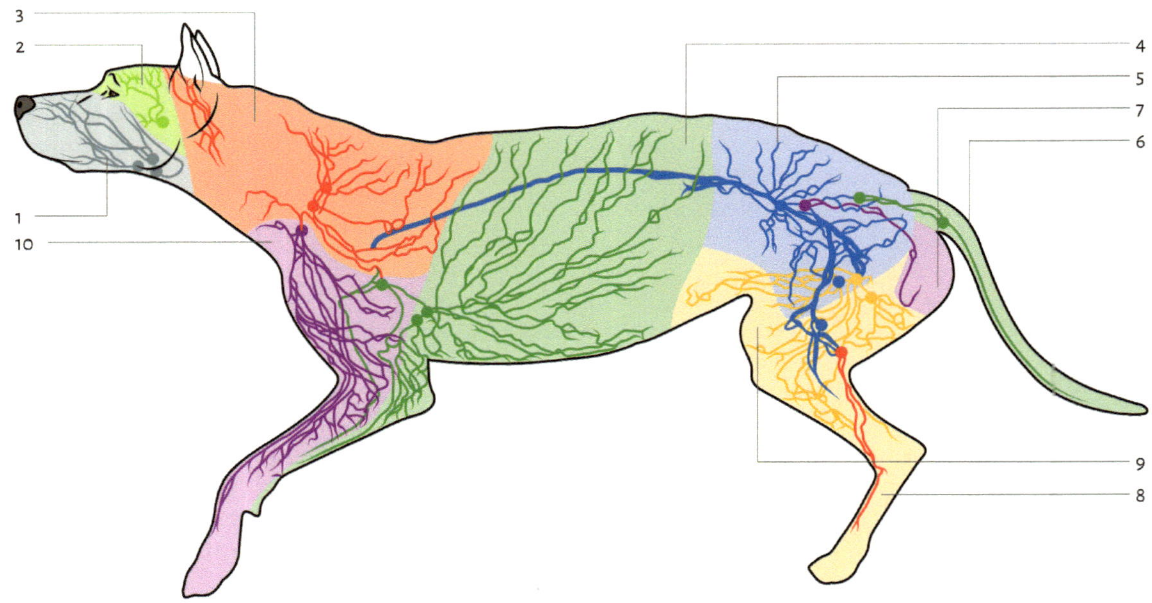

Figure 7. Lymphatic territories in the dog. 1: submandibular; 2: parotid; 3: dorsal superficial cervical; 4: axillary; 5: medial iliac; 6: lateral sacral; 7: hypogastric; 8: popliteal; 9: superficial inguinal; 10: ventral superficial cervical.

Illustration adapted from: Lymphatic Territories (Lymphosomes) in a Canine: An Animal Model for Investigation of Postoperative Lymphatic Alterations. *PLOS ONE*. Hiroo et al. 2013.

the tumour) is not always the centinel lymph node (the one where the tumour drains).

During 2019 and 2020, a few studies revealed that in 25-40% of the patients with mast cell tumours, the centinel lymph node does not correspond with the regional lymph node.

Although the regional lymph node must always be evaluated and aspirated/biopsied, the centinel lymph node should also be taken into consideration according to the lymphatic territories described for the dog (fig. 7). There are different published techniques to identify the centinel lymph node (metilene blue, lymphoscint graphy, etc.).

Additionally, while staging the patient, any enlarged lymph node should be aspirated/biopsied, independently of its location.

In another study, from 2017, the percentage of mast cells in lymph node aspirates from normal dogs, with dermatological disease, or with skin MCTs was compared. The percentage of mast cells was 0% in normal dogs, 0.05% in ones with allergies and 0.4% in MCT.

Computerised Tomography

CT can be useful for surgical planning in the case of complicated surgical cases, due to location or size.

Treatment

Treatment options depend on clinical features, stage, and grade.

The key factors to be considered are:
- is complete excision possible; and
- is local therapy enough or is systemic therapy also necessary.

Surgery

If the **tumour can be treated surgically**, it has traditionally been described that the goal is to resect the tumour with 3 cm lateral margins and a deep layer of fascia (Figure 8).

However, more recent studies have shown that for grades I and II (or low-grade), a lateral margin of 2 cm and a deep fascia layer is sufficient. In another study which included cases with low-grade MCT (Patnaik I and II) with 1 cm depth and 4 mm lateral margin, no recurrence was observed. On the other hand, more aggressive tumours must be excised with a 3 cm margin and a deep layer of fascia (Figure 9).

Consideration should be given to the use of sterile skin staples or haemoclips (e.g. markers visible on radiographs) in deep parts of the tissue bed to mark the area if postoperative radiation therapy is necessary; this is especially recommended for MCT on the body wall.

Before surgery, it is very important to explain to the owners of the patient that on some occasions MCTs may not be completely removed, and if that is the case for their pet, radiotherapy treatment or a second surgery may be necessary. Tumours on the limbs are less likely to be completely removed than trunk tumours.

If the **tumour cannot be treated by surgery** (for example, a large body wall, head/neck, or inguinal tumours):
- punch biopsy should be performed to confirm diagnosis/grade, MI and staging tests should be performed first, to help decide on treatment;
- an oncology consultation may be necessary; or
- considering chemotherapy, receptor inhibition with tyrosine kinase activity and/or radiotherapy may be necessary to shrink the tumour before or instead of surgery (presurgical antineoplastic treatment). Also, the use of Stelfonta® (toglato de tigilanol) might be indicated in some of these cases.

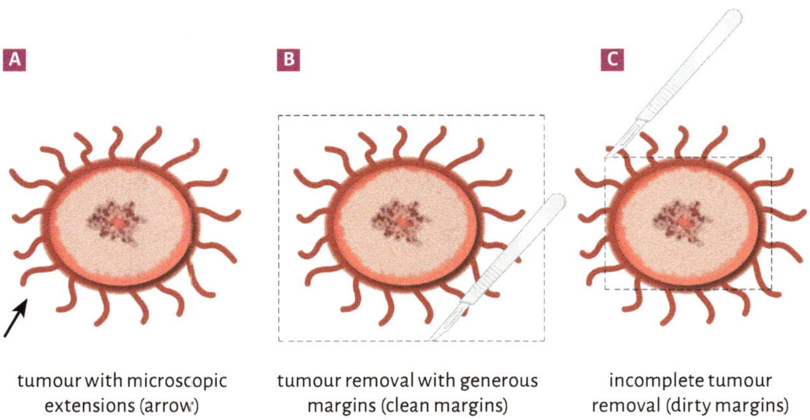

Figure 8. Diagram of a tumour where one part can be observed macroscopically, although microscopically the tumour exceeds those margins (**A**). Diagram of a tumour removed with wide or generous margins, where clean margins are obtained as they include both the macroscopic and microscopic parts of the tumour (**B**). Diagram of a tumour removed with narrow margins, where incomplete or dirty margins are obtained given they only include the macroscopic part, but the microscopic region of the tumour is not removed (**C**).

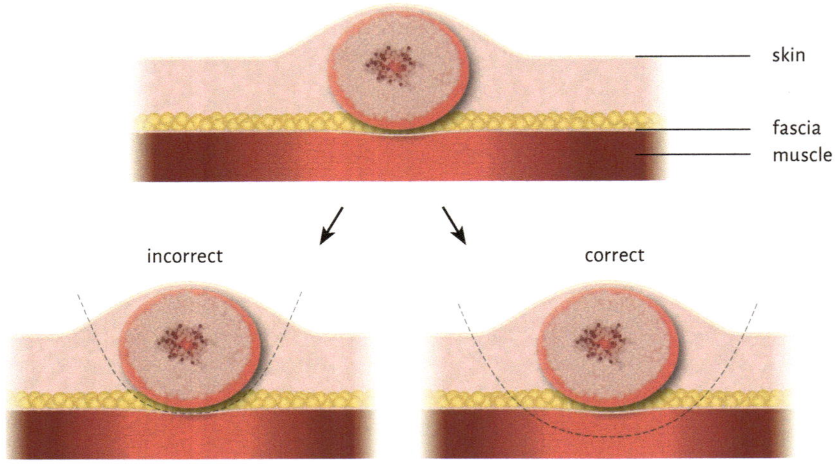

Figure 9. Illustration of the adequate (bottom right corner of diagram) and inadequate (bottom left corner) removal of a mast cell tumour. The part of the tumour visible macroscopically should be removed as well as margins surrounding it and a deep plane of tissue below.

Surgical Biopsy

All resected tissue should be sent to a pathologist for evaluation. Tissue marking with dyes such as India ink or the Davidson Marking System® (Bradley Products) multicolour system can help the pathologist to detect if and where the surgical margins are incomplete; it is best to **ask what method the pathologist uses to evaluate the margins**.

It can be difficult for pathologists to determine exact margins due to tissue shrinkage in formalin, but most will try to provide this information to clinicians. Histological measurement may estimate that the margins are smaller than the disease-free margins due to the problem of tissue shrinking in formalin.

MCT surgical margins should be evaluated in the context of tumour size – for example, the smaller the tumour, the more likely it is to have been completely removed. In tumours on a large body wall or on the extremities, where resection is likely to be incomplete, a biopsy report describing complete margins should be distrusted. Ideally, there should be a minimum distance of 1 cm between the tumour and normal tissue on biopsy (this is considered a complete margin). Any margin less than 5 mm is a "close" margin and there is always concern that the margin may be incomplete near that area.

The evaluation of MCT margins can be complicated due to the presence of discontinuous metastases which are areas deep to the tumour not adjacent to it, which are probably islands of neoplastic cells and can cause tumour recurrence.

- If the **surgical margins are incomplete** (tumour cells extend to the excision margins), the options are:
  - second resection, with scar correction (generally not possible in limb tumours due to inability to close wounds);
  - complementary radiotherapy or electrochemotherapy;
  - follow-up for recurrence (not the best option, but the success and outcome will depend on the tumour grade); and
  - chemotherapy or possible steroids, according to tumour grade.
- If the **surgical margins are close** (for example, less than 5 mm; generally, a margin >1 cm is optimal), the options are:
  - second resection with scar correction;
  - thorough monitoring;
  - adjuvant radiotherapy or electrochemotherapy if the tumour is high-grade and a close margin is suspected, with doubt as to whether there is microscopic disease; and
  - chemotherapy with/without steroids, depending on the tumour grade.
- If the **surgical margins are complete**, frequent check-ups are recommended (once a month for the first 3 months, then every 3 months for the first year, depending on the location and tumour grade) to control possible recurrences and check that no new tumours appear.

A tumour may not recur even after incomplete resection. Several studies have shown that only 20–30% of incompletely removed MCTs will recur. Once tumours recur, they tend to behave more aggressively, so it is generally best to treat tumours as aggressively as possible to prevent recurrence.

It is currently difficult to recommend "doing nothing" after incomplete MCT resection, as radiotherapy is very effective at controlling tumours, but the option of close monitoring to detect whether the tumour reappears may be reasonable for clients who have limited resources for further treatment or in pets that may not be able to withstand additional treatments, particularly in the case of dogs with small (<2 cm) tumours that are grade I or II, according to Patnaik's classification, or low-grade, according to the 2-tier system.

In the case of Patnaik grade III or metastatic grade II tumours, with MI >5/HPF or high-grade 2-tier, incomplete or complete resection should be followed by adjuvant chemotherapy, in addition to treatment of local remnants of the tumour. In some hospitals, chemotherapy (rather than radiotherapy) is recommended for dogs with incompletely removed MCTs. Some studies suggest that chemotherapy can help prevent/delay tumour recurrence (such as the use of prednisone, prednisone + vinblastine, lomustine + prednisone ...):

- with **prednisone**: 23% recurrence
- with **vinblastine and prednisone**: 10% recurrence
- with **lomustine and prednisone**: there was no recurrence of stage I or II incompletely resected grade II mast cell tumours.

Radiotherapy (RT)

Complete surgery is considered the best local treatment, and radiotherapy is advisable when surgery is not sufficient to obtain local control of the tumour. When surgical margin re-excision can not be performed, it can be a very good option to achieve complete margins. However, RT can also be used to treat the regional lymph node.

Ideally, the RT should be planned prior to surgery, rather than as an option after an incomplete excision has been performed. In one study, 96% of dogs with incompletely removed intermediate differentiation (grade II) tumours treated with radiotherapy achieved a year tumour-free survival time and 88% had a 5-year tumour-free survival.

Poorly Differentiated and Metastatic Tumours

For high-grade and metastatic tumours of any grade, treatment of the primary site can help palliate the tumour and improve patient well-being. In a small unpublished study, dogs with poorly differentiated tumours (grade III) treated with radiation therapy and chemotherapy lived longer than dogs treated with chemotherapy alone.

In a 2003 study of dogs with incompletely excised grade III mast cell tumours and no evidence of metastasis, 71% survived for one year after radiotherapy treatment of the tumour bed; this study showed a longer survival period compared to previous reports of dogs with grade III tumours.

Inoperable Tumours

Large tumours are often considered radioresistant because they are likely to have RT-resistant clones in some areas and are more difficult to irradiate. A 2011 study of combined radiotherapy and Palladia® treatment for inoperable tumours showed a survival time of more than one year for these types of tumours.

Radiotherapy can palliate clinical signs and shrink the tumour. Caution should be taken when irradiating large numbers of mast cells, as rapid degranulation with hypotension and anaphylactic shock can occur. It is important to advise owners and administer antihistamines and proton pump inhibitors (omeprazole) beforehand.

Chemotherapy

Chemotherapy can be used in dogs in three ways.

- When **systemic therapy is needed** to treat, delay, or prevent disseminated metastases in high-grade tumours.
- As a neoadjuvant, **before surgery or radiation**. It may be effective to treat large inoperable tumours with chemotherapy to try and reduce their size (preoperative antineoplastic chemotherapy).
- Treat **microscopic disease** when surgery or radiation treatment is not possible.

Its application should be considered in high-grade or metastatic MCTs or tumours with a high MI in any grade, as well as in dogs with clinical signs linked to mast cell degranulation, or in locations that may be associated with a higher incidence of metastasis (scrotum, foreskin, toe). First-line adjuvant protocols usually include vinblastine and prednisone, and in second place, lomustine and prednisone. For other therapeutic agents there are fewer studies available. Table 4 summarises some of the most common chemotherapy protocols and the clinical responses associated with them.

Table 4. Published information regarding the use of chemotherapy for treatment of mast cell tumours.

Active ingredient	Average response rate	Average duration of response
Prednisone	20%	NA
Vincristine	7%	NA
Vinblastine	12–27%*	NA
Prednisone/vinblastine	47%	154 days
Vinorelbine	12%	NA
CCNU (lomustine)	44%	79 days
Vinblastine/CCNU	57%	1 year
Vinblastine/CCNU/ prednisone	65%	Macroscopically: 140 days Adjuvant: 1.5 years
Vinblastine/ cyclophosphamide/ prednisone	78%	18 months
Hydroxyurea	28%	50–60 days
Cyclophosphamide/ vincristine/prednisone/ hydroxyurea	59%	53 days
Paclitaxel	23%	100 days

* dose dependent

Tyrosine Kinase Inhibitors (Palladia®, Masivet®)

Receptors for tyrosine kinase (RTK) are an important group of related surface receptors, the activation of which is involved in cell proliferation, differentiation, and survival (Figure 10). RTK alterations implicated in different cancers have been described.

Palladia® (Toceranib Phosphate)

Palladia® is the **first FDA-approved treatment for cancer in dogs**. It is a RTK that blocks the activation of KIT, both in the wild and mutated types; efficacy is the same in patients with or without c-kit mutations.

A response (complete response, CR, plus partial response, PR) is obtained in 42% of treated patients, 60% if animals with stable disease (SD) are included. However, animals positive for the c-kit mutation have been found to respond better than those without the mutation (82% and 55% response, respectively).

It can be effective for the treatment of many other types of tumours influenced by RTK (such as some types of solid tumours, e.g. thyroid carcinoma, squamous cell carcinoma, etc.). It can also be used to treat atopic dermatitis, as it inhibits mast cell proliferation.

Although in the vast majority of cases the **adverse effects** are mild, they can be serious (even fatal) and specific follow-up tests are required when this drug is administered.

- The most common side effect is digestive upset and possibly gastrointestinal bleeding. Other side effects such as neutropaenia/thrombocytopaenia, alopecia, etc. may also be present.
- Consultation with an oncologist is recommended before administering this drug.

Kinavet/Masivet® (Masitinib Mesylate)

Masitinib is a RTK inhibitor.

Survival increases regardless of mutation status, although it has better outcomes in c-kit positive cases.

In a recent study, 83% of dogs with gross MCT were found to respond to masitinib (38.5% complete response and 43.6% partial response). Average progression and survival times were 79 and 160 days, respectively.

In a 2017 study evaluating masitinib in dogs with metastatic or inoperable MCT, a 50% response rate was observed. Median survival time for responsive cases was 630 days, compared with 137 days for non-responsive ones. Response to masitinib was the most important predictor of survival. Toxicity was observed in 61% of the cases. The adverse effects are similar to those produced by Palladia® (increased ALT and vomiting were the most common).

In addition, the use of **combined protocols** between receptor tyrosine kinase inhibitors and traditional chemotherapy (for example, combinations of vinblastine or lomustine with Palladia®) are currently being studied.

- **Vinblastine and Palladia®**. The tolerated dose of vinblastine when combined with Palladia® was 1.6 mg/m². A protocol using vinblastine at 1.6 mg/m² every 2 weeks combined with Palladia® at 3.25 mg/kg PO every other day was safe and showed a 71% response. However, the authors have suggested that more studies be performed before recommending it.
- **Lomustine and Palladia®**. Palladia® was administered on days 1, 3 and 5 of a 21-day cycle at a dose of 2.75 mg/kg and lomustine was administered every 21 days at 50 mg/m². The dose limitation was neutropaenia. The response rate was 46% (4 complete and 15 partial responses). Overall, it was well tolerated and may be a reasonable treatment option for metastatic or inoperable MCT.

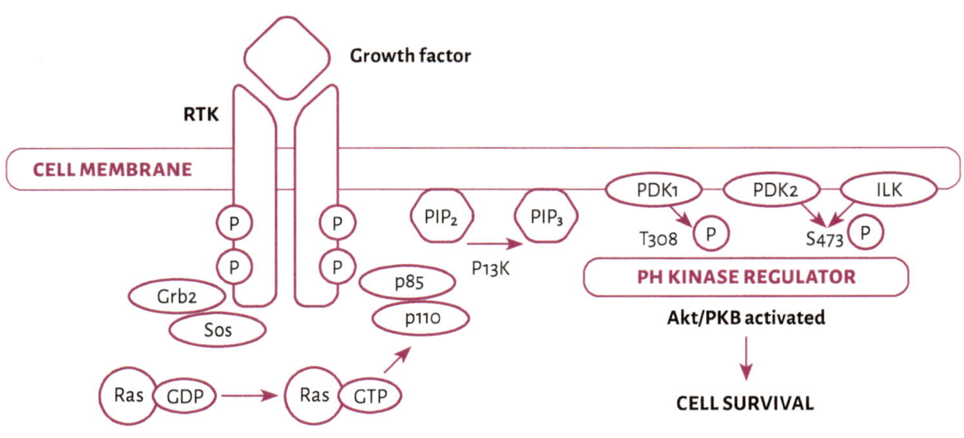

Figure 10. Diagram of a tyrosine kinase receptor (receptor tyrosine kinase, RTK) found in the cell membrane, which is activated by ligand binding, causing activation of different cell pathways at the same time. (Image: Tbatam/CC-BY-SA-3.0).

Local Therapy

Electrochemotherapy

In recent years, there has been a lot of talk about the use of electrochemotherapy for the treatment of some skin tumours, including MCTs.

The treatment **combines the administration of low systemic doses of chemotherapy with the application of local microsecond electrical pulses** that cause a change in permeability in the cell membrane, thereby increasing the permeabilisation of tumour cell membranes. The treated cells uptake a higher concentration of the chemotherapy drug and internalise it in their DNA, which will be damaged. When the cells move to the division phase in the cell cycle, the cell will die. Tumours with higher replication rates are more sensitive than low growth rate tumours.

In a 2017 study its use as a first line of treatment or as an adjunct to surgery was evaluated. The groups treated with both had better disease-free times and it was found to be better for small lesions when used as the sole treatment method. Further research into which are the ideal candidates for this type of treatment and its advantages over other types of therapies is still necessary.

Stelfonta® (Tigilanol Tiglate)

In 2020, the U.S. Food and Drug Administration approved Stelfonta® (tigilanol tiglate injection). It is specifically tailored to address nonmetastatic cutaneous mast cell tumours and nonmetastatic subcutaneous mast cell tumours situated distal to the elbow or hock, provided they are 10 cm^3 or smaller in size. In a randomized controlled clinical trial, it was found that a single injection led to complete tumour resolution in 75% of the treated dogs within 28 days. When accounting for dogs who required retreatment after 28 days due to an incomplete response, a noteworthy 87% of the dogs achieved complete tumour resolution. Ultimately, 96% of the dogs remained free of the disease at the 12-week mark following the initial injection, and within 3 months, complete wound healing was observed in 98.2% of cases.

Treatment with Stelfonta® has been associated with cellulitis and severe tissue sloughing extending away from the treated site resulting in extensive wounds that require additional treatment and prolonged recovery times. Case selection is important, to avoid complications.

Adjuvant Therapy

Dogs with MCT have higher than normal levels of systemic histamine. **Antihistamines** can help control signs associated with elevated histamine levels, such as peritumoural swelling and oedema, and gastric ulceration.

The administration of antihistamines is recommended if:

- there is a visible tumour that will be treated surgically, with chemotherapy or radiotherapy;
- there are signs of digestive upset or ulceration, for example weight loss, vomiting, black stools, or diarrhoea; or
- the patient presents evidence of systemic or regional metastasis.

Antihistamines can be H1 type (diphenhydramine, cyproheptadine) or H2 type (famotidine, ranitidine, cimetidine).

In dogs with signs of gastrointestinal ulceration, the administration of omeprazole, a proton pump inhibitor that is the most potent inhibitor of gastric secretion, should be considered.

Deionised water injections into the tumour bed are not recommended.

Intratumoural injections of steroids, such as triamcinolone, can palliate inoperable tumours (although they are not more beneficial than oral steroids and their routine application is not recommended).

Feline Mast Cell Tumours

MCTs in cats constitute approximately 20% of skin tumours in this domestic species. It is the second most common skin tumour in these animals.

The aetiology of feline MCTs is unknown: they are not associated with FeLV, FIV, FIP, or other viruses. A genetic predisposition has been proposed in Siamese cats as well as an increased frequency in other purebreds.

Clinical Presentation. Types of Feline MCTs

Cutaneous MCT

80% of cutaneous MCTs present as solitary, firm, well-defined, hairless masses, such as a dermal nodule. Up to 20% of cases present with multiple injuries. Tumours can itch, increase in size, and shrink, due to the intermittent release of histamine. The head is the most frequent presentation site, with some studies describing more than a 50% incidence on the head or head and neck, although they can also appear on the body and legs.

They usually **present as small (<0.5 cm) hairless, raised areas on the head or neck**, which are often mistaken for eosinophilic granuloma complexes (EGC) or stings; they may have the appearance of a plaque, but are generally white and well defined. In 25% of cases, the surface may be ulcerated.

In general, they are benign, but some of them will metastasise to regional lymph nodes and systemically. Therefore, evaluation of the regional lymph nodes is important. A **19% rate of metastasis to the spleen in feline cutaneous MCTs** has been described. Consideration should be given to the possibility of performing systemic staging tests if there are clinical signs of systemic disease or signs of regional lymph node metastasis.

Two different forms of cutaneous MCT have been described in cats.

- **Histiocytic**. Uncommon, it occurs in younger animals (average age 2 years). Diagnosis is difficult because only 20% of cells are mast cells, while the rest are histiocytes, lymphocytes, and eosinophils. In some cases, the histiocytic forms return spontaneously. These patients usually present with multiple firm, non-itchy, hairless, and sometimes ulcerated masses, but otherwise cats are healthy. Lesions usually return within 4–24 months.
- **Mast cell**. It is a more frequent form and occurs in adult animals (Figure 11). Histologically resembles canine MCTs. The average age of onset is 10 years. In turn, there are two types.
  - **Compact** (well differentiated), which is the most common (50–90% of cases). Benign and less metastatic.
  - **Diffuse** (anaplastic). Less common, but more malignant.

Siamese cats are predisposed to both types (at least, as described in one study).

Visceral

Visceral MCTs are more common than in dogs – they account for 50% of all feline MCT cases. Cats are usually unwell for several months before the diagnosis is made. In these patients, finding multiple metastases is common. It is often referred to as visceral MCT in the cat **when it is located in the spleen or intestine**. It has also been described in the cranial mediastinum. Signs related to MCT degranulation are more common in visceral or disseminated MCTs than in cutaneous ones.

Splenic

It is the **most common cause of splenomegaly in cats**: the spleen is usually soft to touch and is enlarged, although it can also be nodular. Other differential diagnoses of splenomegaly are lymphoma, haemangiosarcoma, splenitis secondary to infections, myeloproliferative disorders, or hyperplastic nodules, among others. The mean age of presentation is 10 years and there is no breed or sex predisposition.

Clinical signs often include weight loss, bloating, vomiting, and diarrhoea. Between 40–100% of cases have peripheral blood mastocythaemia, 33% have anaemia, 90% have alterations in coagulation and/or hyperglobulinaemia. 50% of bone marrow aspirates and buffy coat smears are positive.

Metastases to the liver (90%), visceral lymph nodes (73%), bone marrow (40%), lung (20%), and intestine (17%) have been described at necropsy of 50 cats with primary splenic MCT.

Intestinal

It is the **third most common primary intestinal tumour in cats** (after lymphoma and adenocarcinoma). It is associated with poor prognosis because the patient commonly develops systemic disease. It can affect the small intestine (most common) or the colon (least common).

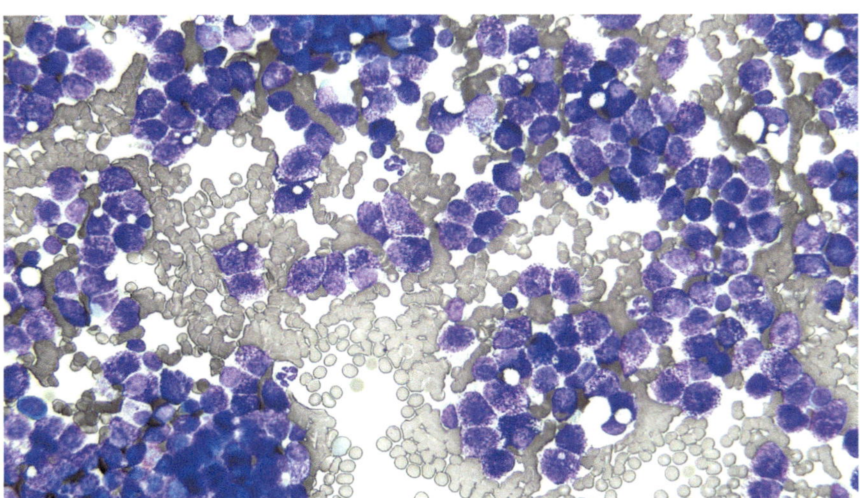

Figure 11. Typical cytological image of a well-differentiated mast cell tumour (mastocytic type) in a cat. An abundant population of round cells with granules visible inside them can be seen.

Intestinal lesions can be single or multiple, be a mass or be disseminated throughout the digestive tract (such as lymphoma): **feline intestinal sclerosing mast cell tumour** is a variant of intestinal mastocytosis that consists of mast cells with severe secondary fibrosis.

The mean age of presentation is 13 years old, and **clinical signs** include weight loss, abdominal effusion, vomiting, and diarrhoea. 33% of patients with this type of MCT have anaemia.

The primary intestinal form almost never presents with peripheral mastocytosis but does cause eosinophilia. It may metastasise to the liver or regional lymph nodes.

Staging

Not all cats require complete staging, so the process should be performed step by step. Minimum staging includes the evaluation of the regional lymph node (palpation, ultrasound, examination, FNA...). Complete staging with regional lymph node aspirate, abdominal ultrasound, and FNA may also include thoracic radiography and buffy coat smear if cats present with:

- multiple lesions
- palpable abdominal abnormalities
- poorly differentiated or histologically poorly differentiated tumours
- visceral (intestinal or splenic) or cranial mediastinal tumours
- mastocythaemia (circulating mast cells in peripheral blood).

Bone marrow aspiration is not indicated in most feline MCTs since, in general, cases with significant bone marrow involvement have widespread disease and a positive result is unlikely to change the patient's management or prognosis. A bone marrow sample may be indicated, for example, when there is a solitary mass and at the same time mastocythaemia is detected.

Staging is recommended for cutaneous MCTs, as some cats with cutaneous MCTs have concurrent splenic MCT; occasionally, splenectomy can result in the disappearance of cutaneous MCTs.

Aspiration by puncture of visceral organs is diagnostic of the splenic or intestinal forms.

Prognostic Factors

So far, these are not as clear as in dogs, since the grading system for cutaneous MCT in dogs is not prognostic for cats.

Proliferation Markers

These are not as well-known as for the dog, but the **mitotic index is the factor that best predicts the prognosis in feline MCTs**.

A high mitotic index is associated with aggressive behaviour. If the mitotic index and Ki-67 are elevated at the same time, it is an indication of high pleomorphism and a worse prognosis. However, no cut-off values have been described for these parameters.

Histological Characteristics

Histological characteristics, such as the degree of pleomorphism, are another of the prognostic factors that must be considered.

KIT Expression

The relationship between KIT expression, KIT gene mutations, histological grade, and prognosis is much less clear than for dogs. 52% of cats are KIT positive. It is not related to the histotype, but a higher positive percentage is usually associated with a higher proliferation index and, therefore, with a worse prognosis, although in another subsequent study no association between KIT and prognosis was found. Therefore, immunoreactivity may be associated with a worse prognosis, but it is not clear from the data available so far.

For splenic MCTs, in 2016 a study was published in which 85% of tumours had KIT expression in the cytoplasm and there were mutations in 20% (not detected in exons 11 and 17). There was no correlation between KIT expression and mutations, nor was the c-kit mutation correlated with tumour differentiation, mitotic activity, or survival.

Treatment

Treatment of Cutaneous MCT

Surgery is the best option for isolated skin MCTs. The small size of the patients and the frequent location on the head and neck limits surgeries with wide margins, although this may not be as important for well-differentiated tumours and/or compact tumours.

When a preoperative biopsy suggests aggressive behaviour, extensive surgery combined with adjuvant therapy should be performed. If the resection is incomplete, watching and waiting is generally recommended, since local recurrence is less frequent than in dogs (0–22% according to various studies, although it will depend on the prognostic factors associated to the tumour and the histopathological description). However, **close follow-up is recommended to rule out metastases** to distant organs or to the regional lymph node.

Electrochemotherapy might be an option for some of these lesions, specially for those tumours localised in areas where surgical margins can be difficult to obtain; the combination of surgery and intraoperatory electrochemotherapy, or electrochemotherapy alone for some cases, can be an alternative.

Some tumours with a diameter of less than 5 mm can be treated with **Sr-90 (strontium) radiotherapy**, which is a single dose treatment effective against MCT in places where surgery is complicated, such as the eyelids or the ear. A recent study showed that more than 95% of cats with small cutaneous MCT treated with this modality had long disease-free periods (more than 5 years).

Splenic MCT Treatment

The treatment of choice is splenectomy. Biopsy of the liver, mesenteric lymph nodes, and small intestine is recommended for staging, even when these areas appear normal.

Long-term survival is possible in cats after splenectomy, even if there is metastasis beyond the spleen (one study describes a median survival of 12–19 months).

Treatment of Intestinal MCT

The prognosis is not as good as in splenic MCT but may improve if surgical excision is achieved with acceptable margins (5–10 cm margin). The median survival time is 3–6 months.

Chemotherapy

To date, not much information is available about the efficacy of treating feline MCT with chemotherapy, either palliatively or as an adjuvant. It is not widely used in these animals if there is no evidence of metastasis to distant organs or regional lymph nodes. It is usually reserved for cats with pleomorphic, locally invasive, or metastatic MCT.

The role of chemotherapy in metastatic visceral MCT is also unclear, but its administration is recommended if there is evidence of MCT in organs other than the spleen. Cases of spontaneous disappearance of metastases after splenectomy have been described.

To date, there is little information in the literature on the efficacy of various chemotherapeutic substances against mastocytosis in cats, although they are usually treated with protocols similar to in dogs (for example, lomustine or vinblastine are used).

The role of steroids in the treatment of feline MCTs has not been demonstrated.

Radiotherapy

There is little literature available on the use of radiotherapy to treat feline MCTs. Few cats are good candidates, because many have multiple tumours or metastases at the time of diagnosis.

Additionally, it is not widely used in feline MCTs since tumour recurrence after incomplete removal of skin tumours may be less frequent than in dogs. Strontium radiation therapy is applied to small lesions on the face/ears.

Receptor Tyrosine Kinase Inhibitors (RTKI)

To date, there is little information regarding the use of RTKI in cats with mast cell tumours. In a 2016 study on cats with different tumour types, including MCT, an acceptable response to treatment with RTKI was observed. Generally, it was well tolerated, with slight gastrointestinal toxicity or myelosuppression, although the appearance of hepatotoxicity can be a problem (10% of cases with proteinuria were described in one study), but the information published in this regard is still scarce.

Supportive Therapy

Anti-H1 and H2, type drugs, which prevent degranulation, can be effective. The use of H1 antagonists is recommended before surgical interventions and in animals with obvious clinical signs of degranulation. The use of H2 antagonists is recommended for cats with possible gastritis or gastrointestinal ulceration secondary to histamine elimination and for cats with disseminated or visceral disease.

Skin Neoplasms in Dogs and Cats

Incidence of Skin Tumours

They are the **most frequently diagnosed neoplasms in domestic animals**, probably because they are easily identified and the skin is constantly exposed to the environment, which predisposes it to neoplastic transformation. Chemical carcinogens, radiation, viruses, etc. may be involved in the development of skin neoplasms.

The skin is a complex structure, composed of several tissues, all of them with the potential for tumour development: epithelial, mesenchymal, neural, and neuroectoderm. Because skin tumours are so diverse, classification is difficult. In a study published in JAVMA in 2011 the clinical records of one million dogs from multiple university veterinary hospitals were analysed through the Veterinary Medical Data Base and it was found that 2% of cases came to the veterinarian's clinic solely for skin tumours.

The risk of developing a skin tumour increases with the age of the patient: 10–15 years-old dogs are at very high risk. This study also described the predisposition of certain breeds of dog to develop certain tumour types.

For cats, in a study that analysed the records of more than 9000 feline skin tumour samples from a veterinary diagnostic laboratory, the study found that only 6.6% of these samples were not neoplastic in nature. The three most common diagnoses of non-neoplastic skin masses were follicular cysts, apocrine gland cysts, and dermoid cysts. Among the remaining samples of neoplastic masses, 52.7% were considered histologically malignant. In this study of cats, the British Blue and Himalayan breeds had a higher percentage of development of skin tumours (benign and malignant), when compared to cats without pedigree. On the other hand, the Persian, Burmese, and Oriental breeds seem to be less predisposed to developing skin tumours. The most frequent types of tumours found in dogs and cats are summarised in Box 2.

Box 2. Common skin tumours in order of frequency

Dog

- **Mast cell tumour**
- **Lipoma**
- **Histiocytoma**
- **Perianal gland adenoma**
- **Sebaceous adenoma/hyperplasia**
- **Squamous cell carcinoma**
- **Melanoma**
- **Fibrosarcoma**
- **Basal cell tumour**
- **Malignant nerve sheath tumours**
- **Papilloma**
- **Sweat gland carcinoma**
- **Sebaceous adenocarcinoma.**

Cat

- **Basal cell tumour**
- **Mast cell tumour**
- **Squamous cell carcinoma**
- **Fibrosarcoma**
- **Apocrine cystadenoma**
- **Lipoma**
- **Haemangiosarcoma**
- **Sebaceous adenoma**
- **Fibroma**
- **Haemangioma**
- **Melanoma**
- **Malignant fibrous histiocytoma.**

Physical Examination

When performing a physical examination, a **careful and thorough palpation** of the patient's skin and tissues is always necessary. In animals with long hair, the hair should be parted to observe the underlying skin. In addition, when this complete skin examination is performed, the feet/nail beds, periocular areas, tips of the ears of cats should always be checked for preneoplastic skin lesions such as comedones, scales or cutaneous erythema.

Once all lesions have been measured and recorded (Figure 12), aspirates should be obtained by **fine needle puncture** of all of them for cytological study (the two techniques for puncture aspiration are described in the following section *Cytological evaluation*).

Once the sample has been obtained, the contents of the needle must be forcefully/rapidly expelled with a syringe onto a glass slide. Smears should be performed quickly, and an attempt should be made to obtain a thin layer of cells for evaluation by the pathologist (Figure 13).

In addition, before submitting the material to the pathologist, it is advisable to review a stained sample on a slide, to ensure that it is a diagnostic sample. Slides should be shipped in a cardboard tray or in a special container for glass slides and,

HISTORY OF VISIBLE TUMOURS

Patient name: ______________________

Owner's name: ______________________

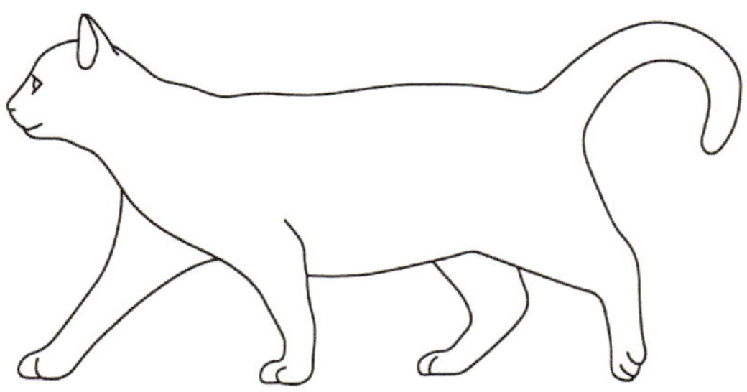

LEFT LATERAL VIEW

	Date	Size	Initials
1			
2			
3			
...			

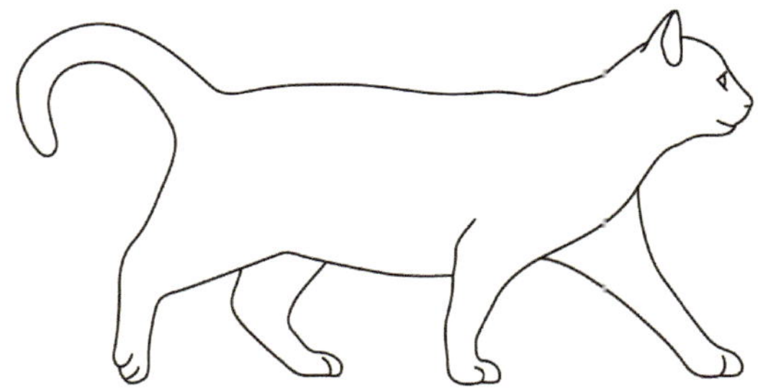

RIGHT LATERAL VIEW

	Date	Size	Initials
1			
2			
3			
...			

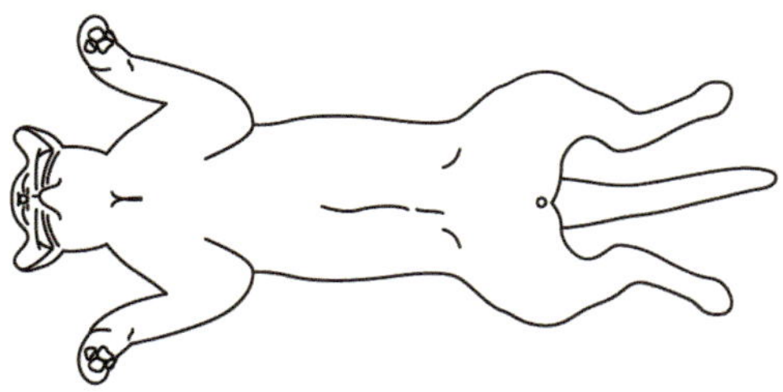

VENTRAL VIEW

	Date	Size	Initials
1			
2			
3			
...			

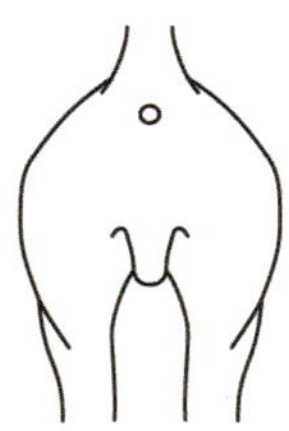

CAUDAL VIEW

	Date	Size	Initials
1			
2			
3			
...			

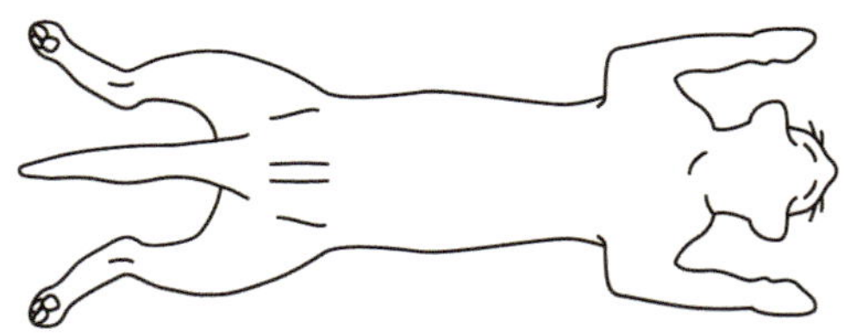

DORSAL VIEW

	Date	Size	Initials
1			
2			
3			
...			

Figure 12. Example of a "body map" document of a cat where location, size and details of each lesion can be noted on each visit to assess the progression of each one (download the template from the following link: https://publication.improveinternational.com).

always, in a container separate from formaldehyde. Biopsy and histological analysis are recommended for skin masses that are growing, changing in appearance, or causing irritation and when cytological analysis does not provide a definitive diagnosis.

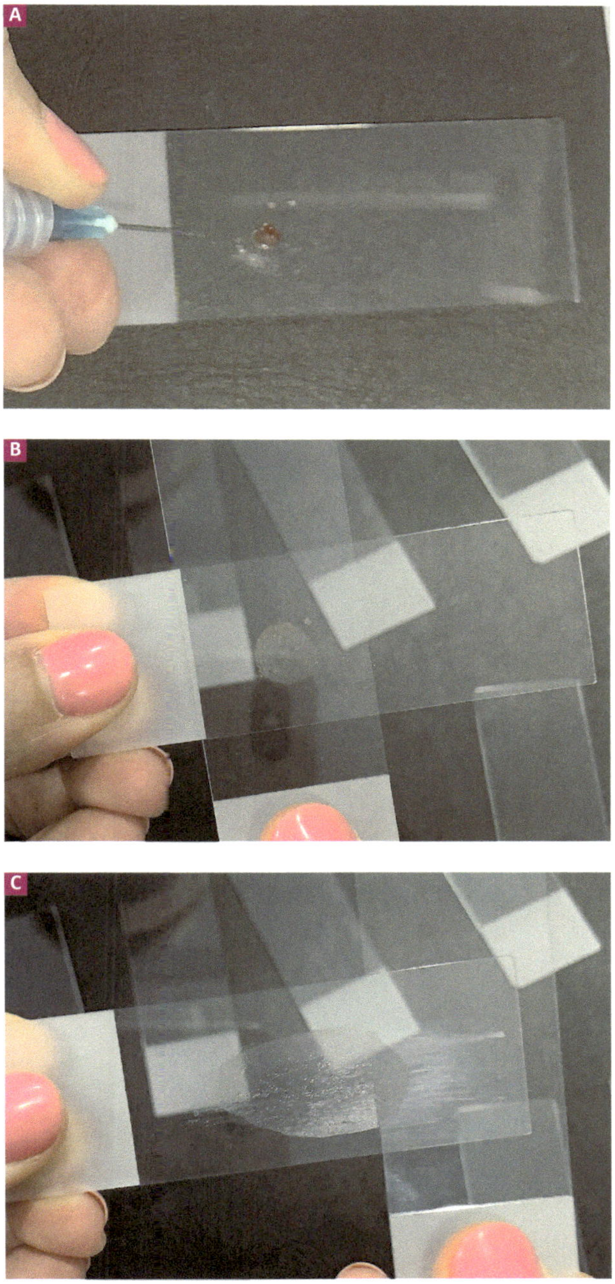

Figure 13. Preparation of cytology from sample obtained from fine needle aspiration. A 5 ml syringe is connected to the needle used for the aspirate with the plunger at the 5 ml mark and the air is expelled quickly so the sample in the needle is expelled onto the slide (**A**). With another slide in a perpendicular position the sample is extended with a medium pressure, covering the whole area without destroying the cells due to excess pressure (**B**). The sample is ready to stain and evaluate under the microscope (**C**).

Description of Skin Tumours

When submitting a cytology or biopsy specimen for histopathologic or cytologic evaluation, a complete description must be included in all cases.

1. **Location**: epidermal, dermo epidermal or subcutaneous. If subcutaneous, whether the tumours are attached to underlying structures should be specified. And the location or locations on the body.
2. **Surface**: state of the epidermis and the hair that covers it; hyperplastic, normal, alopecic, atrophied (thin), ulcerated.
3. **Size**: measurement and annotation of location on the body map.
4. **Colour**: whether the tumour is pigmented or not if it is filled with blood.
5. **Consistency**: firm, soft, variable.
6. **Shape**: smooth, lobed, or cauliflower-like, papillose, fungal.
7. **Growth behaviour**: circumscribed, infiltrating, sessile, pedunculated, elevated (exophytic) or below the surface.

Cytological Evaluation

Cytology by Fine Needle Puncture

Puncture aspiration techniques include the needle-in-syringe technique and the non-syringe technique ("woodpecker").

- The **syringe technique** is recommended for masses that are firm, that are likely to be less exfoliative, and for which it is more difficult to obtain a good sample with just the needle (Figure 14).
- The "**woodpecker**" **technique** is recommended for most skin masses and lymph nodes because it tends to produce less bleeding in tumours (Figure 15).

As outlined in the *Physical Examination* section above, all skin masses and regional/drainage lymph nodes should be aspirated and a sample of each should be stained and clinically evaluated to ensure a diagnostic specimen is sent. Unless the diagnosis is very certain, to sending the samples collected to a clinical pathologist/veterinary laboratory is recommended.

Benign Tumours: Cytology

- homogeneous cell population
- well-differentiated appearance (the cells appear normal; they resemble those of the tissue from which they came)
- little variation in cell or nucleus size
- small nucleus/cytoplasm ratio
- a single nucleolus or no nucleolus visible
- from few to no mitotic figures
- possible secondary inflammation.

Benign masses must be closely monitored for changes in size, consistency, ulceration, or invasiveness.

They should be surgically removed if they bleed or bother the patient, if the tumour grows, or if the cytological diagnosis is doubtful.

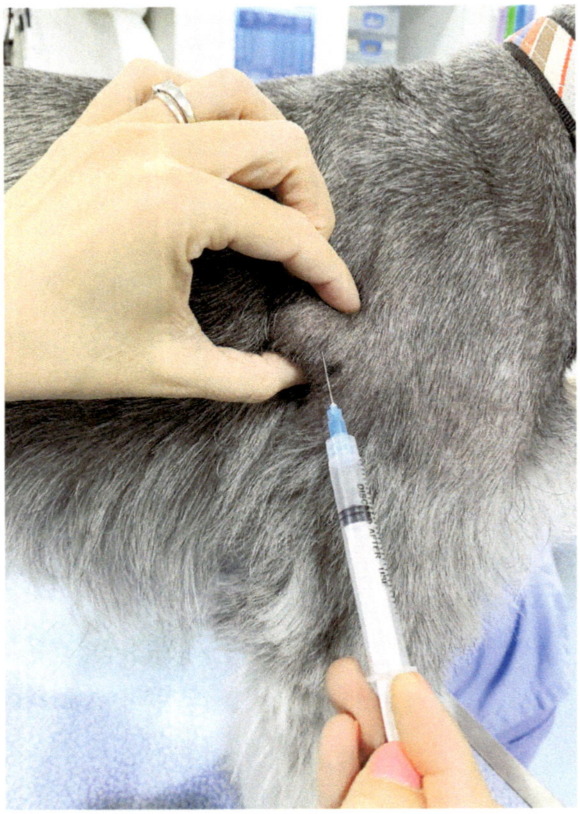

Figure 14. Example of obtaining samples using fine needle aspiration where the syringe is connected to the needle, which is particularly useful in firm masses or those which do not exfoliate easily.

Malignant Tumours: Cytology

- pleomorphic cell population
- poorly differentiated (abnormal cells and different from those of the tissue where they are located)
- significant variation in cell or nucleus size
- high nucleus/cytoplasm ratio
- multiple nucleoli
- numerous mitotic figures
- atypical mitoses.

Some malignant tumours present with secondary inflammation, and it can sometimes be difficult to determine whether it is a tumour or inflammation, particularly in the case of epithelial tumours (there may be false negatives aspirated upon puncture).

Biopsy and/or surgical resection is recommended.

Biopsy Evaluation

Incisional or Excisional Biopsy

The decision to carry out one or the other depends on:

- **size**. If the tumours are too large or locally invasive to be completely removed, a previous incisional biopsy can be obtained to determine a definitive therapeutic plan;
- **ulceration**. Where possible, ulcerated masses should be completely excised (excisional biopsy) for palliative and diagnostic purposes;
- **provisional diagnosis**. If the cytology is diagnostic for a benign tumour, performing, whenever possible, an excisional biopsy is recommended;
- recommendation of other additional treatment (radiotherapy, electrochemotherapy or chemotherapy). In some cases, neoadjuvant treatments before surgical removal of tumours is recommended to try to reduce their

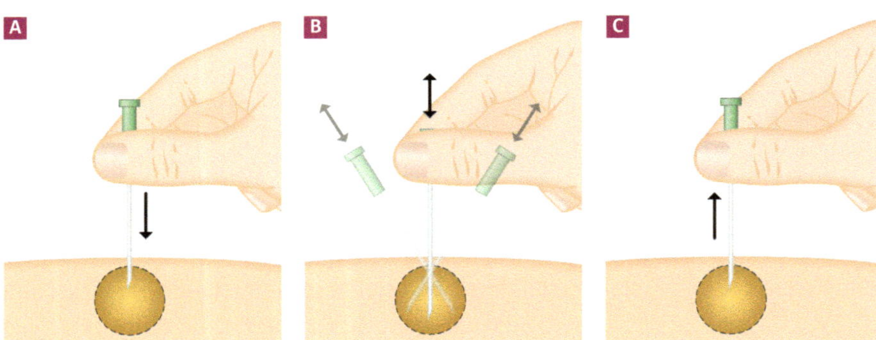

Figure 15. Technique to obtain samples using a fine needle without syringe: the needle is introduced into the lesion (**A**). Once the needle is in the lesion it is redirected in several different directions to obtain a sample from different areas (**B**). The needle is removed from the lesion (**C**).

size and facilitate excision. In these cases, performing an incisional biopsy before treatment to obtain histological information is recommended; and
- if the result of the biopsy influences the type of surgery to be carried out (Figure 16), an incisional biopsy must always be performed first, especially in the case where the type of surgery that may be needed is very aggressive and/or requires reconstructive procedures.

Presurgical Evaluation for Patients Undergoing Excisional Biopsy

The minimum information needed includes:
- complete blood count, biochemistry (and urinalysis as required);
- electrocardiogram; and
- regional lymph node aspirate. This is very important because regional lymph nodes with metastases should be removed concurrently with surgery unless systemic staging shows more distant metastases. In general, if there is lymph node metastasis from a cutaneous tumour, systemic staging (thoracic radiographs – three views – and abdominal ultrasound) is recommended before any treatment.

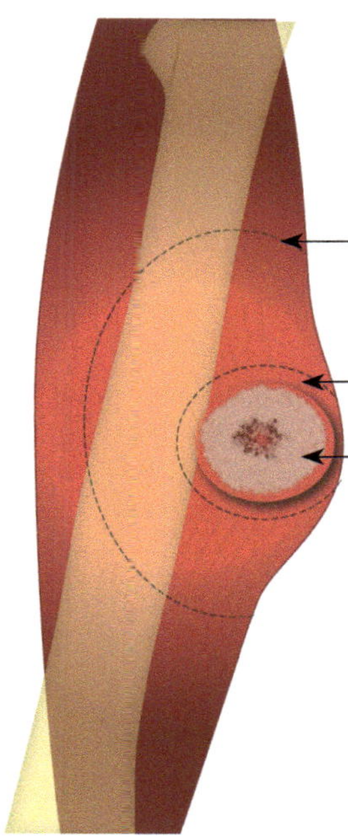

Figure 16. Diagram showing a lesion which demonstrates how to establish margins for intralesional excision within the lesion, marginal excision (around the external margins of the lesion) and a wide or radical excision (where the lesion is included as well as a wide margin around its outer margins).

Additional Tests

Depending on the patient's age, physical condition, provisional diagnosis, or lymph node metastasis status, the following may be recommended:
- diagnosis by sectional imaging (CT, MRI)
- retroviral screening (in cats)
- bone marrow aspirate.

Shipment of the Biopsy Sample

- All **excised tissue should be sent** for histopathological analysis.
- The diagnosis can vary between different lesions in different locations.
- Large lesions should be sliced, to be properly fixed.
- If possible, all margins should be identified (Davison multicolour ink system; suspected incomplete margins should always be identified (usually deep margin); India ink, sutured label, send pot or container separately).
- It is important to always **work with a veterinary pathologist**.
- A detailed clinical history and description should always be provided, as well as the lesion map and the results of the previous puncture aspiration.

Information Provided by Histopathology Report

- definitive diagnosis
- degree of completeness of the margins
- presence of vascular or lymphatic invasion
- mitotic index
- histological grade (if applicable)
- suggestion for evaluation of other molecular markers specific to certain tumour types (e.g., c-kit staining for mast cell tumours, etc).

These findings are used to be able to **stage/classify/provide a prognosis** for certain types of tumours.

It is important to remember that pathology is not always a "black and white" science. Sometimes the pathologist may recommend additional tests (special stains or special procedures) on the tissues that have been sent to help determine what the tumour type is. In almost all cases, these stains are necessary, since, in general, they provide a definitive diagnosis, and are the only way to offer the client the most precise information and the necessary recommendations about the cancer their pet is suffering from.

Special stains are usually antibody stains that identify cell surface antigens/markers for certain cell types (immunohistochemistry). It is important to remember that some tumours, especially in the case of very malignant or anaplastic tumours, can give negative results for all stains and it is possible that sometimes a definitive diagnosis will not be achieved.

Ideally, in most tumours, margins should be more than 2 cm between normal and tumour tissue. At times, it can be difficult for the pathologist to accurately measure the margins since tumours shrink when in formalin. If the margins are close (5 mm), careful monitoring for recurrence and/or possibly additional treatment may be recommended. However, the need for larger or smaller margins is fundamentally determined by the type, grade, and behaviour of the tumour.

Specific Types of Tumours

The most prominent tumour skin changes will be reviewed following the below classification.

1. Epithelial tumours
2. Mesenchymal tumours
3. Round cell tumours
4. Histiocytic neoplasms
5. Secondary skin neoplasms
6. Non-neoplastic tumours.

Epithelial Tumours

Papilloma

Oral papilloma is a benign tumour affecting the dog, which is also called canine oral papillomatosis.

It usually occurs in young dogs (Figure 17), caused by a parvovirus. They are highly contagious from dog to dog and can be transmitted by biting or play. There may be a single lesion or so many that it is not possible to count them.

The lesions are found in the mouth and around it. They have a characteristic cauliflower-shaped exophytic appearance. In most cases, there is spontaneous remission mediated by an infiltration of T lymphocytes, but surgical removal may be recommended if the lesions bleed, are very numerous or large, or if they affect food intake.

While papillomaviruses are known to be involved in oral squamous cell carcinoma (SCC) in humans, it is less clear in dogs. In a 2015 study, oral SCC lesions from dogs were sampled and no evidence of papillomavirus DNA was found, so it appears that papillomaviruses are not a major cause of oral SCC in dogs. However, some dermal papillomas containing papillomavirus have been described. These lesions can form large plaques and transformation to malignant phenotypes (SCC) is possible.

The approach to papillomas may include observation, surgical removal, cryosurgery, electrosurgery, electrochemotherapy or imiquimod 5% cream (Aldara™). In cats, some papillomavirus can cause oral papilloma, viral plaques, bowenoid in situ carcinomas and feline sarcoids. Also, some of them may induce cutaneous basal cell and squamous cell carcinoma (SCC); however, it is not clear whether SCC develops from viral plaques or directly from normal skin.

Infundibular Keratinising Acanthoma

Also known as IKA (infundibular keratinising acanthoma) or keratoacanthoma, affects young dogs and is benign.

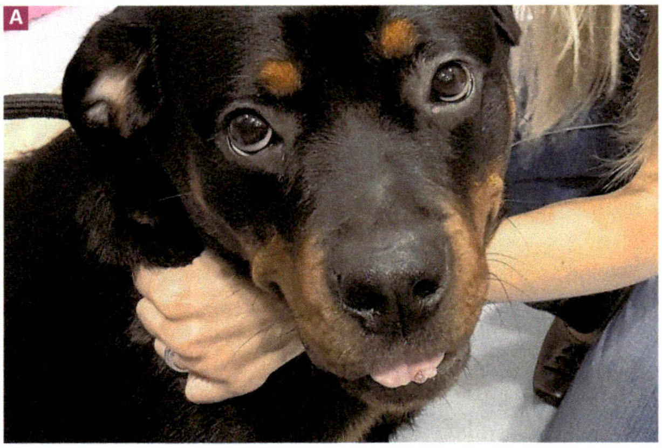

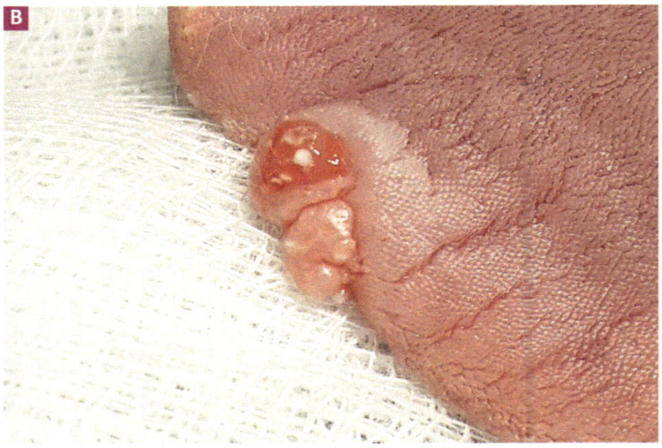

Figure 17. 1-year-old Rottweiler with a lesion on the rostral area of the tongue, compatible with an oral papilloma (**A**). Detail of the lesion shows the typical cauliflower like appearance (**B**).

It usually appears in young to middle-aged dogs (1–10 years), almost always on the back and extremities. Norwegian Elkhound hunting dogs are predisposed to the generalised form (multiple tumours). In other breeds it appears as a single tumour.

Its appearance varies from firm to fluctuating, well defined, dermal, or subcutaneous, with a size of 0.5–4 cm and, in general, with a "pore" opening with an obstruction that can be large. The cystic centre is filled with keratin. It can rupture and cause an abscess.

Isolated injuries are treated surgically. Dogs with multiple lesions are generally resistant to medical treatment and in these cases the use of oral retinoids, such as isotretinoin or etretinate, or intralesional chemotherapy should be considered.

Squamous Cell Carcinoma (SCC)

These tumours can occur in cats and dogs and are malignant. They develop in several locations, with variable behaviour:

SCC of the Oral Cavity

Covered in the Gastrointestinal Neoplasms in Cats and Dogs chapter in this book.

Subungual SCC (Nail Bed)

In the **dog** (Figure 18), it usually occurs in elderly individuals (over 10 years old). Black coated breeds, and dogs weighing over 30 kg (Giant Schnauzer, Scottish Setter, Poodle, Labrador Retriever) are predisposed. Multiple digital SCC can occur simultaneously.

In general, forelimbs are more commonly affected than hindlimbs. On many occasions, the diagnosis is mistaken for a nail infection. Radiographic evidence of toe bone lysis is frequently present (80% of affected dogs), and while regional lymph node metastasis is common, thoracic metastasis is rare.

In **cats**, nail bed carcinomas can be a **metastasis from a primary lung carcinoma**. For this reason, all nail bed carcinomas diagnosed in cats should be accompanied by complementary tests that include thoracic radiographs.

Solar Radiation Induced SCC

In **cats**, animals with a white coat, especially a white face, are predisposed to developing SCC. They are generally localised on the tips of the ears, periocular areas (Figure 19), eyelids and nose.

Regarding **dogs**, they are also more frequent in white coated dogs, such as the Bull Terrier, Pit Bull, Dalmatian, and White English Greyhound breeds (on the ventral abdomen in areas with little hair and fine skin) (Figure 20).

Before SCCs develop, preneoplastic lesions appear: **solar (actinic) keratoses**. These lesions are a sun-induced inflammation of the skin and resemble sunburn. Erythema, oedema, and scaling are seen followed by induration with thickening and wrinkling.

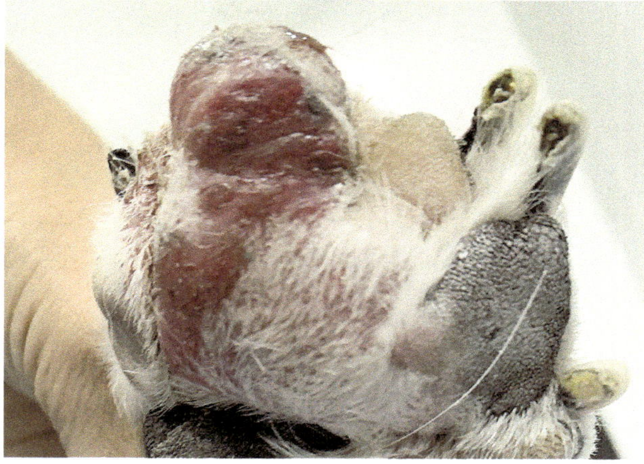

Figure 18. Ulcerative, erosive lesion at the base of the nail, compatible with a squamous cell carcinoma of the nail bed.

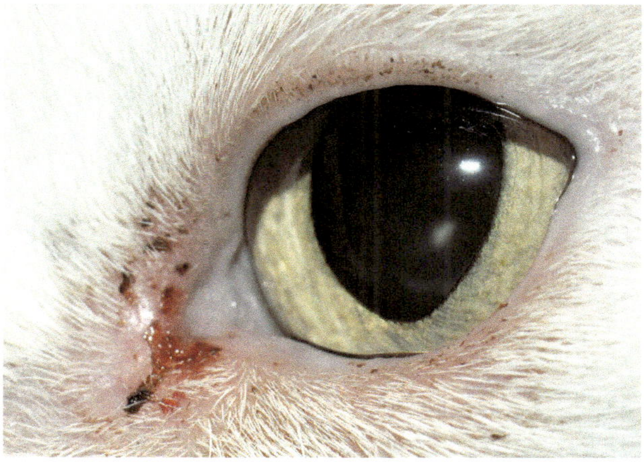

Figure 19. Skin lesion in the lacrimal area of a white cat. The lesion was erythematous and ulcerated and biopsy confirmed a solar induced squamous cell carcinoma.

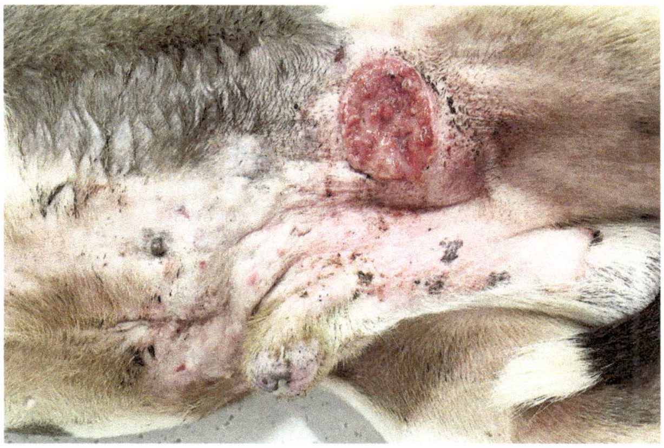

Figure 20. Solar induced squamous cell carcinoma on the abdomen of a dog. The inguinal, abdominal, and part of the ventral thorax regions are affected with oedema, erythema, pustules, and ulcers. In the right inguinal area a larger sized ulcerated lesion can be seen.

Affected animals usually have a history of several years of exposure to the sun (in dogs, sunbathing on their backs, in cats, which are allowed outdoors during the day or sleep in sunny areas of the house).

The **treatment/approach** to these tumours consists of:

- if **localised**, surgical excision;
- **systemic/non-localised**. Systemic treatment is less effective and consists of oral retinoids and oral COX inhibitors (anti-inflammatory and possibly also antineoplastic effects in carcinomas). Other types of chemotherapy, such as carboplatin or tyrosine kinase inhibitors, can be effective in some cases, but they are often resistant to chemotherapy;
- **strontium (Sr-90) radiotherapy** or **electrochemotherapy** can be an effective treatment for cats with sun-induced superficial lesions on the tips of the ears, nasal plane, etc., but which are difficult to remove surgically. ECT is very effective for the treatment of localised cutaneous SCC in cats. However, in the dog, ECT is not as effective than for cats for the treatment of nasal planum SCC;
- **avoiding exposure to the sun** (the animal should stay out of the sun, sunglasses can be used, as well as t-shirts and sunscreen, although they usually lick it off).

Client education on this disease is essential, as animals suffering from solar induction inflammation/neoplasia will continue to suffer from this syndrome throughout their lives. The best thing is prevention, so it is necessary to explain to owners with high-risk animals that they should limit sun exposure as much as possible.

For animals already affected, the typical approach is to remove gross lesions and treat preneoplastic lesions non-surgically (although this is complicated and not always as effective).

Bowen's Disease

Bowen's disease is a **localised carcinoma in the cat**. The lesions do not progress beyond the basal membrane of the skin and usually appear as multiple superficial, crusty lesions on the head, trunk, and extremities. Histopathological analysis is required for diagnosis.

Treatment includes surgery, topical imiquimod, Sr90, radiation therapy, electrochemotherapy, and oral retinoids.

This disease is usually chronic and progresses slowly, however new lesions can appear at any time. It is not caused by the sun, so it can be seen in cats of all colours and can develop anywhere on the body.

Other Cutaneous SCCs

SCCs have a typical appearance of proliferative or ulcerative masses, they can be cauliflower-shaped with a brittle surface, ranging from superficial to crateriform ulcers.

Treatment may include surgery (which is usually the best treatment option), radiotherapy (when the lesions are not surgically removable), electrochemotherapy, or, with very low success, intralesional chemotherapy (platinum drugs).

If the lesions are very superficial (<3/5 mm deep), photodynamics, cryosurgery, electrochemotherapy or plesiotherapy (Sr90) may be good therapeutic options.

SCCs are usually locally invasive; they can metastasise through lymphatic vessels to lymph nodes, nearby skin, lungs, or any other location in the body.

In general, SCC is easily diagnosed with cytology. However, concurrent inflammation is common and may make diagnosis difficult.

Trichoblastoma

Can be found in dogs and cats. They were previously called basal cell carcinomas (Figure 21). They are not induced by ultraviolet light, as is commonly the case in humans.

The average age for developing these tumours is around 6–9 years old for dogs, and 10 years old for cats and it seems that the Kerry Blue Terrier, Spaniel and Poodle breeds, as well as Persian and Himalayan cats are predisposed.

Typically, a single tumour appears on the head and neck, and metastasis is rare. They are firm, round, raised, well demarcated, dermo epidermal, alopecic to ulcerative, and often pigmented (cutaneous or subcutaneous bluish colour).

They are treated by surgical resection, cryosurgery, or electrosurgery. Radiotherapy may be given if removal is not complete or chemotherapy if systemic metastases develop (which is rare).

Sebaceous Gland Tumours

These tumours occur frequently in elderly dogs. There is a breed predisposition in the Cocker Spaniel, Shih Tzu, and Poodle. Patients may only present with one, however, they usually present multiple tumours on different parts of the body, which can be pigmented.

Different types of sebaceous gland tumours have been described.

- **Nodular sebaceous hyperplasia**. Firm raised (but not pedunculated), alopecic, small (2–10 mm). **Very common**.
- **Sebaceous adenoma**. Larger size, less lobulated, it is commonly pigmented (Figure 22).
- **Sebaceous adenocarcinoma**. Larger, firm, poorly defined, ulcerative, metastases are rare.

The approach of choice is to remove the tumour. Oral retinoids can be trialled to treat multiple lesions.

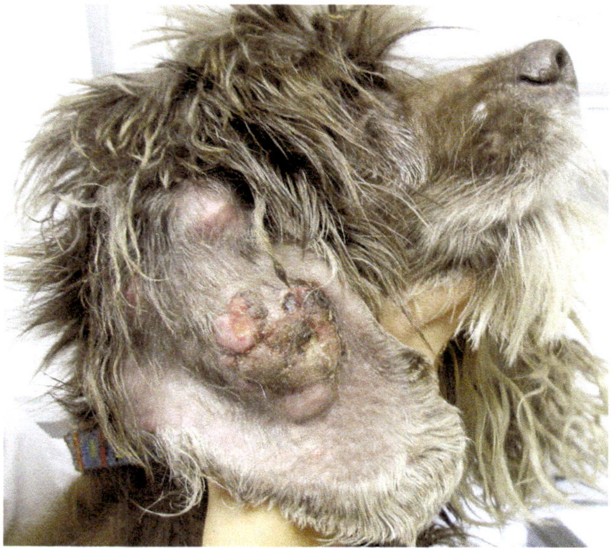

Figure 21. Trichob astoma (basal cell carcinoma) on the ear of a dog.

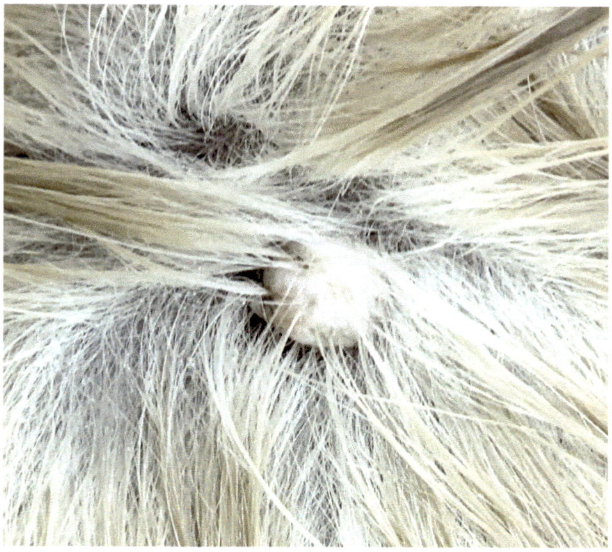

Figure 22. Sebaceous adenoma in a dog.

Hair Follicle Tumours

Include **trichoepitheliomas, pilomatrixomas and trichilemmomas**. This type of tumour is named differently depending on where the cell forms in the hair follicle.

They represent 5% of all canine skin tumours and are very rare in cats.

They are single round or oval tumours, which are well defined, without hair and usually exhibits benign behaviour.

They have an excellent prognosis with surgical removal. In very rare cases, they present metastases to the lymph nodes and lung.

These cases shou d always be monitored, depending on histopathology results.

Apocrine (Sweat) Gland Tumours

These tumours can occur in both dogs and cats. They can be of three types.

- **Apocrine cyst**: often multiple cysts, on the head and neck, which are raised, round, fluctuating, very well defined, and greyish in colour.
- **Apocrine adenoma**: firm, raised, well defined, 1–4 cm.
- **Apocrine (malignant) adenocarcinoma**: firm, infiltrating, poorly defined, often ulcerative, invasive, and metastatic. This type often metastasises through the cutaneous lymphatic vessels and may look like hot spots (moist/exudative).

The approach will depend on the histological type and the location, hence, for cysts wait an see can be recommended. On the other hand, surgery, electrochemotherapy, radiation and even adjuvant chemotherapy might be necessary for more agressive tumours.

Ceruminous Gland Adenocarcinoma

An invasive tumour of the external ear canal; it can affect both ears. It progresses slowly and infrequently develops local and distant metastasis. It causes itching, bleeding, and affected animals often cause self-trauma to the ear.

Cocker Spaniels are predisposed to suffering from this type of tumour. Dogs and cats with chronic infections or inflammation of the external ear canal are also more predisposed to developing them.

Treatment includes total ablation of the external ear canal, to which supplemental radiotherapy may be added when resection is incomplete. Long-term survival is possible with aggressive local treatment. Also, electrochemotherapy might be usefull as a first line therapy for small and difficult to resect tumours, or as intraoperatory/postoperatory adjuvant treatment.

Perianal Gland Tumours

This tumour is modulated by androgens (mainly testosterone); most are adenomas (carcinomas are rare) (Figure 23).

Most patients suffering from this tumour are elderly male dogs. They can appear as a single or multiple tumours, near the anus, although they can also affect the tail and perineum. They can vary from very demarcated to poorly defined, alopecic, and elevated, and can ulcerate as they grow.

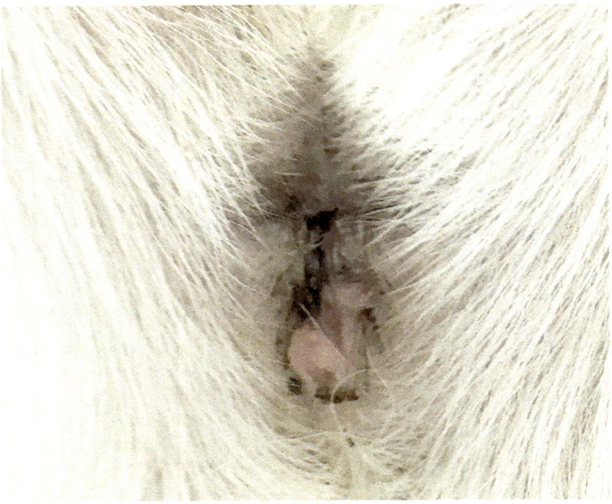

Figure 23. Canine perianal adenoma.

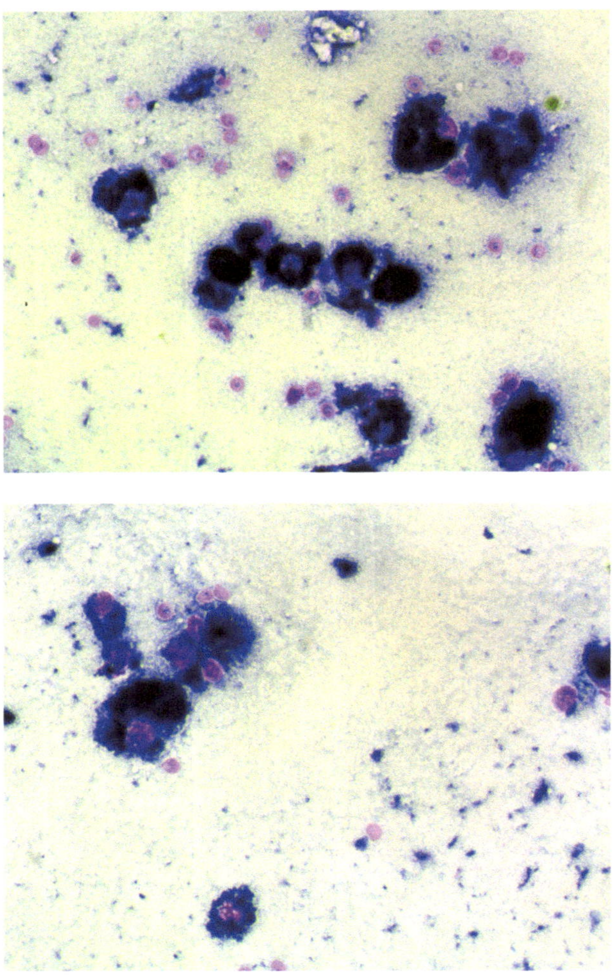

Figure 24. Two cytological images taken of a pigmented cutaneous nodule. The cytology is compatible with a melanoma. Multiple round cells can be seen with abundant melanin pigmentation inside.

The treatment of choice is surgical, with removal of the tumour plus castration or solely castration. In isolated cases, external radiotherapy or electrochemotherapy of perianal adenomas that cover the entire circumference of the anus may be recommended.

If perianal adenomas recur after castration of intact male dogs or if they are seen in castrated males or spayed/intact females, it is important to investigate whether there is an underlying source of androgens (androgen-secreting adrenal gland tumours, cryptorchidism in neutered males).

Mesenchymal Tumours of the Skin and Subcutaneous Tissues

Melanoma

More common in dogs and rare in cats.

Melanoma is often classified as a round cell tumour due to its cytologic appearance (Figure 24) and its biological behaviour. However, melanocytes arise from the neuroectoderm and are technically mesenchymal cells.

Purebred dogs are at higher risk (Terriers, particularly Scottish Terriers, Standard and Miniature Schnauzers, Dobermanns, Rottweilers, Golden Retrievers, and Labrador Retrievers).

Generally, they present as a single tumour, which is usually pigmented, but not always. 20% of melanomas are not pigmented (amelanotic melanomas) (Figure 25).

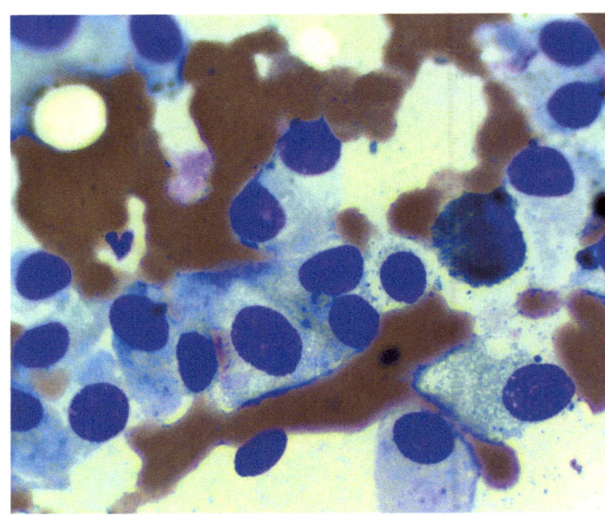

Figure 25. Cytological image of an amelanotic/poorly differentiated melanoma. To the contrary of the appearance in well-differentiated melanomas most tumour cells do not show evidence of granules with melanin pigmentation.

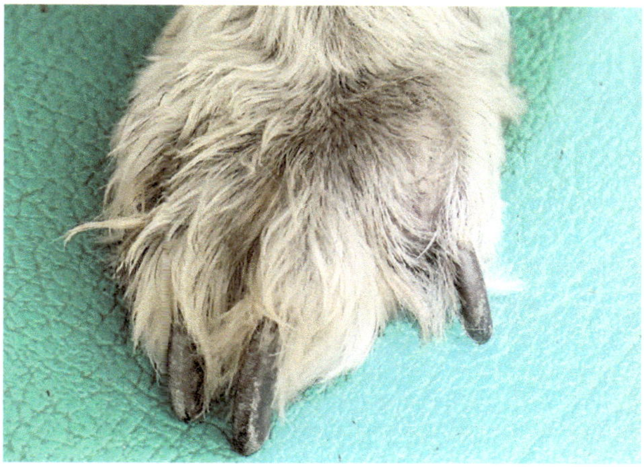

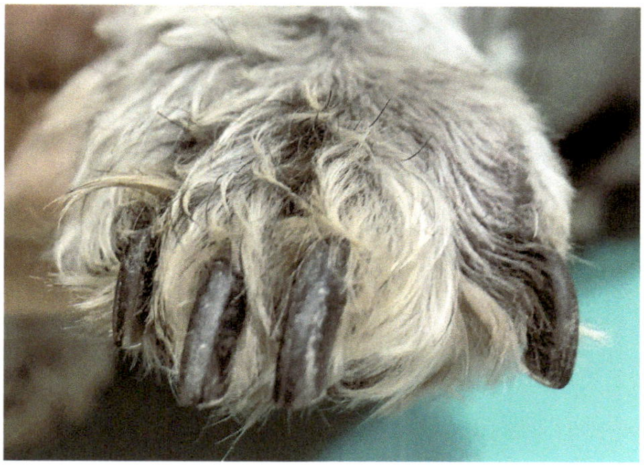

Figure 26. Digital melanoma affecting the base of the nail of the fifth toe and extending towards the fourth on the right forelimb.

There are some locations that are generally associated with tumours with more benign behaviour:

- dogs: on the head or forelimbs;
- cats: almost always on the head (the main differential diagnosis in cats is pigmented trichoblastoma); and
- they usually present as brown or black spots and plaques, but they can also give rise to firm, smooth dome-shaped nodules of around 0.5–2 cm.

In dogs, 90% of digital and mucocutaneous melanomas are malignant, show aggressive local and systemic behaviour, and metastasise to lymph nodes, lungs, and other areas. In general, these tumours grow rapidly, are poorly defined, and are dome-shaped to ulcerative.

In many cases, the diagnosis can be obtained by fine needle aspiration since granules with melanotic pigment are evident. However, in poorly differentiated tumours or amelanotic melanomas, the diagnosis can be more complicated. Benign and malignant forms are distinguished by histological features as well as their location.

Treatment options include excision, which may be followed by chemotherapy, radiotherapy, electrochemotherapy, and/or immunotherapy (melanoma vaccine).

The prognosis is based on the location, histological characteristics, and size of the tumour.

- **Dogs**: dermal melanomas, low mitotic index ≤2 MF in 10 HPF is associated with longer survival periods.
- **Dogs have a worse prognosis than cats**, since they are prone to developing metastases.

Digital melanomas (nail bed) (Figure 26) show an aggressive behaviour and local and distant metastases appear in more than 50% of cases.

Treatment usually consists of amputation of the toe followed by chemotherapy (carboplatin), which can be supplemented with immunotherapy. The one-year survival rate is 42% and 13% at 2 years.

Lipoma

A benign tumour that can occur in dogs and cats, but much more frequently in dogs. Some predisposed breeds are: Dobermann, Labrador Retriever and Miniature Schnauzer dog breeds (Figure 27).

They can be a single or multiple tumours that appear more commonly on the trunk and proximal extremities. They are cupuliform in shape, with a consistency between soft and flaccid, generally 1–30 cm in size, multilobed and located subcutaneously.

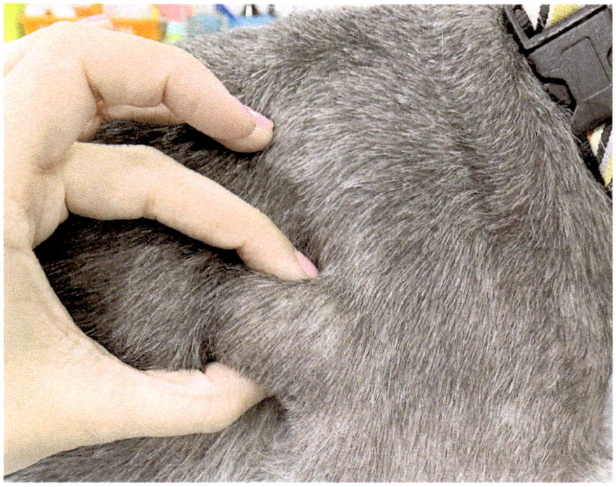

Figure 27. Typical image of a lipoma in a 9-year-old Miniature Schnauzer.

Care must be taken not to confuse other types of tumours with lipomas, since some skin tumours can be surrounded by a layer of fat that can make them appear similar to a lipoma, such as mast cell tumours.

Aspiration should always be performed in various locations on the lipoma and the character of the mass and its behaviour, such as changes in appearance, etc. should be considered.

"Normal" Lipoma
Subcutaneous masses, which generally move freely and they are usually not resected unless they continue to grow rapidly or prevent normal body function/gait, etc.

Regular monitoring of these tumours by the veterinarian and the owner is important, as rapid growth could indicate that a different type of tumour is growing underneath (mast cell, etc.) and should be re-examined. They are very easy to diagnose with a cytology of a fine needle aspirate.

Intermuscular Lipoma
Usually appears as if a hindleg is slowly becoming enlarged, which is due to the presence of a lipoma growing between the muscle bellies (fat does not infiltrate the muscle, as with an infiltrating lipoma). Suspicion of this type of tumour is based on clinical signs and a fine needle aspirate of the mass/limb reveals the presence of fat.

A CT scan is required to reveal the extent of the mass and plan for surgical removal. Surgery is recommended for this tumour type because, when it is left untreated, it can compress normal muscle and nerve tissue. In general, it appears between the semimembranosus and semitendinosus muscles.

Treatment includes surgery, removing the mass. The prognosis is generally excellent.

Infiltrating Lipoma
This type of lipoma infiltrates and should be removed because it is locally invasive. Infiltrating lipoma can be suspected if a "normal" lipoma appears to be firmly attached to the underlying body wall. **The diagnosis is based on the appearance on a CT scan of fat infiltrated in the muscle tissue**.

A fine needle aspirate will reveal fat cells, as in a normal lipoma, and the biopsy will reveal fat infiltrated into the muscle tissue. Treatment consists of surgery and radiotherapy is recommended to prevent/delay local recurrence if surgical removal is incomplete. The long-term prognosis is good if local tumour control is achieved. Even if the tumours are inoperable, they can be controlled with radiotherapy.

Fibroma (Dermatofibroma)
It can affect older cats and dogs. It is a benign tumour.

It appears as a single tumour on the extremities and head, which is well defined, from firm to soft, from cupuliform to pedunculated, from dermo epidermal to subcutaneous.

Treatment may consist of surgery, but it can also be monitored, as it is a benign tumour.

Fibrovascular Papilloma
Also called **acrochordon or skin tag**. It occurs in the dog and is benign.

In general, multiple tumours appear, from filiform to pedunculated, smooth, or hyperkeratotic, soft, and small. In most cases they are located on the extremities or on the ventral thorax.

If their location leads to self-trauma or haemorrhage, removal is recommended. If not, they can be ignored.

Haemangioma
This benign tumour occurs in dogs and rarely in cats.

In general, there are multiple tumours. They are usually found on the ventral abdomen, ventral limbs, or thorax, in dogs, or on the face of cats.

They are usually well defined, firm, fluctuating, round, from bluish to red-black and from dermo epidermal to subcutaneous. Heavy bleeding may occur if the masses rupture. Puncture aspiration reveals blood.

In general, they are **induced by the sun** (in the same breeds as the sun induced SCC) and it is common for multiple tumours to appear due to the "**field cancerisation**" phenomenon due to prolonged exposure to the sun of affected areas.

Surgical removal and biopsy are recommended to rule out dermal haemangiosarcoma, as these tumours look similar (haemangiomas are usually smaller and do not infiltrate the subcutaneous tissue).

Treatment tipically includes surgery, cryotherapy or electrochemotherapy.

Haemangiosarcoma (HSA)
It occurs in both the dog and the cat and is a malignant tumour.

The dermal (Figure 28) and subcutaneous forms have different biological behaviour.

- Dermal HSA is caused by the sun.
- Subcutaneous HSA can be a dermal HSA infiltration or a primary or metastatic tumour (from a splenic/liver etc. tumour).

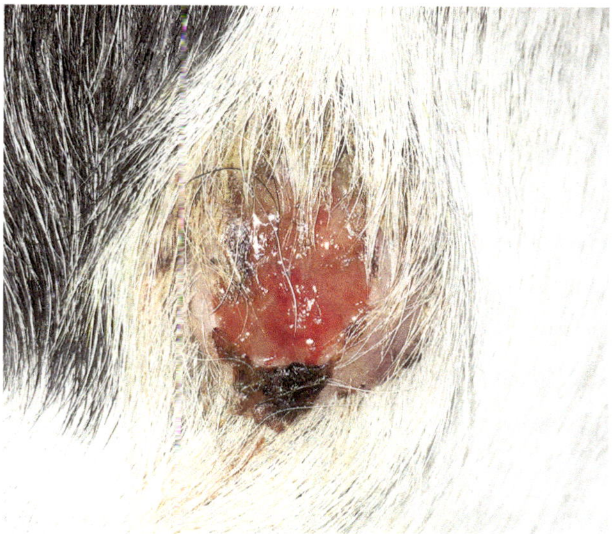

Figure 28. Cutaneous haemangiosarcoma on the right thigh of a dog. It is ulcerated, poorly defined, and attached to deep tissue planes.

HSA can be a single tumour or multiple tumours (metastatic or caused by the sun). Often, necrosis, ulceration, and haemorrhage (which can be massive) are seen. Puncture aspiration reveals blood. The diagnosis via fine needle aspiration can be difficult, as mesenchymal cells are rarely seen on haemangiosarcoma cytology, due to contamination with blood.

It is an invasive and malignant tumour that is often associated with bleeding disorders (acute or chronic DIC and changes in the morphology of red blood cells, such as acanthocytes or schistocytes). In cases of dermal HSA, surgical removal is recommended. If there is infiltration into subcutaneous tissue, complete staging (including abdominal ultrasound, thoracic radiographs, and, if appropriate, an echocardiogram) is recommended to confirm the location of the primary tumour.

The treatment choice is surgical resection. Dermal HSA is treated with only surgery; however, chemotherapy is recommended in all cases of subcutaneous HSA due to its metastatic potential. Radiotherapy can be effective in inoperable cases or tumours which have not been completely removed. Electrochemotherapy can be an alternative for some dermal lesions, or as an adjuvant treatment for margins during or postsurgery.

Prognosis

- **Dermal HSA**: mean survival of 780 days after surgery (dermal HSA does not usually metastasise).
- **Subcutaneous HSA**: mean survival of approximately 300 days if only treated with surgery (most dogs die from metastasis). Survival may be longer if postsurgical chemotherapy is used.

Soft-tissue Sarcoma

This group includes various tumours, which are covered in the corresponding section of this book.

Round Cell Tumours

MCT, transmissible venereal tumour (TVT), lymphoma, and canine and feline plasma cell tumours are discussed in the appropriate sections of this book.

Histiocytic Neoplasms

Canine Cutaneous Histiocytoma

Histiocytomas are benign skin tumours of the Langerhans cells (antigen-presenting cells) of the epidermis (Figure 29).

They affect young dogs (in 50% of cases the animals are less than 2 years old) and the English Bulldog, Scottish Terrier and other Terriers, Boxer and Spaniel-type breeds are predisposed to suffering from them.

They usually present as a single tumour on the head, ears, or extremities, are small (less than 3 cm), firm, dome-shaped or button-shaped, delimited, dermo epidermal (Figure 29) and, in some cases, with superficial ulceration. Owners sometimes describe very rapid growth; in fact, this phase of rapid growth is usually associated with the phase of spontaneous remission within 3 months, which in turn is associated with an infiltration of CD8 cells and T lymphocytes. Histiocytomas have a characteristic cytologic appearance ("fried egg" shaped cells) (Figure 30) and are often infiltrated by lymphocytes when they begin to regress. Diagnosis is easy by fine needle aspiration cytology.

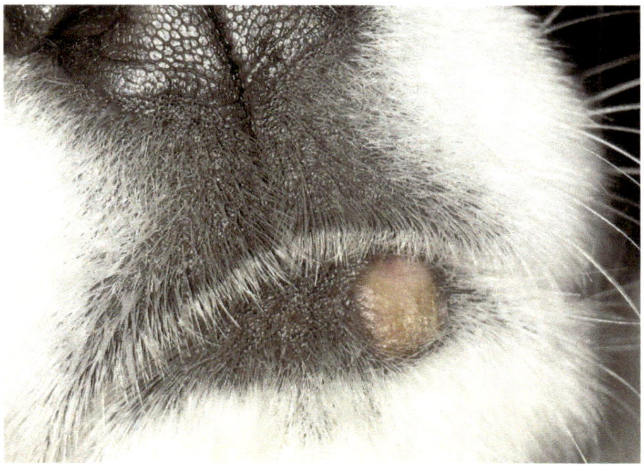

Figure 29. Cutaneous canine histiocytoma. 1-year-old Husky which presents for consultation regarding a cutaneous alopecic lesion which is not ulcerated on the rostral area of the mandible. The cytology from the lesion is shown in Figure 30.

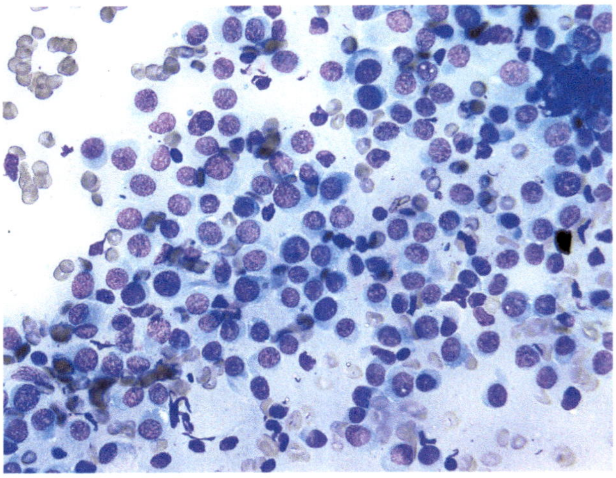

Figure 30. Cytological sample obtained using fine needle aspiration of the lesion in Figure 29. The sample has a high cellularity, with a monomorphic population of round cells which have abundant blue cytoplasm, with a round nucleus and nucleolus which is not visible, without evidence of signs of malignancy. This cytological image is typical of canine histiocytomas.

They are not usually treated and follow up until they resolve is recommended. The possibility of resection should be considered only if they bleed or confirming the diagnosis is necessary.

Other Histiocytic Neoplasms

Histiocytic Sarcoma

The histiocytic sarcoma of the skin is very uncommon. High predisposition in the Bernese Mountain Dog, Rottweiler, Golden Retriever and Smooth-Haired Retriever.

Its forms include:
- isolated tumours
- associated with joints (very common in stifle)
- disseminated organic infiltration (spleen, liver/lungs).

A highly malignant tumour that is treated aggressively with surgery/chemotherapy/radiotherapy and has a poor prognosis (median survival with treatment is approximately 4 months).

Cutaneous Histiocytosis

Immune-mediated skin disease, without age, breed, or sex predisposition.

It produces multiple, erythematous, dermal, or subcutaneous plaques or nodules, fluctuating lesions. It is not a systemic disease.

It may respond to treatment with steroids or other immunosuppressive treatments (cyclosporine, interferon, etc.).

Secondary Skin Neoplasms

These are produced by metastasis of a primary tumour to the skin or due to a paraneoplastic skin disease and are very rare in the dog and cat.

Metastatic lesions from mammary carcinomas and other carcinomas have been observed. In cats, a paraneoplastic syndrome of exfoliative dermatitis associated with a thymoma has been documented.

Its presence is indicative of a serious prognosis since it represents a **disseminated metastatic disease**.

Non-neoplastic Tumours

Cutaneous Cysts

These are non-neoplastic lesions with the epithelial wall and secretory or keratin content and can occur in dogs and cats.

There are three types:
- epidermoid cysts (epidermal cyst)
- dermoid cysts
- follicular cysts.

It is important to remember that all cysts can be complicated by rupture with inflammation/infection.

Epidermoid Cyst (Epidermal Cyst)

Acquired lesions that can be the consequence of trauma. They can be a single or multiple injuries. Round, smooth and delimited in appearance, firm to fluctuating, 0.5–5 cm, often bluish, dermo epidermal to subcutaneous. Located on the head, neck, trunk, proximal extremities (not acral).

Histologically, an epithelial lining is observed without attached structures.

They may break open and release grey to white-brown cheese-like material (like keratin, looks like toothpaste)

Dermoid Cysts

A congenital/hereditary problem which is diagnosed in young animals. It can be an isolated injury or multiple injuries and occurs in Boxers, Kerry Blue Terriers, and the Rhodesian Ridgeback (it is congenital in the latter).

It is normally seen along the lumbar spine and the opening can communicate with the spinal cord in that area.

Histologically, an epithelial lining with cutaneous attachments is observed. Surgical removal is required to prevent myelitis in patients with lesions communicating with the CNS.

Follicular Cysts

Retention of follicular/glandular products due to the lack of the follicular orifice or its obstruction. They are about 2–5 mm, white to yellow, and look like pustules. Histologically, an enormously dilated hair follicle is observed.

Nevi (Nevus)

A demarcated congenital cutaneous anomaly. German Shepherds suffer from a syndrome of multiple collagenic nevi called **nodular dermatofibrosis**, which is genetic and associated with renal adenocarcinomas and uterine leiomyomas.

Keratosis

Firm, raised, delimited areas of excess keratin production. There are four different types:

- seborrhoeic keratoses
- actinic (solar) keratoses
- lichenoid keratosis (Figure 31)
- cutaneous horns (Figure 32).

Calcinosis Circumscripta

Seen in young dogs in 80% of large breeds (very common in German Shepherds).

It has a firm, dome-shaped appearance, 1–10 cm. Initially it is covered with hair and later becomes ulcerative (secretes a calcareous substance) (Figure 33).

It can be isolated or multiple lesions or near pressure points, it is also found on the tongue and base of the ear.

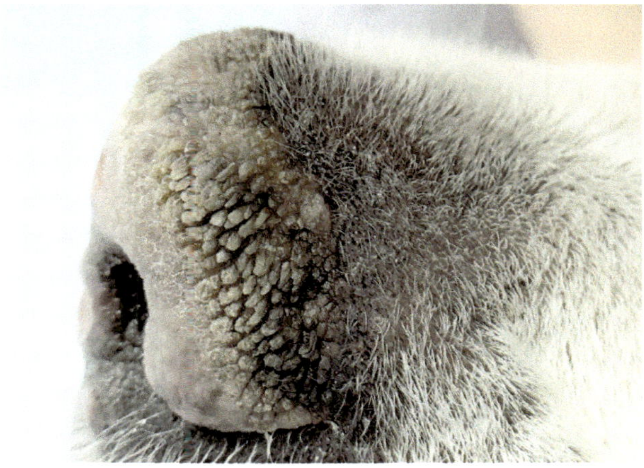

Figure 31. Lichenoid keratosis of the dorsal area of the nasal plane in a dog

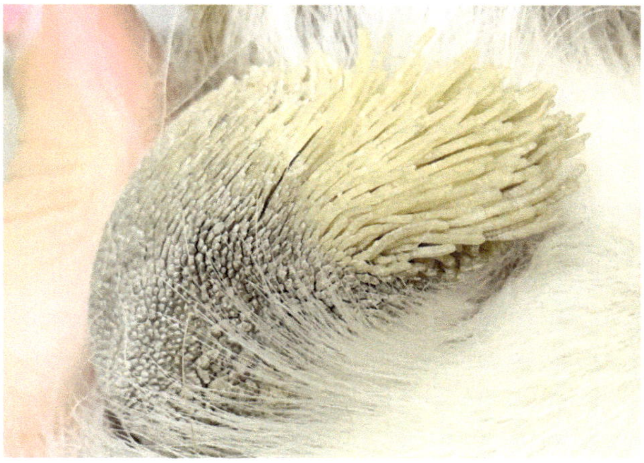

Figure 32. Cutaneous horns present on the plantar pads of a dog.

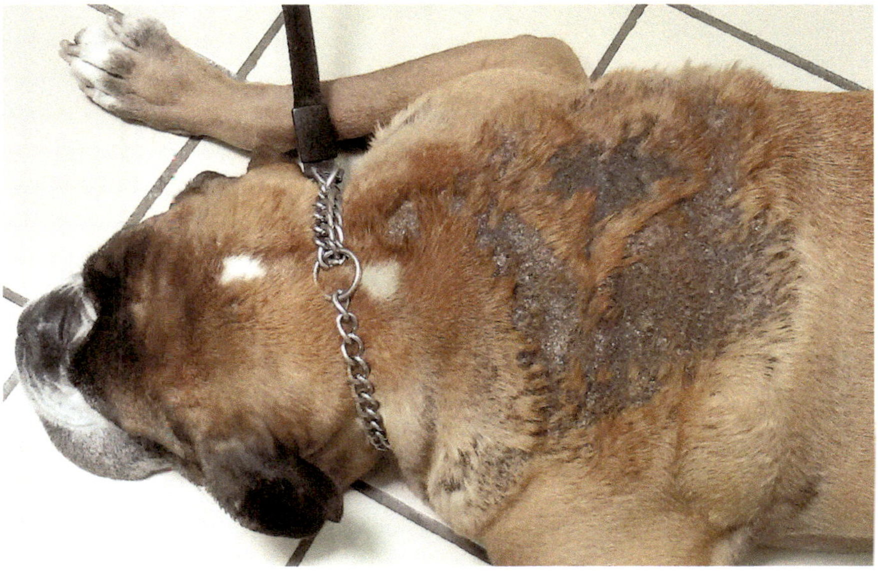

Figure 33. Calcinosis circumscripta on the dorsal area of the neck of a Boxer (Image courtesy of María Dolores Pérez-Alenza).

Soft-tissue Sarcomas

Soft-tissue sarcomas (STS) are a heterogeneous group of tumours that derive from mesenchymal tissue and share a similar presentation, behaviour, and histological characteristics, which is why they are usually included in the same group (Table 5). They are usually solitary masses and are found in the skin and subcutaneous tissue, although they can also be found in deeper tissues. They generally affect middle-aged or older cats and dogs. In the case of dogs, large breeds are more commonly affected and there is no known sex predisposition.

Biological Behaviour

Soft-tissue sarcomas are grouped according to the similarity and common characteristics of their biological behaviour.

1. **They are locally invasive**. They have a soft to firm texture and have a pseudocapsule. They have poorly defined histological margins and infiltrate layers of fascia (Figure 34).
2. **Local recurrence** after conservative surgical excision is common (7–75%).
3. Sarcomas **tend to metastasise through haematic routes**, and metastases often appear in the lungs. Regional lymph node metastasis is rare (except for synovial sarcoma).
4. **Histopathological grade is predictive** of metastasis and local recurrence.
5. The **margins of the excised tumour are predictive** of local recurrence.
6. Bulky tumours (>5 cm) **often respond poorly to chemotherapy and radiation therapy**.
7. STSs do not usually exfoliate easily, and **false negatives are common on cytologic analysis** (23% non-diagnostic and 15% false negatives).

Classification System for STS

Tumours with a higher histological grade are associated with a more aggressive biological behaviour, which is reflected in a greater probability of local recurrence, distant metastasis, and shorter disease-free times (Table 6).

In the case of poorly differentiated tumours, immunohistochemistry can be used to identify the tissue the tumour originated from and confirm a diagnosis of STS.

Patients with STS

Blood tests and urinalysis (with culture if necessary) are usually normal but should always be performed to assess the overall health of the patient.

Table 6. Scoring system for STS to establish tumour grade and metastatic capacity.

Score	Degree of differentiation	Mitotic figures in 10 HPF	Necrosis
1	Normal appearance to mesenchymal tissue	0–9	No
2	Specific histological type	10–19	<50% of tissue examined is necrotic
3	Undifferentiated	>20	>50% of tissue examined is necrotic

- Grade 1 (low-grade): score of ≤4 for the 3 categories; rate of metastasis 10%.
- Grade 2 (intermediate-grade): cumulative score of 5 or 6; rate of metastasis 20%.
- Grade 3 (high-grade): cumulative score of ≥7; rate of metastasis 40%.
- Most soft-tissue sarcomas (>90%) in dogs are of low or intermediate grade.

Table 5. Classification of soft-tissue tumours.

Tissue of origin	Benign tumour	Malignant tumour*	Metastatic potential
Fibroblasts	Fibroma	Fibrosarcoma	Low to moderate
Mucin producing fibroblasts	Myxoma	Myxosarcoma	Low to moderate
Blood vessel pericytes		Haemangiopericytoma	Low
Adipose tissue	Lipoma/infiltrative lipoma	Liposarcoma	Low to moderate
Nerve sheath		Nerve sheath tumour	Low to moderate
Smooth muscle	Leiomyoma	Leiomyosarcoma	Moderate
Synovial cells	Synovial cyst	Synovial cell sarcoma	Moderate to high
Skeletal muscle	Rhabdomyoma	Rhabdomyosarcoma	Moderate
Mixture of various types of mesenchymal cells		Mesenchymoma	Low to moderate

*Some tumours cannot be classified according to place of origin and are called undifferentiated sarcomas.

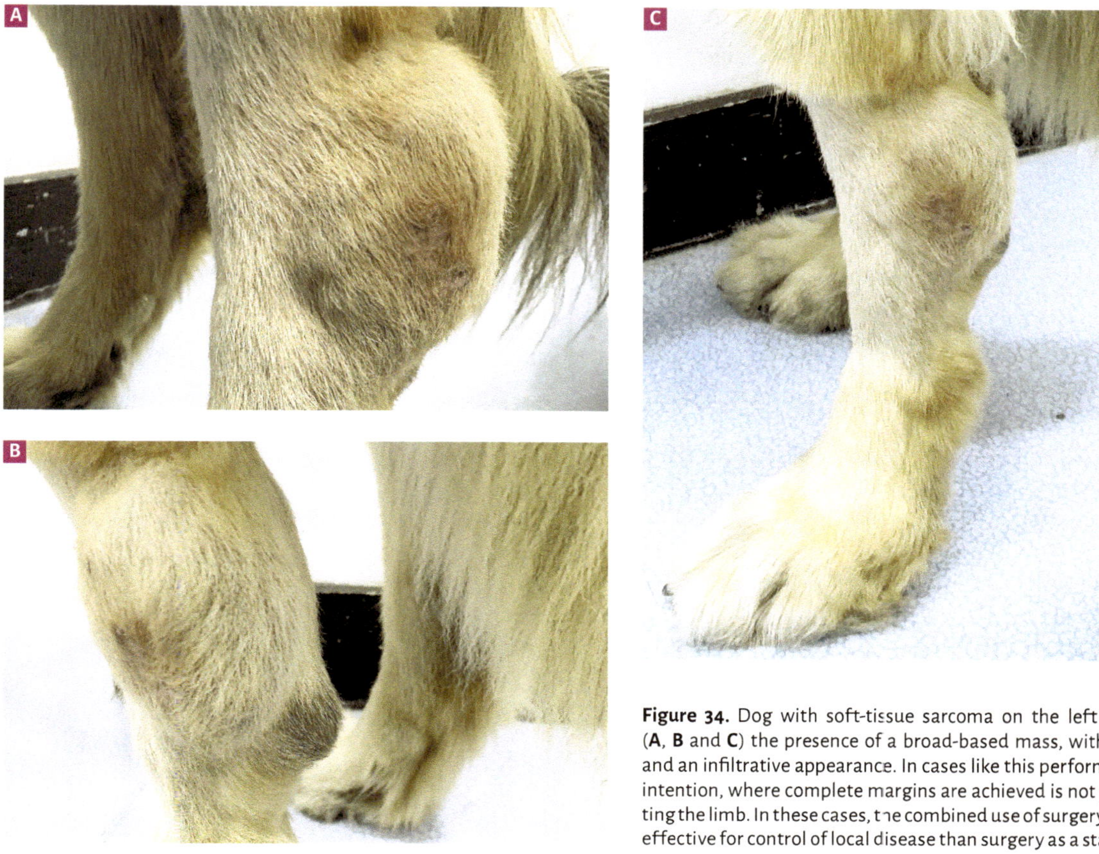

Figure 34. Dog with soft-tissue sarcoma on the left hindlimb. In the images (**A**, **B** and **C**) the presence of a broad-based mass, with poorly defined margins, and an infiltrative appearance. In cases like this performing surgery with curative intention, where complete margins are achieved is not possible without amputating the limb. In these cases, the combined use of surgery and radiotherapy is more effective for control of local disease than surgery as a stand-alone treatment.

Although cytological aspiration is always recommended, these tumours generally do not exfoliate well so it is not always possible to get a diagnosis via fine needle aspiration. However, mesenchymal cells may be obtained that can be suggestive of these neoplasms. Although cytology can be helpful, the definitive diagnosis and the tumour grade is obtained via histopathology (Figure 35).

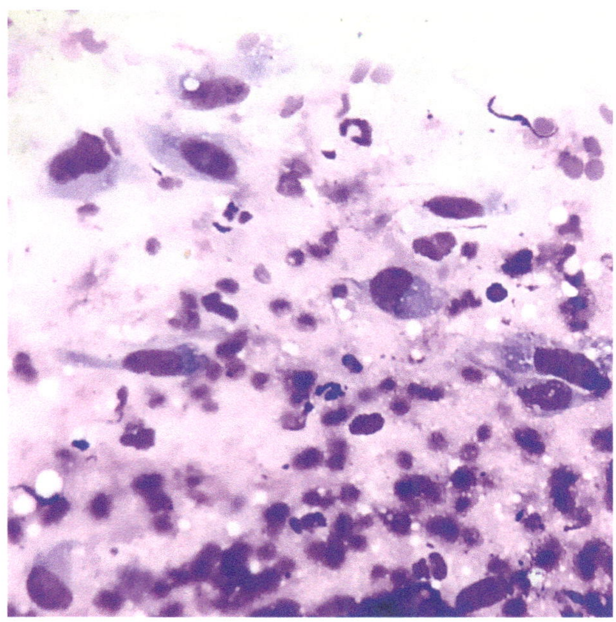

Figure 35. Cytology obtained using fine needle aspiration (FNA) of a soft-tissue sarcoma in a dog. Multiple cells compatible with lineage of mesenchymatous origin can be seen. Note the large deep purple nuclei, heterogenous chromatin, irregular mildly fusiform cytoplasm which tails off. Cytological diagnosis is compatible with a soft-tissue sarcoma.

Radiographs of the tumour area can be helpful in looking at bone destruction, but they are usually normal. However, thoracic radiographs should always be obtained before definitive treatment to rule out metastatic disease.

CT or MRI is always recommended in cases of STS, particularly in the case of body wall tumours or any tumour that requires aggressive resection or radiation therapy, since palpation alone underestimates the magnitude of the tumour.

Soft tissue sarcomas rarely metastasise to the lymph nodes, however, if possible, it is indicated to aspirate the regional lymph node, specially if it is enlarged. Abdominal radiographs/ultrasounds are indicated to complete staging.

An **incisional biopsy** is recommended prior to definitive treatment for some soft-tissue sarcomas, including:

- tumours present in a body wall;
- tumours that are large or locally invasive and appear inoperable (if it is not certain that the entire tumour can be removed, it is best not to try); and
- in cats with suspected injection site sarcomas.

The biopsy should be oriented so that the route by which it has been performed is excised during the definitive surgical intervention.

Treatment for STS

According to a study, in more than 80% of STS surgeries performed in veterinary practices, the surgeon does not know the tumour type or its potential biological behaviour.

Consequently, many of the tumours are not excised with wide margins, which is associated with lower patient survival after surgery.

Surgery

The **most important primary treatment**.

- Aggressive surgery is recommended.
- Margins of 2–3 cm should be obtained laterally and from a layer of tissue below the tumour, without incising it.
- **A sarcome should never be "opened"**. STS have a pseudocapsule.
- Biopsy tracts should be included in the surgical plan.
- The most distal/deepest parts of the tissue in the surgical area should be marked with haemoclips, sterile skin staples, or stainless-steel sutures, if necessary for radiation therapy.
- Marking the resected tissue with sutures or stains to help the pathologist analyse the margins is recommended.
- It is very important to **inform the client about the possibility of incomplete removal of the STS prior to surgery**.

After surgery, the **histological report should be reviewed for the following information**:

- diagnosis and type of tumour
- grade (histological) of the tumour
- presence of lymphatic or vascular invasion
- degree of invasion of normal tissue and reaction of the tissue to the tumour
- suitability of margins (Box 3).

Radiotherapy (RT)

Soft-tissue sarcomas are considered to be relatively radioresistant, but RT is very helpful in local control of the disease, **especially for cases when the margins are incomplete post-surgery**. The prognosis is generally good to excellent for incompletely excised STS (microscopic pathology) treated with a definitive course of radiation therapy. Radiation therapy can also be used as palliative therapy.

Radiation is unlikely to cure untreated primary tumours (30% complete response, 1-year control rates 48–67%, 2-year control rate only 33%). On the other hand, radiation therapy is ineffective as a treatment for large-volume sarcomas associated with certain tumour characteristics, such as relatively slow growth/absence of cells in mitosis, poor oxygenation in some tumours, and other factors.

Box 3. Treatment after surgery based on the surgical margins obtained and tumour grade

If the margins are complete

- **Low-grade tumours: regular check-ups to monitor for recurrence or formation of new tumours (at 1, 3, 6, 9 and 12 months and then at least every 6 months after surgery) and thoracic radiographs to determine if there is thoracic metastasis every 6–12 months.**
- **High-grade tumours: adjuvant chemotherapy should be considered to treat the possible systemic disease.**
- **Doxorubicin or doxorubicin/platinum combination therapy: thoracic radiographs to determine if there are thoracic metastases every 3 months for the first year after surgery and every 3–6 months thereafter.**

If the margins are incomplete

- **Radiation therapy.**
- **Surgical re-excision. The scar should be treated as if it were a new tumour, maintaining the same margins and including all previously biopsied areas.**

Chemotherapy

The role of chemotherapy in veterinary medicine is not yet very clear. **It can have palliative effects in gross tumours** (expected response rate 15–20%), but these are short-lived and as neoadjuvant treatment it can improve the chances of achieving a complete surgery.

Doxorubicin, platinum drugs, and mitoxantrone are effective against STS in these cases:

- along with surgery for high-grade STS (may prevent or delay local recurrence or distant metastasis);
- in patients with pulmonary metastases; and
- in inoperable primary tumours.

Metronomic therapy with cyclophosphamide (10 mg/m²/24h) and piroxicam has previously been described as effective in delaying recurrence times, although in recent years there is much debate about this effect, and if there is any real benefit obtained from this therapy.

Electrochemotherapy (ECT)

It has been proven that ECT could be an effective treatment for an early control of STS recurrence. Additionally, ECT can be used in combination with surgery to treat the tumour nest and margins at the time of surgery. It can also be used to treat the surgical scar postsurgery. The efficacy is still not well established for each setting, but it can definitely be part of a combination treatment for these tumours.

Prognosis

In general, with **proper treatment, many dogs enjoy long-term tumour control** (mean survival >3–6 years). Favourable prognostic factors are a size smaller than 5 cm, superficial location, low histological grade, that it is not fixed and that tumour-free surgical margins are achieved.

If treatment is limited to surgery, the **result depends on the histological grade and the degree of completion of surgical resection**. With aggressive treatment at an early stage, long-term control is more likely to be achieved: recurrence intervals between surgeries tend to shorten and the potential for metastasis may increase with each new tumour recurrence.

The grade is a prognostic factor for recurrence and metastasis. Regarding intratumoural microvascular density, it is not clear whether it is a prognostic factor. High expression of the Ki67 cell proliferation antigen or a high AgNOR score are associated with shorter survival times, although they are not routinely assessed.

The **mitotic index** is considered a prognostic factor to predict recurrence, metastasis, survival time, and disease-free time.

Specific Types of Tumours

Fibrosarcoma

Fibrosarcoma (non oral) is a common type of soft-tissue sarcoma in dogs. It usually affects older patients, and they are more frequently low-grade.

These types of tumours with a "low histological grade, high biological grade" are seen in the oral cavity: **oral fibrosarcoma is the third most common malignant oral tumour in the dog**. It is characterised by a high recurrence rate (57%), although distant metastases are less frequent (0–35% of cases). Achieving local control is most difficult. En bloc excision is very important, but multimodal therapy combining surgery and radiation is the best alternative.

Peripheral Nerve Sheath Tumour

It is the **most common cutaneous and subcutaneous soft-tissue sarcoma in the dog**. It can affect peripheral nerves or nerves adjacent to the brain or spinal cord; the peripheral form responds better to treatment. Tumours that form in the spinal cord often produce clinical signs such as monoparesis/paralysis; they are often difficult to diagnose, and sectional imaging is usually necessary (MRI is the best option).

Peripheral nerve sheath tumours in dogs are typically a single mass. On the rare occasions when a dog develops more than one tumour, it is likely that each is a primary tumour rather than a case of metastasis.

Typical treatment includes surgery, in some occasions combination with radiation therapy or electrochemotherapy might be indicated. Treatment options for tumours localised in the plexus, often include amputation of the affected limb and radiation of the tumour.

Intermuscular and Infiltrating Lipoma

These tumours have been discussed in the section on lipomas in this chapter.

Liposarcoma

Malignant adipocyte tumours that **do not originate from pre-existing lipomas**. They should not be confused cytologically or clinically with lipomas.

They have a good prognosis if appropriate treatment is administered (extensive resection, which may or may not be accompanied by radiotherapy or electrochemotherapy).

Synovial Sarcoma

This is also a sarcoma, but not originated in the skin. Formed in the synovial tissue, joints, the synovial bursa, and the tendon sheaths. Lysis of the bones proximal and distal to the affected joint often appears on radiographs, helping to differentiate synovial sarcoma from osteosarcoma, since osteosarcoma does not usually traverse the joint. Clinically they have an appearance similar to histiocytic sarcomas since both tumours cross the joint space.

It metastasises to regional lymph nodes more frequently than other STSs, although the metastatic capacity is highly dependent on the tumour grade. The best way to diagnose these tumours is by immunohistochemistry.

Leiomyoma/Leiomyosarcoma

Originates in the smooth muscle of the digestive and urogenital tubes or the spleen.

Vaginal leiomyomas are linked to hormones and often protrude from the vulva. Intact female dogs with this tumour should be spayed at the time of surgical removal to avoid recurrence. Female German Shepherds with nodular dermatofibrosis have a high predisposition to vaginal leiomyomas/sarcomas. Benign and malignant smooth muscle tumours have been associated with hypoglycaemia as a paraneoplastic syndrome.

Leiomyosarcomas are malignant tumours with a moderate metastatic potential, depending on the location of the primary tumour. For example, all those affecting the liver are metastatic, those in the spleen metastasise very frequently, and dermal ones do not metastasise.

Surgery is recommended as a treatment for leiomyosarcomas, although recurrences are common.

Myxosarcoma

Infiltrated growths with or without clear delimitation. In general, they affect the subcutaneous tissue.

The indications for the approach and treatment are the same than for the rest of the general STS group.

Rhabdomyosarcoma

A rare tumour in dogs. They are malignant tumours of skeletal muscle and tend to appear in young individuals (Figure 36). They can also appear in the spleen. They are usually associated to high grade tumours with a poor prognosis.

Surgery and/or radiation are the treatment of choice, and chemotherapy might be indicated.

Feline Injection Site Sarcoma

Feline injection site sarcomas (ISS) are **malignant skin tumours of mesenchymal origin that develop in around 1 to 10 of every 10 000 cats**. The term injection site sarcoma is preferred over vaccination site sarcoma because the tumours

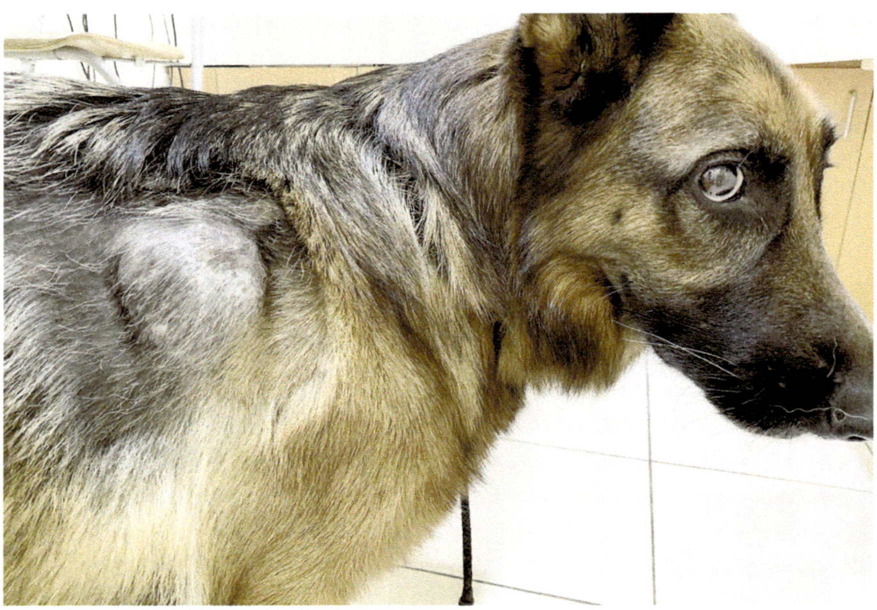

Figure 36. 6-year-old German Shepherd with a mass associated with the upper right part of the thorax. On palpation it was firm, with poorly defined margins and attached to deep places. The histopathological report was compatible with a grade III rhabdomyosarcoma.

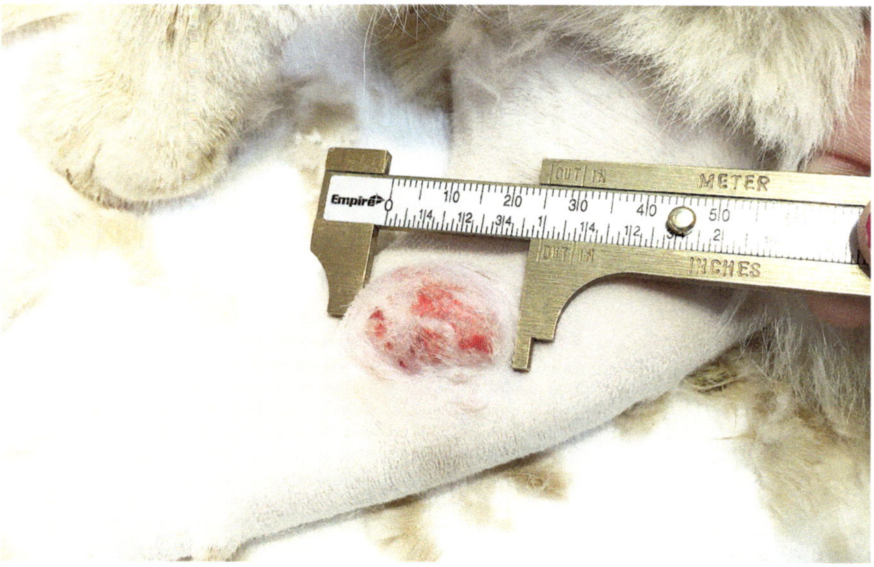

Figure 37. 8-year-old cat with a firm, ulcerated mass, with poorly defined margins and attached to deep planes. This is an example of a soft-tissue sarcoma which is not associated with an injection site.

have been seen to develop after administration of both vaccines and other injectable drugs.

In general, the sarcomas can be classified as:

- **spontaneous and non-postvaccine/injection**: behave like canine soft-tissue sarcomas (Figure 37);
- **postvaccine/associated with injection sites:** biologically they are more locally aggressive and metastasise more easily than non-postvaccine spontaneous tumours; or
- **associated with trauma**: for example, intraocular sarcomas after ocular trauma.

Epidemiology

A **strong association has been described between the administration of vaccines for FeLV and rabies and the subsequent development of soft-tissue sarcomas**. Both are inactivated virus vaccines that contain adjuvant. One study states that 51% of ISS are associated with rabies virus vaccines, 29% with FeLV vaccines, and 20% with FVRCP (rhinotracheitis, circovirus, and panleukopoenia). However, there is no vaccine that is 100% safe, although non-adjuvanted vaccines have been found to be safer, as well as recombinant vaccines over inactivated ones.

Associations have been established with other vaccines and injectable drugs (Luferunon, Program®; methylprednisolone acetate, Depo Medrol®; slow-absorption penicillin drugs); chronic administration of insulin and subcutaneous fluid, as well as microchip implantation and non-absorbable suture material have also been associated with this type of tumour.

According to one study, there is a higher risk of developing an ISS with the number of vaccines administered simultaneously at the same location.

The risk also increases with the use of cold vaccines (fresh from the refrigerator).

Factors that do not increase the incidence of ISS are reusing the syringe, needle gauge, using multidose vials, manufacturer, mixing vaccines in a single syringe, and massaging the area after vaccine administration.

Pathogenesis

The exact pathogenesis is **unknown**. The most widely accepted hypothesis of the possible mechanism of development of ISS is that there are inappropriate, or excessive immunological or inflammatory reactions associated with the presence of components/adjuvants in the vaccine.

The fact that not all cats develop ISS after vaccination suggests that there must be a genetic predisposition.

Diagnosis

The time it takes for the tumour to develop after vaccination has been reported to be between 4 weeks and 10 years, although the average is about 4 years.

- The **anatomical location, shape, and size** (measured with callipers and recorded in three dimensions) of all masses that appear at the injection site should be recorded.
- **Any mass that appears at an injection site should be treated as malignant** until proven otherwise, if it meets any of the following criteria (rule of 1, 2, 3):
  - a mass that increases in size after one month post-injection;
  - the mass diameter is >2 cm; or
  - the mass remains evident for more than 3 months after an injection.
- If a mass meets one or more of the above criteria, a **diagnostic biopsy should be performed before establishing a treatment plan**.

Fine needle aspiration does not usually help to differentiate the injection site reaction from a sarcoma, since both contain inflammatory cells, although it may be useful to rule out other differential diagnoses.

Tissue biopsy is necessary for the definitive diagnosis and differentiation of the postvaccine inflammatory reaction against ISS. Before carrying out a biopsy, the following should be considered.

- The biopsy area should be planned so that this area can be easily removed when the definitive surgery is performed.
- Layers of unaffected tissue should not be invaded with the biopsy.
- When an incisional biopsy is performed, the risk of "seeding" must be controlled by minimising bleeding.
- Use of drains should be avoided because they can be contaminated with tumour cells and cause seeding of tumour cells.
- Excisional biopsy is not recommended.
- If the tumours are very heterogeneous, multiple samples should be taken.

Approach/Staging

(Adapted from VAFSTF guidelines)

If a diagnosis of ISS is made, tumour staging should be performed before the treatment approach is planned. The metastasis rate at the time of initial presentation is relatively low, ranging between 6–23%. Metastasis occurs primarily to the lungs, but can also be seen in regional lymph nodes, skin, and visceral organs.

Steps to follow are:

- **radiographs** including three thoracic views and preoperative laboratory tests;
- **fine needle aspiration of the regional lymph node** if it is accessible;
- **abdominal imaging** (in older cats or tumours in the caudal half);
- **the ISS should be evaluated by CT or MRI** before formulating a treatment plan. There is a discrepancy between the macroscopic evaluation of the margins in practice and the dimensions obtained by CT or MRI, and the tumour is usually understimated on palpation compared to advanced imaging diagnostics;
- **referral to a specialist should always be considered** before performing definitive surgery;
- **the entire excised sample should be sent for histopathological evaluation**. The edges of the sample excised should ideally be identified; this way, the pathologist will be able to evaluate the different margins and inform about whether margins are complete; and
- after tumour removal, a **monthly physical examination** should be recommended for the first 3 months and then at least every 3 months for 1 year after.

Treatment

Because the metastatic rate is relatively low, initially, the treatment is primarily aimed at controlling the local tumour.

Surgery

Surgery is the gold standard for treatment and the **best alternative for curative intent**. ISSs are poorly encapsulated tumours and tend to infiltrate and spread into deep planes, so aggressive and radical surgery is recommended. In practice, that means at least 3 cm (preferably 5 cm) margins in all directions around the tumour and one or two deep planes.

If the tumour involves adjacent bones such as the scapula, spinous processes, or the pelvis, these structures must also be removed. Simple (marginal) excision inevitably leads to local recurrence, which is more difficult to control than the original tumour (Figure 38).

Local recurrence rates range from 30–89% almost always within a year, except if the surgery has 5 cm margins and two fasciae, which brings the recurrence rate down to 14%. Even if histopathological analysis shows complete margins, there is a 20–50% recurrence when surgery alone is performed (data vary between studies).

Pre- and Postoperative Radiation Therapy

Radiation therapy can be used successfully both before and after surgery to increase tumour control. Additionally, radiation therapy can be used in a palliative setting for large and inoperable tumours.

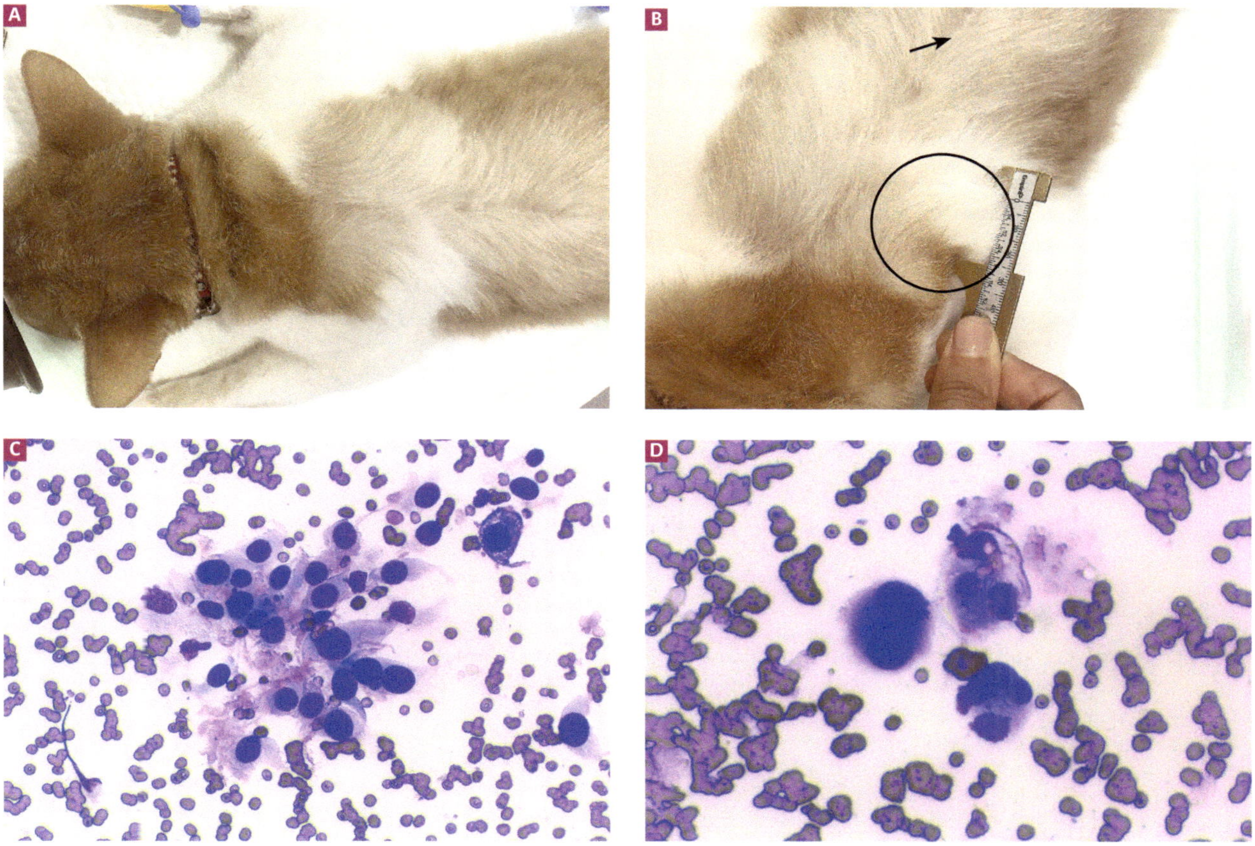

Figure 38. 12-year-old cat with a scar in the interscapular space. Six months before the photo (**A**) was taken the referring veterinarian removed a high-grade injection site fibrosarcoma in the interscapular area. The tumour was removed with incomplete margins and recurred the month after surgery. The recurrence was removed with complete margins and the area was treated with radiotherapy. The cat returned 4 months later for a check-up. In image **B** an arrow indicates where the scar from previous surgeries is, and a circle shows the presence of a new firm mass with poorly defined margins which is suspected to be a recurrence of the injection site sarcoma from the interscapular area. In image **C** a cytological image can be seen of a fine needle aspirate from the mass shown on the cat in image B. It is a cellular sample, where multiple cells compatible with a lineage of mesenchymatous origin can be seen. These cells are large, with a large eccentric nucleus, an elevated N:C ratio, prominent nucleoli, heterogenous chromatin and an irregular, mildly fusiform cytoplasm which tails off. The cytological diagnosis is compatible with a soft-tissue sarcoma. Considering the location and previous history of the patient, it can be concluded that it is a recurrence from the injection site sarcoma previously excised. Image **D** shows the cytological detail from the same patient where giant multinucleated cells can be observed which are typical of sarcomas associated with injection sites.

Despite combining wide surgical margins with radiation therapy, local recurrence is still possible. In one study, it was described that 79% of the cases had local failure, although the disease-free interval time was greater than the cases that only received surgery (1000 days versus 398 days). When palliative RT is performed, survival and disease-free interval time is longer when micro disease cases are treated versus macro disease cases.

Chemotherapy

Traditional Chemotherapy

The relatively low percentage of metastases (25%) argues against the use of systemic chemotherapy but, since ISS are extremely locally invasive with high recurrence rates (and also 1 in 4 cats will develop metastatic diseased), **many oncologists include adjuvant chemotherapy to slow down the progression of the disease and to increase the disease-free interval period**.

Doxorubicin is usually the drug of choice, however, many other alternatives have been used, among others, carboplatin (an encapsulated doxorubicin formulation), mitoxantrone, epirubicin (a combination of doxorubicin and cyclophosphamide), vincristine, ifosfamide, and lomustine in cats with ISS, with responses varying from 0% to more than 50%.

Chemotherapy should not be used as monotherapy, although it may occasionally be considered as palliative treatment. It has a palliative effect in large, inoperable tumours.

If administered before surgery, it can shrink the tumour. On the other hand, systemic chemotherapy can contribute to the delay or prevention of metastasis.

When used in combination with surgery and radiation therapy, **adjuvant chemotherapy can improve clinical outcomes**.

Targeted Therapies

Masitinib (Masivet®): has a demonstrated antiproliferative effect in vitro.

Toceranib phosphate (Palladia®): did not show efficacy for ISS in one study.

Electrochemotherapy (ECT)

As previously mentioned, it has been proven that ECT can be an effective treatment for the **early control of STS** recurrences, hence, it can also be used to control recurrences of ISS.

ECT can be used to treat surgical scars, to treat early recurrences (if indicated for that case); or in combination with surgery.

According to one study, feline ISS excised with incomplete margins but treated with adjuvant ECT might have a longer survival time than cases treated only with surgery.

Prognosis

The most important prognostic indicator in cats treated with multimodal therapy is the completion of surgical margins, associated with local recurrence. The disease-free interval in cats with completely excised tumours is 2–3 years versus 6–10 months for cats with incomplete surgical margins. Cats treated with multiple surgeries have a worse prognosis: after each surgical intervention the tumour generally recurs in around half the time it took for the previous tumour to recur. Recurrent tumours are also more likely to metastasise.

Histological type is also significantly associated with survival time. The histological grade (determined by the mitotic index, the percentage of necrosis and the degree of pleomorphism) has been associated with the possibility of metastasis. On the other hand, the less time that elapses between surgery and radiation, the better survival and disease-free times are achieved.

In general, the cats with the best prognosis are those with the smallest tumours and which have received aggressive treatment (combination of surgery, radiation therapy, and possibly chemotherapy and/or electrochemotherapy). It is very rare for these tumours to be cured with surgery alone.

Box 4. Recommendations for location of vaccination sites in cats

1. No vaccines should be administered in the interscapular space.
2. Rabies: right distal hindlimb.
3. Feline leukaemia virus: left distal hindlimb.
4. FVRCP – right shoulder region as distal as possible.
5. Follow AAFP (American Association of Feline Practitioners) recommendations for vaccination.

Clients should be shown vaccination sites so they can be vigilant and examine the area to aid early detection.

Box 5. Recommendations for the prevention and control of ISS

1. Over vaccinating should be avoided. The indiscriminate use of feline leukaemia vaccines and other vaccines that are not required annually should be stopped. Vaccination of strictly indoor cats is not always recommended.
2. Vaccine injection sites should be standardised, separated and recorded.
3. Only single-dose ampules at room temperature should be used.
4. A detailed vaccine and injection record should be kept for each patient, including point of administration, vaccine/product type, manufacturer, and serial number.
5. The manufacturer should be informed of postvaccine sarcomas.
6. Polyvalent vaccines should not be used (that is, FeLV and FVRCP in the same vaccine).
7. Vaccines without adjuvants should be used.
8. Vaccines should be administered subcutaneously rather than intramuscularly (subcutaneous tumours are easier to detect than intramuscular).
9. If possible, an alternative injection site to the interscapular space should be used (e.g. at the base of the tail).
10. If vaccines are administered in the extremities, it should be done as low as possible and the interscapular area avoided.
11. Cats diagnosed with ISS should not be revaccinated.

Bibliography

- Abadie, J.J., Amardeilh, M.A., Delverdier, M.E. (1999) Immunohistochemical detection of proliferating cell nuclear antigen and Ki-67 in mast cell tumors from dogs. *J Am Vet Med Assoc*, 215, pp. 1629–1634.
- Al-Sarraf, R., Mauldin, G.N., Patnaik, A.K. et al. (1996) A prospective study of radiation therapy for the treatment of grade 2 mast cell tumors in 32 dogs. *J Vet Intern Med*, 10, pp. 376–378.
- Baer, K.E., Helton, K. (1993) Multicentric squamous cell carcinoma in situ resembling Bowen's disease in cats. *Vet Pathol*, 30(6), pp. 535–43.
- Baez, J.L., Hendrick, M.J., Shofer, F.S. et al (2004) Liposarcomas in dogs: 56 cases (1989–2000). *J Am Vet Med Assoc*, 224, pp. 887–891.
- Bailey, D.B., Rassnick, K.M., Erb, H.N. et al (2004) Effect of glomerular filtration rate on clearance and myelotoxicity of carboplatin in cats with tumors. *Am J Vet Res*, 65, pp. 1502–1507.
- Banerji, N., Kanjilal, S. (2006) Somatic alterations of the p53 tumor-suppressor gene in vaccine-associated sarcoma. *Am J Vet Res*, 67, pp. 1766–1772.
- Barber, L.G., Sorenmo, K.U., Cronin, K.L. et al (2000) Combined doxorubicin and cyclophosphamide chemotherapy for nonresectable feline fibrosarcoma. *J Am Anim Hosp Assoc*, 36, pp. 416–421.
- Bergman, P.J. Camps-Palau, M.A., McKnight, J.A. et al (2006) Development of a xenogeneic DNA vaccine program for canine malignant melanoma at the Animal Medical Center. *Vaccine*, 24(21), pp. 4582–5.
- Bergman, P.J., Craft, D.M., Newman, S.J. et al. (2004) Correlation of histologic grading of canine mast cell tumors with Ki67/PCNA/AgNOR/c-Kit scores: 38 cases (2002–2003). *Vet Comp Oncol* 2, p. 98.
- Bergman, P.J., Meleo, K.A., De Lorimier, L.P. et al. (2005) Clinical Use Information of Soft-tissue sarcoma. Veterinary Internet Betwork. Last updated 28.11.
- Book, A.P., Fidel, J., Wills, T. et al. (2011) Correlation of ultrasound findings, liver and spleen cytology, and prognosis in the clinical staging of high metastatic risk canine mast cell tumors. *Vet Radiol Ultrasound*. 52, pp. 548–554.
- Bostock, D.E., Crocker, J., Harris, K. et al. (1989) Nucleolar organiser regions as indicators of post-surgical prognosis in canine spontaneous mast cell tumours. *Br J Cancer*, 59, pp. 915–918.
- Bostock, D.E., Dye, M.T. (1980) Prognosis after surgical excision of canine fibrous connective tissue sarcomas. *Vet Pathol*, 17, pp. 581–588.
- Bostock, D.E., Dye, M.T. (1979) Prognosis after surgical excision of fibrosarcomas in cats. *J Am Vet Med Assoc*, 175, pp. 727–728.
- Bostock, D.E. (1979) Prognosis after surgical excision of canine melanomas. *Vet Pathol*, 16(1), pp. 32–40.
- Bray, J., Polton, G. (2016) Neoadjuvant and adjuvant chemotherapy combined with anatomical resection of feline injection-site sarcoma: results in 21 cats. *Vet Comp Oncol*, 14(2), pp. 147–60.
- Buchholz, J., Wergin, M., Walt, H. et al. (2007) Photodynamic therapy of feline cutaneous squamous cell carcinoma using a newly developed liposomalphotosensitizer: preliminary results concerning drug safety and efficacy. *J Vet Intern Med*, 21(4), pp. 770–5.
- Burton, J.H., Venable, R.O., Vail, D.M. et al. (2015) Pulse-Administered Toceranib Phosphate Plus Lomustine for Treatment of Unresectable Mast Cell Tumors in Dogs. *J Vet Intern Med*, 29(4), pp. 1098–104.
- Campbell, O., de Lorimier, L.P., Beauregard, G. et al. (2017) Presumptive primary pulmonary mast cell tumor in 2 dogs. *Can Vet J*, 58(6), pp. 591–59.
- Camps-Palau, M.A., Leibman, N.F., Elmslie, R., et al. (2007) Treatment of canine mast cell tumours with vinblastine, cyclophosphamide and prednisone: 35 cases (1997–2004). *Vet Comp Oncol*, 5, pp. 156–167.
- Camus, M.S., Priest, H.L., Koehler, J.W. et al. (2016) Cytologic Criteria for Mast Cell Tumor Grading in Dogs With Evaluation of Clinical Outcome. *Vet Pathol*, 53(6), pp. 1117–1123.
- Cancedda, S., Marconato, L., Meier, V. et al. (2016) Hypofractionated radiotherapy for macroscopic canine soft tissue sarcoma: a retrospective study of 50 cases treated with a 5 × 6 GY protocol with or without metronomic chemotherapy. *Vet Radiol Ultrasound*, 57(1), pp. 75–83.
- Cherzan, N.L., Fryer, K., Burke, B. et al. (2023) Factors affecting prognosis in canine subcutaneous mast cell tumors: 45 cases. *Vet Surg*, 52(4):531-537.
- Clark, G.N., Berg, J., Engler, S.J. et al. (1992) Extramedullary plasmacytomas in dog: results of surgical excision in 131 dogs. *J Am Anim Hosp Assoc*, 28: 105–111.
- Cohen, M., Post, G.S., Wright, J.C. (2003) Gastrointestinal leiomyosarcoma in 14 dogs. *JVetIntMed*, 17, pp. 107–110.
- Cooper, M., Tsai, X., Bennett, P. (2009) Combination CCNU and vinblastine chemotherapy for canine mast cell tumours: 57 cases. *Vet Comp Oncol*, 7, pp. 196–206.
- Day, D.G., Couto, C.G., Weisbrode, S.E. et al. (1994) Basal cell carcinoma in two cats. *J AM Anim Hosp Assoc*, 30, pp. 265– 269.
- Dennis, M.M. et al. (2011) Prognostic factors for cutaneous and subcutaneous soft tissue sarcomas in dogs. *Veterinary Pathology*, 48(1), pp. 73–84.
- Dillon, C.J., Mauldin, G.N., Baer, K.E. (2005) Outcome following surgical removal of nonvisceral soft-tissue sarcomas in cats: 42 cases (1992–2000). *J Am Vet Med Assoc*, 227, pp. 1955–1957.
- Diters, R.W., Walsh, K.M. (1984) Feline basal cell tumors: a review of 124 cases. *Vet Pathol*, 21(1), pp. 51–6.
- Dobromylskyj, M.J., Rasotto, R., Melville, K. et al. (2015) Evaluation of Minichromosome Maintenance Protein 7 and c-KIT as Prognostic Markers in Feline Cutaneous Mast Cell Tumours. *J Comp Pathol*, 153(4), pp. 244–50.
- Eisenhauer, E.A., Therasse, P., Bogaerts, J. et al. (2009) New response evaluation criteria in solid tumours: revised RECIST guideline (version 1.1). *Eur J Cancer*, 45(2):228-47.

■ Elmslie, R.E., Glawe, P., Dow, S.W. (2008) Metronomic therapy with cyclophosphamide and piroxicam effectively delays tumor recurrence in dogs with incompletely resected soft tissue sarcomas. *J Vet Intern Med*, 22(6), pp. 1373–9.

■ Endicott, M.M., Charney, S.C., McKnight, J.A. et al. (2007) Clinicopathological findings and results of bone marrow aspiration in dogs with cutaneous mast cell tumours: 157 cases (1999–2002), *Vet Comp Oncol* 5, pp. 31–37.

■ Ettinger, S. (2023) Stelfonta for MCT in 2023: How to Get Started and What We Have Learned So Far. Presented at Fetch dvm360® Conference; Kansas City, Missouri.

■ Ettinger, S.N., Scase, T.J., Oberthaler, K.T. et al (2006) Association of argyrophilic nucleolar organizing regions, Ki-67, and proliferating cell nuclear antigen scores with histologic grade and survival in dogs with soft-tissue sarcomas: 60 cases (1996–2002). *J Am Vet Med Assoc*, 228, pp. 1053–1062.

■ Feinmehl, R., Matus, R., Mauldin, G.N. et al. (1992) Splenic mast cell tumors in 43 cats (1975–1992). *Proc Annu Conf Vet Cancer Soc*, 12, p. 50.

■ Ferrari, R., Di Giancamillo, M., Stefanello, D., et al. (2017) Clinical and computed tomography tumour dimension assessments for planning wide excision of injection site sarcomas in cats: how strong is the agreement? *Vet Comp Oncol*, 15(2), pp. 374–382.

■ Forrest, L.J., Chun, R., Adams, W.M. et al (2000) Postoperative radiotherapy for canine soft-tissue sarcoma. *J Vet Int Med*, 14, pp. 578–582.

■ Fox, L.E., Rosenthal, R.C., Twedt, D.C. et al. (1990) Plasma histamine and gastrin concentrations in 17 dogs with mast cell tumors. *J Vet Intern Med*, 4, pp. 242–246.

■ Fournier, Q., Thierry, F., Longo, M. et al. (2021) Contrast-enhanced ultrasound for sentinel lymph node mapping in the routine staging of canine mast cell tumours: A feasibility study. *Vet Comp Oncol*, 19(3):451-462.

■ Frost, D., Lasota, J., Miettinen, M. (2003) Gastrointestinal stromal tumors and leiomyomas in the dog: a histopathologic, immunohistochemical, and molecular genetic study of 50 cases. *Vet Pathol*, 40, pp. 42–54.

■ Fulcher, R.P., Ludwig, L.L., Bergman, P.J. et al. (2006) Evaluation of a two-centimeter lateral surgical margin for excision of grade I and grade II cutaneous mast cell tumors in dogs. *J Am Vet Med Assoc* 228, pp. 210–215.

■ Garrett, L.D., Craig, C.L., Szladovits, B. et al. (2007) Evaluation of buffy coat smears for circulating mast cells in healthy cats and ill cats without mast cell tumor-related disease. *J Am Vet Med Assoc*, 231, pp. 1685–1687.

■ Garrett, L.D. (2014) Canine mast cell tumors: diagnosis, treatment, and prognosis. *Veterinary Medicine: Research and Reports*, Volume 2014. ISSN: 2230–2034 (Online).

■ Gerritsen, R.J., Teske, E., Kraus, J.S. et al. (1998) Multi-agent chemotherapy for mast cell tumours in the dog. *Vet Q*, 20, pp. 28–31.

■ Ghisleni, G., Roccabianca, P., Ceruti, R. et al. (2006) Correlation between fine-needle aspiration cytology and histopathology in the evaluation of cutaneous and subcutaneous masses from dogs and cats. *Vet Clin Pathol*, 35(1), pp. 24–30.

■ Gieger, T.L., Theon, A.P., Werner, J.A. et al. (2003) Biologic behavior and prognostic factors for mast cell tumors of the canine muzzle: 24 cases (1990–2001). *J Vet Intern Med*, 17, pp. 687–692.

■ Gill, V.L., Bergman, P.J., Baer, K.E. et al. (2008) Use of imiquimod 5 % cream (Aldara) in cats with multicentric squamous cell carcinoma in situ: 12 cases (2002–2005). *Vet Comp Oncol*, 6(1), pp. 55–64.

■ Goldschmidt, M.H., Liu, SMS., Shofer, F.S. (1992) Feline dermal melanoma: a retrospective study. *Vet Derm*, 2, pp. 285–291.

■ Gordon, S.S., McClaran, J.K., Bergman, P.J. et al. (2010) Outcome following splenectomy in cats. *J Feline Med Surg* 12, pp. 256–261.

■ Grant, J., North, S., Lanore, D. (2016) Clinical response of masitinib mesylate in the treatment of canine macroscopic mast cell tumours. *J Small Anim Pract*. [Epub ahead of print]

■ Grimes, J.A., Secrest, S.A., Wallace, M.L. et al. (2020) Use of indirect computed tomography lymphangiography to determine metastatic status of sentinel lymph nodes in dogs with a pre-operative diagnosis of melanoma or mast cell tumour. *Vet Comp Oncol*, 18(4):818-824.

■ Hahn, K.A., Endicott, M.M., King, G.K. et al (2007) Evaluation of radiotherapy alone or in combination with doxorubicin chemotherapy for the treatment of cats with incompletely excised soft-tissue sarcomas: 71 cases (1989–1999). *J Am Vet Med Assoc*, 231:742–745.

■ Hahn, K.A., King, G.K., Carreras, J.K. (2004) Efficacy of radiation therapy for incompletely resected grade-III mast cell tumors in dogs: 31 cases (1987–1998). *J Am Vet Med Assoc*, 224, pp. 79–82.

■ Hahn, K.A., Legendre, A.M., Shaw, N.G. et al. (2010) Evaluation of 12- and 24-month survival rates after treatment with masitinib in dogs with nonresectable mast cell tumors. *Am J Vet Res*, 71, pp. 1354–1361.

■ Halsey, C.H., Powers, B.E., Kamstock, D.A. (2010) Feline intestinal sclerosing mast cell tumour: 50 cases (1997–2008). *Vet Comp Oncol*, 8, pp. 72–79.

■ Hammond, G.M., Gordon, I.K., Theon, A.P. et al. (2007) Evaluation of strontium Sr 90 for the treatment of superficial squamous cell carcinoma of the nasal planum in cats: 49 cases (1990–2006). *J Am Vet Med Assoc*, 231(5), pp. 736–41.

■ Harper, A., Blackwood, L. (2017) Toxicity and response in cats with neoplasia treated with toceranib phosphate. *J Feline Med Surg*, 19(6), pp. 619–623.

■ Hartmann, K., Day, M.J., Thiry, E., Lloret, A., Frymus, T., et al. (2015) Feline injection-site sarcoma: ABCD guidelines on prevention and management. *J Feline Med Surg*, 17(7), pp. 606–13.

■ Hauck, M.L. (2013) Tumors of the skin and subcutaneous tissues. In: Withrow, S. and Vail, D. *Small Animal Clinical Oncology*, Saunders, 5th Ed, pp. 304–320.

■ Hayes, H.M. Jr, Wilson, G.P. (1977) Hormone-dependent neoplasms of the canine perianal gland. *Cancer Res*, 37(7 Pt 1), pp. 2068–71.

■ Hendrick, M.J. (1999) Feline vaccine-associated sarcomas. *Cancer Invest*, 17, pp. 273–277.
■ Henry, C.J., Brewer, W.G. Jr, Whitley, E.M. et al. (2005) Veterinary Cooperative Oncology Group (VCOG). Canine digital tumors: a veterinary cooperative oncology group retrospective study of 64 dogs. *J Vet Intern Med*, 19(5):720–4.
■ Hergt, F., von Bomhard, W., Kent, M.S. et al (2016) Use of a 2-tier histologic grading system for canine cutaneous mast cell tumors on cytology specimens. *Vet Clin Pathol*, 45(3), pp. 477–83.
■ Hershey, A.E., Dubielzig, R.R., Padilla, M.L., et al. (2005) Aberrant p53 expression in feline vaccine-associated sarcomas and correlation with prognosis. *Vet Pathol*, 42, pp. 805–811.
■ Hershey, A.E., Sorenmo, K.U., Hendrick, M.J. et al (2000) Prognosis for presumed feline vaccine-associated sarcoma after excision: 61 cases (1986–1996). *J Am Vet Med Assoc*, 216, pp. 58–61.
■ Hillman, L.A., Garrett, L.D., de Lorimier, L.P. et al. (2010) Biological behavior of oral and perioral mast cell tumors in dogs: 44 cases (1996–2006). *J Am Vet Med Assoc* 237, pp. 936–942.
■ Ho, N.T., Smith, K.C., Dobromylskyj, M.J. (2017) Retrospective study of more than 9000 feline cutaneous tumours in the United Kingdom: 2006–2013. *J Feline Med Surg*.
■ Holtermann, N., Kiupel, M., Hirschberger (2017) The tyrosine kinase inhibitor toceranib in feline injection site sarcoma: efficacy and side effects. *J. Vet Comp Oncol*, 15(2), pp. 632–640.
■ Hosoya, K., Kisseberth, W.C., Alvarez, F.J. et al. (2009) Adjuvant CCNU (lomustine) and prednisone chemotherapy for dogs with incompletely excised grade 2 mast cell tumors. *J Am Anim Hosp Assoc* 45, pp. 14–18.
■ Howard, E.B., Sawa, T.R., Nielsen, S.W. et al. (1969) Mastocytoma and gastroduodenal ulceration. Gastric and duodenal ulcers in dogs with mastocitoma. *Pathol Vet*, 6, pp. 146–158.
■ Hume, C.T., Kiupel, M., Rigatti, L. et al. (2011) Outcomes of dogs with grade 3 mast cell tumors: 43 cases (1997–2007). *J Am Anim Hosp Assoc*, 47, pp. 37–44.
■ Isotani, M., Ishida, N., Tominaga, M. et al. (2008) Effect of tyrosine kinase inhibition by imatinib mesylate on mast cell tumors in dogs. *J Vet Intern Med*, 22(4), pp. 985–958.
■ Jas, D., Soyer, C., De Fornel-Thibaud, P. et al. (2015) Adjuvant immunotherapy of feline injection-site sarcomas with the recombinant canarypox virus expressing feline interleukine-2 evaluated in a controlled monocentric clinical trial when used in association with surgery and brachytherapy. *Trials in Vaccinology*. Volume 4, pp. 1–8.
■ Kalaher, K.M , Anderson, W.I., Scott, D.W. (1990) Neoplasms of the apocrine sweat glands in 44 dogs and 10 cats. *Vet Rec*, 20;127(16), pp. 400–3.
■ Kandefer-Gola, M., Madej, J.A., Dzimira, S. et al. (2015) Comparative analysis of markers of cell proliferation in canine mast cell tumours according to current classifications. *Pol J Vet Sci*, 18(2), pp. 241–7.
■ Kass, P.H., Spangler, W.L., Hendrick, M.J. et al. (2003) Multicenter case-control study of risk factors associated with development of vaccine-associated sarcomas in cats. *J Am Vet Med Assoc*, 223, pp. 1283–1292.
■ Rassnick, K.M.; Rodriguez, C.O., Khanna, C. et al. (2006) Results of a phase II clinical trial on the use of ifosfamide for treatment of cats with vaccine-associated sarcomas. *American Journal of Veterinary Research*, Vol. 67, No. 3, pp. 517–523.
■ Kisseberth, W.C., Vail, D.M., Yaissle, J. et al (2008) Phase I clinical evaluation of carboplatin in tumor-bearing cats: a veterinary cooperative oncology group study. *J Vet Intern Med*, 22, pp. 83–88.
■ Kitchell, B.K., Orenberg, E.K., Brown, D.M. et al. (1995) Intralesional sustained-release chemotherapy with therapeutic implants for treatment of canine sun-induced squamous cell carcinoma. *Eur J Cancer*, 31A(12), pp. 2093–8.
■ Kiupel, M., Webster, J.D., Bailey, K.L. et al. (2011) Proposal of a 2-tier histologic grading system for canine cutaneous mast cell tumors to more accurately predict biological behavior. *Vet Pathol*, 48, pp. 147–155.
■ Kiupel, M., Webster, J.D., Kaneene, J.B. et al. (2004) The use of KIT and tryptase expression patterns as prognostic tools for canine cutaneous mast cell tumors. *Vet Pathol* 41, pp. 371–377.
■ Kobayashi, T., Hauck, M.L., Dodge, R. et al. (2002) Preoperative radiotherapy for vaccine-associated sarcoma in 92 cats. *Vet Radiol Ultrasound*, 43, pp. ,473–479.
■ Krick, E.L., Billings, A.P., Shofer, F.S. et al. (2009) Cytological lymph node evaluation in dogs with mast cell tumours: association with grade and survival. *Vet Comp Oncol* 7, pp. 130–138.
■ Kuntsi-Vaattovaara, H., Verstraete, F.J., Newsome, J.T. et al. (2003) Resolution of persistent oral papillomatosis in a dog after treatment with recombinant canine oral papillomavirus vaccine. *Vet Comp Oncol*, 1(1), pp. 57–63
■ Kuntz, C.A., Dernell, W.S., Powers, B.E. et al. (1997) Prognostic factors for surgical treatment of soft-tissue sarcomas in dogs: 75 cases (1986–1996). *J Am Vet Med Assoc*, 211, pp. 1147–1151.
■ Lachowicz, J.L., Post, G.S., Brodsky, E. (2005) A phase I clinical trial evaluating imatinib mesylate (Gleevec) in tumor-bearing cats. *J Vet Intern Med*, 19, pp. 860–864.
■ LaDue, T., Price, G.S., Dodge, R. et al. (1998) Radiation therapy for incompletely resected canine mast cell tumors. *Vet Radiol Ultrasound*, 39, pp. 57–62.
■ Lana, S.E., Ogilvie, G.K., Withrow, S.J. et al. (1997) Feline cutaneous squamous cell carcinoma of the nasal planum and the pinnae: 61 cases. *J Am Anim Hosp Assoc*, 33(4), pp. 329–32.
■ Laprie, C., Abadie, J., Amardeilh, M.F. et al. (2001) MIB-1 immunoreactivity correlates with biologic behaviour in canine cutaneous melanoma. *Vet Dermatol*, 12(3), pp. 139–47.
■ Lapsley, J., Hayes, G.M., Janvier, V. et al. (2021) Influence of locoregional lymph node aspiration cytology vs sentinel lymph node mapping and biopsy on disease stage assignment in dogs with integumentary mast cell tumors. *Vet Surg*, 50(1):133-141.
■ Lascelles, B.D., Parry, A.T., Stidworthy, M.F. et al. (2000) Squamous cell carcinoma of the nasal planum in 17 dogs. *Vet Rec*, 147(17), pp. 473–6.

■ Lawrence, J., Forrest, L., Adams, W., et al (2008) Four-fraction radiation therapy for macroscopic sarcomas in 16 dogs. *J Am Anim Hosp Assoc*, 44(3), pp. 100–8.

■ LeBlanc, A.K., Daniel, G.B. (2007) Advanced imaging of veterinary cancer patients. *Vet Clin Small Anim Pract*, 37, pp. 1059–1077.

■ Liao, J.C., Gregor, P., Wolchok, J.D. et al. (2006) Vaccination with human tyrosinase DNA induces antibody responses in dogs with advanced melanoma. *Cancer Immun*, 6, p. 8.

■ Liptak, J.M., Forrest, L.J. (2013) Soft tissue sarcomas. In: Withrow, S. and Vail, D. *Small Animal Clinical Oncology*. Saunders, 5h Ed., pp. 356–380.

■ Liptak, J.M., Dernell, W.S., Ehrhart, E.J. et al. (2004) Retroperitoneal sarcomas in dogs: 14 cases (1992–2002). *J Am Vet Med Assoc*, 224, pp. 1471–1477.

■ Litster, A.L., Sorenmo, K.U. (2006) Characterisation of the signalment, clinical and survival characteristics of 41 cats with mast cell neoplasia. *J Feline Med Surg* 8, pp. 177–183.

■ London, C.A., Thamm, D.H. (2013) Mast Cell Tumors in Withrow S and Vail D. *Small Animal Clinical Oncology*. Saunders, 5th Ed., pp. 335–355.

■ London, C.A., Dubilzeig, R.R., Vail, D.M. et al. (1996) Evaluation of dogs and cats with tumors of the ear canal: 145 cases (1978–1992). *J Am Vet Med Assoc*, 208(9), pp. 1413–8.

■ London, C.A., Galli, S.J., Yuuki, T. et al. (1999) Spontaneous canine mast cell tumors express tandem duplications in the proto-oncogene c-kit Exp. *Hematol*, 27, pp. 689–697.

■ London, C.A., Kisseberth, W.C., Galli, S.J. et al. (1996) Expression of stem cell factor receptor (c-kit) by the malignant mast cells from spontaneous canine mast cell tumours. *J Comp Pathol*, 115, pp. 399–414.

■ London, C.A., Malpas, P.B., Wood-Follis, S.L. et al. (2009) Multi-center, placebo-controlled, double-blind, randomized study of oral toceranib phosphate (SU11654), a receptor tyrosine kinase inhibitor, for the treatment of dogs with recurrent (either local or distant) mast cell tumor following surgical excision. *Clin Cancer Res*, 15, pp. 3856–3865.

■ Lowe, R., Gavazza, A., Impellizeri, J.A. et al. (2017) The treatment of canine mast cell tumours with electrochemotherapy with or without surgical excision. *Vet Comp Oncol*, 15(3), pp. 775–784.

■ Lucroy, M.D., Edwards, B.F., Madewell, B.R. (2000) Veterinary photodynamic therapy. *J Am Vet Med Assoc*, 216(11), pp. 1745–51.

■ Lucroy, M.D., Hill, F.I., Moore, P.F. et al. (1998) Cutaneous papillomatosis in a dog with malignant lymphoma following long-term chemotherapy. *J Vet Diagn Invest*, 10(4), pp. 369–71.

■ Luong, R.H., Baer, K.E., Craft, D.M. et al (2006) Prognostic significance of intratumoral microvessel density in canine soft-tissue sarcomas. *Vet Pathol*, 43, pp. 622–631.

■ Macy, D.W. (1986) Canine and feline mast cell tumors: Biologic behavior, diagnosis, and therapy, *Sem Vet Med Surg (Sm Anim)*, 1, pp. 72–83.

■ Maglennon, G.A., Murphy, S., Adams, V. et al. (2008) Association of Ki67index with prognosis for intermediate-grade canine cutaneous mast cell tumours. *Vet Comp Oncol*, 6, pp. 268–274.

■ Mann, F.A., Pace, L.W. (1993) Marking margins of tumorectomies and excisional biopsies to facilitate histological assessment of excision completeness. *Sem Vet Med Surg (Small Anim)*, 8, pp. 279–283.

■ Marconato, L., Comastri, S., Lorenzo, M.R. et al. (2007) Postsurgical intra-incisional 5-fluorouracil in dogs with incompletely resected, extremity malignant spindle cell tumours: a pilot study. *Vet Comp Oncol*, 5(4), pp. 239–49

■ Marconato, L., Stefanello, D., Solari, F. (2023) Subcutaneous mast cell tumours: A prospective multi-institutional clinicopathological and prognostic study of 43 dogs. *VetRecord*, 193(1), pp. 8-15.

■ Marino, D.J., MacDonald, J.M., Matthiesen, D.T. et al. (1993) Results of surgery and long term follow-up in dogs with ceruminous gland adenocarcinoma. *J Am Anim Hosp Assoc*, 29, pp. 560–563.

■ Marino, D.J., MacDonald, J.M., Matthiesen, D.T. et al. (1994) Results of surgery in cats with ceruminous gland adenocarcinoma. *J Am Anim Hosp Assoc*, 30, pp. 54–58.

■ Marino, D.J., Matthiesen, D.T., Stefanacc , J.D. et al. (1995) Evaluation of dogs with digit masses: 117 cases (1981–1991). *J Am Vet Med Assoc*, 207(6), pp. 726–8.

■ Marks, S.L., Song, M.D., Stannard, A.A. et al. (1992) Clinical evaluation of etretinate for the treatment of canine solar-induced squamous cell carcinoma and preneoplastic lesions. *J Am Acad Dermatol*, 27(1), pp. 11–6.

■ Martano, M., Morello, E., Buracco, P. (2011) Feline injections-site sarcoma: past, present, and future perspectives. *Vet J*, 188, pp. 136–141.

■ Martano, M., Morello, E., Ughetto, M. et al. (2005) Surgery alone versus surgery and doxorubicin for the treatment of feline injection-site sarcomas: a report on 69 cases. *Vet J*, 170, pp. 84–90.

■ McEntee, M.C., Samii, V.F., Walsh, P. et al. (2004) Postoperative assessment of surgical clip position in 16 dogs with cancer: a pilot study. *J Am Anim Hosp Assoc*, 40, pp. 300–308.

■ McEntee, M.C., Steffey, M., Dykes, N.L. (2008) Potential utility of surgical hemoclips in radiation treatment planning. *Vet Rad Ultrasound*, 49, pp. 395–399.

■ McKnight, J.A., Mauldin, G.N., McEntee, M.C. et al. (2000) Radiation treatment for incompletely resected soft-tissue sarcomas in dogs. *J Am Vet Med Assoc*, 217, pp. 205–210.

■ McNiel, E.A., Prink, A.L., O'Brien, T.D. (2004) Evaluation of risk and clinical outcome of mast cell tumours in pug dogs. *Vet Comp Oncol*, 4, pp. 2–8.

■ Michels, G.M., Knapp, D.W., DeNicola, D.B. et al. (2002) Prognosis following surgical excision of canine cutaneous mast cell tumors with histopathologically tumor-free versus nontumor-free margins: a retrospective study of 31 cases. *J Am Anim Hosp Assoc*, 38, pp. 458–466.

■ Mikaelian, I., Wong, V. (2003) Follicular stem cell carcinoma: histologic, immunohistochemical, ultrastructural, and clinical characterization in 30 dogs. *Vet Pathol*, 40(4), pp. 433–44.

■ Mochizuki, H., Motsinger-Reif, A., Bettini, C. et al. (2017) Association of breed and histopathological grade in canine mast cell tumours. *Vet Comp Oncol*, 15(3), pp. 829–839.
■ Moirano, S.J., Lima, S.F., Hume, K,R, et al. (2017) Association of prognostic features and treatment on survival time of dogs with systemic mastocytosis: A retrospective analysis of 40 dogs. *Vet Comp Oncol*.
■ Monti, P., Barnes, D., Adrian, A. et al. (2018) Synovial cell sarcoma in a dog: A misnomer - Cytologic and histologic findings and review of the literature. *Vet Clin Path*, 47, pp. 181–18.
■ Morrison, W.B., Starr, R.M. (2001) Vaccine-associated feline sarcomas. *J Am Vet Med Assoc*, 218, pp. 697–702.
■ Müller, N., Kessler, M. (2017) Curative intent radical en bloc resect on using a minimum of a 3 cm margin in feline injection-sitesarcomas: a retrospective analysis of 131 cases. *J Feline Med Surg*.
■ Mullins, M.N., Dernell, W.S., Withrow, S.J. et al. (2006) Evaluation of prognostic factors associated with outcome in dogs with multiple cutaneous mast cell tumors treated with surgery with and without adjuvant treatment: 54 cases (1998–2004). *J Am Vet Med Assoc*, 228, pp. 91–95.
■ Munday, J.S., French, A., Harvey, C.J. (2015) Molecular and immunohistochemical studies do not support a role for papillomaviruses in canine oral squamous cell carcinoma development. *Vet J*, 204(2), pp. 223–5.
■ Munday, J.S., Hanlon, E.M., Howe, L. et al. (2007) Feline cutaneous viral papilloma associated with human papillomavirus type 9. *Vet Pathol*, 44(6), pp. 924–7.
■ Murphy, S., Sparkes, A.H., Smith, K.C. et al. (2004) Relationships between the histological grade of cutaneous mast cell tumours in dogs, their survival and the efficacy of surgical resection. *Vet Rec* 154, pp. 743–746.
■ Mutsaers, A.J. (2007) Chemotherapy: new uses for old drugs. *Vet Clin North Am Small Anim Pract*, 37, pp. 1079–1090.
■ Mutz, M.L., Boudreaux, B.B., Royal, A, et al. (2017) Cytologic comparison of the percentage of mast cells in lymph node aspirate samples from clinically normal dogs versus dogs with allergic dermatologic disease and dogs with cutaneous mast cell tumors. *J Am Vet Med Assoc*, 251(4), pp. 421–428.
■ Nemanic, S., Milovancev, M., Terry, J.L. et al. (2016) Microscopic Evaluation of Peritumoral Lesions of Feline Injection Site Sarcomas Identified by Magnetic Resonance Imaging and Computed Tomography. *Vet Surg*, 45(3), pp. 392–401.
■ Nicholls, P.K., Stanley, M.A. (1999) Canine papillomavirus-A centenary review. *J Comp Pathol*, 120(3), pp. 219–33.
■ Northrup, N C., Harmon, B.G., Gieger, T.L. et al. (2005) Variation among pathologists in histologic grading of canine cutaneous mast cell tumors. *J Vet Diagn Invest*, 17, pp. 245–248.
■ Ozaki, K., Yamagami, T., Nomura, K. et al. (2002) Mast cell tumors of the gastrointestinal tract in 39 dogs. *Vet Pathol*, 39, pp. 557–564.
■ Patnaik, A.K., Ehler, W.J., MacEwen, E.G. (1984) Canine cutaneous mast cell tumor: morphologic grading and survival time in 83 dogs. *Vet Pathol*, 21, pp. 469–474.
■ Pestili de Almeida, E.M., Piché, C., Sirois, J. et al (2001) Expression of cyclo-oxygenase-2 in naturally occurring squamous cell carcinomas in dogs. *J Histochem Cytochem*, 49(7), pp. 867–75.
■ Pisani, G., Millanta, F., Lorenzi, D. et al. (2006) Androgen receptor expression in normal, hyperplastic and neoplastic hepatoid glands in the dog. *Res Vet Sci*, 81(2), pp. 231–6.
■ Poirier, V.J., Adams, W.M., Forrest, L.J. et al. (2006) Radiation therapy for incompletely excised grade II canine mast cell tumors. *J Am Anim Hosp Assoc*, 42, pp. 430–434.
■ Preziosi, R., Sarli, G., Paltrinieri, M. (2004) Prognostic value of intratumoral vessel density in cutaneous mast cell tumors of the dog. *J Comp Pathol*, 130, pp. 143–151.
■ Rakich, P.M., Latimer, K.S., Weiss, R. (1989) Mucocutaneous plasmacytomas in dogs: 75 cases (1980–1987). *J Am Vet Med Assoc*, 194(6), pp. 803–10.
■ Rassnick, K.M., Bailey, D.B., Flory, A.B. et al. (2008) Efficacy of vinblastine for treatment of canine mast cell tumors. *J Vet Intern Med* 22, pp. 1390–1396.
■ Rassnick, K.M., Moore, A.S., Williams, L.E. et al. (1999) Treatment of canine mast cell tumors with CCNU (lomustine). *J Vet Intern Med*, 13, pp. 601–605.
■ Rassnick, K.M., Rodriquez, C.O., Khanna, C. et al. (2006) Results of a phase II clinical trial on the use of ifosfamide for treatment of cats with vaccine-associated sarcomas. *Am J Vet Res*, 67, pp. 517–523.
■ Rassnick, K.M., Ruslander, D.M., Cotter, S.M. et al. (2001) Use of carboplatin for treatment of dogs with malignant melanoma: 27 cases (1989–2000). *J Am Vet Med Assoc*, 218(9), pp. 1444–8.
■ Rassnick, K.M., Williams, L.E., Kristal, O. et al. (2008) Lomustine for treatment of mast cell tumors in cats: 38 cases (1999–2005). *J Am Vet Med Assoc*, 232, pp. 1200–1205.
■ Rassnick, K.M. (2004) Medical management of soft-tissue sarcomas. *Vet Clin North Am Small Anim Pract*, 33, pp. 517–531.
■ Reimer, S.B., Séguin, B., DeCock, H.E. et al. (2005) Evaluation of the effect of routine histologic processing on the size of skin samples obtained from dogs. *Am J Vet Res*, 66(3), pp. 500–5.
■ Risselada, M., Mathews, K.G., Griffith, E. (2015) Surgically planned versus histologically measured lateral tumor margins for resection of cutaneous and subcutaneous mast cell tumors in dogs: 46 cases (2010–2013). *J Am Vet Med Assoc*, 247(2), pp. 184–9.
■ Robinson, W.P., Elliott, J., Baines, S.J. et al. (2017) Intramuscular mast cell tumors in 7 dogs. *Can Vet J.*, 58(9), pp. 931–935.
■ Rochat, M.C., Mann, F.A., Pace, L.W. et al. (1992) Identification of surgical biopsy borders by use of India ink. *J Am Vet Med Assoc*, 201, pp. 873–878.
■ Rodríguez, F., Herráez, P., Rodríguez, E. (1995) Metastatic pilomatrixoma associated with neurological signs in a dog. *Vet Rec*, 137(10), pp. 247–8.
■ Romanelli, G., Marconato, L., Olivero, D. et al. (2008) Analysis of prognostic factors associated with injection-site sarcomas in cats: 57 cases (2001–2007). *J Am Vet Med Assoc*, 232, pp. 1193–1199.
■ Romansik, E.M., Reilly, C.M., Kass, P.H. et al. (2007) Mitotic index is predictive for survival for canine cutaneous mast cell tumors, *Vet Pathol*, 44, pp. 335–341.

■ Russell, K.N., Mehler, S.J., Skorupski, K.A. et al. (2007) Clinical and immunohistochemical differentiation of gastrointestinal stromal tumors from leiomyosarcomas in dogs: 42 cases (1990–2003). *J Am Vet Med Assoc*, 230, pp. 1329–1333.
■ Saba, C. (2017) Vaccine- associated feline sarcoma: current perspectives. *Vet Med (Auckl)* 8, pp. 13–20.
■ Sabattini, S., Barzon, G., Giantin, M. et al. (2017) Kit receptor tyrosine kinase dysregulations in feline splenic mast cell tumours. *Vet Comp Oncol*, 15(3), pp. 1051–61.
■ Sabattini, S., Scarpa, F., Berlato, D. et al. (2015) Histologic grading of canine mast cell tumor: is 2 better than 3? *Vet Pathol*, 52(1), pp. 70–3.
■ Sato, A.F., Solano, M. (2004) Ultrasonographic findings in abdominal mastcell disease: a retrospective study of 19 patients. *Vet Radiol Ultrasound*, 45, pp. 51–57.
■ Scase, T.J., Edwards, D., Miller, J. et al. (2006) Canine mast cell tumors: correlation of apoptosis and proliferation markers with prognosis. *J Vet Intern Med*, 20, pp. 151–158.
■ Schultheiss, P.C., Gardiner, D.W., Rao, S. et al. (2011) Association of histologic tumor characteristics and size of surgical margins with clinical outcome after surgical removal of cutaneous mast cell tumors in dogs. *J Am Vet Med Assoc*, 238, pp. 1464–1469.
■ Schultheiss, P.C. (2006) Histologic features and clinical outcomes of melanomas of lip, haired skin, and nail bed locations of dogs. *J Vet Diagn Invest*, 18(4), pp. 422–5.
■ Scott, D.W., Anderson, W.I. (1990) Canine sebaceous gland tumors: a retrospective analysis of 172 cases. *Canine Pract*, 15, p. 19.
■ Scott, D.W., Miller, W.H., Griffin, C.E. (2001) Neoplastic and nonneoplastic tumors. In: Scott DW, Miller WH, Griffin CE, ed. *Small animal dermatology*. Philadelphia: Saunders, p. 1236.
■ Scott, H.W., Parris, W.C.V., Sandidge, P.C. et al. (1983) Hazards in operative management of patients with systemic mastocytosis. *Ann Surg*, 197, pp. 507–514.
■ Seguin, B., Besancon, M.F., McCallan, J.L. et al. (2006) Recurrence rate, clinical outcome, and cellular proliferation indices as prognostic indicators after incomplete surgical excision of cutaneous grade II mast cell tumors: 28 dogs (1994–2002). *J Vet Intern Med*, 20(4), pp. 933–940.
■ Seguin, B., Leibman, N.F., Bregazzi, V.S. et al. (2001) Clinical outcome of dogs with grade-II mast cell tumors treated with surgery alone: 55 cases (1996–1999). *J Am Vet Med Assoc*, 218, pp. 1120–1123.
■ Seitz, S.E., Foley, G.L., Marretta, S.M. (1995) Evaluation of marking materials for cutaneous surgical margins. *Am J Vet Res*, 56, pp. 826–833.
■ Selting, K.A., Powers, B.A., Thompson, L.J. et al. (2005) Outcome of dogs with high-grade soft-tissue sarcomas treated with and without adjuvant doxorubicin chemotherapy: 39 cases (1996–2004). *J Am Vet Med Assoc*, 227, pp. 1442–1448.
■ Sfiligoi, G., Rassnick, K.M., Scarlett, J.M. et al. (2005) Outcome of dogs with mast cell tumors in the inguinal or perineal region versus other cutaneous locations: 124 cases (1990–2001). *J Am Vet Med Assoc*, 226, pp. 1368–1374.
■ Simko, E., Wilcock, B.P., Yager, J.A. (2003) A retrospective study of 44 canine apocrine sweat gland adenocarcinomas. *Can Vet J*, 44(1), pp. 38–42.
■ Simon, D., Ruslander, D.M., Rassnick, K.M. (2002) Combination of Orthovoltage Radiation Therapy and Con-Current Low-Dose Doxorubicin for Incompletely Excised Soft-Tissue Sarcomas in 39 Dogs. 12th ECVIM-CA/ESVIM Congress.
■ Simpson, A.M., Ludwig, L.L., Newman, S.J. et al. (2004) Evaluation of surgical margins required for complete excision of cutaneous mast cell tumors in dogs. *J Am Vet Med Assoc*, 224, pp. 236–240.
■ Smith, D.A., Knottenbelt, M.K. (1988) Spontaneous regression of intracutaneous cornifying epithelioma in a dog. *J Small Anim Pract*, 29, p. 201.
■ Smith, S.H., Goldschmidt, M.H., McManus, M. (2002) Comparative review of melanocytic neoplasms *Vet Pathol*, 39(6), pp.651–78.
■ Smrkovski, O.A., Essick, L., Rohrbach, B.W. et al. (2015) Masitinib mesylate for metastatic and non-resectable canine cutaneous mast cell tumours. *Vet Comp Oncol*, 13(3), pp. 314–21.
■ Spangler, W.L., Culbertson, M.R. (1992) Prevalence and type of splenic diseases in cats: 455 cases (1985–1991). *J Am Vet Med Assoc*, 201(5), pp. 773–6.
■ Spangler, W.L., Kass, P.H. (2006) The histologic and epidemiologic bases for prognostic considerations in canine melanocytic neoplasia. *Vet Pathol*, 43(2), pp. 136–49.
■ Stanclift, R.M., Gilson, S.D. (2008) Evaluation of neoadjuvant prednisone administration and surgical excision in treatment of cutaneous mast cell tumors in dogs. *J Am Vet Med Assoc*, 232, pp. 53–62.
■ Stannard, A.A., Pulley, L.T. (1975) Intracutaneous cornifying epithelioma (keratoacanthoma) in the dog: a retrospective study of 25 cases. *J Am Vet Med Assoc*, 167(5), pp. 385–8.
■ Stefanello, D., Morello, E., Roccabianca, P. et al. (2008) Marginal excision of low-grade spindle cell sarcoma of canine extremities: 35 dogs (1996–2006). *Vet Surg*, 37, pp. 461–465.
■ Stefanello, D., Valenti, P., Faverzani, S. et al (2009). Ultrasound-guided cytology of spleen and liver: a prognostic tool in canine cutaneousmast cell tumor. *J Vet Intern Med*, 23, pp. 1051–57.
■ Stell, A.J., Dobson, J.M., Langmack, K.J. (2001). Photodynamic therapy of feline superficial squamous cell carcinoma using topical 5-aminolaevulinic acid. *Small Anim Pract*, 42(4), pp. 164–9.
■ Stone, J.M., Jacky, P.B., Prieur, D.J. (1991) Chromosomal fragile site expression in boxer dogs with mast cell tumors. *Am J Med Genetics*, 40, pp. 223–229.
■ Suami, H., Yamashita, S., Soto-Miranda, M.A. et al. (2013) Lymphatic Territories (Lymphosomes) in a Canine: An Animal Model for Investigation of Postoperative Lymphatic Alterations. *PLOS ONE* 8(7): e69222.
■ Ter Haar, G., van der Gaag, I., Kirpensteijn, J. (1998): Canine intestinal leiomyosarcoma. *Vet Q*, 20, pp. S111–S112.
■ Thamm, D.H., Mauldin, E.A., Vail, D.M. (1999) Prednisone and vinblastine chemotherapy for canine mast cell tumor—41 cases (1992–1997). *J Vet Intern Med*, 13, pp. 491–497.

■ Thamm, D.H., Vail, D.M. (2001) Mast cell tumors. In: Withrow, S.J., MacEwen, E.G. editors. *Small animal clinical oncology*, ed 3. Philadelphia: WB Saunders, pp. 261–282.
■ Théon, A.P., Barthez, P.Y., Madewell, B.R. et al. (1994) Radiation therapy of ceruminous gland carcinomas in dogs and cats. *J Am Vet Med Assoc*, 205(4), pp. 566–9.
■ Théon, A.P., Madewell, B.R., Shearn, V.I. et al. (1995) Prognostic factors associated with radiotherapy of squamous cell carcinoma of the nasal plane in cats. *J Am Vet Med Assoc*;206(7), pp. 991–6.
■ Théon, A.P., VanVechten, M.K., Madewell, B.R. (1996) Intratumoral administration of carboplatin for treatment of squamous cell carcinomas of the nasal plane in cats. *Am J Vet Res*, 57(2), pp. 205–10.
■ Thompson, J.J., Pearl, D.L., Yager, J.A. et al. (2011) Canine subcutaneous mast cell tumor: characterization and prognostic indices. *Vet Pathol*, 48, pp. 156–168.
■ Tobler, K., Lange, C., Carlotti, D.N. et al. (2008) Detection of a novel papillomavirus in pigmented plaques of four pugs. *Vet Dermatol*, 19(1), pp. 21–5.
■ Treggiari, E., Valenti, P., Porcellato, I. et al. (2023) Retrospective analysis of outcome and prognostic factors of subcutaneous mast cell tumours in dogs undergoing surgery with or without adjuvant treatment. *Vet Comp Oncol*, 21(3):437-446.
■ Turrel, J.M., Farrelly, J., Page, R.L. et al. (2006) Evaluation of strontium 90 irradiation in treatment of cutaneous mast cell tumors in cats: 35 cases (1992–2002). *J am Vet Med Assoc*, 228(6), pp. 898–901.
■ Vaccine-Associated Feline Sarcoma Task Force (2005) The current understanding and management of vaccine-associated sarcomas in cats. *J Am Vet Med Assoc*, 226, pp. 1821–1842.
■ Vail, D.M., von Euler, H., Rusk, A.W. et al. (2012) A randomized trial investigating the efficacy and safety of water-soluble micellar paclitaxel (Paccal Vet) for treatment of nonresectable grade 2 or 3 mast cell tumors in dogs. *J Vet Intern Med*, 26(3), pp. 598–607.
■ Vail, D.M., Withrow, S.J., Schwarz, P.D. (1990) Perianal adenocarcinoma in the canine male: a retrospective study of 41 cases. *J Am Anim Hosp Assoc*.
■ Van der Linde-Sipman, J.S., de Wit, M.M., van Garderen, E. et al. (1997) Cutaneous malignant melanomas in 57 cats: identification of (amelanotic) signet-ring and balloon cell types and verification of their origin by immunohistochemistry, electron microscopy, and in situ hybridization. *Vet Pathol*, 34(1), pp. 31–8.
■ Van der Linde-Sipman, J.S., van den Ingh, T.S. (2000). Primary and metastatic carcinomas in the digits of cats. *Vet Q*, 22(3), pp. 141–5.
■ Van Lelyveld, S., Warland, J., Miller, R. (2015) Comparison between Ki-67 index and mitotic index for predicting outcome in canine mast cell tumours. *J Small Anim Pract*, 56(5), pp. 312–9
■ Vascellari, M., Melchiotti, E., Bozza, M.A. et al. (2003) Fibrosarcomas at presumed sites of injection in dogs: characteristics and comparison with non–vaccination site fibrosarcomas and feline postvaccinal fibrosarcomas. *J Vet Med A Physiol Pathol Clin Med*, 50, pp. 286–291.
■ Vascellari, M., Melchiotti, E., Mutinelli, F. (2006) Fibrosarcoma with typical features of postinjection sarcoma at site of microchip implant in a dog: histologic and immunohistochemical study. *Vet Pathol* 43, pp. 545–548.
■ Vascellari, M., Mutinelli, F., Cossettini, R. et al. (2004) Liposarcoma at the site of an implanted microchip in a dog. *Vet J*, 168, pp. 188–190.
■ Villamil, J.A., Henry, C.J., Bryan, J.N. et al. (2011) Identification of the most common cutaneous neoplasms in dogs and evaluation of breed and age distributions for selected neoplasms. *J Am Vet Med Assoc*, 239(7), pp. 960–5.
■ Warland, J., Amores-Fuster, I., Newbury, W. et al. (2014) The utility of staging in canine mast cell tumours. *Vet Comp Oncol*, 12(4), pp. 287–98.
■ Webster, J.D., Yuzbasiyan-Gurkan, V., Kaneene, J.B. et al. (2006) The role of c-KIT in tumorigenesis: evaluation in canine cutaneous mast cell tumors. *Neoplasia*, 8, pp. 104–111.
■ Webster, J.D., Yuzbasiyan-Gurkan, V., Thamm, D.H. et al. (2008) Evaluation of prognostic markers for canine mast cell tumors treated with vinblastine and prednisone. *BMC Vet Res*, 4, p. 32.
■ Weisse, C., Shofer, F.S., Sorenmo, K. (2002) Recurrence rates and sites for grade II canine cutaneous mast cell tumors following complete surgical excision. *J Am Anim Hosp Assoc*, 38, pp. 71–73.
■ White, C.R., Hohenhaus, A.E., Kelsey, J. et al. (2011) Cutaneous MCTs: Associations with spay/neuter status, breed, body size, and phylogenetic cluster. *J Am Anim Hosp Assoc*, 47, pp. 210–216.
■ White, S.D., Rosychuk, R.A., Scott, K.V. et al. (1993) Use of isotretinoin and etretinate for the treatment of benign cutaneous neoplasia and cutaneous lymphoma in dogs. *J Am Vet Med Assoc*, 202(3), pp. 387–91.
■ Wobeser, B.K., Kidney, B.A., Powers, B.E. et al. (2007) Agreement among surgical pathologists evaluating routine histologic sections of digits amputated from cats and dogs. *J Vet Diagn Invest*, 19(4), pp. 439–43.
■ Wobeser, B.K., Kidney, B.A., Powers, B.E. et al. (2007) Diagnoses and clinical outcomes associated with surgically amputated canine digits submitted to multiple veterinary diagnostic laboratories. *Vet Pathol*, 44(3), pp. 355–61.
■ Zabielska-Koczywąs, K., Wojtalewicz, A., Lechowski, R. (2017) Current knowledge on feline injection-site sarcoma treatment. *Acta Vet Scand*, 59(1), p. 47.
■ Zeiss, C.J., Johnson, E.M., Dubielzig, R.R. (2003) Feline intraocular tumors may arise from transformation of lens epithelium. *Vet Pathol*, 40, pp. 355–362.

Test

Answers on Page 200

1. **An 8-year-old Boston Terrier dog is brought to the practice and on physical examination 3 nodules on the trunk of about 5 mm in diameter are detected, these are subcutaneous, soft/firm in consistency, well defined and not ulcerated. The owner explains that they have been present for more than a year and that they have not changed much, that only occasionally does one of them increase and decrease in size a little. Considering the breed, history, and clinical findings, what type of tumour would you suspect?**
   a. Lipoma because it is the most common skin tumour in dogs.
   b. Mast cell tumour, probably low-grade.
   c. Basal cell tumour because of the breed, location, and age.
   d. Mast cell tumour, probably high-grade because it changes in size.

2. **When approaching skin tumours on a dog or cat, what should always be done?**
   a. Aspiration of the nodule/s detected.
   b. Mapping the body to record all the lesions and nodules with their measurements.
   c. Performing a complete physical examination looking for any other nodules or signs of a possible concurrent problem.
   d. All the above are correct.

3. **After seeing a dog with a history of an excised mast cell tumour it is important to call the laboratory to ask for information that would allow the owner to be given an approximate prognosis, what parameter is essential?**
   a. Surgical margins and mitotic index.
   b. The mitotic index value and the presence of c-kit mutation.
   c. The histological grade and surgical margins.
   d. The presence of c-kit mutation and surgical margins.

4. **Which chemotherapy protocol described has been associated with an increase in survival in cases of soft-tissue sarcomas, when chemotherapy has been administered after surgery with a curative intent?**
   a. Doxorubicin.
   b. Cyclophosphamide and piroxicam.
   c. Palladia®.
   d. None.

5. **What is the most predictive prognostic factor in feline mast cell tumours?**
   a. Mitotic index.
   b. Presence or absence of c-kit mutation.
   c. Histological grade.
   d. Ki-67. value.

6. **A cat with skin lesions on multiple toes is brought to the practice. The owner explains that it started on one toe and now there are injuries on several and the animal is limping and licking itself constantly. What test should not be missed in the diagnostic approach?**
   a. Radiographs of the affected toes.
   b. Thoracic radiographs.
   c. Cytology of any of the lesions.
   d. Blood tests.

7. **A dog presents with marked hypoglycaemia. which of the following differentials would not form part of the list?**
   a. Hepatic tumour.
   b. Insulinoma.
   c. Haemangiosarcoma.
   d. Leiomyosarcoma.

8. **Which statement is correct?**
   a. Palladia® + vinblastine may have a synergistic effect when treating canine MCT.
   b. Palladia® + vinblastine cannot be combined in dogs that are c-kit negative for the mutation.
   c. Palladia® + vinblastine is a recommended therapeutic option over a single agent vinblastine protocol.
   d. Palladia® + vinblastine have been combined to treat non-operable canine MCT, with a response rate of 71%.

9. **A 12-year-old male mixed breed dog is presented with a large mass on the left hindlimb, firm on palpation and with poorly defined margins, with deep attachments and which is not moveable. Fine needle aspiration reveals lipid cells without characteristics of malignancy:**
   a. Intermuscular lipoma.
   b. Liposarcoma.
   c. Intramuscular lipoma.
   d. An MRI or CT is needed to determine if it is an intramuscular or intermuscular lipoma.

10. Which of the following stains can be used to help differentiate a mast cell tumour?

a. Cytokeratin.
b. Vimentin.
c. Methylene blue.
d. Toluidine blue.

11. Which of the following statements is correct regarding injection site associated fibrosarcomas in cats?

a. The anatomical location of the tumour is not a prognostic factor.
b. Complete removal of the tumour does not help extend disease-free and survival periods.
c. Histologically, vaccine-associated sarcomas are usually characterised by an inflammatory infiltrate of lymphocytes and macrophages, with aluminum particles occasionally detected in some macrophages.
d. The combination of chemotherapy using adriamycin and cytoxan has been shown to be effective as the sole treatment for non-surgical fibrosarcomas, with some complete responses observed.

12. Which of the following immunohistochemical stains is not correctly associated with the cell type you are able to identify?

a. CD 18 – histiocytic.
b. S 100 – smooth muscle.
c. CD 31 – endothelial.
d. Synaptophysin – neuroendocrine.

13. Prognostic factors related to the success of treatment for injection site associated sarcomas include:

a. Time from vaccination to tumour development: the prognosis is worse when there is a short interval.
b. Radical surgical excision significantly increases disease-free time compared to a first marginal excision.
c. There is no significant difference in the time to first recurrence between cats where a first radical or marginal excision is performed.
d. Cats with tumours located in the extremities do not show significant differences in time to first recurrence compared to tumours in other locations.

14. Which of the following statements regarding skin tumours in dogs and cats is false?

a. Skin tumours tend to be more aggressive in dogs than in cats.
b. Skin tumours are the second most diagnosed tumour in the dog, after lymphoid tumours.
c. Squamous cell carcinoma of the nail bed is more common in dogs than cats.
d. The mitotic index is predictive of malignant behaviour in cutaneous melanoma of the dog, but not in the cat.

15. A 9-year-old Labrador presents at the clinic for evaluation of multiple cauliflower-shaped masses affecting the corner of the mouth. Which of the following questions regarding the dog's history would be most helpful in determining the patient's clinical condition?

a. Are there other young dogs in the home with similar lesions?
b. Is the dog receiving any type of immunosuppressive medication?
c. Has there been any lameness, shortness of breath, or gastrointestinal signs?
d. How long have the injuries been present and what has their growth rate been?

16. Of the following factors, which has been shown to be a negative prognostic indicator for canine cutaneous melanoma?

a. Inguinal location.
b. Miniature Schnauzer.
c. High mitotic index.
d. CD18 positive on immunohistochemistry.

Clinical Case

Peanut is an 11-year-old castrated Pug. Four months ago, he had a dental cleaning and the referring veterinarian found a rostral mandibular mass with the following characteristics (Figure 1).

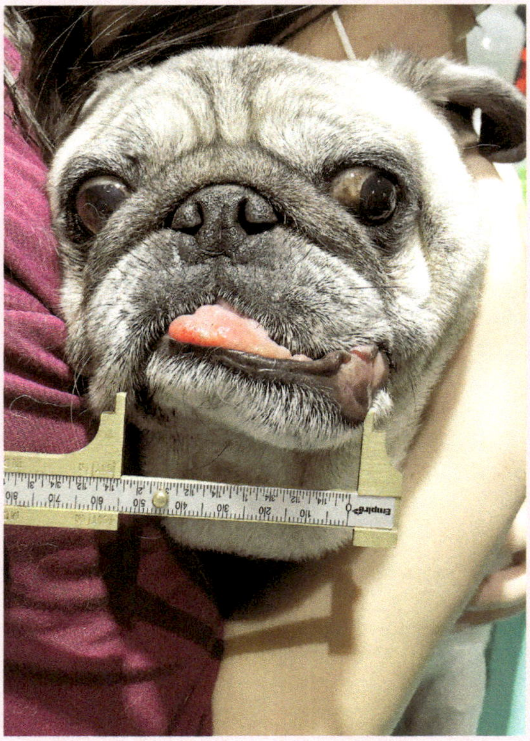

- About 5 cm in size.
- Unpigmented.
- Poorly delimited.
- Adhered to deep planes.
- Moving the incisors rostrally and to the right.

Peanut did not present any other symptoms.

1. What are the differential diagnoses?

2. What minimum diagnostic tests should be performed?

a. Incisional biopsy, lymph node DNA, haematology and presurgical biochemistry.
b. Tumour biopsy and thoracic radiographs.
c. FNA (tumour and regional lymph node if possible), oral radiographs (ideally CT if possible) and biopsy if FNA is non-diagnostic.
d. Tumour and lymph node FNA, thoracic radiographs and abdominal ultrasound.

3. If, when performing a fine needle aspiration of the tumour, a sample like the one shown in the images in Figure 2 is obtained, what diagnosis should be suspected?

a. Round cell tumour.
b. It is not a tumour, it is an inflammatory process.
c. It is a tumour of epithelial origin.
d. It is a tumour of mesenchymal origin.

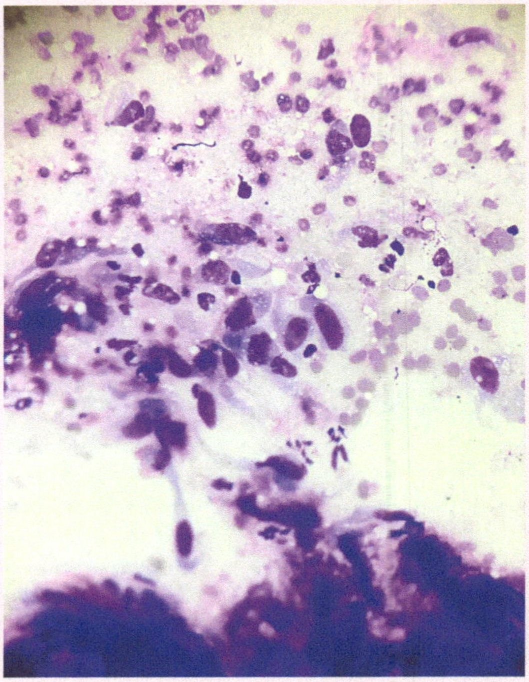

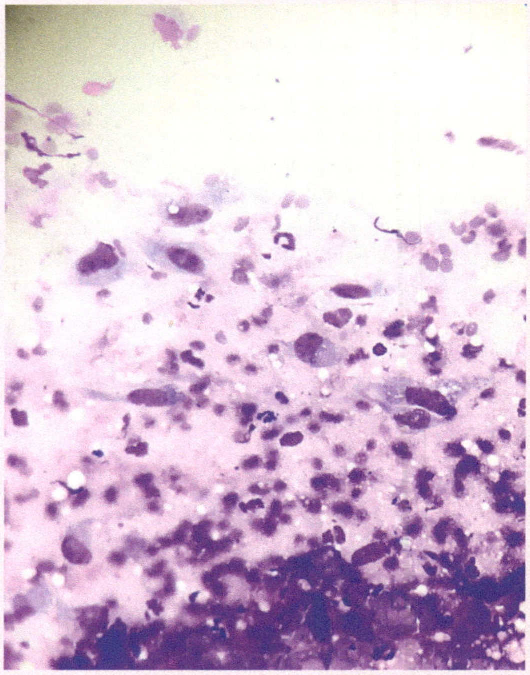

The biopsy results were consistent with a soft-tissue sarcoma, with a low mitotic index (2 MF X 10 HPF). The diagnosis was compatible with oral fibrosarcoma.

4. Considering the histopathology results, what is the general recommendation of treatment for this tumour type, with curative intent?

a. Aggressive surgery (partial rostral mandibulectomy) and radiation if the margins are incomplete.
b. Conservative surgery since it is a low-grade sarcoma.
c. Preoperative metronomic chemotherapy to reduce tumour size.
d. Radiation: once a week for 4 consecutive weeks.

5. Do these oral tumours have any notable features?

a. Canine oral fibrosarcomas are characterised by their slow growth and low rate of metastasis.
b. Canine oral fibrosarcomas are characterised by a low histological grade and low-grade tumour behaviour.
c. Patients with oral fibrosarcomas usually present at diagnosis with pulmonary metastases, which are the main cause of euthanasia in these cases.
d. Canine oral fibrosarcomas are characterised by a low histological grade and high-grade tumour behaviour.

Correct Answers:

Test

1. b
2. d
3. c
4. d
5. a
6. b
7. c
8. d
9. d
10. d
11. c
12. b
13. b
14. b
15. b
16. c

Clinical Case

1. **What are the differential diagnoses?**
   The most common oral tumours in dogs:
   - melanoma
   - squamous cell carcinoma
   - epuli
   - sarcoma
   - osteosarcoma.

2. **Which minimum diagnostic tests should be performed?**
   c. FNA (tumour and regional lymph node if possible), oral radiographs (ideally CT if possible) and biopsy if FNA is non-diagnostic.

3. **If, when performing a fine needle aspiration of the tumour, a sample like the one shown in the following images is obtained, what diagnosis should be suspected?**
   d. It is a tumour of mesenchymal origin.

4. **Considering the histopathology results, what is the general recommendation of treatment for this tumour type, with curative intent?**
   a. Aggressive surgery (partial rostral mandibulectomy) and radiation if the margins are incomplete.

5. **Do these oral tumours have any notable features?**
   d. Canine oral fibrosarcomas are characterised by a low histological grade and high-grade tumour behaviour.

Notes

Neoplasms of the Nervous System: Diagnosis, Treatment, and Prognosis

Mónica Clemente

Nervous system (NS) neoplasms **occur relatively frequently in dogs (incidence of 1–3% on postmortem) and cats**. In dogs, tumours of the nervous system are more frequent in the brain than in the spinal cord or peripheral nerves and appear with a frequency and histopathological distribution similar to those described in human medicine. While in cats tumours are relatively less common, and most are meningiomas and lymphomas.

Primary tumours of the nervous system originate from neuroectodermal, ectodermal, and/or mesodermal cells normally present in or associated with the brain, spinal cord, or peripheral nerves. Secondary tumours affecting the nervous system can originate from surrounding structures, such as bones and muscles, or they can result from haematogenous metastasis from a primary tumour to another organ.

Metastases from CNS tumours are rare, but can occur through cerebrospinal fluid (CSF), especially if the tumours are located near the subarachnoid space or ventricular cavities (e.g. in choroid plexus papilloma's, neuroblastoma, or medulloblastoma). Tumours can also spread to surrounding tissues, especially bones, by direct extension.

In 1993, the World Health Organization (WHO) endorsed a comprehensive classification of neoplasms affecting the CNS. The classification of brain tumours is based on the premise that each type of tumour results from the abnormal growth of a specific cell type. To the extent that the behaviour of a tumour correlates with the basic cell type, tumour classification dictates the choice of therapy and predicts prognosis.

The 2007 WHO classification system classified CNS tumours in domestic species into eight categories. However, in veterinary medicine this classification is histological and does not consider factors such as prognosis, which has not been rigorously investigated in domestic species as it has in humans. In 2016 an update of the WHO classification was published, breaking the old principle of diagnosis based solely on the microscopic appearance and incorporating molecular parameters into the classification of tumours of the central nervous system. In 2021, a new update of this classification was carried out. This revision introduces major changes that advance the role of molecular diagnosis in CNS tumour classification while it maintains the other established approaches to tumour diagnosis such as histology and immunohistochemistry (Table 1).

Table 1. WHO classification of tumours of the central nervous system (2021). Provisional entities are in italics.

Tumours
Gliomas, glioneuronal tumours, and neuronal tumours
Adult-type diffuse gliomas
Astrocytoma, IDH-mutant
Oligodendroglioma, IDH-mutant, and 1p/19q-codeleted
Glioblastoma, IDH-wildtype
Pediatric-type diffuse low-grade gliomas
Diffuse astrocytoma, *MYB*- or *MYBL1*-altered
Angiocentric glioma
Polymorphous low-grade neuroepithelial tumour of the young
Diffuse low-grade glioma, MAPK pathway-altered
Pediatric-type diffuse high-grade gliomas
Diffuse midline glioma, H3 K27-altered
Diffuse hemispheric glioma, H3 G34-mutant
Diffuse pediatric-type high-grade glioma, H3-wildtype and IDH-wildtype
Infant-type hemispheric glioma
Circumscribed astrocytic gliomas
Pilocytic astrocytoma
High-grade astrocytoma with piloid features
Pleomorphic xanthoastrocytoma
Subependymal giant cell astrocytoma
Chordoid glioma
Astroblastoma, *MN1*-altered
Glioneuronal and neuronal tumours
Ganglioglioma
Desmoplastic infantile ganglioglioma/ desmoplastic infantile astrocytoma
Dysembryoplastic neuroepithelial tumour
Diffuse glioneuronal tumour with oligodendroglioma-like features and nuclear clusters
Papillary glioneuronal tumour
Rosette-forming glioneuronal tumour
Myxoid glioneuronal tumour
Diffuse leptomeningeal glioneuronal tumour
Gangliocytoma
Multinodular and vacuolating neuronal tumour
Dysplastic cerebellar gangliocytoma (Lhermitte-Duclos disease)
Central neurocytoma
Extraventricular neurocytoma
Cerebellar liponeurocytoma
Ependymal tumours
Supratentorial ependymoma
Supratentorial ependymoma, *ZFTA* fusion-positive
Supratentorial ependymoma, *YAP1* fusion-positive
Posterior fossa ependymoma
Posterior fossa ependymoma, group PFA
Posterior fossa ependymoma, group PFB
Spinal ependymoma
Spinal ependymoma, *MYCN*-amplified
Myxopapillary ependymoma
Subependymoma

Tumours
Choroid plexus tumours
Choroid plexus papilloma
Atypical choroid plexus papilloma
Choroid plexus carcinoma
Embryonal tumours
Medulloblastoma
Medulloblastomas, molecularly defined
Medulloblastoma, WNT-activated
Medulloblastoma, SHH-activated and *TP53*-wildtype
Medulloblastoma, SHH-activated and *TP53*-mutant
Medulloblastoma, non-WNT/non-SHH
Medulloblastomas, histologically defined
Other CNS embryonal tumours
Atypical teratoid/rhabdoid tumour
Cribriform neuroepithelial tumour
Embryonal tumour with multilayered rosettes
CNS neuroblastoma *FOXR2*-activated
CNS tumour with *BCOR* internal tandem duplication
CNS embryonal tumour
Pineal tumours
Pineocytoma
Pineal parenchymal tumour of intermediate differentiation
Pineoblastoma
Papillary tumour of the pineal region
Desmoplastic myxoid tumour of the pineal region, *SMARCB1*-mutant
Cranial and paraspinal nerve tumours
Schwannoma
Neurofibroma
Perineurioma
Hybrid nerve sheath tumour
Malignant melanotic nerve sheath tumour
Malignant peripheral nerve sheath tumour
Paraganglioma
Meningiomas
Meningioma
Mesenchymal, non-meningothelial tumours
Soft-tissue tumours
Fibroblastic and myofibroblastic tumours
Solitary fibrous tumour
Vascular tumours
Hemangiomas and vascular malformations
Hemangioblastoma
Skeletal muscle tumours
Rhabdomyosarcoma
Uncertain differentiation
Intracranial mesenchymal tumour, FET-CREB fusion-positive
CIC-rearranged sarcoma
Primary intracranial sarcoma, *DICER1*-mutant
Ewing sarcoma
Chondro-osseous tumours
Chondrogenic tumours
Mesenchymal chondrosarcoma
Chondrosarcoma
Notochordal tumours
Chordoma (including poorly differentiated chordoma)
Melanocytic tumours
Diffuse meningeal melanocytic neoplasms
Meningeal melanocytosis and meningeal melanomatosis
Circumscribed meningeal melanocytic neoplasms
Meningeal melanocytoma and meningeal melanoma
Haematolymphoid tumours
Lymphomas
CNS lymphomas
Primary diffuse large B-cell lymphoma of the CNS
Immunodeficiency-associated CNS lymphoma
Lymphomatoid granulomatosis
Intravascular large B-cell lymphoma
Miscellaneous rare lymphomas in the CNS
MALT lymphoma of the dura
Other low-grade B-cell lymphomas of the CNS
Anaplastic large cell lymphoma (*ALK+/ALK–*)
T-cell and NK/T-cell lymphomas
Histiocytic tumours
Erdheim-Chester disease
Rosai-Dorfman disease
Juvenile xanthogranuloma
Langerhans cell histiocytosis
Histiocytic sarcoma
Germ-cell tumours
Mature teratoma
Immature teratoma
Teratoma with somatic-type malignancy
Germinoma
Embryonal carcinoma
Yolk sac tumour
Choriocarcinoma
Mixed germ cell tumour
Tumours of the sellar region
Adamantinomatous craniopharyngioma
Papillary craniopharyngioma
Pituicytoma, granular cell tumour of the sellar region, and spindle cell oncocytoma
Pituitary adenoma/PitNET
Pituitary blastoma
Metastases to the CNS
Metastases to the brain and spinal cord parenchyma
Metastases to the meninges

CNS: central nervous system; IDH: isocitrate dehydrogenase; NK: natural killer; PitNET: pituitary neuroendocrine tumour; SHH: sonic hedgehog.

Depending on their location, tumours that affect the spinal cord can be divided into intramedullary, intradural-extramedullary, and extradural (Figure 1). Some of these tumours can originate in one compartment and spread to another, which is why they are called mixed compartment tumours. In the cranial cavity those that are in the centre of the brain parenchyma are called intra-axial and if they are outside the parenchyma, they are termed extra-axial (Figure 2).

The **grade**, following the WHO classification (Table 2), is **one of the most important factors in predicting response to therapy and survival**. The new WHO system is particularly useful in this regard. The WHO classification provides a parallel, grade classification system for each tumour type. In this classification, most of the named tumours are of a single defined grade.

- **Grade 1**. Low proliferation potential: possible cure with surgery.
- **Grade 2**. Infiltrative/low proliferation: may recur or progress despite surgery.
- **Grade 3**. Histological evidence of malignancy: adjuvant therapy is required.
- **Grade 4**. Cytological malignancy/necrosis/mitosis.

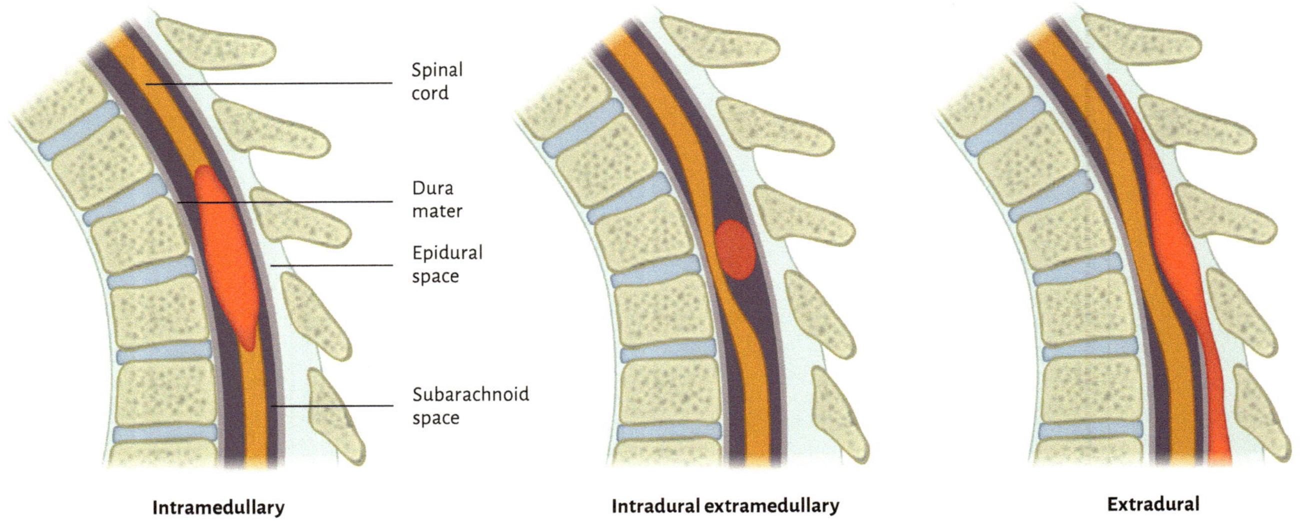

Figure 1. Tumours which affect the spinal cord can be categorised into intramedullary, intradural extramedullary and extradural types, depending on their location.

Table 2. CNS WHO grades of selected types, covering entities for which there is a new approach to grading, an updated grade, or a newly recognised tumour that has an accepted grade.

Tumour	Grade
Astrocytoma, IDH-mutant	2, 3, 4
Oligodendroglioma, IDH-mutant, and 1p/19q-codeleted	2, 3
Glioblastoma, IDH-wildtype	4
Diffuse astrocytoma, MYB- or MYBL1-altered	1
Polymorphous low-grade neuroepithelial tumour of the young	1
Diffuse hemispheric glioma, H3 G34-mutant	4
Pleomorphic xanthoastrocytoma	2, 3
Multinodular and vacuolating neuronal tumour	1
Supratentorial ependymoma[a]	2, 3
Posterior fossa ependymoma[a]	2, 3
Myxopapillary ependymoma	2
Meningioma	1, 2, 3
Solitary fibrous tumour	1, 2, 3

Grade is based on natural history and for some tumour types, definite grading criteria and understanding of natural history are not yet known. Note the use of Arabic numerals.
[a] For morphologically defined ependymomas.

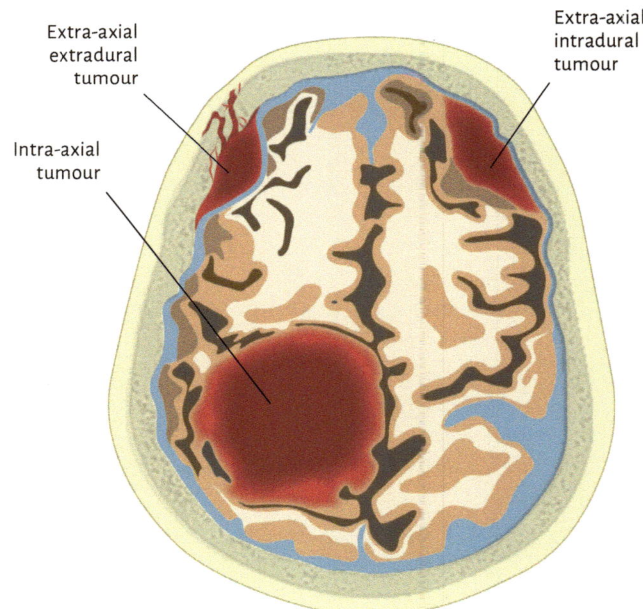

Figure 2. In the cranial cavity, tumours which are within the encephalic parenchyma are called intra-axial, while those outside the parenchyma are called extra-axial.

Brain Tumours

Primary tumours of the nervous system in dogs and cats occur more frequently in the brain than in the spinal cord or peripheral nerves. Primary brain tumours originate from the brain parenchyma (glial cells and neurons), cells that form the inner and outer lining of the brain (ependyma and meninges respectively), as well as from the vascular elements (choroid plexus).

In both **dogs and cats, the most common tumours are meningiomas** (Box 1).

The extension of primary tumours of the nasal cavities into the cranial vault through the cribriform plate is relatively common. On the other hand, it is less frequent that tumours originating from the middle or inner ear canal will spread/invade the brain.

Primary brain tumours can occur in any breed or sex, in both dogs and cats, but are more common in middle-aged or geriatric animals (>5 years). The mean age of presentation in dogs is 9 years old and 10 in cats.

Dolichocephalic (German Shepherd, Collie) are considered predisposed breeds for the development of meningiomas, as well as brachycephalic breeds which are prone to developing gliomas. Both Golden Retrievers and Boxers are predisposed to develop brain tumours.

Box 1. Most common brain tumours in dogs and cats

The most common primary brain tumours in dogs

- **Meningiomas.**
- **Gliomas (astrocytomas, oligodendrogliomas).**
  - **— Astrocytomas (Figure 3).**
  - **— Oligodendrogliomas (Figure 4).**
- **Undifferentiated sarcomas.**
- **Pituitary tumours.**
- **Ventricular tumours (choroid plexus papillomas and ependymomas).**

Other tumours have been previously described: gangliocytomas, neuroblastomas, pinealomas, craniopharyngiomas, and medulloblastomas, but they are rare.

The most common intracranial tumours in cats

- **Meningiomas.**
- **Lymphoma.**
- **Astrocytoma.**

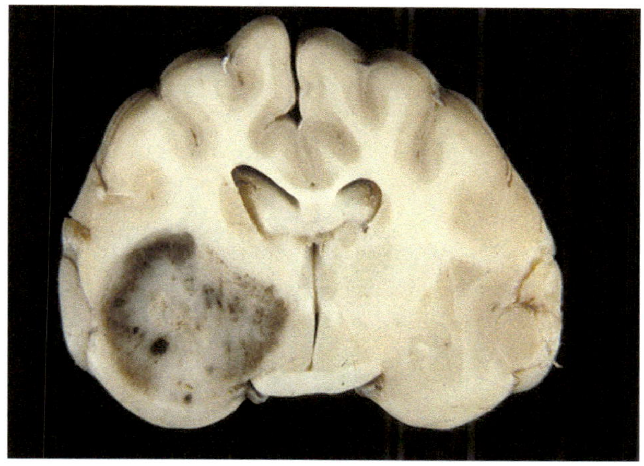

Figure 3. Macroscopic appearance of an astrocytoma.

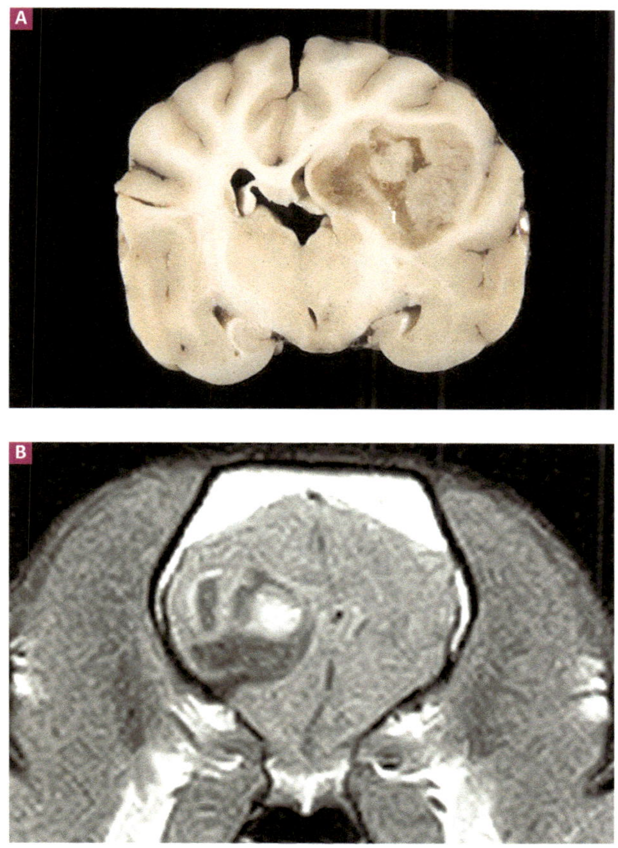

Figure 4. Section of the brain of a dog where an oligodendroglioma can be seen (**A**). Appearance of an oligodendroglioma on MRI (**B**).

Meningioma

Meningiomas are **primary tumours originating in the CNS meninges**, which are frequently located in the cerebral convexities and in the spinal subarachnoid space, although they can also be located in the optic nerves. They probably originate from the arachnoid cells of the head.

The mean age of presentation is 10 years old, although they have been described in animals between 1–16 years of age.

Macroscopically, meningiomas in dogs and cats are discrete, firm and elastic, lobular, grey, or pink extramedullary masses. They are usually well encapsulated (especially in cats) and attached to the underlying dura, displacing the brain without invading it. However, in the dog, the borders of the tumours can be difficult to distinguish from oedematous brain tissue, and **meningiomas are invasive in nearly 30% of cases**. Hyperostosis reactions or proliferation of the calvary bone in contact with the mass can be generated in response to the pressure of the meningioma (especially in cats).

They are usually slow-growing neoplasms and can progress without neurological signs until they have reached a considerable size. The neurological signs they cause are the result of compression rather than invasion of brain tissue. The presence of **seizures is the most common neurological sign**.

Most cases in cats are benign, and relatively easy to remove surgically. In contrast, between 18% and 27% of canine meningiomas are malignant and invade the Virchow-Robin space. In general, the term benign should be used with caution when discussing meningiomas in dogs.

Computerised tomography (CT) (Figure 5) or magnetic resonance (MRI) appearance might provide a diagnostic suspicion; however, the definitive diagnosis is only achieved by excisional biopsy, which in turn serves as treatment; or CT-guided biopsy. Various tumours such as histiocytomas, meningioangiomatosis, idiopathic pachymeningitis, or even focal meningitis or radiculoneuritis can have an appearance similar to some meningiomas on MRI and CT.

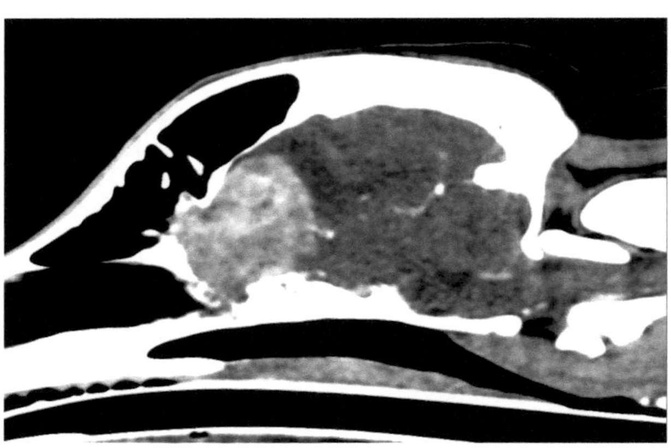

Figure 5. Appearance of a meningioma on CT.

As in human medicine, these tumours express progesterone receptors (79–100% of cases) without their role being very clear. In both species, lower progesterone expression has been shown to correlate with early recurrence and a high proliferation rate. All express VEGF, PCNA, and Ki67. In other studies, >90% of cases express VEGFR1 and 2 and EGFR1 and expression is associated with the prognosis.

Gliomas

Gliomas include **tumours whose precursor cells are constituents of the central nervous parenchyma**: astrocytes, oligodendrocytes, ependymocytes, etc. They usually affect older animals but have also been described in young animals. Brachiocephalic breeds are most predisposed.

Neurological signs depend on the location of the tumour, the degree of peritumoural oedema, and the presence of associated bleeding. Most are in the brain and diencephalon, with 28% of them located in the cerebellum. 35% of cases show abnormal p53 expression, 23% express EGFR, and 84% are GFAP positive.

Secondary Metastasis/Neoplasia

Secondary CNS neoplasms are **increasingly being identified in dogs and cats**, although they are less common in feline species.

Of the intracranial tumours evaluated histopathologically in a study between 1986 and 1990, 65% were secondary tumours, compared to only 28% intracranial tumours examined between 1951 and 1986.

The incidence of secondary brain tumours may be increasing because, nowadays, more animals with systemic neoplasms are being treated more aggressively, with multimodal therapies that prolong their survival, allowing more time for intracranial metastasis to develop.

Another possibility is that, the incidence of secondary brain tumours may have been previously underestimated because it had not been consistently evaluated in diagnostic tests.

Historically, carcinomas have been the most common type of secondary tumour in the brain, followed by sarcomas. In a large study that included 177 cases with secondary intracranial neoplasias, the mean age of presentation was almost 10 years, and most of the neoplasms were located in the telencephalon. The most frequent tumour was haemangiosarcoma (29%) followed by pituitary tumours (25%), lymphomas (12%) and carcinomas (12%).

Clinical Pathology and Clinical Signs

The presence of a brain tumour should be suspected in dogs with:

- appearance of seizures after 5 years of age; and
- signs of progressive brain dysfunction.

A **definitive diagnosis is only obtained by biopsy or necropsy**. CT and MRI is helpful to localise the lesion, but, on some ocasions, the findings obtained with these diagnostics, might be confused with local inflammation and cerebral infarcts.

The severity of clinical signs mainly depends on the growth rate and the location of the tumour, peritumoural oedema, intracranial pressure, and compensatory mechanisms within the brain.

One study revealed that, in over 50 % of the cases, the primary tumour occupied several anatomical areas of the brain. These patients might be diagnosed with multifocal disease during neurological examination.

Seizures are the most common clinical symptom, which occurs in around 50–60% of cases. Tumours arising from the outside part of the cerebral parenchyma will cause a mass effect, as they will gradually compress normal brain tissue. The progression of the symptoms associated with the tumour are usually slow, because the mass effect is initially compensated. Hence, on many occasions, the initial behaviour changes are associated with the "advanced age" of the animal, which can delay the tumour diagnosis. When the normal compensatory mechanisms of the brain are exhausted (the volume of cerebrospinal fluid [CSF] and blood decrease), the clinical signs can develop acutely or subacutely.

In cats, up to 20% of the cases will present clinical signs that are not attributable to the tumour (without neurological symptoms), including lethargy and anorexia. According to some studies, up to 20% of the tumours are diagnosed as an incidental finding.

Neurological signs include, in addition to seizures, vestibular signs, obtundation, coma, ataxia, etc., depending on the location of the tumour. In cases of large tumours, cerebral herniation and death from cardiorespiratory arrest can occur.

Diagnosis

As for all neurological problems, the **anatomical location of the injury** needs to be determined. A correct localisation allows the best diagnostic method to be selected.

The definitive diagnosis of a brain tumour cannot be made without a biopsy. However, an approximate presumptive diagnosis can be made based on diagnostic imaging techniques.

Diagnostic imaging techniques

The best method to detect CNS neoplasias is MRI. MRI allows the lesion to be located, and the extension of the tumour to be defined. Before performing large imaging studies, **clinical staging of the patient is indicated**. In all animals with suspected neoplasia, it is necessary to obtain a blood profile (complete blood count and biochemistry), thoracic radiographs and abdominal ultrasound to rule out a primary tumour, metastatic disease and to evaluate the general medical condition of the patient.

At the intracranial level, multilobular osteochondrosarcomas and some meningiomas can be identified by plain radiography. In one study, it was shown that almost 23% of patients diagnosed with a primary brain tumour also had another tumour of a different type. Therefore, performing a **complete staging** in these patients that includes abdominal ultrasound and thoracic radiographs is always recommended.

In a recent retrospective study with 15 dogs with glioma, CT and MRI were compared and it determined that the accuracy for prediction of tumour grade (high or low) was 46% for CT and 53% for MRI. Likewise, the accuracy for prediction of tumour type was 53% for CT and 60% for MRI. Therefore, **both CT and MRI are valid for the evaluation of gliomas**, although not 100% sensitive or specific.

Furthermore, a 2018 study showed that tumour volume determined by MRI was not associated with the outcome of surgery or adjuvant therapy for dogs with glioma, and **the tumour grade can only be established by biopsy**. Given the low-moderate prediction of glioma diagnosis with CT or MRI, histopathology is still necessary to obtain an accurate diagnosis of canine brain tumours.

In general, **the two most widely used diagnostic tests are CT and MRI**. The latter is, in general, the method of choice. Using MRI, it is possible to obtain sections in different planes, as well as different sequences, in order to visualise the characteristics of the tumour. No tumour has a unique imaging pattern, therefore, MRI is not a 100% sensitive diagnostic method. However, common features for different tumours have been described. By using different sequences, the presence of invasion of surrounding tissues can be detected, although it is much more complicated to determine if there is invasion in the nervous system.

Although there are exceptions, and certain tumours may present differently, there are several characteristics that allow general differentiation of meningiomas from gliomas.

- **Meningiomas** commonly reveal a **broad-based extra-axial fixation** (growing from the periphery of the brain inward or axially), exhibit **well-defined margins, and acquire contrast uniformly**. Meningiomas tend to displace rather than invade parenchymal tissue. Some meningiomas may present with calcifications, a characteristic that can be seen on a CT scan without contrast. The **dural tail sign** (Figure 6) is a feature often observed on MRI, where a tail associated with the meninges with an increase in the acquisition of contrast extends from the main mass. Meningiomas can also have a cystic component.
- **Gliomas** normally originate in **intra-axial locations** (from within the brain substance outwards) and frequently **do not have very well-defined borders** (they tend to infiltrate rather than displace the tissue) and normally **do not acquire contrast well** and if they do, it is non-uniform. The phenomenon of ring enhancement, which consists of a ring of increased contrast acquisition surrounding an area with little contrast, is not a pathognomonic sign and has been associated with neoplastic and non-neoplastic diseases. Although in many cases it is associated with gliomas.

Choroid plexus tumours and ependymomas tend to be **intraventricularly** located and **acquire contrast uniformly**.

In medicine, MRI is 65–96% effective in predicting the diagnosis. In general terms, the degree of oedema is usually associated with the degree of malignancy, as well as the degree of increase in contrast acquisition in intra-axial masses.

CSF Analysis

Many experts continue to question the usefulness of this technique in the diagnosis of intracranial tumours. Most cases with tumours have **alterations in the CSF, but these are usually non-specific**, such as an increase in the number of cells in almost 27–58% of cases and a mixed cell pleocytosis. In between 10–30% of cases with intracranial tumours, the CSF sample is found to be normal.

In the case of **choroid plexus carcinomas** (Figure 7), it is **usually more useful**, since protein concentrations of >100 mg/dl tend to be more suggestive of carcinomas compared to papillomas.

In case of suspicion of an intracranial tumour, diagnostic imaging techniques should be carried out before obtaining CSF.

Treatment

Treatment of intracranial tumours can be approached definitively or palliatively.

Unfortunately, the available data regarding different histological tumours is missing, since many clients decide not to treat, and radiation or chemotherapy is administered without knowing the tumour type.

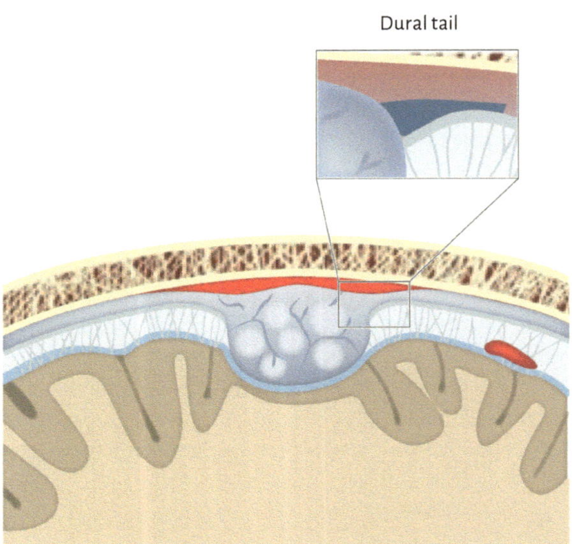

Figure 6. Diagram showing the dural tail seen in meningiomas, which can be seen on MRI.

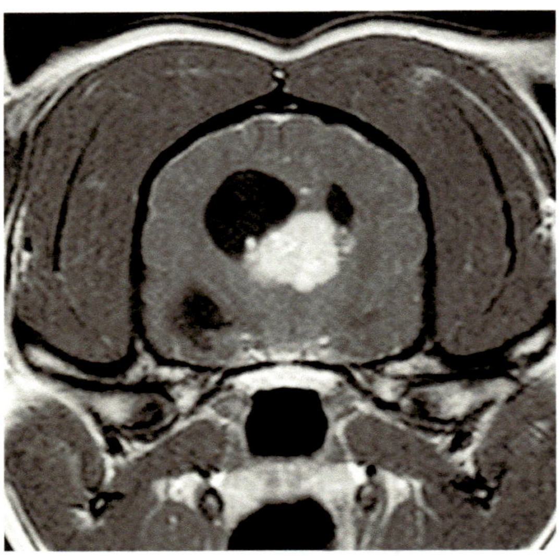

Figure 7. MRI of a choroid plexus tumour.

Definitive Treatment

The treatment indicated for most intracranial tumours is surgery, radiation therapy or a **combination of surgery with radiotherapy**.

Surgery

The surgery offers:

- **immediate decompressive effect**, facilitating the improvement of clinical signs;
- **histopathological diagnosis**; and
- in some cases, **complete resection is achieved**.

Some of these tumours respond to chemotherapy, such as lymphoma, hence, chemotherapy might prevent recurrence, even if resection is not complete. Most meningiomas in cats are resectable, while in dogs, surgical resection can be more complicated, as almost 30% of them are invasive. Cortical and cerebellar tumours are easier to remove by surgery, whereas brain stem tumours are almost impossible to remove. In the case of gliomas, surgery is usually more complicated due to the invasive nature of these types of tumours, and it is difficult to distinguish between healthy brain tissue and neoplasia.

The surgical treatment of secondary tumours depends on the tumour type; some, such as multilobular osteochondrosarcoma, generally have a fairly good prognosis. The **immediate postoperative period is critical**, as it can be associated with severe complications, including elevated intracranial pressure.

Radiotherapy

RT equipment has advanced to the predominant use of linear accelerators, including IMRT and SRT, since they are better for sparing normal tissues, hence, decreasing the risk for toxiciy. Radiotherapy treatments for intracranial tumours have evolved in veterinary medicine over the years. RT can be successful for the treatment of primary and secondary brain tumours, when used alone or combined with surgery. The information regarding efficacy per histologic type is scant, due to the lack of histologically diagnosed tumours.

The **brain cannot tolerate large doses of radiation**, the total dose is limited by adverse effects. Despite the fact hypofractionated protocols have been described, using 2–3 doses per week, or even a single weekly dose, often daily doses are used as in human medicine. This avoids side effects, such as delayed brain toxicity, which is caused with higher doses, typical of hypofractionated protocols. According to some studies, up to 15% of dogs were euthanised due to these complications.

The most important thing to avoid complications in these protocols is the **total dose**, the **dose per fraction** and the **amount of brain tissue to be radiated**. Complications associated with radiation therapy for CNS tumours have been described, the most common being **radiation brain necrosis**.

Multiple studies that have included intracranial masses treated with RT as an only therapy have reported MST between 7 to 23 months. MST for extra-axial masses, most of them suspected as meningiomas, ranges from 9–19 months; while MST for intra-axial masses ranges from 9–13 months. According to some studies, extra-axial tumours might have a better prognosis than intra-axial tumours.

Considering the variable outcomes associated with RT and surgery, at the moment there is not a clear superior choice between these two treatment modalites, when used alone for canine meningiomas. RT is also useful as an adjuvant therapy of canine meningiomas, combined with surgery, with MST between 16–30 months.

Palliative Treatment

In cases in which the owners choose not to treat these patients with conventional therapies, a combination of **glucocorticoids** and **anticonvulsant therapy** can be administered to control the symptoms (Table 3). Glucocorticoids help control peritumoural oedema and CSF production, as well as decrease the permeability of tumour capillaries and tumour blood volume.

The use of **phenobarbital and potassium bromide are recommended as first options** and **benzodiazepines in emergencies**, although some authors prefer the use of other types of anticonvulsant drugs because, in cases of brain tumours, they observe a greater degree of sedation when using phenobarbital (for example, zonisamide or levetiracetam).

Table 3. Active ingredients used in palliative treatment of brain tumours.

Active ingredient		Dose
Glucocorticoids	Methylprednisolone	· 30 mg/kg single dose IV
	Prednisone/ prednisolone	· 0.5–1 mg/kg divided into two doses
Anticonvulsant therapy	Phenobarbital	· **Starting dose:** 5 mg/kg as necessary IV (up to 20 mg/kg total) · **Maintenance:** 2–3 mg/kg BID
	Potassium bromide	· **Starting dose:** 70 mg/kg BID PO · **Maintenance:** 20 mg/kg BID PO
	Benzodiazepines: diazepam and midazolam (more effective in emergencies)	· 0.5 mg/kg as necessary IV · 2 mg/kg as necessary rectally
	Zonisamide/ levetiracetam	

Chemotherapy

Chemotherapy is **not a general choice of treatment for brain tumours**, because the blood-brain barrier prevents or reduces the passage of many drugs and limits their effect.

In both human and veterinary medicine, drug development in neuro-oncology for neoplasms of the central nervous system (CNS) remains a challenge. Medications can be administered peripherally (that is, orally or intravenously) or locally (into the tumour). Each of these routes has advantages and disadvantages. As with treatment for non-CNS cancers, side effects (gastrointestinal, myelosuppression) can occur.

The nervous system is a privileged location, protected by the **blood-brain barrier**, which means that many agents developed for peripheral administration do not penetrate the CNS due to particle size, charge, or lack of lipid solubility. Furthermore, abnormal vasculature, increased interstitial pressure, and inherent mechanisms of tumour resistance (methyl guanine-methyl transferase [MGMT], P-glycoprotein, etc.) within cerebral neoplasms reduce the efficacy of many chemotherapeutic agents. Each of these problems alone, and all of them together, are reasons for the limited success of therapeutic agents directed against CNS tumours, despite promising data obtained using cell lines and animal models.

Historically, chemotherapy for brain tumours has been limited by the need for drugs that can cross the blood-brain barrier (Figure 8). There are several articles where compounds such as lomustine, carmustine and, temozolomide or hydroxyurea. They are highly fat-soluble agents, which cross the barrier.

Lomustine

With **lomustine, special care must be taken**, since the same enzymes that metabolise the compound into antineoplastic active substances are responsible for the metabolism and transformation of phenobarbital.

To avoid reduced efficacy in patients treated with lomustine, seeking alternative medications for seizure control is recommended. Although these agents are not generally recommended for use in patients with meningiomas, one publication describes the successful use of lomustine which, together with prednisone, facilitated a 13-month survival time.

The lomustine dose range is broad and the protocol commonly used consists of 60–90 mg/m² every 3 weeks in dogs and 50–60 mg/m² every 4–6 weeks in cats.

Hydroxyurea

One **potentially promising treatment** involves the antineoplastic agent hydroxyurea, which is used in human and veterinary

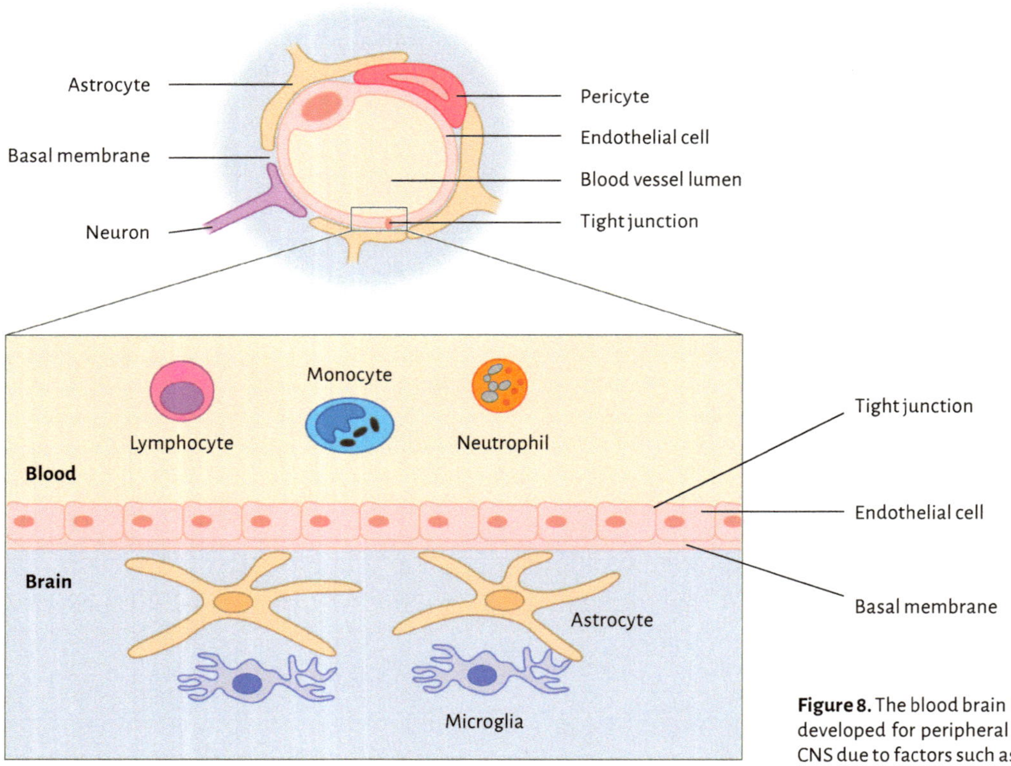

Figure 8. The blood brain barrier means that many medications developed for peripheral administration do not penetrate the CNS due to factors such as size, charge, or lack of fat solubility.

medicine for the long-term treatment of chronic myelogenous leukaemia and polycythaemia vera.

This drug **inhibits DNA synthesis without interfering with RNA and protein synthesis**, thereby causing the death of cells in the S phase of the cell cycle. **Adverse effects are minimal** and rarely include myelosuppression as well as nail shedding (this is the main dose-limiting toxicity).

Hydroxyurea has been shown to slow the growth of meningioma cell cultures in vitro, as well as in vivo with transplanted tumours in mice. These favourable results have been seen with hydroxyurea in human patients with meningioma, but there are no controlled veterinary studies until now. However, the drug is often used in veterinary neurology as a relatively inexpensive, non-invasive treatment. It is an **oral medication** that can be offered in conjunction with surgery and radiation for recurrent tumours or in addition to palliative therapy.

Dogs with MRI-confirmed meningiomas in which hydroxyurea was used as sole therapy (20 mg/kg/day) had survival times of 7 to 8 months, compared to 3 months in dogs treated with palliative therapy alone. Two dogs that underwent surgical aspiration of intracranial meningioma with ultrasound received hydroxyurea (50 mg/kg three times weekly) once tumour recurrence was detected at 499 and 1405 days postoperatively. Both dogs were alive at the time of publication, with a median survival time of 42 months after starting treatment. A review of six cats with tentorial meningiomas described the use of hydroxyurea (20 mg/kg/day) without associated complications. All cats died or were euthanised due to tumour progression in the 6–30-month follow-up time.

Temozolomide

It is used in melanoma and gliomas in humans and, **in dogs, there is only one study concerning lymphoma**, in which the safe dose and the most frequent side effects were defined.

The dose is between 60–100 mg/m² orally per day for 5 consecutive days, repeating the cycle after 3 weeks, and side effects are infrequent. In human medicine it is used at a higher dose, but dogs are more sensitive and do not tolerate the doses that are administered to people.

New Therapies

There are numerous aberrant signalling pathways involved in tumour progression identified in meningiomas and other brain tumours, especially in human medicine, but also in veterinary medicine. This deregulated cell signalling and how it is related to proliferation, survival, invasion, and angiogenesis in meningioma cell cultures has been identified. In particular, PDGF and its receptors (PDGFR) are frequently expressed in meningiomas, regardless of the histological grade. Activation of PDGFR is believed to result in aberrant cell signalling either through one of two pathways: PI3K Akt or Ras-MAPK pathways.

Many new agents are being investigated that target PDGF, VEGF and other components of the MAPK pathway with variable activity, such as imatinib, sunitinib, etc. Specifically, in veterinary medicine, all meningiomas express VEGF, PCNA and Ki-67 with >90% expressing VEGFR-1&2 and EGFR-1 This expression is related to grade and prognosis.

There are several case reports responding to targeted therapies in medicine, including therapy with bevacizumab, a VEGF inhibitor. Meningiomas are hypervascular and the inhibition of this vascularisation with compounds such as bevacizumab, which blocks VEGF, may be behind the responses observed. VEGF has been clearly shown to contribute centrally to tumour angiogenesis. It has also been found that the level of VEGF expression in meningiomas appears to correlate with tumour grade. Finally, inhibition of tumour angiogenesis also reduces peritumoural oedema, which contributes to the development of clinical signs produced by the presence of meningiomas and to morbidity.

It appears that dual inhibition of VEGF and PDGF receptors in recurrent or progressive meningiomas can lead to stabilisation of the disease and is being studied in human medicine. Palladia®, the most widely used RTKI drug in veterinary medicine, has a molecular structure almost identical to sunitinib and crosses the blood-brain barrier.

There are no control studies with this drug in veterinary medicine regarding treatment of intracranial tumours, but given the responses seen in other tumours and the scientific basis in the case of some brain tumours, it is a drug whose use should be further researched. Not only as a single agent but its possible combination with traditional chemotherapy as used in human medicine (for example, in gliomas, with sunitinib and metronomic temozolomide) needs to be investigated.

To finish the section on treatment of CNS tumours, Table 4 includes a summary of the most relevant studies regarding the success of various treatment protocols.

Spinal Tumours

Spinal tumours can be divided into primary and secondary, according to their tissue of origin. **Primary ones are the most frequent**.

- **Primary**: include tumours that originate from the parenchyma of the spinal cord (neurons, glial cells ...) or associated tissue (meningeal/ependymal).

Table 4. Summary of most relevant studies on the success of various CNS tumour treatments in dogs and cats.

Treatment	Tumour type	Number of cases	Survival time	Publication
Corticoids	Meningiomas	13	75 days (1–405 days)	Foster ES et al. JVIM. 1988
	Astrocytomas	7	77 days (7–150)	Foster ES et al. JVIM. 1988
	Brain tumours (unspecified)	45	6 days	Heidner GL et al. JVIM. 1991
		8	81 days	Turrel JM et al. JAVMA. 1981
		8	59 days	Turrel JM et al. JAVMA. 1984
Surgery	Canine meningioma	14	80 days	Axlund TW et al. JAVMA. 2002
		4	88 days (63–203)	Kostolich M et al. Vet Surg. 1987
		10	98 days	Niebauer GW et al. JAVMA. 1991
		17	254 days	Greco JJ et al. JAVMA. 2006
	Feline meningioma	10	650 days (60–900)	Lawson DC et al. JAVMA. 1984
		4	485	Niebauer GW et al. JAVMA. 1991
		17	830 (540–1410)	Gallagher JG et al. JAVMA. 1993
		34	685	Troxel et al. JVIM. 2003
		42	630 (40–1140)	Niebauer GW et al. JAVMA. 1991
Radiotherapy	Primary tumours (unspecified)	16	225 days	Turrel JM et al. Proc VCS. 1986
		14	345 days	Evans SM et al. JVIM. 1993 (ortovoltaje)
		4	322 days	Turrel JM et al. JAVMA. 1984
		25	140 days	Heidner GL et al. JVIM. 1991
		29	250 days	Spugnini EP et al. Vet Radiol & US
		15	344 days	LeCouteur R et al. Int J Rad Oncol.
	Canine extramedullary tumours	35	370 days	Brearly et al. JVIM. 1999
Surgery and radiotherapy	Meningiomas	12	610 days	Axlund TW et al. JAVMA. 2002
		20	1150 days	Theon A et al. JAVMA. 2000
		6	441 days	Brearly MJ et al. JVIM. 1999
Surgery and lomustine		3	552 days	Bilderback et al. ACVIM. 2006
Lomustine		1	13 months	Jung Di et al. JVMS. 2006
Hydroxyurea		?	8 months	Dewey et al. VIN.
Surgery and hydroxyurea	Relapsed meningioma	2	42 months	Graco et al. JAVMA. 2006

- **Secondary**: include primary or secondary vertebral tumours, malignant peripheral nerve sheath tumours, metastases to the extradural space or the parenchyma of the cord (intramedullary metastases).

When classifying these tumours, their relationship with the meninges is considered: **extradural, intradural/extramedullary, or intramedullary**. In a study of nearly 400 spinal tumours in dogs, 48% were extradural, 13% were intradural/extramedullary, 6% were intramedullary, and 33% were mixed compartment (affecting multiple sites). The most common type of tumour varies between sheath tumours, osteosarcoma, and meningioma, depending on the study. In cats, however, the most common tumour in all publications is lymphoma, which can be in any of the compartments, including the brain. The location of the tumour in some or all of the compartments can help to define the type of tumour present (Box 2).

Dogs and cats older than 5 years of age, are predisposed. However, there are some tumour types that affect younger animals, such as nephroblastomas (3 months to 6 years) or **germ-cell tumours** (younger than 2 years). There is no sex predisposition, and large breed dogs are more predisposed to develop vertebral tumours. Boxer dogs were overrepresented in one study of intraspinal meningiomas, and both Boxers and other brachycephalic breeds are predisposed to tumours of glial origin.

Spinal tumours **usually cause progressive signs of myelopathy**, but they can also present with acute or subacute spinal cord dysfunction. The acute presentation of clinical signs may be due to a pathological fracture of a vertebra invaded by the tumour, acute haemorrhage or necrosis of the tumour, or rapid tumour growth causing damage to the spinal cord (this usually occurs in the intramedullary types).

The **most frequent clinical sign** for most spinal tumours is **ataxia and paresis**, which can affect one or all four limbs, depending on their location. The presence of pain is not constant. Animals with intramedullary tumours do not have signs of pain since there are no nociceptive receptors at this level. But vertebral tumours, pathological fractures or nerve compression can cause intense, localised pain. The duration of the signs of the spinal problem can vary from a day to up to a year.

Box 2. Most frequent types of spinal tumours according to location

Extradural

- **Primary**
  - **Vertebral**
    - **Dogs: OSA> CSA, myeloma, FSA, HSA.**
    - **Cats: OSA> LSA> FSA, undifferentiated sarcoma, plasmacytomas.**
  - **Non-vertebral**
    - **Dogs: OSA, HSA or LSA.**
    - **Cats: LSA.**
- **Secondary**
  - **Carcinomas (prostate and mammary the most common).**
  - **Lipomas, myelolipomas, infiltrative lipomas, and liposarcomas have also been described extradurally.**
  - **Meningiomas are usually intradural, like those of the peripheral nerve sheath, but cases with an extradural presentation have been described.**

Intradural/extramedullary

- **Meningiomas (the most common).**
- **Peripheral nerve sheath tumours.**
- **Nephroblastomas (in young dogs).**
- **Lymphoma.**

Intramedullary

- **Parenchymal (glial cell) tumours: astrocytomas, oligodendrogliomas, ependymoma, germ cell tumour.**
- **Metastasis: haemangiosarcoma, lymphoma, carcinoma.**

Diagnosis

The minimum database for a patient with a suspected spinal cord neoplasia is identical to that for a brain tumour patient. Although the laboratory results rarely provide a definitive diagnosis regarding the aetiology of the neoplasia, on some occasions they can be helpful offering information about paraneopalstic syndromes, other tumours such as lymphoma or multiple myeloma

For the diagnosis of vertebral tumours, **radiographs can be very useful**. Survey radiographs may reveal primary vertebral tumours, metastasis, fractures, but are frequently normal. In cats, lytic lesions are most commonly seen in nonlymphoid neoplasms. The animal must be sedated and well positioned and at least two projections are needed. The most common radiographic finding in vertebral neoplasms is osteolysis.

In cases of vertebral tumours, the intraosseous pattern predominates, although there may also be osteoproliferation with loss of defined edges of the bone cortices, depending on the type of tumour. The predominant pattern in nerve sheath tumours is osteolysis, which is easily identified by plain radiography.

In cases where the animal presents with multifocal pain, full-spine radiographs should be performed to identify bone lesions that could suggest metastasis.

Myelography is a technique that allows location of a tumour and a more specific list of possible differential diagnoses to be developed. In addition, with myelography, the entire spine can be evaluated, which can be useful in multifocal tumours or when the neurological examination suggests more than one location. Sometimes the finding of a characteristic pattern may be enough to locate the tumour, clarify possible differential diagnoses, and plan surgery. When it comes to extradural tumours, the neurological signs are due to spinal cord compression, hence, the size of the tumour might be large enough to be detected on radiographs. Although, if these are not observed, it does not mean that they are not present.

Using **CT** more information can be obtained to help narrow down a list of differentials, because it delimits the myelography findings and determines the location within the vertebral canal. In fact, CT is more sensitive for localisation than MRI.

As with brain tumours, **MRI** is the modality of choice for the evaluation of spinal tumours, however, CT combined with myelography can be helpful for determination of the longitudinal and axial location of many tumours.

Magnetic resonance imaging allows sections in different planes and different sequences to be obtained to help define the macroscopic characteristics of the tumour. As previously discussed regarding the brain tumours, vertebral and spinal cord tumours often display MRI characteristics that allow for presumptive diagnosis, but the definitive diagnosis can only be obtained with histopathology, as there is an overlap between the features of some tumours and non-neoplastic lesions.

In tumours of vertebral origin, or which are superficial, an attempt can be made to obtain a sample by fine needle aspiration for evaluation by **cytology**. Biopsy of tumours affecting the vertebrae or the spinal cord is required for definitive diagnosis. Generally, the biopsy is taken at the time of surgery; however, needle biopsy can be performed using image-guided techniques.

Cerebrospinal fluid analysis is frequently performed combined with imaging, although it is a sensitive but not specific diagnostic test. Lymphomas are an exception, since more than 60% of the patients with lymphoma can be diagnosed based on the CSF analysis.

Treatment

The approach in the treatment of these tumours is, in general, similar to that of intracranial tumours and has a poor prognosis if management is palliative. There is **very little information about the treatment and prognosis of these tumours** except in the case of feline lymphomas, for which it is somewhat better described, but there is evidence that **multimodal treatment** is necessary, and the more types of therapy used, the better the results obtained.

In the case of vertebral tumours, normally decompression can favour the temporary disappearance of symptoms, but the usual presence of lysis at the time of diagnosis complicates the surgical techniques which can be performed.

The only vertebral tumour with a **better prognosis is the plasma cell tumour**, with survival times of more than 1 year in many cases treated with chemotherapy. For the rest of tumours (OSA, CSA, FSA...) the combination of chemotherapy and surgery is generally unrewarding, with survival times of less than 3–4 months.

Tumours of Cranial, Paraspinal and Peripheral Nerves

Peripheral nerve tumours (known as peripheral nerve sheath tumours [PNST]) are uncommon in dogs and rare in cats. PNST are divided into benign and malignant, based on microscopic features. The majority of PNST in dogs are malignant, and the benign type are more common in cats compared with dogs.

They represent **27% of all canine nervous system neoplasms**, with a mean age of presentation of 8.7 years old (3–13). The most common location is between C6–T2 and they can affect cranial nerve V (±III).

These tumours arise in any cranial nerve, spinal nerve root, or somatic or autonomic peripheral nerve.

The metastatic potential is considered low. However, some other secondary tumours can involve the peripheral nerves.

The clinical symptoms are related to the tumour location. PNST in dogs more commonly involve the nerve roots or the nerves of the brachial and lumbar plexi, hence, it is relatively common that the main presenting complaint is chronic lameness. However, if the PNST affects another nerve, the clinical signs will be related to that location; PNST of the trigeminal nerve causes masticatory problems (unilateral), Horner's syndrome, etc.

Diagnosis

A **palpable mass is seen in 30% of cases affecting the brachial plexus. Electromyography (EMG) is abnormal in 100% of cases**. EMG is useful to locate and characterise these tumours, and even to predict whether there is invasion of the medullary canal.

Ultrasound is more sensitive than palpation for mass detection, however, MRI is the ideal diagnostic technique for use in these cases. Using **MRI**, a diffuse nodule is usually appreciated instead of a thickening or mass, and they are usually T2 hyperintense/T1 isointense. Performing **cytology** using FNA will not provide a definitive diagnosis, but it can confirm the presence of a neoplasm. On **CT**, 83% of the masses acquire contrast with 54% presenting a ring sign. Masses as small as 1 cm can be seen, and detection of possible invasion of the thorax is made easier.

Treatment

Surgery is still the preferred treatment for dogs and cats, as long as the tumour is resectable with margins. Treatment continues to focus on local control of the lesion and **surgical resection, with both chemotherapy and radiotherapy have been used**. The success of treatment depends on the location of the lesion, as well as histopathology. Peripheral tumours have a better prognosis with surgical resection compared to plexus tumours, which have a disease-free time of about 7.5 months, with an average survival time of 12 months. Nerve root tumours have a disease-free time of 1 month (0–14) and an average survival time of 5 months.

The response to stereotactic radiosurgery treatment of intracranial peripheral nerve sheath tumours was evaluated. The mean survival time was prolonged (745 days), and patients tolerated treatment well, as there were no signs of obvious acute adverse effects. Although evidence of delayed adverse effects or tumour progression was not available because few animals were examined postmortem.

Radiotherapy for the treatment of PNST has been reported to be more effective than surgery for the treatment of dogs that presented nerve root and vertebral canal invasion.

Trigeminal PNST can be treated with surgery or radiation, although some untreated dogs can live over one year without treatment. Radiation seems to be superior to palliative and surgical treatment, also resolving the neurological signs.

Bibliography

- Adamo, P.F., Cantile, C., Steinberg, H. (2003) Evaluation of progesterone and estrogen receptor expression in 15 meningiomas of dogs and cats. *Am J Vet Res*, 64(10), pp. 1310–1318.
- Adamo, P.F., Forrest, L.F., Dubielzig, R. (2004) Canine and feline meningiomas: diagnosis, treatment, and prognosis. *Compend Contin Educ Pract Vet*, 27, pp. 951–966.
- Axlund, T.W., McGlasson, M.L., Smith, A.N. (2002) Surgery alone or in combination with radiation therapy for treatment of intracranial meningiomas in dogs: 31 cases (1989–2002). *JAVMA*, 221(11), pp. 1597–1600.
- Bagley, R.S., Gavin, P.R., Moore, M.P. et al. (1999) Clinical signs associated with brain tumours in dogs: 97 cases (1992–1997). *JAVMA*, 215(6), pp. 818–819.
- Bagley, R.S. (2010) Spinal neoplasms in small animals. *Vet Clin North Am Small Anim Pract*, 40(5), pp. 915–27.
- Bailey, C.S., Higgins, R.J. (1986) Characteristics of cisternal cerebrospinal fluid associated with primary brain tumours in the dog: a retrospective study. *JAVMA*, 188(4), pp. 414–417.
- Benjamin, D. et al. (2011) Magnetic resonance imaging features of intracranial astrocytomas and oligodendrogliomas in dogs. *Veterinary Radiology & Ultrasound*, Vol. 52, No. 2, pp 132–141.
- Bentley, R.T. (2015) Magnetic resonance imaging diagnosis of brain tumours in dogs. *Vet J*, 205(2), pp. 204–16.
- Berg, J.M. (2004) Canine meningiomas, other approaches: hydroxyurea and ultrasonic aspiration. Proc 23rd *ACVIM*.
- Besalti, O., Caliskan, M., Can, P. et al. (2016) Imaging and surgical outcomes of spinal tumours in 18 dogs and one cat. *J Vet Sci*, 17(2), pp. 225–34.
- Bley, C.R., Sumova, A., Roos, M. et al. (2005) Irradiation of brain tumours in dogs with neurologic disease. *J Vet Intern Med*, 19, pp. 849–854.
- Brearley, M.J., Jeffery, N.D., Phillips, S.M. et al. (1999) Hypofractionated radiation therapy of brain masses in dogs: a retrospective analysis of survival of 83 cases (1991–1996). *J Vet Intern Med*, 13, pp. 408–412.
- Brehm, D.M., Vite, C.H., Steinberg, H.S., et al. (1995) A retrospective evaluation of 51 cases of peripheral nerve sheath tumours in the dog. *J Am Anim Hosp Assoc*, 31(4), pp. 349–59.
- Cervera, V., Mai, W., Vite, C.H. et al. (2011) Comparative magnetic resonance imaging findings between gliomas and presumed cerebrovascular accidents in dogs. *Vet Radiol Ultrasound*, 52(1), pp. 33–40.
- Chow, K.E., Tyrrell, D., Long, S.N. (2015) Early postoperative magnetic resonance imaging findings in five dogs with confirmed and suspected brain tumours. *Vet Radiol Ultrasound*, 56(5), pp. 531–9.10.
- Dewey, C.W. (2009) Hydroxyurea and meningiomas. *Veterinary Information Network*. Accessed February 2009 at www.vin.com.
- Dickinson, P.J., Sturges, B.K., Kass, P.H. et al. (2006). Characteristics of cisternal cerebrospinal fluid associated with intracranial meningiomas in dogs: 56 cases (1985–2004). *JAVMA*, 228(4), pp. 564–567.
- Evans, S.M., Dayrell-Hart, B., Powlis, W. et al. (1993) Radiation Therapy of canine brain masses. *J Vet Intern Med*, 7(4), pp. 216–9.
- Forterre, F., Fritsch, G., Kaiser, S. et al. (2006) Surgical approach for tentorial meningiomas in cats: a review of six cases. *J Feline Med Surg*, 8, pp. 227–233.
- Forterre, F., Tomek, A., Konar, M., et al. (2007) Multiple meningiomas: clinical, radiological, surgical, and pathological findings with outcome in four cats. *J Feline Med Surg*, 9(1), pp. 36–43.
- Friedman, W.A., Foote, K.D. (2003) Linear accelerator-based radiosurgery for vestibular schwannoma. *Neurosurg Focus*, 14(5), pp. 1–8.
- Gordon, L.E., Thacher C., Matthiesen D.T. et al. (1994) Results of craniotomy for the treatment of cerebral meningioma in 42 cats. *Vet Surg*, 23(2), pp. 94–100.
- Greco, J.J., Aiken, S.A., Berg, J.M. et al. (2006) Evaluation of intracranial meningioma resection with a surgical aspirator in dogs: 17 cases (1996–2004). *JAVMA*, 229(3), pp. 394–400.
- Hansen, K.S., Zwingenberger, A.L., Théon, A.P. (2016) Treatment of MRI-Diagnosed Trigeminal Peripheral Nerve Sheath Tumors by Stereotactic Radiotherapy in Dogs. *J Vet Intern Med*, 30(4), pp. 1112–20.
- Hu, H., Barker, A., Harcourt-Brown, T. (2015) Systematic Review of Brain Tumor Treatment in Dogs. *J Vet Intern Med*, 29(6), pp. 1456–63.
- John, F., Deeken, Löscher, W. (2007) The Blood-Brain Barrier and Cancer: Transporters, Treatment, and Trojan Horses. *Clin Cancer Res*, 13, pp. 1663
- Jung, D.I., Kim, H.J., Park, C. et al. (2006) Long-term chemotherapy with lomustine of intracranial meningioma occurring in a miniature Schnauzer. *J Vet Med Sci*, 68(4), pp. 383–86.
- Kippenes, H., Gavin, P.R., Bagley, R.S. et al. (1999) Magnetic resonance imaging features of tumours of the spine and spinal cord in dogs. *Vet Radiol Ultrasound*, 40(6), pp. 627–33.
- Koblik, P.D., LeCouteur, R.A., Higgins, R.J. et al. (1999) CT-guided brain biopsy using a modified Pelorus mark III stereotactic system: experience with 50 dogs. *Vet Radiol Ultrasound*, 40(4), pp. 434–40.
- Kollova, A., Lisca, K.R., Novotna, J. et al. (2007) Gamma knife surgery for benign meningioma. *J Neurosurg*, 107(2), pp. 325–36.
- Konstantinidou, A.E., Korkolopoulou, P., Mahera, H. et al. (2003) Hormone receptors in non-malignant meningiomas correlate with apoptosis, cell proliferation and recurrence-free survival. *Histopathology*, 43(3), pp. 280–90.
- Lamb, C.R., David, F.H. (2012) Advanced imaging: use and misuse. *J Feline Med Surg*, 14(7), pp. 483–97
- Lester, N.V., Hopkins, A.L., Bova, F.J. et al. (2001) Radiosurgery using a stereotactic headframe system for irradiation of brain tumours in dogs. *JAVMA*, 219(11), pp. 1562–67.
- Levy, M.S., Kapatkin, A.S., Patnaik, A.K. et al. (1997) Spinal tumours in 37 dogs: Clinical outcome and long-term survival (1987–1994). *J Am Anim Hosp Assoc*, 33(4), pp. 307–312.

■ Louis, D.N., Perry, A., Reifenberger, G. et al. (2016) The 2016 World Health Organization Classification of Tumors of the Central Nervous System: a summary. *Acta Neuropathol*, 131, pp. 803–20.
■ Lu, D., Pocknell, A., Lamb, C.R. et al. (2003) Concurrent benign and malignant multiple meningiomas in a cat: clinical, MRI and pathological findings. *Vet Rec*, 152(25), pp. 780–82.
■ Luttgen, P.J., Braund, K.G., Brawner, W.R. et al. (1980) A retrospective study of twenty-nine spinal tumours in the dg and the cat. *J. Small Anim Pract*, 21(4), pp. 213–26.
■ MacLellan, J.D., Arnold, S.A., Dave, A.C. et al. (2018) Association of magnetic resonance imaging-based preoperative tumor volume with postsurgical survival time in dogs with primary intracranial glioma. *J Am Vet Med Assoc*, 252(1), pp. 98–102.
■ Marioni-Henry, K. Van Winkle, T.J., Smith, S.H. et al. (2008) Tumors affecting the spinal cord of cats: 85 cases (1980–2005). *J Am Vet Med Assoc*, 232(15), pp. 237–43.
■ Marioni-Henry, K. (2010) Feline spinal cord diseases. *Vet Clin North Am Small Anim Pract*, 40(5), pp. 1011–28.
■ Matiasek, L.A., Platt, S.R., Adams, V. et al. (2009) Ki-67 and vascular endothelial growth factor expression in intracranial meningiomas in dogs. *J Vet Intern Med*, 23(1), pp. 146–51
■ McEntee, M., Dewey, C. (2012) Tumors of the nervous system. In: Withrow, S.J., MacEwen, E.G., eds. *Small Animal Clinical Oncology*. Philadelphia: WB Saunders, pp. 583–96.
■ Modha, A., Gutin, P.H. (2005) Diagnosis and treatment of atypical and anaplastic meningiomas: a review. *Neurosurgery*, 57(3), pp. 538–50
■ Parry, A.T., Harris, A., Upjohn, M.M. et al. (2010) Does choice of imaging modality affect outcome in dogs with thoracolumbar spinal conditions? *J Small Anim Pract*, 51(6), pp. 312–7
■ Petersen, S.A., Sturges, B.K., Dickinson, P.J. et al. (2008) Canine intraspinal meningiomas: imaging features, histopathologic classification, and long-term outcome in 34 dogs. *J Vet Intern Med*, 22(4), pp. 946–53.
■ Polizopoulou, Z.S., Koutinas, A.F., Souftas, V.D. et al. (2004) Diagnostics correlation of CT-MRI and histopathology in 10 dogs with brain neoplasms. *J Vet Med* A Physiol Pathol Clin Med, 51(5), pp. 226–31.
■ Schrell, U.M., Rittig, M.G. Anders M, et al. (1997) Hydroxyurea for treatment of unresectable and recurrent meningiomas. I. Inhibition of primary human meningioma cells in culture and in meningioma transplants by induction of the apoptotic pathway. *J Neurosurg*, 86(5):845–852.
■ Schrell, U.M., Rittig, M.G., Anders, M. et al. (1997) Hydroxyurea for treatment of unresectable and recurrent meningiomas. II. Decrease in the size of meningiomas in patients treated with hydroxyurea. *J Neurosurg*, 86(5), pp. 840–44.
■ Schwartz, M., Lamb, C.R., Brodbelt. D.C. et al. (2011) Canine intracranial neoplasia: clinical risk factors for development of epileptic seizures. *J Small Anim Pract*, 52(12), pp. 632–7.
■ Sessums, K., Mariani, C.L. (2007) Analysis of KI-67, matrix metallinoproteinase 2 and cathepsin B in canine intracranial meningiomas. *J Vet Intern Med*, 21(3), pp. 640–641.
■ Snyder, J.M., Shofer, F.S., Van Winkle, T.J. et al. (2006) Canine intracranial primary neoplasia: 173 cases (1986–2003). *J Vet Intern Med*, 12(3), pp. 669–75.
■ Spugnini, E.P., Thrall, D.E., Price, G.S. et al. (2000) Primary irradiation of canine intracranial masses. *Vet Radiol Ultrasound*, 41(4), pp. 377–380.
■ Stadler, K.L., Ruth, J.D., Pancotto, T.E. et al. (2017) Computed Tomography and Magnetic Resonance Imaging Are Equivalent in Mensuration and Similarly Inaccurate in Grade and Type Predictability of Canine Intracranial Gliomas. *Front Vet Sci*, 4, p. 157.
■ Stoica, G., Levine, J., Wolff, J. (2011) Canine Astrocytic Tumors: A Comparative Review. *Veterinary Pathology*, 48(1), pp. 266–275.
■ Sturges, B.K., Dickinson, P.J., Bollen, A.W. et al. (2008) Magnetic resonance imaging and histological classification of intracranial meningiomas in 112 dogs. *J Vet Intern Med*, 22(3), pp. 586–95
■ Theon, A.P., LeCouteur, R.A., Carr, E.A. et al. (2000) Influence of tumor cell proliferation and sex-hormone receptors on effectiveness of radiation therapy for dogs with incompletely resected meningiomas. *JAVMA*, 216(5), pp. 701–7.
■ Tomek, A., Cizinauskas, S., Doher, M. et al. (2006) Intracranial neoplasia in 61 cats: localisation, tumour types and seizure patterns. *J Feline Med Surg*, 8, pp. 243–53.
■ Troxel, M.T., Vite, C.H., Massicotte, C. et al. (2004) Magnetic resonance imaging features of feline intracranial neoplasia: retrospective analysis of 46 cats. *J Vet Intern Med*, 18(2), pp. 176–89.
■ Troxel, M.T., Vite, C.H., Van Winkle, T.J. et al. (2003) Feline intracranial neoplasia: retrospective review of 160 cases (1985–2001). *J Vet Intern Med*, 17(6), pp. 850–59.
■ Yamanaka, R., Saya, H. (2009) Molecularly targeted therapies for glioma. *Ann Neurol*, 66(6), pp. 717–29.
■ Zwingenberger, A.L., Pollard, R.E., Taylor, S.L. et al. (2016) Perfusion and Volume Response of Canine Brain Tumors to Stereotactic Radiosurgery and Radiotherapy. *J Vet Intern Med*, 30(3), pp. 827-835.

Test

1. **Which of the following statements is true regarding meningiomas?**
   a. They are the most common brain tumour in dogs and cats. In general, they are slow growing and, therefore, usually take time to cause neurological signs.
   b. They are the most common tumour in the dog and the second most common in the cat, they grow rapidly and are metastatic.
   c. These tumours are rare in cats and dogs. Cerebral lymphoma is more common than meningioma.
   d. They are benign tumours which are very rare.

2. **Which of the following medications is not used for brain tumours?**
   a. Doxorubicin.
   b. Lomustine.
   c. Hydroxyurea.
   d. Temozolomide.

3. **Which of the following tumours can be detected with simple radiography?**
   a. Noncalcified meningioma.
   b. Astrocytoma.
   c. Multilobular osteochondrosarcoma.
   d. CNS lymphoma.

4. **Regarding central nervous system tumours:**
   a. A CNS tumour should be suspected in any dog over 9 years of age with neurological signs.
   b. MRI is diagnostic for certain brain tumours.
   c. The definitive diagnosis is only obtained by histopathology.
   d. Lomustine, mitoxantrone, and temozolomide are some chemotherapy drugs that cross the blood-brain barrier and are useful for treating CNS tumours.

5. **Primary canine brain tumours are generally considered:**
   a. Biologically malignant, but cytologically benign.
   b. Biologically malignant and cytologically malignant.
   c. Biologically benign and cytologically benign.
   d. Biologically benign, but cytologically malignant.

Answers on Page 220

6. **Regarding the clinical presentation of extradural spinal cord tumours versus intradural-extramedullary:**
   a. Extradural tumours present with a longer duration of clinical signs, whereas intradural-extramedullary tumours have a faster clinical progression.
   b. The clinical signs of extradural tumours worsen with physical exercise, whereas intradural-extramedullary tumours do not.
   c. Extradural tumours are not associated with spinal hyperaesthesia, whereas intradural-extramedullary tumours are painful.
   d. Extradural tumours present with intermittent paresis, whereas intradural-extramedullary tumours present with constant paresis.

7. **Regarding brain tumours, which of the following statements is false?**
   a. Gliomas are more common in brachycephalic breeds and meningiomas in dolichocephalic breeds.
   b. The most common clinical sign are seizures.
   c. In certain cases of cerebral meningioma, the diagnosis can be confirmed by evaluating the obvious signs on MRI.
   d. At the intracranial level, multilobular osteochondrosarcomas and some meningiomas can be identified by plain radiography.

8. **What is the most common metastatic brain tumour in dogs?**
   a. Carcinoma.
   b. Melanoma.
   c. Histiocytic sarcoma.
   d. Haemangiosarcoma.

9. **An 11-year-old Boxer presents with a history of a presumptively diagnosed glioma based on history, symptoms, age, breed, location, and appearance on MRI. The owners are not interested in radiotherapy. What could be a good alternative for this patient?**
   a. Treatment with nonsteroidal anti-inflammatory drugs for their anti-COX2 and anticonvulsant effects to control clinical signs.
   b. Without surgery, it is estimated that this patient will only survive between 2–4 weeks due to the rapid progression of this tumour type.
   c. Temozolomide with or without a combination of Palladia®.
   d. Lomustine and prednisone.

10. **For a dog diagnosed with central nervous system lymphoma:**
    a. Fat-soluble medications should be administered.
    b. CHOP protocol is the gold standard treatment.
    c. The prognosis is guarded, and CNS lymphoma is resistant to chemotherapy drugs; it is only sensitive to radiation.
    d. Administration of drugs that are not expelled by P-glycoprotein.

CLINICAL CASE

Brutus Schneider is an 11-year-old male German Shepherd. He is brought to the practice and the owner comments that he has been "tripping over" for a month, which has progressed to walking in wide circles to the right side and possible loss of vision.

On physical examination, he is bright and alert, walks in circles to the right, and has a greasy eye discharge in both eyes. All other parameters are normal.

Neurological examination

- Mental status is obtunded.
- Posture: tilts the head to the right.
- Normal cranial nerve examination.
- Walks in large circles to the right.
- Normal spinal reflexes in all limbs.
- Postural reactions absent in the left thoracic limb and delayed in the left pelvic limb.
- There is no pain on spinal palpation.

Considering the information provided so far:

1. **What are the main problems and what is the neurolocation of the lesion?**
    a. Right prosencephalon.
    b. Cerebellum.
    c. Left prosencephalon.
    d. Spinal cord.

2. **What complementary diagnostic tests should be recommended and in what order?**
    a. Blood tests, thoracic radiographs, abdominal ultrasound, MRI.
    b. MRI and blood tests.
    c. Blood tests, radiographs of the thorax and cranium, abdominal ultrasound.
    d. Thoracic radiographs, abdominal ultrasound, and MRI.

3. **In the tests carried out, no anomalies were found. An MRI is performed, and the results reveal a broad-based mass between the skull and the temporal brain lobe; the base is wider in the skull area, with a "dural tail sign". Considering the history, breed, location, and results of tests performed, what is the most likely diagnosis?**
    a. Glioma.
    b. Metastasis of a primary tumour outside the CNS.
    c. Meningioma.
    d. Lymphoma.

4. **Considering the diagnosis, what treatment option should be recommended?**
    a. Surgical removal.
    b. Chemotherapy protocol with Madison-Wisconsin (CHOP).
    c. Temozolomide chemotherapy.
    d. Anti-inflammatory and antibiotic treatment.

Correct Answers:

Test

1. a
2. a
3. c
4. c
5. a
6. b
7. c
8. d
9. c
10. a

Clinical Case

1. a
2. a
3. c
4. a

NOTES

Fundamentals of Radiation Oncology: Principles and Practices

Mónica Clemente

The History of Radiation

Radiotherapy has been used in veterinary medicine since the discovery of X-rays by Roentgen in 1895. **The first data on the use of radiotherapy by veterinarians to treat animal pathologies dates back to 1906**. Richard Eberlein, physician, and veterinarian, published on the subject and he is considered the father of veterinary radiotherapy. Years later, in 1927, the Roentgen Foundation was created through a collaboration between the University of Veterinary Medicine in Vienna and the Rockefeller Foundation. Alois Pommer (an Austrian veterinarian) was director of this institution and published extensively in Europe regarding the effects of radiotherapy in animals.

Through collaborations with the University of Pennsylvania, one of Pommer's alumni, MA Emmerson, became the first radiotherapy veterinarian in the United States and founded the Radiotherapy Service at the university.

During this time, radiotherapy was used to treat chronic skin infections and inflammatory processes and its use was less complex than today. However, Alois Pommel had already published results for treatment of sarcomas and carcinomas. During those early years, animals were restrained using immobilisation devices, but over time anaesthesia was used to immobilise them.

In the early days of radiotherapy, low-energy or orthovoltage X-rays (few thousand volts) were used, which had minimal tissue penetration capacity. Later the Cobalt 60 bomb was incorporated, whose gamma (γ) ray radiation (with an energy of 1.6 MeV) penetrates deeper.

In the 50s, linear electron accelerators (LINAC) emerged that produce both high-energy X-rays and allowed the power to be adjusted from 1.5 to 25 MeV, as well as electrons which served to treat superficial tumours. The protocols have been optimised over the years and the use of linear accelerators began in 1960 at the University of Cambridge.

Throughout these years, radiotherapy in veterinary medicine and medicine has evolved with scientific advances in physics, oncology, and computing, improving both the equipment and the precision, quality, and specifics of treatments. This has led to the use of new radiotherapy modalities:

- **DCRT**: three-dimensional radiation therapy
- **IMRT**: intensity-modulated radiation therapy
- **IGRT**: image-guided radiation therapy
- **VMAT**: volumetric modulated arc therapy.

Radiation in Medicine

It is estimated that more than 50% of cancer patients in human medicine will require radiotherapy treatment for tumour control or as palliative therapy at some point in the evolution of tumours of the head and neck, prostate, breast, brain, lung, bladder, or thyroid.

Other uses of radiation therapy are:

- bone marrow ablation
- lymphoma treatment.

Radiotherapy is often used in combination with surgery and chemotherapy and is one of the three pillars of cancer treatment.

Radiation in Veterinary Medicine

Today, radiation has become an **indispensable type of therapy for the adequate treatment of many tumours**, such as nasal tumours. In addition, as mentioned, it is essential in the use of multimodal therapy combined with surgery, chemotherapy, etc.

Fortunately, today there is a wider availability and greater knowledge in veterinary medicine, in general. Additionally, there are Board Certified Veterinary Radiation Oncologists and the radiation centres are more accessible; moreover, the cost is more affordable.

At present, animals subjected to radiation receive safe, quick anaesthesia, with short duration drugs, so that the entire treatment process generally takes less than half an hour (daily treatment 5–10 minutes).

Finally, there is now a better understanding of tumour biology and tumour radiosensitivity, which helps to plan more effective treatment plans.

Biological Basis

Radiation therapy is a type of cancer treatment that **uses ionising radiation to kill tumour cells in the part of the body where it is applied** (local treatment). Radiotherapy works on the tumour, destroying the malignant cells and preventing them from growing and reproducing. This action can also be exerted on normal tissues, however, tumour tissues are generally more sensitive to radiation and cannot repair the damage produced as efficiently as normal tissue can, hence they are destroyed, blocking the cell cycle.

What is Radiation?

All matter is made up of atoms that, in turn, are made up of a nucleus of protons and neutrons and have a cloud of electrons around them (Figure 1).

Radiation interacts with biological matter, mobilising orbiting electrons, which produces "ionisation."

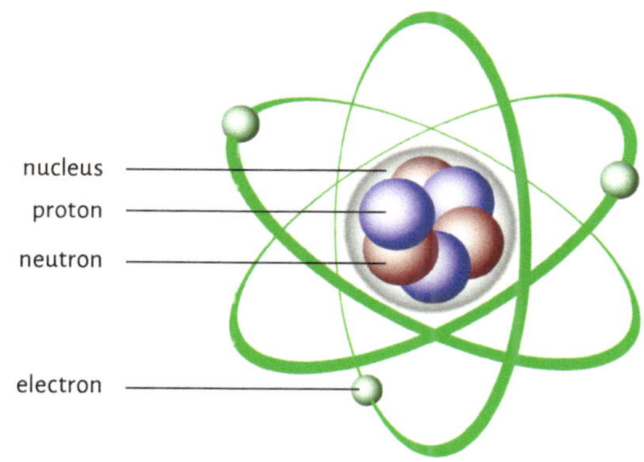

Figure 1. Diagram of an atom with the nucleus composed of protons (blue) and neutrons (red) and the orbits surrounding the nucleus that contain electrons (green).

What is a Photon?

X and γ-rays are part of the continuous spectrum of electromagnetic radiation (EM), of which radio waves, heat, visible light and ultraviolet are also part (Figure 2).

All types of EM radiation are packets of energy called photons. The amount of energy in each photon defines its position in the electromagnetic spectrum (for example, photons in X-rays carry more energy than photons in visible light).

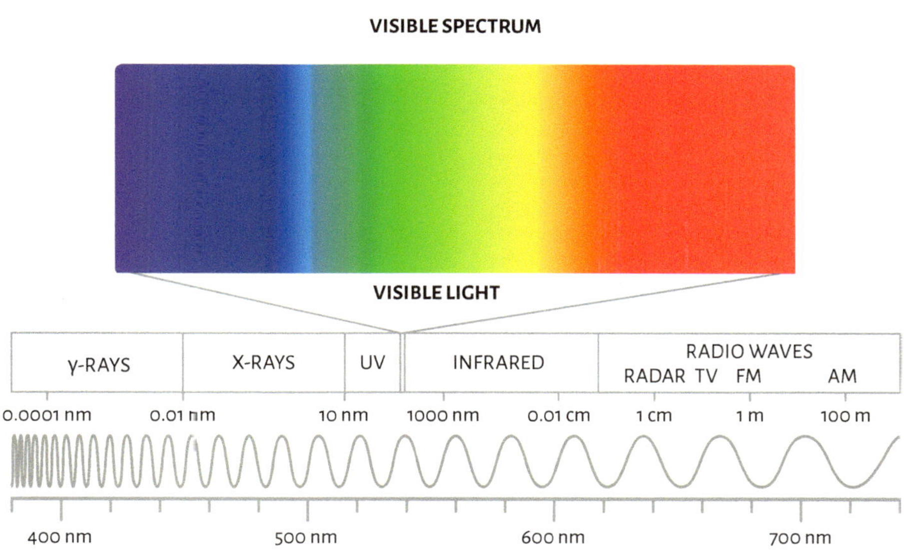

Figure 2. Diagrammatic representation of the electromagnetic spectrum (energy distribution of electromagnetic waves). The electromagnetic spectrum ranges from short length radiation waves such as γ and X-rays, through ultraviolet radiation, visible light, and infrared radiation to long length electromagnetic waves, such as radio waves.

Ionising Radiation

Types

Electromagnetic (photons):

- **X-rays** (man-made)
- **γ-rays** (radioactive emission ^{60}Co).

Particles:

- **electrons**
- **protons**
- **α particles**
- **neutrons**.

X-rays are produced when an accelerated electron collides with a tungsten target and then decelerates, producing a spectrum of radiation. Filtering this radiation is necessary to avoid its scattering if it is to be used clinically (Figure 3).

γ-rays are produced as a radioactive emission from radioactive isotopes (^{60}Co) (Figure 4).

How Does It Work?

Photons

The process of cell death due to X or γ rays begins with the **appearance of ionisation in the tissues**: the radiation photons have enough energy to interact with the atoms of the tissues, producing the ejection of an electron from its orbit and leaving the positively charged atom.

When photons from X-rays interact with tissue, three processes take place:

- photoelectric effect
- Compton effect (the most important)
- pair production.

Compton Effect

The Compton effect is the **most important tissue energy deposition mechanism**. It transmits energy with an effect like a "billiard ball": the photon collides with an electron in the outer orbit of an atom and passes part of its energy to it, so that the photon is deflected and the electron escapes from the orbit leaving the atom with a positive charge (Figure 5). The deflected photon can continue to cause this effect on more atoms. The electron, which has a certain range in tissue, can damage DNA so that cells cannot divide.

The electron can cause direct chemical damage to DNA molecules, but most of the damage is produced by high-energy free radicals originating in the proximity of DNA molecules by the interaction of the electron with water, a very abundant intracellular compound.

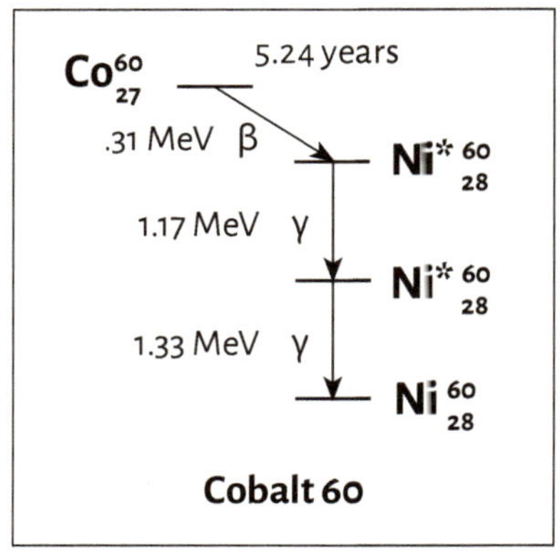

Figure 4. Generation of γ-rays from radioactive cobalt isotopes.

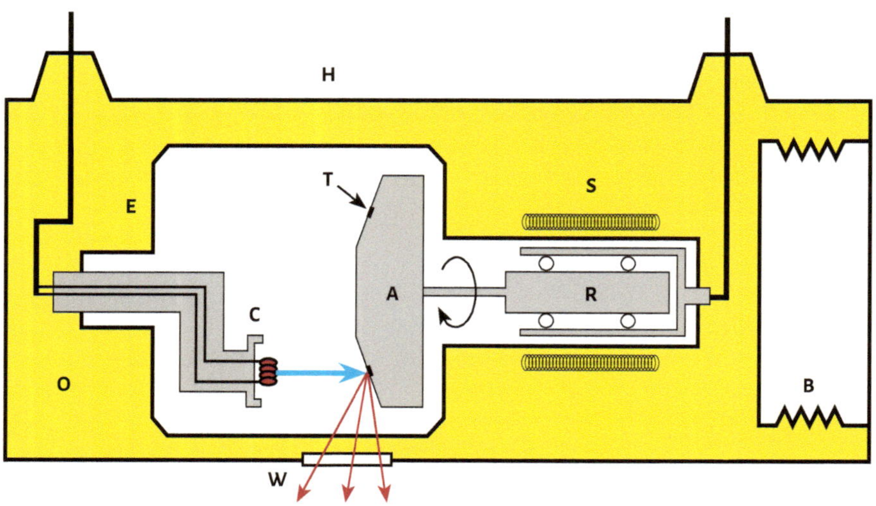

Figure 3. Diagram of an X-ray machine and how it works. A: anode, B: expansion bellows (provides space for cooling oil to expand), C: cathode and heating coil, E: tube envelope, H: tube housing, O: dielectric cooling oil, R: rotor, S: induction stator, T: anode electron target, W: tube window made of aluminium or beryllium, blue arrow: electron beam, red arrows: X-rays. (ChumpusRex - CC BY-SA 3.0).

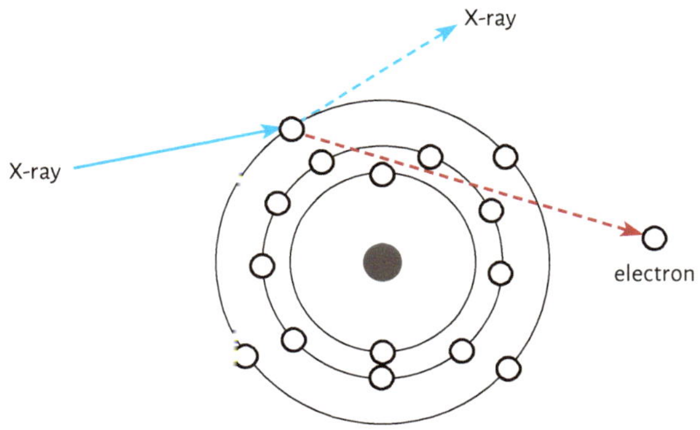

Figure 5. Diagram illustrating the Compton effect. An X-ray hitting an electron in the outer orbit of the atom can be seen, causing deviation of the electron and at the same time redirection of the X-ray.

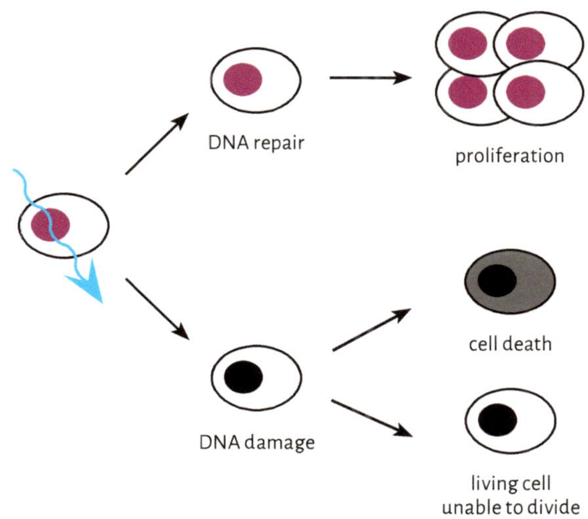

Figure 6. Diagram showing the effect of ionising radiation on a cell. Top part: the cell can repair the damage caused and continue to proliferate. Bottom part: the DNA is damaged by the ionising radiation and can cause cell death (upper) or a cell which enters a quiescent state where it does not die but is unable to divide (lower).

Particles-Electrons

Electrons are different from photons: they scatter, so the beam must be collimated to the surface of the body. In addition, they have some mass, so the **possibility of interaction with atoms is greater than that of photons**. They are used for **superficial treatment** since they are characterised by a rapid decrease in energy with depth. Their use is ideal to avoid critical deeper important organs/structures.

Effect of Ionising Radiation

Photons and electrons can cause **direct damage to cellular DNA**, which is the target for ionising radiation. In general, it must be taken into consideration that ionising radiation:

- may or may not interact with a particular cell
- this interaction may or may not cause damage
- the cell may or may not be able to repair this damage (Figure 6).

Direct Effect

The electron interacts directly with DNA. This circumstance corresponds to 30% of the damage that ionising radiation causes.

Indirect Effect

The electron creates free radicals from water molecules near the DNA and these interact with the DNA, causing 60% of the cell damage (Figure 7).

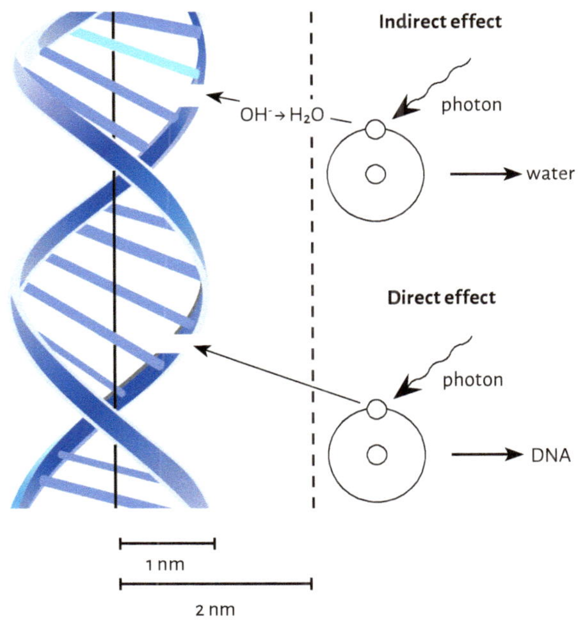

Figure 7. Diagram showing the direct and indirect effect of the electrons accelerated towards cellular DNA. The photons collide with the electrons in the outer layer of the nucleus and the accelerated electrons produce two types of effect: indirect (above), where the electron forms OH^- free radicals which interact with DNA (the electron does not cause the damage itself); and direct (below), where the electron causes direct damage to DNA.

Types of Radiotherapy

Depending on the Distance from the Source

Depending on the distance to the radiation source, two types of treatments can be distinguished.

Brachytherapy

Interstitial (radioactive needles and various tissue implants):

- iridium 192
- radium 226
- caesium 137
- others.

Surface (**plesiotherapy**), with strontium 90:

- indicated only for superficial lesions (incipient squamous cell carcinomas – SCC – or benign mast cell tumours in cats, superficial ocular tumours such as SCC or melanoma);
- high doses are administered: 100–150 Gy per point, 80 Gy for the cornea;
- patients are not radioactive after treatment; and
- protects normal tissue because it has minimal penetration.

Intracavitary (**radioactive suspensions that are infused into body cavities**). Patients will be radioactive for a variable time, depending on the type used.

Systemic radiation therapy consists of the **oral or intravenous administration of the radioactive compound with the aim of reaching the target organ** (radioactive iodine in thyroid diseases, for example). The patient will remain radioactive for a variable time after administration.

Teletherapy or External Radiotherapy

The irradiation source is at a certain distance from the patient in large equipment, such as the **cobalt unit**, the **linear accelerator and the Stereotactic Body Radiation Therapy** (**SBRT**). In this type of treatment, which is **the most common**, patients are anaesthetised daily (Figure 8). Radiation can be γ-rays, X-rays, electrons, or protons.

Conventional external radiotherapy is **three-dimensional radiation therapy** (**3D RT**). Radiosurgery, stereotactic radiation therapy, intensity-modulated radiation therapy (IMRT) and total body irradiation (TBI) also belong to this type of radiation therapy.

Depending on the Time Sequence

Depending on the time sequence with respect to other cancer treatments, radiotherapy can be:

- **exclusive radiotherapy**. The only type of cancer treatment the patient receives is radiation therapy. An example is the treatment of early prostate cancer in human medicine;
- **adjuvant radiotherapy**, as an adjunct to another type of treatment, surgery. It can be neoadjuvant if it is performed before surgery, but it is usually used mainly after (postoperative) (Box 1); or
- **concomitant, concurrent, or synchronous radiotherapy**, which is performed simultaneously with another treatment, generally chemotherapy, mutually enhancing each other.

Depending on the Purpose of Radiotherapy

Depending on its purpose, radiation therapy can be:

- **radical or curative**. This type uses high radiation doses, close to the limit of tolerance of normal tissues, to eliminate the tumour. This type of treatment is usually long and laborious planning is needed to avoid the possible toxicity caused in normal tissues; or
- **palliative**. In this type, lower radiation doses are used; the goal is to improve the symptoms of the cancer patient,

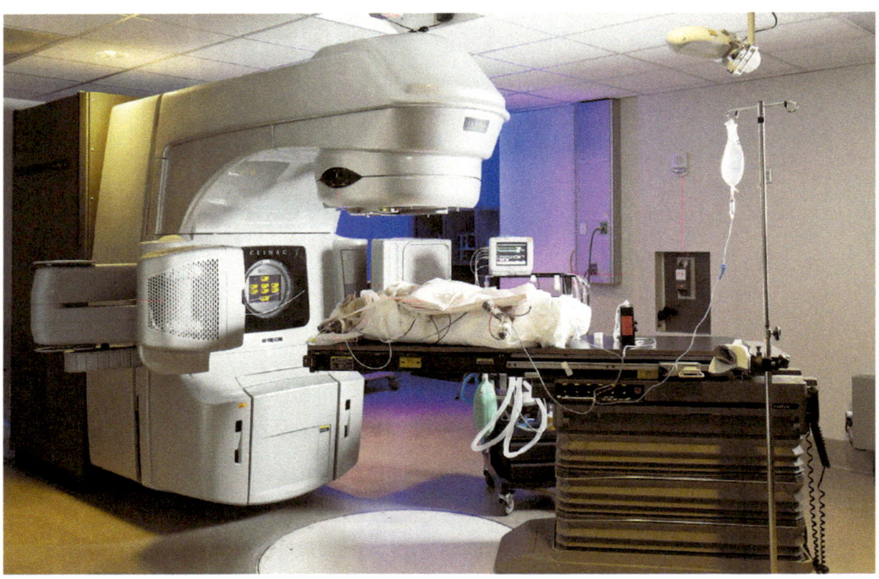

Figure 8. Example of a source of external radiotherapy or teletherapy where the patient is at a distance from the source of the radiation.

with simple planning and short treatment duration, as well as few side effects. Generally, the goal is to eliminate the pain.

Objectives

Radiotherapy aims to
- deliver an amount of radiation to a given tumour volume with minimal damage to surrounding normal tissues, **resulting in tumour eradication**; and
- exploit the difference in response to biological damage between tumour and normal tissue:
  - maximise tumour control
  - minimise the effect on normal tissue.

In general, the primary goal of radiotherapy is to obtain long-term local or locoregional control of a tumour. However, on other occasions it is used in the short term to alleviate clinical signs in cases where the disease is advanced and the prognosis is poor (alleviate pain, for example in OSA or metastatic bone lesions, full body radiation for lymphoma treatment and the treatment of non-neoplastic problems such as arthritis ...).

Use of Radiotherapy (RT) in Veterinary Medicine

Almost any tumour can be irradiated (Box 2). An individualised treatment plan is made for each patient in which the following should be considered:
- **patient situation**
- **owner expectations**
- **treatment objective** (tumour control against adverse effects).

Dose and Fractionation

The response to radiation depends on the **total administered/absorbed dose**. The radiation dose is **measured in grays (Gy)**. One Gy equals 1 Joule absorbed per kg of tissue. As mentioned previously, there is a direct and indirect effect by which cell damage that radiation induces occurs and **cytotoxicity is directly related to the radiation dose**; higher doses of radiation will cause more cell death. (Figure 9). In addition, the percentage of tumours controlled is higher the higher the dose. So why not eradicate all tumours? The answer lies in the **tolerance levels of normal tissues**. Is it possible to avoid irradiating normal tissues?
- Normal tissues are irradiated through necessity: RT must pass through healthy tissues before reaching or after passing through the tumour.
- Margins of normal tissues purposely irradiated:
  - microscopic disease
  - small variations in the position of the patient.

Box 1. Advantages and disadvantages of pre- or postoperative adjuvant therapy

Preoperative
- Advantages:
  - treatment of a smaller area, with less involvement of normal tissue
  - it can decrease tumour size, facilitating surgery
  - lower risk of metastasis due to sterilisation of surgical margins
  - hypoxia decreases the radiation effect.
- Disadvantages:
  - surgery is delayed until the side effects of radiation are solved
  - it can increase complications after surgery.

Postoperative
- Advantages:
  - surgery removes the tumour immediately (lower risk of metastasis)
  - radiation therapy is highly effective in microscopic disease
  - surgery provides more information about the tumour (histopathology report with margin completion, grade...).
- Disadvantages:
  - a larger area is irradiated
  - the surgical scar may not correspond properly with the base of the tumour
  - waiting until the surgical wound heals to avoid complications is necessary.

Box 2. Considerations prior to radiotherapy treatment in veterinary medicine

When is it appropriate?
- any disease with a solitary presentation
- pre- or postsurgery
- to alleviate pain.

When is it inappropriate?
- systemic involvement (distant metastasis ...), although there may be exceptions where it is recommended (for example, to alleviate pain, etc.)
- unwanted or intolerable side effects.

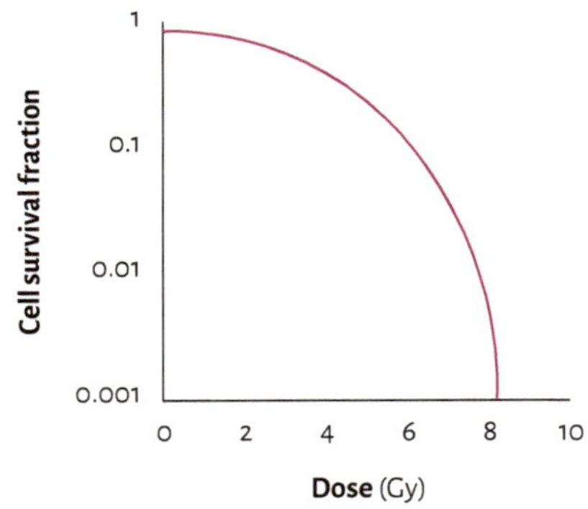

Figure 9. Dose response curve. As the radiation dose increases, the cell survival fraction is reduced.

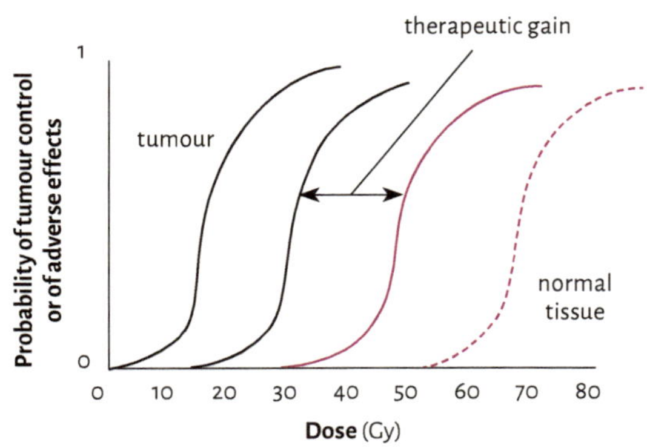

Figure 10. This graph represents the therapeutic index or "gain". The tumour curve is represented in black and that of normal tissue in pink. The greater the dose of radiation, the greater the probability of tumour control and the possibility of causing late onset side effects also increases. The therapeutic gain is the distance between the tumour curve and the normal tissue curve. The greater this distance, the greater the therapeutic gain. Ideally there should be a high therapeutic index, where there is tumour control with few late side effects.

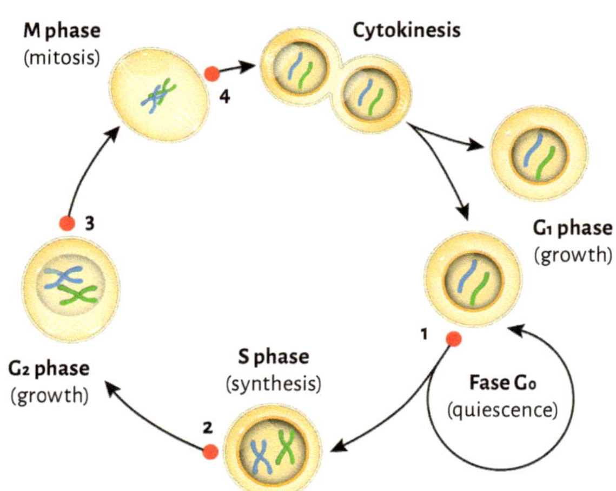

Figure 11. Diagram of the cell cycle.

Here the **concept of the therapeutic index** arises: to what extent does the tumour respond to a certain level of normal tissue damage? (Figure 10). Ideally:

- there should be less than 5% severe complications
- the tumour dose/response curve is to the left of that of normal tissue on the graph.

Variables That Affect the Efficacy of Treatment

Treatment-related factors:

- total dose
- dose per fraction
- time over which the treatment is administered
- type of radiation (photons, electrons, orthovoltage...).

Tumour related factors:

- tumour type
- tumour heterogeneity
- tumour volume (microscopic or macroscopic)
- tumour location (spinal, nasal plane ...)
- tumour hypoxia.

The total radiation dose is divided into multiple treatments, and each of these treatments is called fraction. **Fractionation** allows the administration of a larger total dose, while minimising damage to healthy tissues. The fractionation of the total dose is based on four biological principles that occur between fraction and fraction and are known as "**the four R's**":

- **repair** of tissue damage
- **redistribution** of cells in the cell cycle
- **repopulation** of the tumour and healthy tissues
- **reoxygenation**.

Repair of DNA Damage

Fractionation allows **healthy cells and tissues to repair themselves between fractions**.

Repair occurs in both healthy tissues and in the tumour. Neoplastic cells can also repair in between fractions, but are less efficient at repairing sublethal damage before the next dose.

Redistribution of Cells in the Cell Cycle

Cells are **more sensitive** to radiation when they are in the **G2/M phases of the cell cycle** (the most sensitive phase during mitosis) (Figure 11).

Cells in S phase are radioresistant. The cells that survive after a dose of radiation tend to synchronise in the S phase of the cycle, and then, the cells are redistributed to more sensitive phases before the next fraction is delivered. The redistribution occurs both in healthy tissue and in the tumour.

Tumour Repopulation and Healthy Tissues

Tissue regeneration or recruitment of germ cells (stem cells) **increases the normal tolerance of healthy tissue to radiation therapy**. This repopulation also occurs in the tumour, but will initially be slower for neoplastic cells. Accelerated repopulation in tumour tissue can occur if there are intervals or delays in treatment or it is of very long duration. Therefore, delays in treatment should be avoided.

Reoxygenation

Most of the DNA damage caused by radiation therapy is mediated by **oxygen free radicals** created in oxygenated tissues. Oxygen enhances the effects of radiation therapy by fixing DNA damage causing an irreversible damage that cannot be repaired. Hypoxic cells are 2 to 3 times more radioresistant than cells irradiated in the presence of oxygen. Tumours frequently have both, hypoxic and oxygenated areas. The radiation fraction eliminates the more sensitive, well-oxygenated cell population.

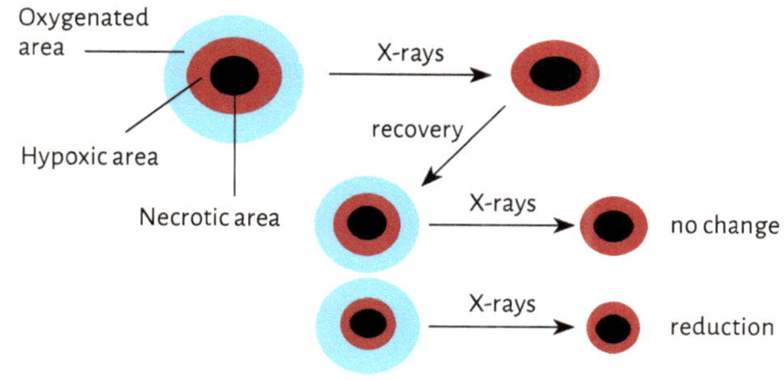

Figure 12. Diagram showing the effect of reoxygenation on irradiated tissue. Blue area: normal oxygenation; red area: hypoxic; black area: necrotic. The oxygenated areas are most sensitive to radiation. With a dose of radiation, the oxygenated area disappears, the hypoxic areas have greater access to oxygen and are converted into an oxygenated area, and, therefore, are more sensitive to radiation.

Tumour Hypoxia

Tumours have abnormal vasculature:

- irregular architecture
- incomplete endothelium
- lack of functional lymphatic vessels.

Some of the hypoxic tumour cells are reoxygenated, in between fractions, because there is more oxygen available, as other cells that were consuming oxygen have been eliminated. Reoxygenation favours greater sensitivity of cells that had previously been in a hypoxic situation to subsequent radiotherapy fractions (Figure 12). Reoxygenation only occurs in tumour tissues since healthy tissues are well oxygenated.

In summary, the total dose and fractionation will largely depend on the type of tumour, tolerance to radiation of the surrounding tissues, and the goal of treatment (definitive or palliative).

Healthy Tissue Reaction and Side Effects

Radiation side effects are classified as early or late:

- **late effects** are seen in tissues with a slower proliferation rate, such as bone, lung, heart, kidney, spinal cord, or connective tissue;
- **early or acute effects** are seen in tissues with a rapid proliferation rate, such as oral and nasal mucosa, gastrointestinal tract, skin, cornea, and conjunctiva.

The **interactions between radiation and tissue**, and the possible side effects, are predictable and expected.

The **severity, duration, and time of appearance of side effects** depend on the type and volume of tissue that is irradiated and the treatment itself (total dose, dose/fraction, treatment plan).

Early or Acute Side Effects

- Appear **days or weeks** after the first RT fraction.
- Are **temporary**.
- **Improve with time**, and the tissues with rapid proliferation rates are affected the most (oral and nasal mucosa, gastrointestinal tract, skin, cornea, and conjunctiva).
- Some of the most common early or acute effects are summarised in Table 1.

Table 1. Most common early or acute side effects of radiotherapy.

Location	Acute effects
Skin	Acute desquamation, alopecia
Oral cavity	Mucositis, halitosis, hypersalivation
Nasal cavity	Mucositis, nasal discharge
Eyes	Blepharitis/blepharospasm, corneal ulcer, conjunctivitis, uveitis
Feet	Nail loss, pad detachment, deformed new nail growth
Neck region	Tracheitis, oesophagitis, pharyngitis
Pelvic region	Cystitis, urethritis, colitis, proctitis
Thoracic region	Pleuritis, pericarditis, pneumonitis

Late Side Effects

- Can develop **months to years after** radiation therapy is completed.
- **Fibrosis and necrosis** are the most common findings in late responding tissues, such as the brain, spinal cord, liver, kidney, and bone; although the risk is low if radiation is well planned, as previously described.
- Late side effects are usually due to the damage caused to vascular support structures or connective tissues, they are **progressive, permanent, and irreversible**.
- The risk of these side effects is **less than 5%**.
- Late side effects (Table 2) are the complication that determines the radiation dose that can be used.

Table 2. Most common late side effects of radiotherapy.

Location	Late effects
Skin	Fibrosis and contraction, non-healing ulcers, leukotrichia, alopecia
Bone	Osteoradionecrosis, secondary tumours, bone sequestration
Limb	Neuropathy, muscular fibrosis, and contraction
Spinal cord	Myelopathy, infarction
Neck region	Hypothyroidism, oesophageal stenosis, tracheitis
Oral cavity	Periodontal disease, xerostomia, bone necrosis
Gastrointestinal tract	Intestinal stenosis/constriction, rarely perforation
Abdominal organs	Fibrosis and reduced functionality
Eyes	Cataracts, keratoconjunctivitis sicca, severe persistent uveitis
Brain	Encephalopathy, fibrosis, oedema, altered mental state

Palliative Radiotherapy

When definitive radiation therapy is not an option, the goal of radiation is to **alleviate clinical signs** associated with the disease, trying to **restore an acceptable quality of life** with minimal risk to the patient. This approach is known as **palliative radiation therapy**. Normally, it does not prolong survival, but it improves the quality of life.

It is usually not recommended for patients that have a life expectancy longer than six months, due to the high possibility of side effects. In this type of radiotherapy, **fewer fractions are used with a higher dose per fraction**. It is recommended when administering a definitive treatment is not an option or in those cases in which there is no longer a possibility of cure (for example, patients with non-resectable/"treatable" metastatic disease), but the primary tumour is producing clinical signs.

One good example of its use is for **pain control** in patients with limb osteosarcoma. In cases in which the patient is not a surgical candidate, or the owners have declined other treatments, pain control can be achieved after two fractions and can last up to two months.

Obstructing tumours of the upper respiratory tract, such as lymphoma of the larynx, have also been successfully treated in cats.

Another type of tumour with a good response to this protocol is oral melanoma, for which, generally, the dose is divided into 3–4 fractions. Up to 80% of tumours respond to this type of treatment.

Frequently used protocols include doses of 5–10 Gy administered in fractions 1–2 times per week. Examples of fractional treatments include four 8 Gy fractions administered once a week, five doses of 4 Gy fractions administered once a day or weekly, one dose of 10 Gy or five 6 Gy fractions once a week.

Many of these tumours, treated with palliative radiation, are large and require a **large radiation field**; administering high-dose fractions to a large volume of tissue increases the risk of late side effects.

Giving a single low-intensity fraction per week will rarely elicit a long-lasting response, as tumour cells will have more time to repair cell damage and proliferate between treatments. Therefore, high doses of radiation are administered to optimise cell destruction, with an increased risk of side effects or long-term toxicities that are accepted as part of treatment.

In many cases, the administration of palliative RT is not intended to prolong the life of the animal, but to improve its quality, so these patients will not live long enough to experience permanent side effects. In addition, a protocol with higher doses per fraction decreases the frequency of anaesthesia, which will benefit dogs with heart or kidney problems, or metastasis.

Definitive Radiotherapy

Definitive treatment with radiotherapy is **frequently used in veterinary medicine**, with multiple applications in cancer patients.

Typically, it involves 12–21 individual doses with a lower radiation dose (for example, 3 Gy fractions) for each treatment, compared to palliative-type radiation therapy, but a higher total dose (for example, 48–63 Gy) than palliative.

The total number of treatments and the total dose administered varies depending on the species, type of tumour, its location and different protocols used in different institutions, as well as other factors.

These type of protocols that use a lower dose per fraction and a higher total dose provide the **best opportunity for good local tumour control, minimising the risk of late side effects**. When designing these types of protocols, it is important to consider the **risks and possible complications** associated with the use of **daily general anaesthesia**. This type of radiation therapy can be used alone or in conjunction with surgery, chemotherapy, or other supportive treatments.

Tumours Located in the Head and Neck

This group of tumours is the **most frequently treated with radiotherapy** due to the difficulty achieving surgical margins in these areas.

Aggressive surgery can imply a loss of function or may not be aesthetically tolerated by the owners. Radiation therapy alone or as an adjunct to less aggressive surgery can provide similar or even better results.

Oral Tumours

Ameloblastoma (acanthomatous epulis) is one of the most sensitive to radiotherapy treatment, which achieves local control close to 90%.

Squamous cell carcinomas can also be treated with radiotherapy, with different results. Local tumour control one year after radiotherapy treatment varies between 34 and 72%. In smaller lesions with a rostral location, better long-term tumour control is usually achieved, unlike larger lesions located more caudally in the oral cavity. **Surgery combined with radiotherapy** increases the chances of achieving a cure for the tumour. Tonsillar squamous cell carcinomas have a poor prognosis because metastases are common and occur rapidly early in the disease.

Oral fibrosarcomas are very difficult to control locally, although they do not usually metastasise. Radiation therapy as the only treatment in this tumour type is rarely curative and is used most frequently after surgery. Even after surgical resection and postoperative radiation, the recurrence rate is high.

Feline oral tumours tend to respond worse to radiation:

- squamous cell carcinoma (SCC) is the most common tumour and is extremely difficult to treat. Most of the results obtained with the different radiotherapy protocols described in the literature have been unsatisfactory; and
- oral fibrosarcomas are the second most frequent tumour in felines, and the results have not been very satisfactory either, mainly due to their size and that surgery is not usually a viable option before radiotherapy.

Nasal and Sinus Tumours

Radiation therapy has been used for many years to treat nasal and sinus tumours, **since surgery as the sole treatment does not offer good results** in most dogs with nasal tumours.

Radiation therapy allows treatment to be administered locally to the tumour, but side effects on the eyes, oral mucosa, and brain are frequent, depending on the location/extent of the tumour and the type of radiation used.

Median nasal tumour survival time after radiation therapy is approximately one year. *A priori*, the best results have been described in cases in which, after receiving radiotherapy, the residual tumour has been surgically removed approximately three months after irradiation. This protocol was associated with serious side effects including rhinitis and bone necrosis, but median survival times were close to four years. In practice, post-radiation surgery is not usually performed. However, second radiation cycles are being applied in cases of disease recurrence, as long as the benefits outweigh the possibility of side effects.

Feline nasal tumours can also be successfully treated with radiotherapy. Nasal lymphoma responds well to radiation therapy in cats. Patients treated with radiotherapy tend to have long survival times (approximately 10–15 months) with manageable and acceptable adverse effects.

Tumours of the Central Nervous System

These tumours can also be treated with radiation, **which is especially advantageous in cases where surgery is not a possibility**.

The best results are obtained in pituitary adenomas and meningiomas. Pituitary tumours usually have a good response, and the median survival time can range from 1–2 years. Neurological symptoms tend to resolve more frequently than those derived from hormonal disorders.

Cats with pituitary tumours can also be treated with radiotherapy with median survival times of up to two years, but problems due to tumour-associated endocrinopathies take longer to improve. Cases in which meningiomas are treated can have long survival times, of between five and sixteen months.

Responses are more difficult to predict in intra-axial tumours. This is partially because the tumour type is often unknown unless a biopsy is obtained.

In summary, if all **brain tumours are included, the average survival time is around two years**.

Cutaneous or Subcutaneous Mast Cell Tumours

Radiation therapy may be considered as the **main treatment for these tumours** (**less frequently**) or as an **adjunct to incomplete surgical resection** (**more frequently**). Resection is considered to be incomplete when malignant cells extend from the margins of the specimen referred for histopathology.

In anatomical locations where it is anticipated that surgery will not allow a complete resection (for example the extremities, muzzle, perineal area ...), radiotherapy is a valid option.

In cases of low-grade mast cell tumours in which minimal tumour volume needs to be treated (microscopic disease or incomplete margins), local tumour control at one year is approximately 90%. Radiotherapy allows a large area around the tumour to be treated, as well as the locoregional lymph node.

Soft-tissue Sarcomas

Soft-tissue sarcomas are infiltrative tumours and are locally invasive. Several tumours (haemangiopericytoma, fibrosarcomas, nerve sheath tumours, etc.) are grouped into the category of soft-tissue sarcomas, since they present the same biological behaviour: they are **locally aggressive** and show **low to moderate metastatic potential**, unless the histological grade is high. Even with wide margins of healthy tissue around the tumour, complete surgical resection is not obtained in all cases.

Although radiotherapy with curative intent is used in the treatment of soft-tissue sarcomas, it is almost always used in combination with surgery. Surgical resection of the tumour followed by radiation therapy achieves local tumour control of up to 80–90%. Hypoxia, slow cell growth, and the relative insensitivity of sarcoma cells to radiation make it more difficult to treat large-volume tumours.

Soft-tissue Sarcomas in Cats

The treatment of soft-tissue sarcomas in **feline patients** is more complicated than in canine patients. Most of these tumours are associated with injection sites and their behaviour is usually extremely locally aggressive, with a relatively low (20%) metastatic potential.

The most important factor when treating these tumours is **achieving tumour-free margins** with the surgical resection: the ideal surgical margins are two deep tissue planes and 5 cm of healthy tissue around the tumour; which is extremely difficult to achieve in all cats.

Using radiotherapy in partially excised tumours or with macroscopic disease is not usually beneficial for the animal, although cats with surgical margins smaller than 5 cm followed by radiotherapy treatment can have good survival times and it may even be curative.

Thyroid Carcinomas

The treatment of choice for non-invasive/non metastatic thyroid carcinomas is surgical resection; however, for those that are non-resectable because they are invading the surounding tissues, radiation therapy can be the treatment of choice with or without combination with systemic treatment (such as target therapy/chemotherapy).

Local tumour control is achieved at three years in 72% of patients treated with radiation therapy.

If vascular invasion or metastasis is present, radiotherapy is generally not recommended; although the metastases of this tumour can grow slowly and, on some occasions, the performance of a palliative protocol can be evaluated.

Anal Sac Carcinomas

Anal sac carcinomas are one of the exceptions to the rule of not treating tumours with high metastatic potential, since, although tumours invade locoregional lymph nodes located in the abdomen early in the course of the disease, metastases in other locations usually take longer to occur.

The combination of surgical removal of the affected lymph nodes and the primary tumour, followed by radiotherapy to treat these areas, plus or minus chemotherapy, **can achieve survival times greater than one and a half years**.

Oral Melanomas

Radiotherapy plays an important role in the maintenance and treatment of canine and feline oral melanomas. It can be used as primary treatment or as adjunctive therapy to surgery, with a **response rate of 82–94%**. When treating macroscopic disease, there is usually a rapid response and a decrease in tumour volume within several weeks.

The disease-free period varies from 5–8 months, with recurrences of 26% in cases of postsurgical microscopic treatment and 45% in animals treated with macroscopic disease. The median survival time is 5–12 months, but these data vary greatly depending on tumour type (grade), clinical stage, size, radiation protocol used, etc.

Other Internal Tumours

Other internal tumours can be treated. However, special care needs to be taken when the treatment plan is calculated, in order to avoid complications associated with the irradiation of other vital organs/structures. This is usually achieved by using the smallest possible treatment field and ensuring that the tumour is located in the same field at each treatment. Smaller fractional doses are often used to minimise the onset of late side effects, such as bladder or intestinal fibrosis.

Prostate and bladder tumours can respond well to radiotherapy. However, prostate tumours tend to have a high metastatic potential, hence, achieving a good local tumour control is not enough to increase survival. A wide variety of other tumours can be treated with curative radiation therapy (Box 3).

Box 3. Which factors should be taken into account when considering radiotherapy treatment of an internal tumour?

- **Only tumours with little potential for metastasis should be irradiated.**
- **Tumours in which a complete surgical resection is not or has not been possible should be treated.**
- **Radiotherapy should be used only when the tissues around the tumour can tolerate enough radiation to kill tumour cells.**

Radiotherapy as Part of a Multimodal Treatment

Although radiation therapy can be used as the sole treatment, it is **much more effective when used in combination with surgery or chemotherapy**. There are various modalities when considering these treatments.

Radiation and Surgery

This combination is generally used when surgery alone is not adequate for local control of the lesion, because it is difficult to remove cells from the tumour periphery with surgery. Both treatments combined may be more effective than when used alone.

Postoperative Radiotherapy

This is the **most common combination** and attempts to eliminate residual cancer cells and microscopic disease (Figure 13).

Radiation therapy is known to be most effective when there is microscopic disease, because the presence of O_2 in the cells maximises radiation-generated DNA damage. Larger tumours or those in macroscopic disease have hypoxic areas in which the action of RT is impeded.

Preoperative Radiotherapy

This combination is being **studied more and more**. As previously explained, arguments in favour of administering radiation therapy prior to surgery include:

- **smaller field to irradiate**, since after surgery the incision must be included in the field and this can be especially large, as in cases of feline injection site sarcoma;
- inactivation of a large number of **peripheral tumour cells**; and
- **reduction of tumour size**, which makes the surgical approach easier.

Intraoperative Radiotherapy

This modality of radiotherapy has been used to treat **carcinomas of the bladder and prostate**.

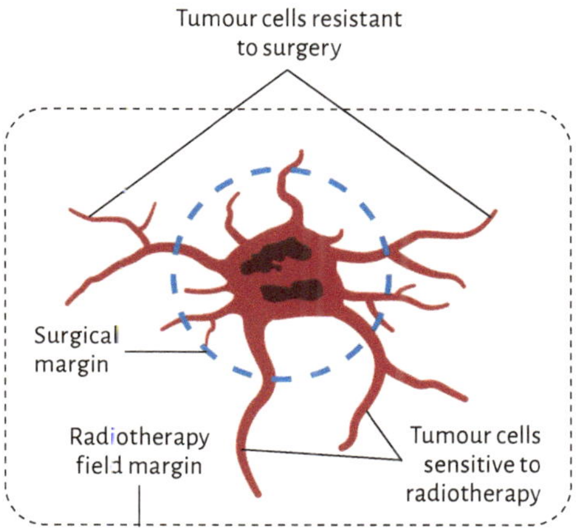

Figure 13. Diagram which shows that a tumour can have microscopic areas which generally remain outside the surgical margin. If only surgery is performed resistant cells can remain outside the surgical margin and radiation can eliminate these cells which remain after incomplete surgery.

In cases of bladder tumours, better results can be obtained when surgery is combined with medical therapies (or medical therapy as the only treatment), so this modality is **not used routinely**.

Radio- and Chemotherapy

Chemotherapy **treats micrometastases** in tumours with metastatic potential and serves as a **radiosensitiser** (it is more than just an additive effect).

Some drugs, such as platinum derivatives, doxorubicin, and gemcitabine are considered radiosensitisers because they can increase the effectiveness when they are administered together.

RT and chemotherapy can be used together to improve local control in chemosensitive tumours. Chemotherapy also serves to sensitise hypoxic cells to radiation. Likewise, it is used in induction protocols for lymphoma.

Bibliography

- Argyle, D.J., Brearley, M.J., Turek, M.M., Roberts. L. (2008) *Decision Making in Small Animal Oncology*, 1st ed. Wiley-Blackwell, pp. 77–92.
- Arthur, J.J., Kleiter, M.M., Thrall, D.E., Pruitt, A.F. (2008) Characterization of normal tissue complications in 51 dogs undergoing definitive pelvic region irradiation. *Vet Radiol Ultrasound*, 49(1), pp. 85–9.
- Adams, W.M., Miller, P.E., Vail, D.M. et al. (1998) An accelerated technique for irradiation of malignant canine nasal and paranasal sinus tumors. *Vet Radiol Ultrasound*, 39, pp. 475–81.
- Adams, W.M., Bjorling, D.E., McAnulty, J.E. et al. (2005) Outcome of accelerated radiotherapy alone or accelerated radiotherapy followed by exenteration of the nasal cavity in dogs with intranasal neoplasia: 53 cases (1990–2002). *J Am Vet Med Assoc*, 227, pp. 936–41.
- Axlund,T.W., McGlasson, M.L., Smith, A.N. (2002) Surgery alone or in combination with radiation therapy for treatment of intracranial meningiomas in dogs: 31 cases (1989–2002). *J Am Vet Med Assoc*, 221, pp. 1597–600.
- Bacon, N.J., Dernell, W.S., Ehrhart, N. et al. (2007) Evaluation of primary re-excision after recent inadequate resection of soft tissue sarcomas in dogs: 41 cases (1999–2004) *J Am Vet Med Assoc*, 230(4), pp. 548–54.
- Bateman, K.E., Catton, P.A., Pennock, P.W. et al. (1994) 0–7–21 radiation therapy for the treatment of canine oral melanoma. *J Vet Intern Med*, 8, pp. 267–72.
- Bley, C.R., Sumova, A., Roos, M. et al. (2005) Irradiation of brain tumors in dogs with neurologic disease. *J Vet Intern Med*, 19, pp. 849–54.
- Bregazzi, V.S., LaRue, S.M., McNiel, E. et al. (2001) Treatment with a combination of doxorubicin, surgery, and radiation versus surgery and radiation alone for cats with vaccine-associated sarcomas: 25 cases (1995–2000). *J Am Vet Med Assoc*, 218, pp. 547–50.
- Brooks, M.B., Matus, R.E., Leifer, C.E. et al. (1988) Chemotherapy versus chemotherapy plus radiotherapy in the treatment of tonsillar squamous cell carcinoma in the dog. *J Vet Intern Med*, 2, p. 206.
- Cohen, M., Wright, J.C., Brawner, W.R. et al. (2001) Use of surgery and electron beam irradiation, with or without chemotherapy, for treatment of vaccine associated sarcomas in cats: 78 cases (1996–2000). *J Am Vet Med Assoc*, 219, pp. 1582–9.
- Connell, P.P., Martel, M.K., Hellman, S. (2005) Principles of radiation oncology. In: DeVita, V.T. Jr, Hellman, S., Rosenberg, S.A. editors. *Cancer: principles and practice of oncology*, 7 ed. Philadelphia: Lippincott Williams & Wilkins.
- Cronin, K., Page, R.L., Spodnick, G. et al. (1998) Radiation therapy and surgery for fibrosarcoma in 33 cats. *Vet Radiol Ultrasound*, 39, pp. 51–6.
- Dow, S.W., LeCouteur, R.A., Rosychuk R.A.W. et al. (1990) Response of dogs with functional pituitary macroadenomas and macrocarcinomas to radiation. *J Small Anim Pract*, 31, pp. 287– 94.

■ Evans, S.M., Shofer, F. (1988) Canine Oral nontonsillar squamous cell carcinomas: prognositc factors for recuuence and survival following orthovoltage radiation therapy. *Vet Radiol*, 29, pp. 133–37.

■ Evans, S.M., Dayrell-Hart, B., Powlis, W. et al. (1993) Radiation therapy of canine brain masses. *J Vet Intern Med*, 7, pp. 216–9.

■ Fidel, J., Schiller, I., Hauser, B. et al. (2006) Histiocytic Sarcomas in Flat Coated Retrievers: a Summary of 37 Cases (November 1998–March 2005). *Comparative Oncology*, 4, pp. 63–74.

■ Forrest, L.J., Chun, R., Adams, W.M. et al. (2000) Postoperative radiotherapy for canine soft tissue sarcoma. *J Vet Intern Med*, 14, pp. 578–82.

■ Frimberger, A.E., Moore, A.S., LaRue, S.M. et al. (1997) Radiotherapy of incompletely resected, moderately differentiated mast cell tumors in the dog: 37 cases (1989–1993). *J Am Anim Hosp Assoc*, 33, pp. 320–4.

■ Gillette, E.L., McChesney, S.L., Dewhirst, M.W. et al. (1987) Response of canine oral carcinomas to heat and radiation. *Int J Radiat Oncol Biol Phys*, 13, pp. 1861–7.

■ Green, E.M., Adams, W.M., Forrest, L.J. (2002) Four fraction palliative radiotherapy for osteosarcoma in 24 dogs. *J Am Anim Hosp Assoc*, 38, pp. 445–51.

■ Haney, S.M., Beaver, L., Turrel, J. et al. (2009) Survival analysis of 97 cats with nasal lymphoma: a multiinstitutional retrospective study (1986–2006). *J Vet Intern Med*, 23, pp. 287–94.

■ Henry, C.J., Brewer, W.G. Jr., Tyler, J.W. et al. (1998) Survival in dogs with nasal adenocarcinoma: 64 cases (1981–1995). *J Vet Intern Med*, 12, pp. 436–9.

■ Hillers, K.R., Lana, S.E., Fuller, C.R. et al. (2007) Effects of palliative radiation therapy on nonsplenic hemangiosarcoma in dogs. *J Am Anim Hosp Assoc*, 43, pp. 187–92.

■ Jones, P.D., de Lorimier, L.P., Kitchell, B.E. et al. (2003) Gemcitabine as a radiosensitizer for nonresectable feline oral squamous cell carcinoma. *J Am Anim Hosp Assoc*, 39, pp. 463–7.

■ Knapp-Hoch, H.M., Fidel, J.L., Sellon, R.K. et al. (2009) An expedited palliative radiation protocol for lytic or proliferative lesions of appendicular bone in dogs. *J Am Anim Hosp Assoc*, 45, p. 24.

■ LaRue, S.M., Gillette, E.L. (2007) Radiation Therapy. In: Withrow, S.J. and Vail, D.M. (eds). *Small animal Clinical Oncology*, 4 ed. Philadelphia: Elsevier, pp. 193–210.

■ LaDue, T.A., Dodge, R., Page, R.L. et al. (1999) Factors influencing survival after radiotherapy of nasal tumors in 130 dogs. *Vet Radiol Ultrasound*, 40, pp. 312–7.

■ LaDue, T., Price, G.S., Dodge, R. et al. (1998) Radiation therapy for incompletely resected canine mast cell tumors. *Vet Radiol Ultrasound*, 39, pp. 57–62.

■ Mayer, M.N., Greco, D.S., LaRue, S.M. (2006) Outcomes of pituitary tumor irradiation in cats. *J Vet Intern Med*, 20, pp. 1151–4.

■ McEntee, M.C. (2006) Veterinary Radiation Therapy: Review and Current State of the Art. *Journal of the American Animal Hospital Association*, 42, pp. 94–109.

■ McEntee, M.C., Page, R.L. (2001) Feline vaccine-associated sarcomas. *J Vet Intern Med*, 15, pp. 176–82.

■ McKnight, J.A., Mauldin, G.N., McEntee, M.C. et al. (2000) Radiation treatment for incompletely resected softtissue sarcomas in dogs. *J Am Vet Med Assoc*, 217, pp. 205–10.

■ Mueller, F., Poirier, V., Melzer, K. et al. (2005) Palliative radiotherapy with electrons of appendicular osteosarcoma in 54 dogs. *In Vivo*, 19, pp. 713–6.

■ Pack, L., Roberts, R.E., Dawson, S.D. et al. (2001) Definitive radiation therapy for infiltrative thyroid carcinoma in dogs. *Vet Radiol Ultrasound*, 42, pp. 471–4.

■ Postorino-Reeves, N.C. T.J., Withrow, S.J. (1993) Oral squamous cell carcinoma in the cat. *J Am Vet Med Assoc*, 202, pp. 438–441.

■ Proulx, D.R., Ruslander, D.M., Dodge, R.K. et al. (2003) A retrospective analysis of 140 dogs with oral melanoma treated with external beam radiation. *Vet Radiol Ultrasound*, 44, pp. 352–9.

■ Ramirez, O., Dodge, R.K., Page, R.L. et al. (1999) Palliative radiotherapy of appendicular osteosarcoma in 95 dogs. *Vet Radiol Ultrasound*, 40, pp. 517–22.

■ Theon, A.P., Rodriguez, C., Griffey, S. et al. (1997) Analysis of prognostic factors and patterns of failure in dogs with periodontal tumors treated with megavoltage irradiation. *J Am Vet Med Assoc*, 210, pp. 785–8.

■ Theon, A.P., Rodriguez, C., Madewell, B.R. (1997) Analysis of prognostic factors and patterns of failure in dogs with malignant oral tumors treated with megavoltage irradiation. *J Am Vet Med Assoc*, 210, pp. 778–84.

■ Theon, A.P., Madewell, B.R., Harb, M.F. et al. (1993) Megavoltage irradiation of neoplasms of the nasal and paranasal cavities in 77 dogs. *J Am Vet Med Assoc*, 202, pp. 1469–75.

■ Theon, A.P., Peaston, A.E., Madewell, B.R. et al. (1994) Irradiation of nonlymphoproliferative neoplasms of the nasal cavity and paranasal sinuses in 16 cats. *J Am Vet Med Assoc*, 204, pp. 78–83.

■ Theon, A.P., Feldman, E.C. (1998) Megavoltage irradiation of pituitary macrotumors in dogs with neurologic signs. *J Am Vet Med Assoc*, 213, pp. 225–31.

■ Theon, A.P., Marks, S.L., Feldman, E.S. et al. (2000) Prognostic factors and patterns of treatment failure in dogs with unresectable differentiated thyroid carcinomas treated with megavoltage irradiation. *J Am Vet Med Assoc*, 216, pp. 1775–9.

■ Thrall, D.E. (1984) Orthovoltage radiotherapy of acanthomatous epulides in 39 dogs. *J Am Vet Med Assoc*, 184, pp. 826–9.

■ White, R., Walker, M., Legendre, A.M. et al. (1990). Development of brachytherapy technique for nasal tumors in dogs. *Am J Vet Res*, 51(8), pp. 1250–6.

■ Whiteley, M.B., Kestenman, D.B., Feeney, D.A. (1991) A bibliography of veterinary radiotherapy. *Veterinary radiology & ultrasound*, volume 32, issue 1, pp. 35–47.

■ Williams, L.E., Gliatto, J.M., Dodge, R.K. et al. (2003) Carcinoma of the apocrine glands of the anal sac in dogs: 113 cases (1985–1995). *J Am Vet Med Assoc*, 223, pp. 825–31.

Test

Answers on Page 240

1. **When irradiating a nasal tumour with a protocol of curative intent, which of the following early side effects are generally observed?**
   a. Cerebral atrophy and oronasal fistula.
   b. Mucositis and conjunctivitis.
   c. Mucositis and blindness of the eye included in the field of treatment.
   d. Leukotrichia and hair loss.

2. **When administering a curative intent radiation therapy protocol, the following should be considered:**
   a. That late onset side effects should not be greater than 5%.
   b. That late onset side effects should not be greater than 15%.
   c. That early side effects last no more than 3 weeks.
   d. That the early side effects do not continue after the treatment protocol is finished.

3. **Which of the following statements is correct?**
   a. Feline lymphomas respond well to radiotherapy, with long survival times.
   b. Meningiomas are benign tumours that respond completely to radiotherapy.
   c. Radiotherapy is the most effective method of treating non-surgical high-grade mast cell tumours.
   d. The treatment of choice for melanomas is curative radiation therapy, with low doses daily for 3–4 weeks.

4. **Based on the principles of radiation biology, which of the following is most likely to reduce the incidence of late side effects when the colon is irradiated?**
   a. Decreased total radiation dose.
   b. Decreased dose per fraction.
   c. Increased time interval between fractions.
   d. Administration of the same dose in fewer fractions.

5. **Which of the following statements is an advantage of preoperative radiation for the maintenance of skin/subcutis soft-tissue tumours?**
   a. It reduces surgical complications.
   b. It decreases the incidence of late adverse effects due to radiotherapy.
   c. There are a lower number of radio-resistant hypoxic cells in the treatment field.
   d. It decreases the severity of acute adverse effects of radiation.

6. **Which of the following answers is theroretically one of the advantages of intensity modulated radiation therapy (IMRT) over standard external conformational radiation for the treatment of canine nasal tumours?**
   a. There is a smaller volume of tissue exposed to ionising radiation with IMRT.
   b. Acute radiation effects are much less likely with IMRT, but late adverse effects are still possible.
   c. A higher radiation dose can be delivered in planning target volume (PTV) with IMRT.
   d. With IMRT there is a lower risk of incidence of radiation-related secondary neoplasms.

7. **Which of the following factors predicts poor local tumour control and reduced survival in dogs with malignant oral melanoma that are treated with radiation?**
   a. Rostral location of the tumour.
   b. Presence of microscopic disease.
   c. Regional lymph node metastasis.
   d. Radiographic evidence of tumour lysis.

8. **What are the R's of radiation?**
   a. Repopulation, repair, reoxygenation and redistribution.
   b. Reorganisation, repair and reoxygenation.
   c. Repair, reoxygenation and redistribution.
   d. Reorganisation, repair, reoxygenation and redistribution.

9. **In which phase of the cell cycle are tumour cells most radiosensitive?**
   a. S phase.
   b. M phase.
   c. G phase.
   d. M and S phases.

10. **Palliative radiotherapy can be helpful because:**
   a. Due to treatment design, there is little risk of late side effects.
   b. It provides pain control in some patients where surgery is not a therapeutic option.
   c. In this type of radiation, fewer fractions are used with lower doses per fraction.
   d. It is used because it prolongs survival time and quality of life.

Clinical Case

Bella is a 9-year-old neutered female Labrador Retriever. She presents at the practice with a history of left unilateral epistaxis lasting more than 2 months which does not respond to antibiotics or anti-inflammatory drugs.

A CT scan and biopsy are performed, and the histopathology results confirm the presence of a nasal carcinoma (Figure 1).

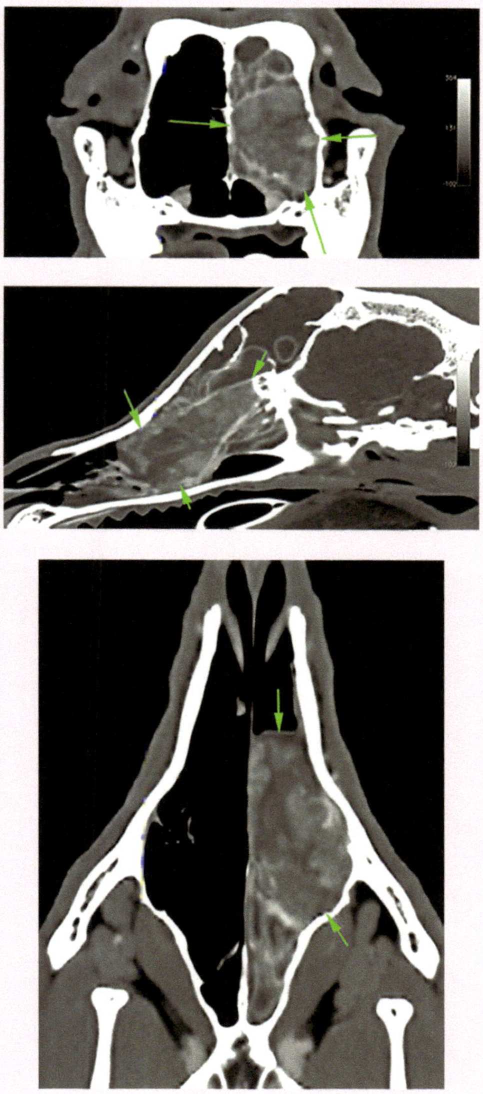

Figure 1. CT images of Bella showing a tumour mass (green arrows). The histopathological study confirmed that it was a nasal carcinoma.

The owners' comment that they have heard that radiotherapy is the best treatment method for nasal tumours.

Questions:

1. **What should be identified on the CT scan to plan the treatment and give a prognosis, taking the clinical stage into account (see table on the following page)?**
   a. There is no evidence of bone invasion, there is no soft tissue involvement but there is involvement of the cribriform plate. Definitive radiation therapy can be given, but the prognosis is worse than without cribriform plate involvement.
   b. There is no evidence of bone invasion, it does not involve the cribriform plate, and there is no soft tissue involvement, which gives it a better prognosis when treated with definitive radiotherapy.
   c. Unilaterally confined lesion, which invades the region of the orbit, which is associated with a worse prognosis.
   d. Unilaterally confined lesion that invades the orbital region, which does not affect prognosis.

2. **What additional complementary tests should be performed before making a decision?**
   a. No further tests are necessary because these tumours have a low metastasis rate.
   b. CT scan of thorax.
   c. Blood tests and thoracic CT because, although the rate of metastasis is low, these tests can help to better determine the prognosis.
   d. Mandibular node aspirate and thoracic radiographs or CT because, although the rate of metastasis is low, they can help to better determine the prognosis.

3. **What would be the ideal type of radiotherapy protocol?**
   a. Radiation therapy with curative intent.
   b. Radiation therapy with palliative intent.
   c. Accelerated protocol to try to shrink the tumour quickly.
   d. Radiation therapy is not indicated in this case.

4. **If the owner cannot afford the chosen protocol or travel, what other radiotherapy options are available?**
   a. Fractionated protocol with curative intent.
   b. Radiation therapy is not indicated in this case due to advanced disease.
   c. Palliative intent protocol with response in 70–80% of cases.
   d. Reductive surgery and curative radiotherapy.

5. What side effects can be expected due to the localisation of the mass for each of the different protocols?

a. Definitive: 65–95% severe acute toxicity in some cases.
b. Palliative: 35% slight acute toxicity.
c. Left eye involvement in a definitive protocol but would not have serious side effects in a palliative protocol.
d. All the answers are correct.

World Health Organisation (WHO) classification system	Théon	Adams	Revised Adams
T: primary tumour · T0: no evidence of primary tumour · T1: tumour confined to one nasal passage with no bone involvement or minimal destruction · T2: bilateral tumour and/or moderate bone destruction · T3: tumour invading surrounding tissues **N: regional lymph nodes (RLN)** · N1: no evidence of RLN involvement · N2: mobile ipsilateral lymph nodes · N3: fixed lymph nodes **M: distant metastasis** · M1: no evidence of distant metastasis · M2: identification of distant metastasis (including lymph nodes)	· Stage 1. Unilateral or bilateral neoplasia confined to the nasal passage without involvement of the frontal sinuses · Stage 2. Bilateral neoplasia which spreads to the frontal sinuses with erosion of the nasal passage bone	· Stage 1. Confined to one nasal passage, paranasal and frontal sinus, no bone involvement beyond turbinates · Stage 2. Bone involvement (beyond turbinates) with no evidence of involvement of orbit, subcutaneous/ submucosal tissue · Stage 3. Involvement of the orbit or presence of a tumour in subcutaneous or submucosal tissue · Stage 4. Involvement of the nasopharynx or cribriform plate with osteolysis	· Stage 1. Confined to one nasal passage, paranasal sinus or frontal sinus, with no bone involvement beyond the turbinates · Stage 2. Any bone involvement (beyond turbinates), but no evidence of orbit/ subcutaneous/submucosal mass · Stage 3. Orbit involved, or nasopharyngeal or subcutaneous or submucosal tumour · Stage 4. Tumour causing lysis of the cribriform plate
CLINICAL RELEVANCE			
Primary tumour stage (T value) is not predictive of the clinical outcome in any study evaluated	Probability of recurrence when radiographic findings are considered: stage 2 tumours are 2.3 times more likely to recur than stage 1 tumours	· Prediction of interval without recurrence and survival based on computed tomography (CT) findings: stage 1 and 2 tumours have a better clinical prognosis compared to stage 3 and 4 tumours · Probable reduction of days without recurrence and survival in dogs in stage 4 in a large cohort · Days without recurrence and survival in a study using palliative radiotherapy (stages 1 and 2 were greater than stages 3 and 4)	Findings based on CT: likely reduction in the days without recurrence and survival in stage 4. There is a greater correlation with clinical outcome than in stage 4 of the original Adams classification. Involvement of the cribriform plate is predictive of a shorter survival time (6.7 months average). Stage 1 has the longest average survival time (23.4 months)

Notes

Correct Answers:

Test

1. b
2. a
3. a
4. b
5. c
6. c
7. d
8. a
9. b
10. b

Clinical Case

1. **What should be identified on the CT scan to plan the treatment and give a prognosis, taking the clinical stage into account?**
   b. There is no evidence of bone invasion, it does not involve the cribriform plate layers, and there is no soft tissue involvement, which gives it a better prognosis when treated with definitive radiotherapy.

2. **What additional complementary tests should be performed before making a decision?**
   d. Mandibular node aspirate and thoracic radiographs or CT because, although the rate of metastasis is low, they can help to better determine the prognosis.

3. **What would be the ideal type of radiotherapy protocol?**
   a. Radiation therapy with curative intent *.

4. **If the owner cannot afford the chosen protocol or travel, what other radiotherapy options are available?**
   c. Palliative intent protocol with response in 70–80% of cases **.

5. **What side effects can be expected due to the localisation of the mass from one protocol and the other?**
   d. All the answers are correct.

Clarifications to answers to questions 3 and 4:

*** With curative radiation therapy (megavoltage >41 Gy):**

- Between 46–90% of cases show reduction in tumour size.
- The median survival time is 8–19.7 months.
- With a protocol of 10 fractions of 4.2 Gy, 68% of patients are alive after one year and 44% after two years.

**** Palliative protocol of 4 fractions of 8 Gy each:**

- 66–80% show a complete response with respect to respiratory symptoms.
- Average response time of 120 days, although most recur.
- Survival of 6–8 months (25% per year).

Notes

Ocular Neoplasms

Carolina Naranjo Freixa

Ocular neoplasms can occur in the eyeball or its adnexa (eyelids, conjunctiva, nictitating membrane, lacrimal glands, and orbit). These neoplasms can be primary or secondary. Primary neoplasms are much more frequent than secondary ones (metastatic or multicentric process).

Neoplasms of the Eyelid

The eyelids are a continuation of the skin and, therefore, can be affected by the same tumours. Tumours with a predisposition for occurrence in the head and neck are those which are most frequently diagnosed on the eyelids: cutaneous histiocytoma, melanocytoma, sebaceous tumours, viral papillomas, trichoblastoma etc. The behaviour of these tumours on the eyelid is like that of other areas of skin.

In dogs, most neoplasms are benign (approximately 3:1 ratio of benign to malignant tumours). Sebaceous adenoma, squamous papilloma, sebaceous adenocarcinoma, melanocytoma, malignant melanoma, histiocytoma, mast cell tumour, and a variety of other tumours are described in order of frequency. Epithelial tumours are also considered more frequent than mesenchymal ones (5:1 ratio). Dogs over ten years old suffer from them most frequently and no sex predisposition is reported. The upper eyelid is affected more frequently than the lower one, although the difference is minimal.

In cats, eyelid neoplasms are relatively rare compared to dogs (prevalence of 1.5–2% of cats presented in a veterinary hospital), although they are malignant more frequently (91% of eyelid tumours). The most frequently described types include, in decreasing order: squamous cell carcinoma (28% of eyelid neoplasms), mast cell tumour (26%), haemangiosarcoma (14%), adenocarcinoma (9%), peripheral nerve sheath tumour (7%), lymphoma (7%), apocrine hydrocystoma (7%), and haemangioma (2%) (Newkirk et al., 2009). Of these, lymphomas, adenocarcinomas, squamous cell carcinomas, and peripheral nerve sheath tumour tend to recur and can result in death or the euthanasia of the cat. In this same study, more tumours were detected in male cats than in females.

In addition, non-neoplastic tumours associated with certain conditions can be observed: eosinophilic granuloma in cats and dogs, granulomas due to *Leishmania* spp. in cats and dogs, pyogranulomas associated with *Staphylococcus* spp. or *Streptococcus* spp. in dogs, cutaneous or systemic histiocytosis in the dog, cutaneous nodular fasciitis in the dog, or mesenchymal hamartomas of the lateral canthus in dogs (Kafarnik et al., 2010).

Melanocytic Tumours of the Skin and Eyelid Margin in the Dog

Melanocytic tumours represent 20% of eyelid tumours in dogs and are mainly comprised of:

- **benign melanocytoma**. Most frequent, between 62 and 87% of melanocytic eyelid tumours; and
- **malignant melanoma**. Between 13 and 38% of melanocytic eyelid tumours.

The distinction between melanocytoma and malignant melanoma is made using mitotic count (three or more mitoses in 10 HPF [high-power fields] indicate a malignant melanoma).

Melanocytic masses are observed in the superficial dermis of the eyelid or the lid margin and are composed of spindle, polygonal or round cells which in most cases contain abundant intracytoplasmic pigment. Neoplastic cell aggregates can be seen in the epidermis and follicular epithelium (junctional activity).

In breeds such as the Vizsla and Dobermann (especially those with a white colour-diluted coat), multifocal melanocytomas are described in the palpebral margin, although this behaviour can also be observed in other breeds (Figure 1). Occasional metastases from malignant melanomas have been reported from the eyelid to the lung and liver (Wang & Kern, 2015).

Mast Cell Tumours of the Eyelid in Cats

Cutaneous mast cell tumours are the second most common skin neoplasm in cats and have a predilection for areas of the head and neck, so they are occasionally seen on the eyelid. In a previous study, mast cell tumours were the **second most frequent tumours on the cat's eyelid**, diagnosed in 26% of reported cases (Newkirk et al., 2009).

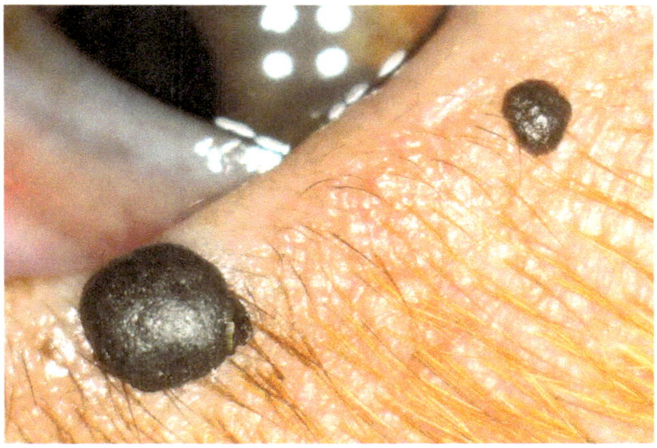

Figure 1. Multiple melanocytomas on the lower eyelid of a Nova Scotia Duck Tolling Retriever. (Image courtesy of Dr Gerlinde Janssens).

As cutaneous mast cell tumours can be multiple in cats, the involvement of the eyelids can be concomitant with other skin masses. In a study of eyelid neoplasms in cats, mast cell tumours occurred in younger cats, compared to the rest of the neoplasms observed (Newkirk et al., 2009).

Regarding their morphology, macroscopically they are raised, sessile, smooth, alopecic, whitish to pinkish masses, which are occasionally ulcerated. The size may vary over time.

Microscopically, they are usually well-differentiated mast cell tumours, although atypical or histiocytic tumours may occur.

In a retrospective study, most of the tumours (96%) that were resected using surgery, some together with adjuvant therapies, did not recur locally, even though in almost 50% of cases local resection was not complete. Only one cat had local recurrence, and another developed additional mast cell tumours in other areas of the skin that did not respond to chemotherapy. No metastases to regional lymph nodes or abdominal viscera were detected (Montgomery et al., 2010).

Apocrine Cystadenomas/Apocrine Hydrocystomas in the Cat

Typical in adult to senior Persian cats, although they can be observed in other breeds, they are multifocal periocular masses that appear pigmented (Figure 2).

They are thought to originate from the apocrine glands of the skin of the eyelid or the eyelid margin (glands of Moll). There is some debate as to whether they are true neoplasms or simply associated with inflammation and cystic retention of secretion. There are studies that show proliferative activity with a proliferation marker (Ki67) which, combined with the absence of significant inflammation around these masses, suggests that they are authentic neoplasms (Cantaloube et al., 2004; Giudice et al., 2009).

Macroscopically, they are raised masses, typically alopecic, smooth, fluctuating, and dark, so the main differential is melanocytic tumours, although these are very rare on cat's eyelids.

Cytological examination is usually not conclusive, although it does show a brownish (basophilic) fluid with few vacuolated macrophages, multinucleated giant cells, and epithelial cells with granular cytoplasm.

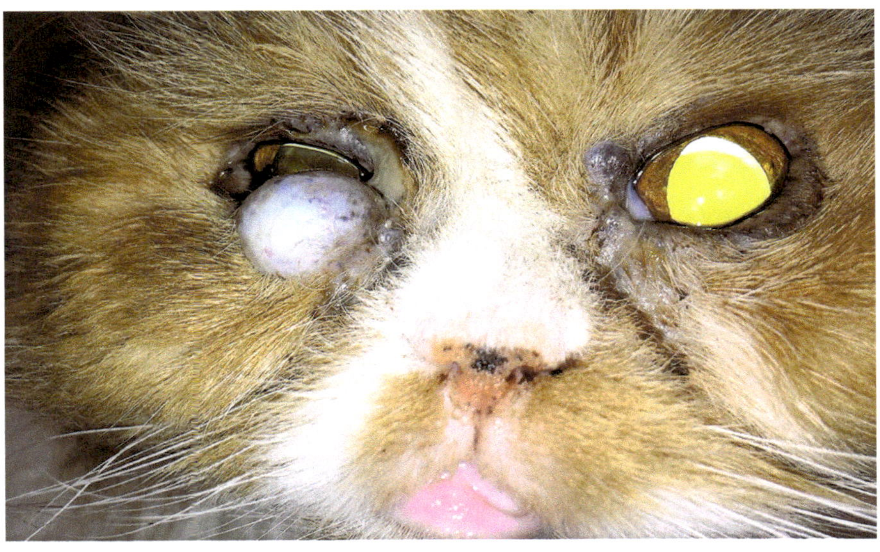

Figure 2. Multiple bilateral apocrine cystadenomas on the eyelids of a Persian cat. (Image courtesy of Dr Gerlinde Janssens).

Histologically, one or more cysts lined with single or double cuboidal epithelium (like the epithelium of apocrine glands) are observed, without excessive cytological atypia, which can form papillary structures, and contain a dense eosinophilic to brownish material in the lumen, with abundant macrophages intermingled and clear vacuoles in the periphery.

These tumours tend to recur locally and, in addition, can occur in other locations on the eyelids of the same eye, or the opposite eye.

Peripheral Nerve Sheath Tumour in the Cat

These tumours are **rare on the eyelids of cats** (7% of eyelid neoplasms in the study by Newkirk et al., 2009), although they may tend to occur on the eyelid rather than in other locations. Adult to senior cats tend to suffer from them, with no documented breed or sex predisposition, and most occur on the upper eyelid (Hoffman et al., 2005; Newkirk et al., 2009).

Macroscopically, they are firm, raised, variably alopecic tumours that can ulcerate. They frequently invade the adjacent conjunctiva.

Microscopically, they are low-grade spindle cell tumours (grade I) organised in two patterns (Figure 3):

- **Antoni A**: spindle cells densely packed so that the nuclei form palisades; or
- **Antoni B**: random distribution of cells, which are loosely arranged within a myxoid stroma.

Immunohistochemically they are positive for vimentin, S100, collagen IV, and laminin, and they are negative for GFAP and smooth muscle actin.

They are locally infiltrative tumours, with **very high local recurrence rates** (up to 100% in the studies by Hoffman et al., 2005, and Newkirk et al., 2009), with an average of three recurrences per cat, therefore resection with wide margins is recommended, which sometimes requires enucleation/exenteration (5/6 cats in the study by Hoffman et al., 2005), but they do not usually metastasise.

Neoplasms of the Eyelid Margins

Meibomian Gland Tumours in the Dog

The **most frequent tumours of the eyelid margin in the dog**. Macroscopically, they are exophytic tumours and frequently papillary, pink, or beige, although some are pigmented (for which the differential diagnosis is established with melanocytic tumours), which protrude from the palpebral margin of the dog. They can ulcerate as well as cause irritation of the ocular surface.

Histologically, they can be classified into

- **meibomian gland adenomas**: most neoplastic cells are well differentiated (sebaceous cells);
- **meibomian gland epitheliomas**: most neoplastic cells

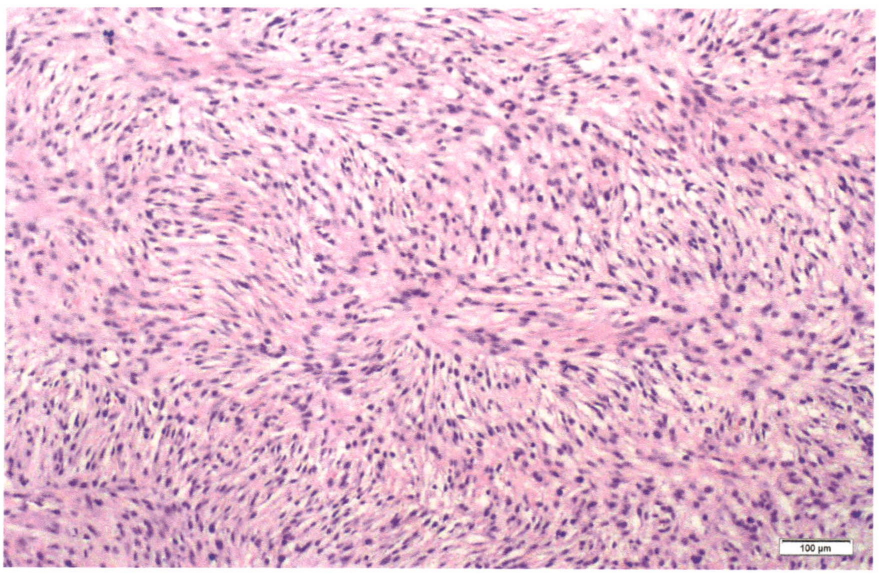

Figure 3. Peripheral nerve sheath tumour on the eyelid of a cat. Area of high cellular density. Haematoxylin/eosin (HE) stain.

are basaloid reserve cells (less differentiated), with a smaller proportion of differentiated sebaceous cells. They are more frequently pigmented than adenomas and tend to extend deeper into the dermis of the eyelid. They usually have a high mitotic index, although atypia and pleomorphism are minimal; and

- **meibomian gland carcinomas**: very rare. In theory, they are more anaplastic, invasive, and atypical than the previous types.

They are usually associated with a lipogranuloma (chalazion), composed of macrophages and multinucleated giant cells with abundant intra- and extracellular lipid material (Figure 4). This inflammation is produced by the foreign body reaction that causes the release of lipids from the sebaceous tumour cells and can occupy a considerable volume of the whole lesion.

The prognosis for this type of tumour is good, since complete local resection is usually curative. Epitheliomas can occasionally recur. Carcinomas are locally invasive, but metastases are rare.

Squamous Cell Carcinoma of the Eyelid Margin in the Cat

Squamous cell carcinoma of the eyelid margin in cats, also called multifocal squamous cell carcinoma, is **considered the most frequent tumour of the eyelid margin and skin of the eyelids in cats**. It usually occurs in white-coated cats, so ultraviolet light is believed to be involved in its pathogenesis.

The lower eyelid is usually affected more frequently than the upper one. In a previous study of eyelid neoplasms in cats, squamous cell carcinomas occurred in cats which were significantly older than those with other eyelid tumours (Newkirk et al., 2009).

Macroscopically, they tend to form poorly defined masses or even diffuse lesions and most commonly appear as ulcerated areas on the skin of the eyelid and eyelid margin.

They normally involve the eyelid margin and extend into the skin. They are considered part of a complex in which dysplastic epithelium with multifocal squamous cell carcinoma is observed, since there may be simultaneous or asynchronous areas of neoplastic transformation in various areas affected by ultraviolet radiation. The conjunctiva shows areas of dysplasia, but not necessarily neoplasia. Examination of the epidermis and follicular epithelium at the tumour margin reveals areas of dysplasia.

In the conjunctiva, primary squamous cell carcinoma (SCC) is less common (usually secondary to eyelid tumours), but it is usually highly invasive and can infiltrate into the eyeball. Ruling out metastatic SCC is necessary since tumours in the lung and middle ear can metastasise to the conjunctival area.

The prognosis is guarded since, although they do not metastasise until the disease is quite advanced (regional lymph nodes and lung), they are highly invasive locally and local recurrence is very frequent and can therefore result in the euthanasia of the cat in a high percentage of cases (78%). In addition, *ex novo* tumours may appear in other areas of the skin and/or conjunctiva due to their actinic/solar origin. Median survival time is approximately seven months after diagnosis.

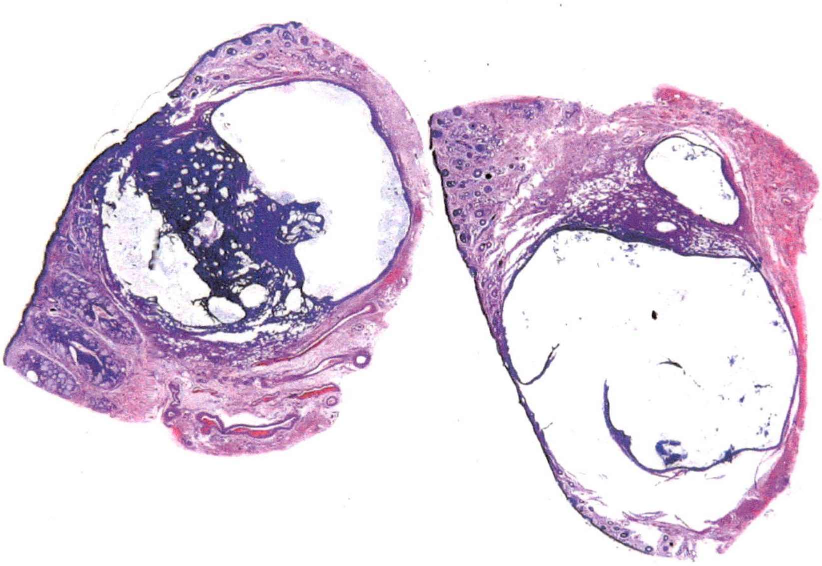

Figure 4. Epithelioma of the meibomian gland with an associated lipogranuloma (chalazion), which is forming a large cavitated area on the eyelid margin of the dog. Submacroscopic image, HE stain.

Squamous Cell Carcinoma in the Dog (Eyelid Margin and Conjunctiva)

Much less frequent than in cats, both in the palpebral margin and in the conjunctiva.

Conjunctival and Nictitating Membrane Neoplasms

A wide variety of tumours are described in the conjunctiva of dogs and cats, including squamous cell carcinomas, melanocytic tumours, haemangiomas and haemangiosarcomas, papillomas, lymphomas, histiocytomas, and transmissible venereal tumour (Komnenou et al., 2015).

Non-tumourous masses can be seen in the conjunctiva, including nodular granulomatous episcleritis (NGE) in the dog, eosinophilic conjunctivitis (also called proliferative) in the cat, sterile conjunctival granulomas or those associated with *Leishmania* spp. (dogs and cats) and *Onchocerca* spp. (dogs), dermoids in dogs and cats, orbital fat prolapse in dogs, and miscellaneous cysts in dogs (epithelial inclusion cysts, dacryops, canaliculops).

Conjunctival Malignant Melanoma and Melanocytoma in the Dog

Most melanocytic tumours in the conjunctiva of the dog are malignant according to histological criteria (81% of malignant melanomas versus 19% of melanocytomas). Most affected dogs have a variably pigmented conjunctiva. These tumours are seen in adult dogs and are common in Retrievers, Rottweilers, and Cocker Spaniels; Weimaraners are believed to be predisposed (Collins et al., 1993).

Macroscopically they are tumours that vary from pink to variably pigmented. They are seen most frequently in the nictitating membrane (61%), the bulbar conjunctiva (22%) and the palpebral conjunctiva (17%).

Histologically, they are differentiated into melanocytomas or malignant melanomas, according to the mitotic count: the cut-off point is established between 3 and 4 mitotic figures in 10 HPF:

- **melanocytoma**: highly pigmented, typically composed of round cells, with a lower proportion of spindle cells. Junctional activity can be observed. Neoplastic or dysplastic melanocytic cell aggregates are not usually seen in the conjunctival epithelium away from the mass;
- **malignant melanoma**: usually more infiltrative and less well defined, they can be multifocal and present variable pigmentation (some are completely amelanotic). Neoplastic cells usually present atypical cytological characteristics: prominent nucleolus, abundant mitosis, and a high N:C ratio. Junctional activity is frequently seen (which can help identify an amelanotic tumour but is not a predictive feature of tumour behaviour). In addition, intraepithelial dysplastic or neoplastic melanocytic cells are seen distant from the primary mass (Figure 5).

Immunohistochemically, these tumours are positive for vimentin, Melan-A, S-100, PNL-2 and other melanocytic markers.

Malignant melanomas usually recur locally (it is estimated that approximately 50% present local recurrence, between three

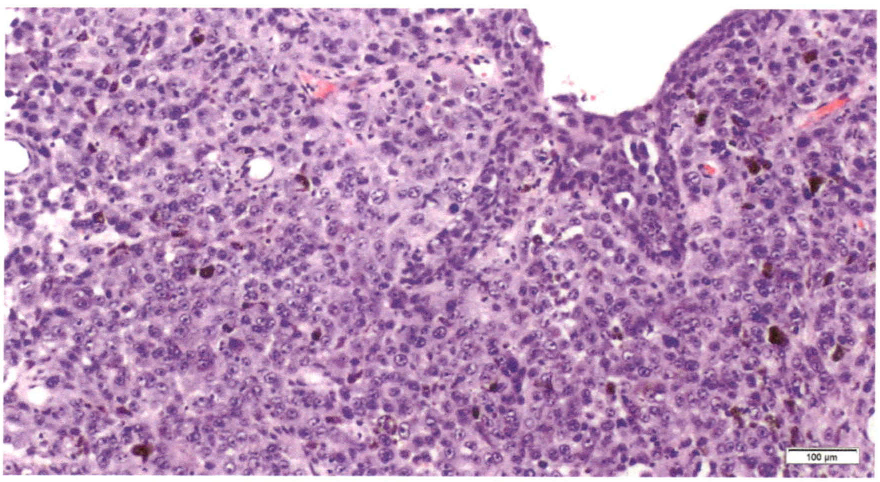

Figure 5. Malignant melanoma of the conjunctiva in a dog, which is partially pigmented. Intraepithelial nests of neoplastic cells can be seen (junctional activity). HE stain.

and seven months after surgery), frequently distant from the primary mass or even multifocally in the conjunctiva (the foci of junctional activity away from the main mass can give rise to these *ex novo* masses in areas other than the initial neoplasm).

The tumour can recur locally even after resection of the nictitating membrane and can invade the subconjunctival and orbital tissue. Metastases are described in between 10 and 33% of cases (between five and sixteen months after surgery) and it has been speculated that tumours of the palpebral conjunctiva have a greater tendency to metastasise (Collins et al., 1993; Reilly et al., 2005; Wang and Kern, 2015). The mitotic index is not considered predictive of the probability of local recurrence or metastasis.

Due to the multifocal and invasive potential of malignant conjunctival melanoma, aggressive surgery (enucleation/exenteration) is recommended after the first recurrence.

Conjunctival Melanoma in the Cat

In cats, conjunctival melanomas are always considered malignant. They occur in adult to senior cats, with no particular breed or sex predisposition. The bulbar conjunctiva is the most frequently reported primary site, from where they spread widely into the orbit, followed by the nictitating membrane and the palpebral conjunctiva.

Macroscopically, they are variably delineated masses, and their colour varies from dark brown to pinkish (Figure 6).

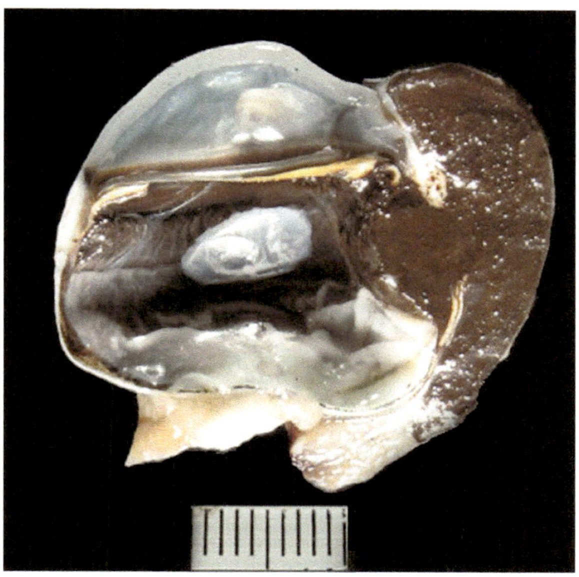

Figure 6. Conjunctival malignant melanoma in a cat, infiltrating the sclera and invading the uvea on one side of the eyeball.

Microscopically, most are composed of round cells and also vary greatly regarding degree of pigmentation, with amelanotic variants being described. The presence of multinucleated cells is characteristic (61% of cases).

Conjunctival melanomas in cats are locally aggressive, they recur locally (between 31 and 75% of cases according to studies) and enucleation or exenteration is necessary to obtain tumour-free surgical margins. Even so, they metastasise relatively frequently (mandibular lymph nodes, abdomen etc., between 23 and 75% of cases) (Patnaik and Mooney, 1988; Schobert et al., 2010; Wang and Kern, 2015). A mortality rate of 61% in cases is described, with a mean survival time of eleven months (range 0.5 to 36 months).

Conjunctival Haemangioma and Haemangiosarcoma (Cat and Dog)

These tumours occur in the conjunctiva, typically in non-pigmented areas, which together with the higher prevalence in **active, outdoor** breeds (in dogs) suggests a role of ultraviolet radiation in the development of these tumours (haemangioma in the Basset Hound, Boxer, English Springer Spaniel, and English Setter and haemangiosarcoma in the Dalmatian; these breeds usually have little or no pigmented conjunctiva and periocular skin.) These tumours are **more common in dogs than in cats**.

In both dogs and cats, adult to geriatric animals are most frequently affected. Haemangiomas are described as more prevalent than haemangiosarcomas, in both dogs and cats. In dogs, the risk of developing haemangiosarcoma (versus haemangioma) increases with exposure to ultraviolet light. In rare cases, they can be bilateral. In cats, a tendency to affect more males than females has been described (Pirie et al., 2006; Newkirk et al., 2009), while in dogs no sex predisposition has been described.

In dogs, the site where they develop most frequently is the leading edge of the nictitating membrane (non-pigmented, 38% of cases, Figure 7), followed by the temporal bulbar conjunctiva (31% of cases), without infiltrating deeper planes. In cats, the nictitating membrane is the most frequently affected site. Ultraviolet radiation is considered to be involved in the pathogenesis of these tumours (due to the location of the lesions, minimal conjunctival pigmentation, dogs from areas with high levels of exposure to ultraviolet light and hunting or sporting breeds). In one study, all cases of haemangiosarcoma and 81% of conjunctival haemangiomas in dogs occurred in unpigmented areas (Pirie et al., 2006).

Macroscopically, they appear as exophytic focal masses, pink to red or brownish, smooth or multilobed, shiny and friable. Haemangiosarcomas tend to be larger than haemangiomas.

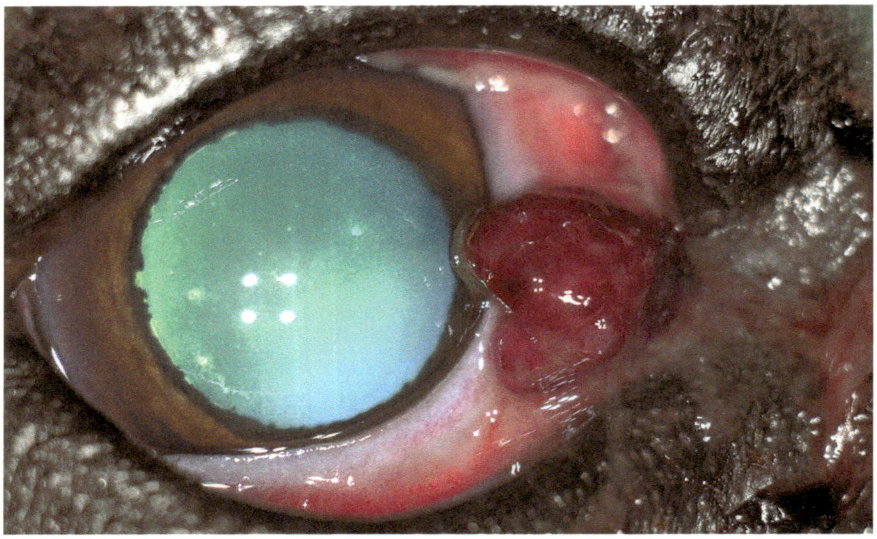

Figure 7. Haemangiosarcoma of the nictitating membrane of the right eye in a dog. (Image courtesy of Dr Gerlinde Janssens).

Microscopically, haemangiomas consist of multiple vascular channels lined by spindle cells with few atypical features, and a low mitotic index. Haemangiosarcomas tend to present more solid areas (less differentiation towards vascular channels), neoplastic cells tend to present atypical characteristics and tend to be more locally infiltrative. Immunohistochemically, these tumours are positive for vimentin, Factor VIII, and CD31.

The prognosis for these tumours is good. Although in cases in which the excision is not complete, they may recur locally (especially haemangiosarcomas, which may require enucleation for complete removal; there is a recurrence rate of 10% for haemangiomas and 55% for haemangiosarcomas, regardless of the reported surgical margins), these vascular tumours do not usually metastasise, so complete resection is usually curative. The recurrence time ranges between 0.75 and 24 months after surgery.

Conjunctival Mast Cell Tumour in the Dog

Mast cell tumours are described occasionally in dogs and very rarely in cats. Macroscopically, they are firm, raised, smooth, beige coloured masses, which can fluctuate. The distribution of tumours in the conjunctiva (bulbar, palpebral, or nictitating membrane) is homogeneous.

Microscopically, they are similar to those seen on the skin and generally appear well differentiated, although low, intermediate, and high-grade tumours are seen. Although the same grading criteria can be applied to these tumours as in the skin, there are no studies that validate these criteria in conjunctival samples, since the grading systems currently applied (Patnaik et al., 1984; Kiupel et al., 2011) are exclusively validated for dermal tumours (for example, the Patnaik et al. scale includes the extent of invasion in the dermis, but the conjunctiva does not have a dermis.)

The prognosis is good, since complete resection is curative and even tumours which are incompletely resected may not recur. Occasionally, they may recur if the excision is not complete. The prognosis is considered independent of the grade, the location in the conjunctiva and the margins (Fife et al., 2011). To date, they have not been reported to metastasise.

Conjunctival Lymphoma (Cat and Dog)

Occasionally lymphomas can be observed in the conjunctiva of dogs and cats and can present in a consultation for an ophthalmological problem. Although most are associated with systemic presentation, it is speculated that some of these lymphomas may be primary (Vascellari et al., 2005; Olbertz et al., 2013; Wiggans et al., 2014).

Macroscopically, they usually form discrete masses or cause diffuse thickening of the conjunctiva, which is greyish to pinkish, typically unilateral, although a bilateral case has been described in a cat (Radi et al., 2004). In a recent article that includes cases in dogs (5) and cats (3) (McCowan et al., 2014), all diffuse lesions were nasal, and all focal lesions were temporal. Lymphadenopathy may be seen in some cases, but in others the conjunctival problem may be the only clinical abnormality.

Microscopically, cases of small, intermediate, and large cells are described. In the dog some are epitheliotropic, while in the cat they are considered non-epitheliotropic.

Immunohistochemically, most canine tumours are CD3 positive (T-cell type), although MALT-type B tumours have been described (Hong et al., 2011) and the majority of reported feline lymphomas are positive for B-cell markers (CD20, CD79 or PAX 5), including Hodgkin-like lymphoma (Holt et al., 2006; McCowan et al., 2014; Olbertz et al., 2013).

The prognosis is variable and in some reported cases, long follow-up periods are described without recurrence of clinical signs after local excision. McCowan et al. (2014) suggests that conjunctival lymphomas in younger dogs (two cases in 3-year-olds) may have a better prognosis than those that occur in adult dogs (three cases), although the numbers are too low to draw conclusions from. Reported cases of MALT-type lymphoma suggest an indolent behaviour (Hong et al., 2011).

Indolent behaviours of these lymphomas have also been described in cats, although in some cases systemic involvement and short survival periods have been reported. In a recent study of presumed primary ocular lymphoma, metastases to regional lymph nodes of conjunctival lymphoma were reported in a dog and a cat (Wiggans et al., 2014), although the prognosis was concluded to be better than for uveal lymphomas (also presumably primary) presented in the same study.

Conjunctival Papillomas in the Dog: Viral, Squamous, and Reactive

Viral papillomas can be detected in the conjunctiva of the dog. Canine oral papillomavirus (COPV) has been detected in these lesions. Although some lesions may spontaneously regress, excision is recommended if they cause irritation, especially to the cornea. The histological appearance is similar to that described in viral papillomas of the skin and other mucosa, with evidence of cytopathic damage and marked keratinisation.

Squamous papillomas are seen in the conjunctiva of dogs and consist of well-delineated, pedunculated, papillary exophytic masses originating on the conjunctival surface (Figure 8). They occur with no association with other tumours or underlying inflammation. They usually occur in older dogs as compared with viral papillomas and are smaller than these (Beckwith-Cohen et al., 2015). Their cause is unknown, and they are not associated with papillomavirus.

Histologically, the papillae end at an acute angle ("spearhead") and are lined by a squamous, non-keratinised stratified epithelium (unlike squamous papillomas in the skin), with occasional goblet cells and no dysplastic or anaplastic features. The presence of pigmentation is variable.

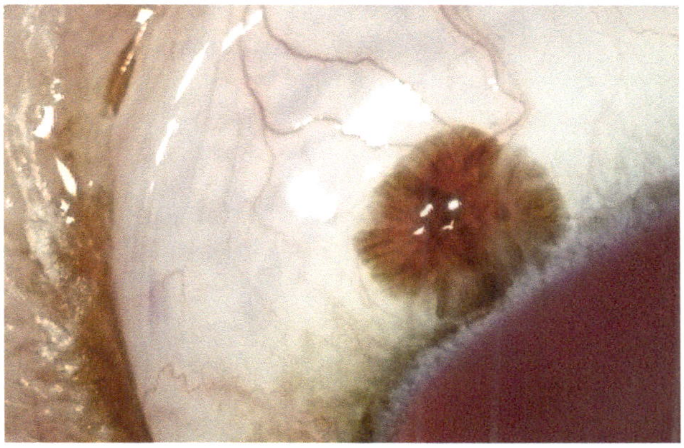

Figure 8. Squamous papilloma of the bulbar conjunctiva in a dog. In this case the tumour appears pigmented. (Image courtesy of Dr Gerlinde Janssens).

The prognosis is excellent after local resection since they do not recur or cause problems in distant locations.

Reactive papillomas usually occur on the palpebral margin in dogs, and form a localised, exophytic, arborising mass with a basal pedicle and papillary projections with rounded edges. They are usually associated with a meibomian gland tumour or an underlying area of inflammation.

Conjunctival Surface Adenocarcinoma in the Cat

An infrequent but highly infiltrative tumour that originates in the superficial conjunctival epithelium, forming delicate exophytic papillary projections, as well as a more invasive portion in the substantia propria of the conjunctiva composed of acini and tubules.

Although it is not reported in the literature as such, in the few cases observed a highly malignant behaviour is detected, with local invasiveness and frequent and rapid metastases to regional lymph nodes and lung.

Nictitating Membrane Gland Tumours (Cat and Dog)

Nictitating membrane gland tumours are described in both dogs and cats, although they are more frequent in the former. They usually occur in older animals, without a defined breed or sex predisposition.

In both species, most are adenocarcinomas, although adenomas (only in dogs, including mixed tumours and complex adenomas) and squamous cell carcinomas have also been described (Dees et al., 2016).

Macroscopically, they are firm, pink tumours that expand the nictitating membrane, and can spread to the orbit and cause exophthalmia, enophthalmos, or strabismus (Figure 9). Immunohistochemically, they are positive for cytokeratin.

They are usually locally invasive and require aggressive surgery (removal of the nictitating membrane or even enucleation or exenteration) since they can recur locally, but metastases are rarely reported. In a recent study, it is estimated that they recur in 11.3% of dogs, while metastases occur in 8.1% (Dees et al., 2016). It is suspected that these tumours may present greater malignancy in cats, although reported cases are very rare. The same study (Dees et al., 2016) estimates that in cats the recurrence rate is 30% and metastases occur in 40% of them.

Corneal Neoplasms

Corneal neoplasms are **rare in cats and dogs**. Squamous cell carcinomas, melanocytomas, squamous papillomas, lymphoma, and vascular tumours (haemangiomas/haemangiosarcomas) are described. Some non-neoplastic masses that are described include NGE, abscesses, and epithelial inclusion cysts.

Squamous Cell Carcinoma in the Dog

Although squamous cell carcinomas can invade the cornea secondary to a limbal, conjunctival, or eyelid tumour, they can also present as a primary tumour in the cornea. In this case, the tumour usually appears in the central (axial) area of the cornea in dogs that have a history of irritation/exposure and chronic keratitis (pigmentary keratitis, keratoconjunctivitis sicca, entropion, distichiasis etc.). Most occur in brachycephalic dogs, especially Pugs, of middle to old age. A possible relationship with topical treatment with immunomodulators (cyclosporine or tacrolimus) has been speculated. Cyclosporine disrupts apoptosis and inhibits T-lymphocyte activation. Associated keratoconjunctivitis sicca is diagnosed in 38% of dogs and chronic superficial keratitis (or pannus) is diagnosed in 15% of cases. The effect of ultraviolet light is not clear in these cases.

Macroscopically, a pinkish mass with an irregular surface is observed (Figure 10), although it may be more diffuse (less nodular). These masses are usually in the axial cornea and in some cases they can be bilateral.

Histologically, approximately 20% of tumours are carcinomas in situ (cells do not infiltrate beyond the basement membrane) or low-grade carcinomas and are usually not highly invasive into the corneal stroma, typically remaining in the superficial third of the stroma. In the mass itself, dysplastic changes transitioning to cellular atypia and anaplasia are observed. They are usually accompanied by severe superficial chronic keratitis, associated with irritation or exposure (chronic inflammation, epithelial hyperplasia and keratinisation, neovascularisation, and pigmentation).

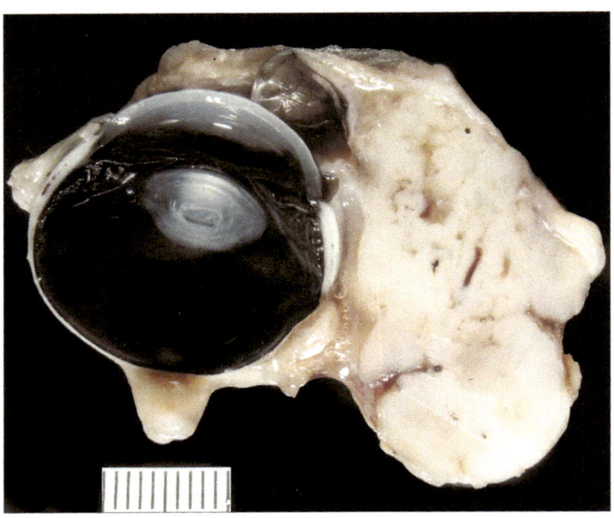

Figure 9. Adenocarcinoma of the gland of the nictitating membrane in a dog.

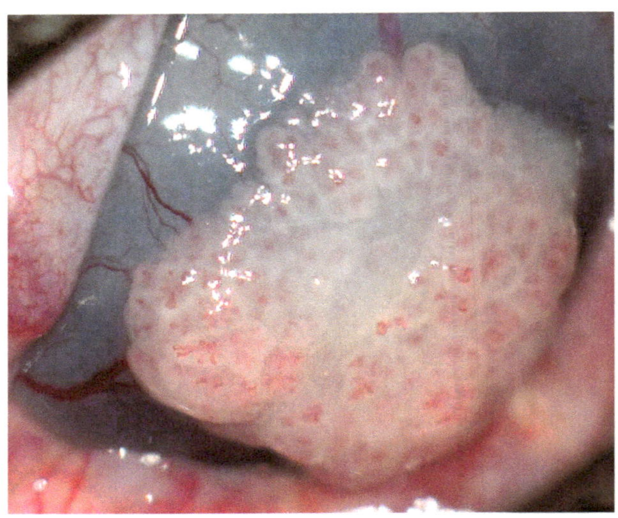

Figure 10. Squamous cell carcinoma of the cornea of a dog. Well vascularised mass with papillary surface. (Image courtesy of Dr Gerlinde Janssens).

Metastases associated with this tumour have not been described and lamellar keratectomy or enucleation (in very extensive cases) are curative. Tumours can recur locally if resection is not complete and may occasionally appear in other areas of the cornea (Dreyfus et al., 2011).

Limbal or Epibulbar Melanocytoma (Cat and Dog)

These tumours are **common in dogs and rare in cats**. In dogs, it is estimated that between 15 and 34% of ophthalmologic melanocytic neoplasms originate in the limbus (Wang and Kern, 2015). The tumour shows a predilection for German Shepherds and Retrievers and is suspected to be hereditary (recessive). It is described as a tumour with a bimodal presentation: there is a peak of incidence at two years of age (in this age range the tumour usually grows rapidly and reaches larger sizes) and another in elderly animals (slow-growing tumours). They are believed to originate from limbic melanocytes.

Macroscopically, they are highly pigmented masses that expand the limbus area and can infiltrate the adjacent cornea, sclera and/or conjunctiva and occasionally invade intraocular structures. The most affected area is usually the dorsal arch between the dorsomedial and ventrolateral limbus (Figure 11).

Histologically, they are composed of well-differentiated, uniform, round, and densely pigmented melanocytes, with a smaller proportion of equally pigmented spindle cells.

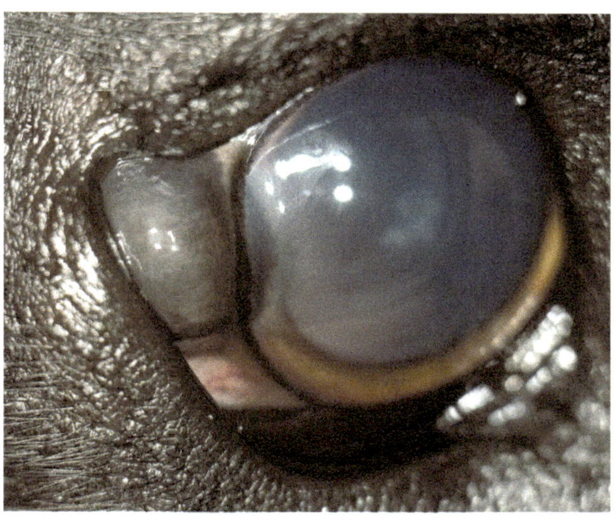

Figure 11. Limbal melanocytoma, temporal limbus of the right eye of a dog (Image courtesy of Dr Gerlinde Janssens).

The differential diagnosis includes the spread of a uveal melanocytic tumour or a conjunctival melanoma. In the first instance, the clinical examination is very important. Furthermore, uveal melanocytomas tend to have a higher proportion of spindle cells than epibulbar melanocytomas. Malignant uveal melanomas present atypical histological characteristics. In the case of conjunctival melanomas, the history is important to determine where the tumour started if it is very extensive. In addition, in the conjunctiva, melanocytic tumours can present prominent atypia. The behaviour of this tumour in dogs is described as benign, although recurrence rates of 30% are also described after excision. For this reason, local excision with adjuvant therapies is usually performed, although they can grow very large (especially in young dogs) and require enucleation for complete resection. Metastases are not described.

A case has recently been described in which there was a concomitant limbal melanocytoma with ocular melanosis and a conjunctival melanocytoma in the contralateral nictitating membrane. In addition, this dog had numerous benign pigmented foci in the conjunctiva, sclera, and orbital tissue, suggesting that a peculiar distribution of melanocytes may have predisposed this dog to develop multiple pigmented lesions (Dees et al., 2013).

In cats, they are mostly benign tumours, with only local infiltration, although isolated cases of generalised metastases have been described.

Uveal Neoplasms

Although many intraocular tumours are benign, they tend to grow and cause complications in the eyeball, the most common being glaucoma (with associated pain); therefore, in these cases enucleation is usually performed to avoid this pain.

Uveal Melanocytic Tumours in the Dog

Uveal melanocytic tumours are the **most common primary neoplasm in the dog's eye**, and the iris is the most common area where ocular melanocytic tumours originate (only 4% of canine ocular melanocytic tumours originate in the choroid). They usually occurs in adult to geriatric dogs. The histopathological terminology used for these tumours is as follows:

- **melanocytoma**: benign melanocytic neoplasm
- **malignant melanoma**: malignant melanocytic neoplasm.

Uveal melanocytomas are the most common primary intraocular tumour in dogs and are more common than malignant melanomas. Likewise, anterior uveal melanocytomas are much more frequent (94% of cases) than choroidal melanocytomas (6%).

Macroscopically, they are tumours that invade the iris and/or the ciliary body and frequently invade the equatorial sclera and the peripheral cornea (Figure 12). Occasionally, they can diffusely infiltrate the iris and ciliary body without forming a discrete mass, which is why they can be confused with uveitis or ocular melanosis.

In the choroid, they usually form a mass that grows towards the inside of the eyeball and frequently cause retinal detachment. Melanocytomas can occur in densely pigmented eyes or originate in the context of ocular melanosis.

Histologically, melanocytomas show a double population of cells in variable proportions. Round, swollen cells are described, with abundant pigment that obliterates the rest of the nuclear characteristics. In addition, a second population of spindle cells is observed, which usually contain less pigment. In general, as tumour malignancy increases, the ratio of spindle cells to round cells increases. Melanocytomas differ from malignant melanomas by showing four or fewer mitotic figures in 10 HPF; finding a higher mitotic count is indicative of malignant melanoma.

The behaviour of uveal melanocytomas is considered benign, in so much as they invade ocular and even periocular structures, but enucleation (or exenteration) is usually curative. Rarely, recurrence of the tumour in the orbit, which can be in the form of malignant melanoma, has been described.

In the uvea, **malignant melanomas** are less common than melanocytomas (approximately 25% of anterior melanocytic neoplasms and 3% of choroidal melanocytic neoplasms). Also, a malignant melanoma can grow within a uveal melanocytoma.

Macroscopically, they may have the same appearance as melanocytomas, although they tend to be less pigmented (Figure 13).

Histologically, these tumours present anaplastic features such as anisocytosis, karyomegaly, irregular nuclei, and prominent nucleoli. They are typically less pigmented than melanocytomas, although this does not have to be the case. They are defined by the presence of more than four mitotic figures in 10 HPF.

Immunohistochemically, they have been described as Melan-A positive, although it is expected that they are also positive for other melanocyte markers.

The prognosis for malignant melanomas is guarded, since they have metastatic potential and present reduced survival compared to control populations and dogs with melanocytoma.

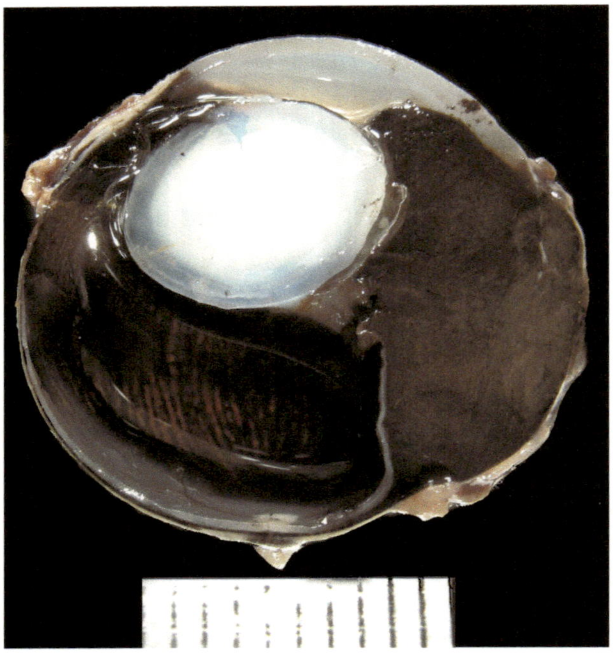

Figure 12. Anterior uveal melanocytoma derived from the iris and the ciliary body and spreading towards the peripheral choroid on one side of the eyeball. The tumour is displacing the lens.

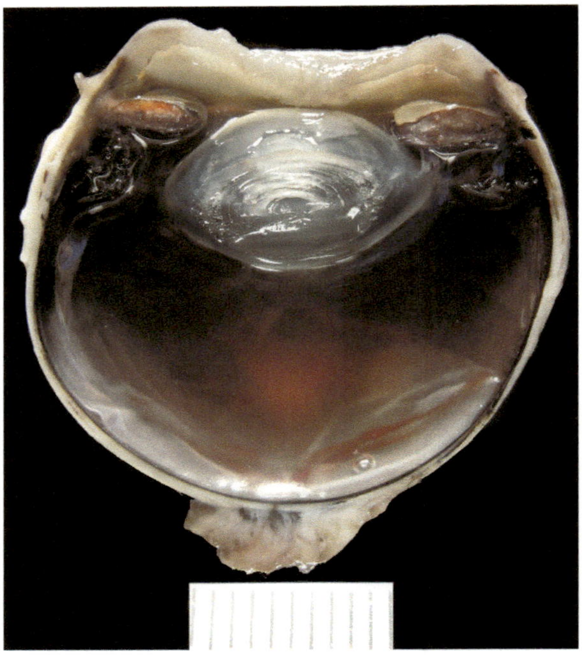

Figure 13. Anterior uveal malignant melanoma. The neoplasm thickens and expands the two iris leaflets, which also display paler areas coinciding with the less pigmented areas of the tumour

In any case, the metastatic potential is considered low (between 4 and 10% of cases). Histological criteria such as necrosis, degree of pigmentation, presence of neoplastic cells in the cornea, iridocorneal angle or episclera, are not considered predictive of the biological behaviour of this type of tumour. It must also be considered that melanomas (mainly of the nailbed, but also skin and oral cavity) can metastasise to the eye and their distribution and morphology can be very similar to those of primary malignant melanomas.

Uveal Melanocytic Tumours in the Cat

In cats, the terminology used is usually **feline diffuse iris melanoma** (FDIM). It is the most common primary intraocular tumour in cats. No breed or sex predisposition is described, and it usually occurs in adult and elderly cats.

The clinical history usually describes areas of multifocal pigmentation in the iris with gradual progression, which grow in extension or in number until they reach coalescence, thicken the iris, and invade structures of the iridocorneal angle, ciliary body, and peripheral choroid, practically destroying all the structures of the eyeball.

Macroscopically, they can present as the dark spots described clinically to thickening of the iris (which appears dark brown), ciliary body and choroid (Figure 14).

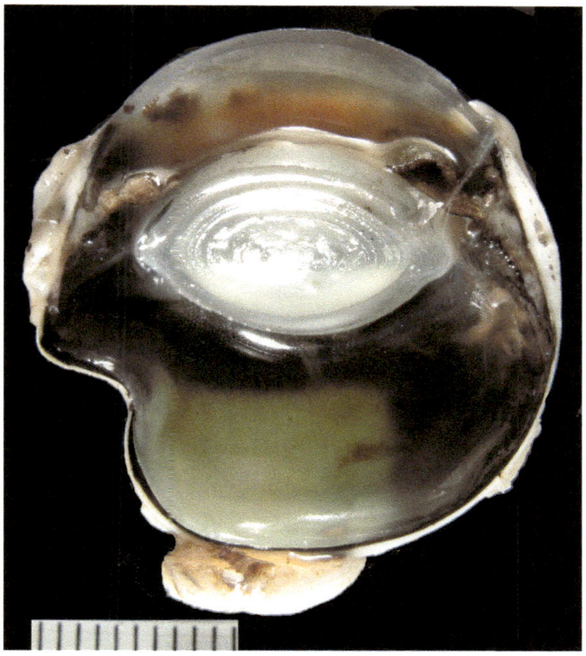

Figure 14. Feline diffuse iris melanoma. The iris appears thickened, with areas of growth which also extend towards the ciliary body.

Occasionally, tumours are described in which discrete solid masses are formed (in the iris, ciliary body, or choroid), so not all cases are strictly diffuse. A recent study (Fragola et al., 2018) indicates that some iridociliary cysts in cats may present with a clinical appearance similar to neoplasia (in particular, diffuse melanoma of the iris). It indicates that some of these cysts may be densely pigmented, not transilluminate, and cause distortion of the iris, which can give them the appearance of a pigmented neoplasm.

Histologically, four stages are distinguished with a certain prognostic value. Until recently, the extension within the eye was the only criterion that could be used to anticipate the cases in which metastasis could develop:

- **iris melanosis**: benign-looking melanocytes (without cellular atypia) are observed that line the anterior surface of the iris, forming multiple layers without infiltrating the stroma. It is not considered neoplastic (Figure 15 A);
- **early FDIM**: melanocytes acquire atypical characteristics (neoplasia) as they invade the iris stroma, although at this stage they are confined to this structure (Figure 15 B);
- **intermediate FDIM**: neoplastic melanocytes extend to the iridocorneal angle and slightly into the ciliary body (anterior aspect);
- **extensive FDIM**: the tumour extensively invades the iris, iridocorneal angle, and ciliary body and may extend into the peripheral choroid and equatorial sclera.

Histologically, FDIMs vary widely in morphology, from densely to sparsely pigmented, composed of round, polygonal, or spindle cells, with balloon cell variants, giant and anaplastic cells, and with variability of cytological criteria for malignancy (anisocytosis, anisokaryosis, karyomegaly, multinucleation, intranuclear pseudoinclusions, abnormal mitotic figures). There are also amelanotic variants that can be confused with inflammation due to the diffuse nature of the tumour. Histologically, amelanotic tumours may have to be differentiated from lymphoma (with immunohistochemistry, they are positive for Melan-A and PNL2.)

The progression of the disease is highly variable: in some cases, it is rapid, while in others it can progress for years (metastasis can occur one to three years after enucleation). It is difficult to establish the proportion of cases that develop metastases, since these animals are not usually referred for necropsy, and they may die from other causes (especially cases with slow progression and in elderly cats), although it has been described that it can be of between 19 (Wiggans et al., 2016) and 63% of cases (Patnaik and Mooney, 1988). As a result the decision as to when to perform an enucleation can be difficult.

Until recently, the only microscopic feature that correlated with biological behaviour was spread within the eyeball, such that early tumours have survival times similar to cats without this tumour, while extensive tumours have reduced survival times possibly associated with the presence of metastases (Kalishman et al., 1998). Cats with glaucoma at enucleation also have reduced survival (Kalishman et al., 1998). Other histological parameters that have been described related to a worse prognosis are a high mitotic index and the presence of neoplastic cells in the scleral venous plexus (Duncan and Peiffer, 1991). A recent article (Wiggans et al., 2016) has described four histological parameters that are associated with reduced survival: the presence of more than seven mitoses in 10 HPF, the presence of intratumoural necrosis, the extension of the neoplasm into the choroid and the extrascleral extension of the tumour. When metastases occur, they are usually in the abdominal cavity (liver), followed in incidence by pulmonary metastases, although extensive metastases have been described, including to the bones (Planellas et al., 2010). In cases of extensive FDIM, the tumour may also recur in the orbit.

Feline atypical melanoma is a rare tumour of the cat's eyeball. It is a tumour composed of multifocal masses throughout the uvea but is not centred on the iris.

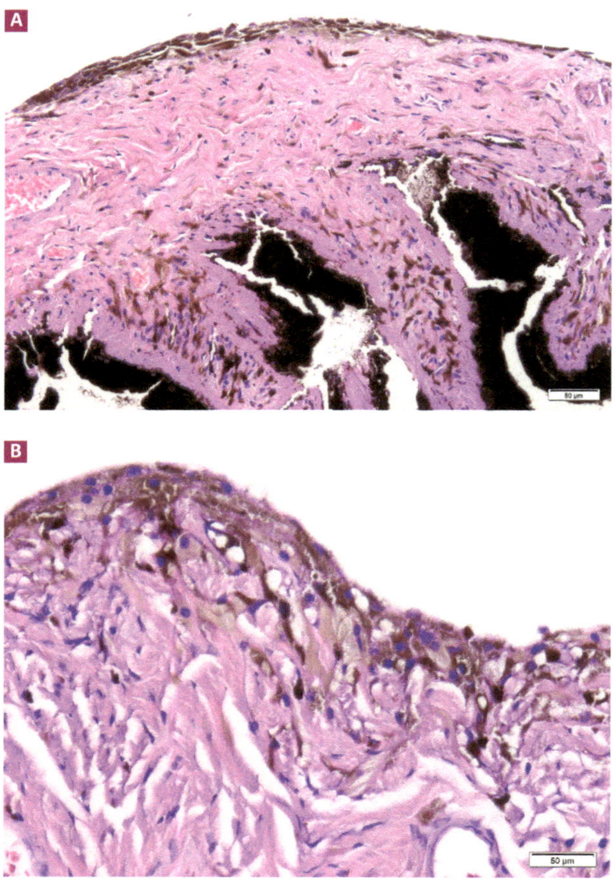

Figure 15. A. Melanosis, multiple layers of melanocytes without cytological atypia carpet the anterior surface of the iris without invading the stroma. **B**. Early diffuse melanoma of the iris. The pigmented cells start to infiltrate the subjacent iridal stroma. HE stain.

Histologically, this tumour is composed of densely pigmented round cells, with a nucleus that does not present significant atypia (homogeneous chromatin without prominent nucleolus). In addition, tumour cell aggregates are seen in the retinal pigment epithelium, in the sub-retinal space, and in the retina. Despite the cell characteristics, these tumours frequently metastasise.

Iridociliary Epithelial Tumours in the Dog

Iridociliary epithelial tumours are the second most common primary intraocular tumour in the dog. They usually occur in middle-aged dogs and no sex predilection is observed, although breed predisposition is reported in Golden Retrievers and Labrador Retrievers. These tumours originate from the pigmented or nonpigmented ciliary body epithelium and, less frequently, from the pigmented posterior epithelium of the iris.

Clinically and macroscopically, they are observed as a well-delineated mass in the posterior or anterior chamber and are most frequently whitish to pink (Figure 16). When pigmented, the main differential diagnosis is an anterior uveal melanocytic tumour.

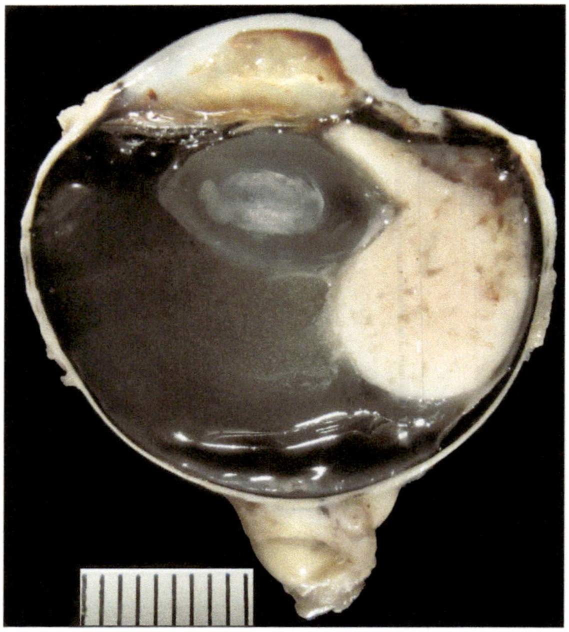

Figure 16. Iridociliary adenoma in a dog. A well-defined, whitish mass can be seen, which arises from the ciliary body and cradles the lens to one side of the eye. In this eye asteroid hyalosis can also be seen in the vitreous.

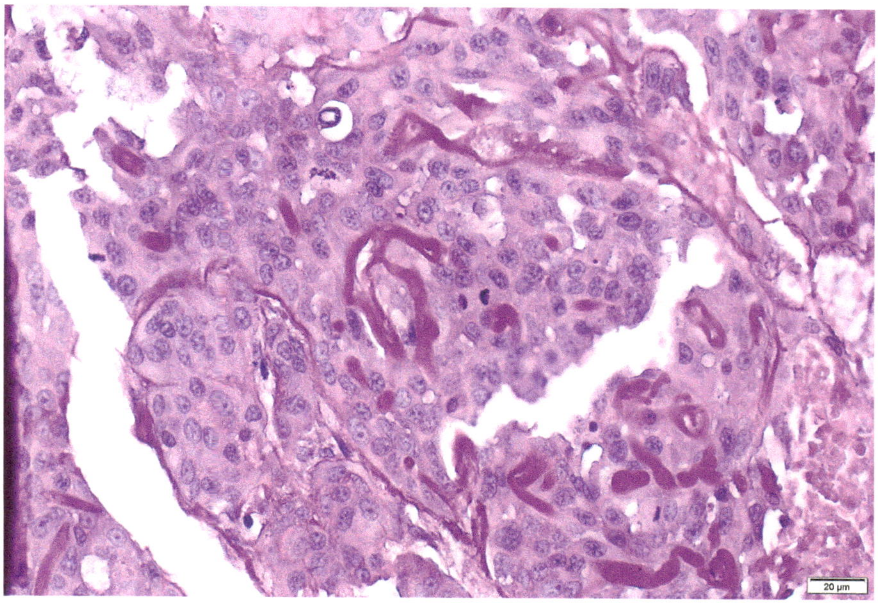

Figure 17. Iridociliary adenoma in a dog. Robust basal membranes stained with an intense magenta colour can be seen between atypical cells. PAS (periodic acid-Schiff) stain.

According to the degree of invasion they are divided into:

- **non-uveoinvasive iridociliary adenoma**: the tumour is confined to the posterior or anterior chamber, without substantially invading the uvea;
- **uveoinvasive iridociliary adenoma**: the tumour invades the uveal stroma but does not invade the sclera; and
- **iridociliary adenocarcinoma**: the tumour invades the uvea and sclera, in approximately 15% of cases. They can have more anaplastic cytological features.

Histologically, these tumours are predominantly nonpigmented in 90% of cases (although approximately 50% show some pigmented cells). Different histological patterns are observed, forming palisades trabeculae, solid tumours, and anaplastic variants. Approximately 60% of these tumours show thick, branching PAS-positive basement membranes between tumour cells (Figure 17). Approximately 50% show the presence of hyaluronic acid, which can be detected by Alcian blue staining, allowing them to be distinguished from metastatic tumours.

Immunohistochemically, these tumours are positive for vimentin and NSE, with variable staining for S100. Benign tumours are negative for cytokeratin and the expression of this marker increases as the invasiveness of the neoplasm progresses. The expression of TERT (telomerase catalytic subunit) also increases with increasing tumour malignancy (Dubielzig et al., 1993; Klosterman et al., 2006).

Despite the different degrees of invasiveness described, the behaviour of all these variants is similar. The tumour itself can cause secondary glaucoma, which is the main reason affected eyes require enucleation. Even so, they are considered benign tumours, since adenomas do not metastasise and, although some cases of metastatic adenocarcinoma are reported, they probably represent examples of pleomorphic adenocarcinomas. Biopsies of these tumours are performed for diagnostic and/or therapeutic purposes, but the recurrence rate is high because complete excision is rarely achieved. In addition, postoperative complications such as synechiae to the incision site and the presence of neoplastic cells in this incision area are described (Beckwith-Cohen et al., 2015).

The histological and behavioural characteristics of **pleomorphic adenocarcinoma** differ from the other variants. It is much less frequent than the rest and usually occurs in eyes with a history of chronic eye problems, such as uveitis or glaucoma. It has recently been described in cases where eyes have previously been injected with gentamicin (Duke et al., 2013).

These tumours invade practically all the structures of the eyeball, and even the orbit, as well as invading vascular structures. Histologically, the cells are extremely anaplastic. Pleomorphic adenocarcinoma has a high risk of metastasis.

As described for iridociliary tumours, pleomorphic adenocarcinoma, which presents increased malignancy, is usually positive for vimentin and for cytokeratin. This pattern serves to distinguish them from metastatic carcinomas to the eye.

Iridociliary Tumours in the Cat

In cats, iridociliary tumours represent the fourth most common primary intraocular tumour. They usually occur in adult cats, without breed or sex predisposition.

Macroscopically, they usually fill the posterior chamber, surrounding the lens, and can infiltrate the iris, ciliary body, and anterior chamber. The sclera is only invaded occasionally. They are usually whitish to beige in colour and can have numerous cavitated areas.

Histologically, they are almost always composed of nonpigmented epithelial cells, in a typical solid sheet formation, and only rarely do they form trabeculae. In approximately 30% of cases, metaplastic bone can be seen in the tumour. They are designated adenocarcinoma (versus adenoma) when the tumour invades the sclera, as in canine tumours.

PAS staining can be performed to reveal the basement membranes that separate tumour cells into small trabeculae and nests, although these basement membranes are not as robust as in canine iridociliary tumours. In some cases, the tumour appears predominantly cystic. Most neoplasms are vimentin-positive and only occasionally stain positive for cytokeratin.

The behaviour of these tumours is benign, and enucleation is curative.

Medulloepithelioma in the Dog

This tumour belongs to the primitive neuroectodermal family of tumours or PNET. Medulloepithelioma has characteristics in common with iridociliary adenoma (it also originates in the neuroectoderm) and shares characteristics with retinoblastomas in people.

These tumours are **rare in dogs and extremely rare in cats**. They are described in young animals, although they can be diagnosed in middle-aged individuals.

Macroscopically, these tumours originate in the ciliary body, occupy the posterior chamber, and can spread to infiltrate the retina. They are whitish and may present papillary or botryoid extensions towards the anterior chamber, forming small nodules.

Histologically, a survival pattern is usually observed around the vasculature, with extensive necrosis away from the blood vessels. The main feature is the formation of rosettes, which can form multiple layers. The individual cells are elongated with an elongated, hyperchromatic nucleus. Formation of bone, cartilage, skeletal muscle, and brain-like tissue may be seen, and in this case they are called teratoid medulloepitheliomas. Immunohistochemically they are positive for TERT, with limited positivity for vimentin and cytokeratin.

The behaviour of medulloepithelioma is defined as locally invasive, although metastases are very rare.

Uveal Lymphoma (Cat and Dog)

In dogs, it is the third most common intraocular tumour and the first if only secondary tumours are considered. Involvement of ocular structures during the course of multicentric lymphoma (37% of dogs with multicentric lymphoma) is considered common (Krohne et al., 1994). Ocular signs are the second most common in dogs with lymphoma after lymphadenopathy. Bilateral involvement is seen more frequently in dogs than in cats (in these bilateral cases the eyes are not necessarily enucleated).

A recent publication (Lanza et al., 2018) indicates the possibility of presumed solitary ocular lymphoma, and in this study up to 61% of dogs had no systemic involvement at the time of diagnosis and these cases did not progress after diagnosis.

In cats, it represents the second most common intraocular neoplasm (the round cell variant of post-traumatic sarcoma, which has specific histological characteristics, is not included) and the most common metastatic tumour. Although the FIV/FeLV status of cats is often not specified on biopsy sheets, it is not thought that uveal lymphoma has a particular association with these viruses. Recently, ocular signs have been observed in 48% of cats at the time of lymphoma diagnosis (Nerschbach et al., 2013), including anterior and posterior uveitis, corneal problems and retrobulbar masses, although this study did not reach either a cytological or histopathological diagnosis in cases with intraocular involvement.

Macroscopically, the anterior uvea (iris and ciliary body) is affected more frequently than the posterior one, and this tumour can present in a nodular (Figure 13) or diffuse form, with a light beige to whitish coloration. If the involvement is diffuse, it can be confused with uveitis. Ocular signs associated with the haematological abnormalities seen in dogs with lymphoma (anaemia, thrombocytopaenia, disseminated intravascular coagulation) may be seen, manifesting primarily as intraocular haemorrhage.

Microscopically, a population of monomorphic round cells is observed that infiltrate and mainly invade the iris and ciliary body, but can invade the retina, the choroid, the limbal area of the cornea, the optic nerve and the peripheral scleral and/or orbital nerves. A morphological variant has recently been described in which the retina is preferentially (although not exclusively) affected (Malmberg et al., 2017). This variant is considered rare, representing approximately 1% of cases of ocular lymphoma in dogs and cats. A lymphoplasmacytic inflammatory infiltrate intermixed with tumour cells is observed in approximately half of the cases; the relationship between inflammation and neoplasia is currently unclear.

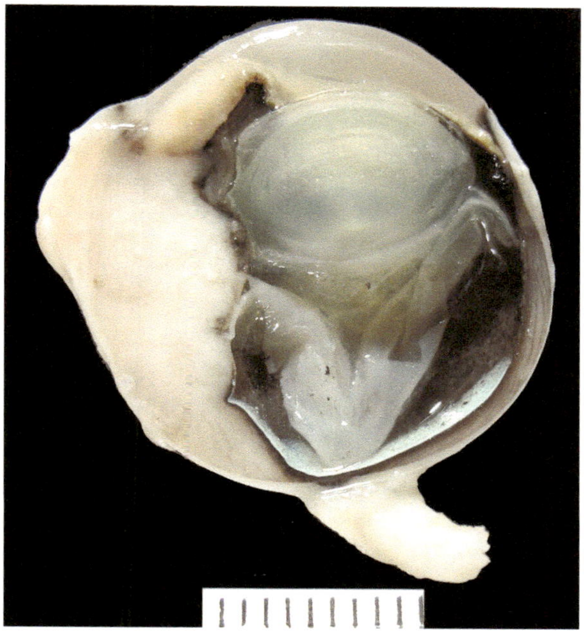

Figure 18. Uveal lymphoma in a cat. A white mass expands and distorts the iris, ciliary body, and choroid on one side of the eyeball. Retinal detachment can be seen.

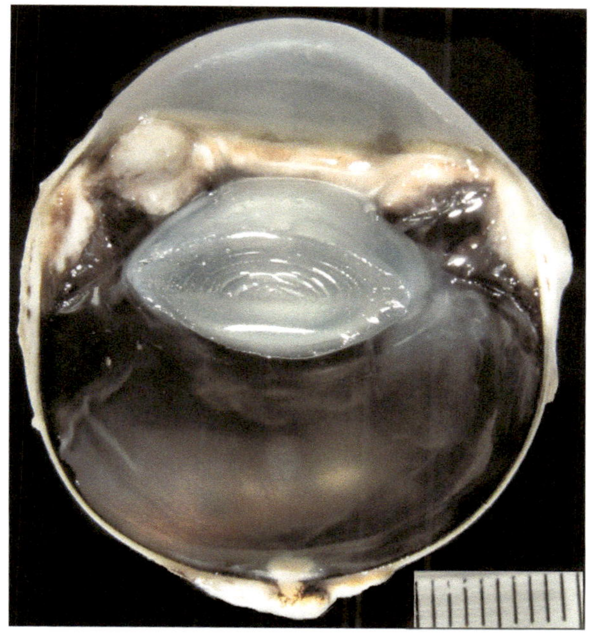

Figure 19. Histiocytic sarcoma expanding and distorting the anterior uvea in a Bernese Mountain Dog.

Immunohistochemically, lymphocyte markers can be used to diagnose this tumour and differentiate it from other round cell tumours (often amelanotic melanoma). Thus, antibodies such as CD20, CD79a, and PAX5 are used to identify B-cell lymphomas, while CD3 is used to identify T-cell lymphomas (one antibody from each lineage is usually used.) Both phenotypes are described affecting intraocular structures (Ota-Kuroki, 2014; Lanza et al., 2018).

The prognosis is variable. In cases in which the ocular involvement is part of a systemic process, the prognosis is guarded. In dogs, the survival of patients with ocular clinical signs is 60–70% of the survival of those without. In addition, dogs with concomitant uveitis and intraocular haemorrhage should be considered clinical stage V (WHO) (Krohne et al., 1994).

To the contrary, recent studies indicate the possibility of presumed primary ocular lymphomas, which is why the current staging system is being questioned (Ota-Kuroki et al., 2014; Wiggans et al., 2014; Lanza et al., 2018). In one of them (Wiggans et al., 2014), dogs with presumed primary intraocular lymphoma developed neurological signs regardless of the presence of neoplastic cells in the optic nerve at the time of enucleation.

In the study by Lanza et al. (2018), on the other hand, dogs that did not present systemic involvement at the time of diagnosis did not show progression of the disease after enucleation and had a significantly longer median survival time than dogs in which there were systemic clinical signs (769 days versus 103 days). There were no differences in survival according to lymphoma subtype (phenotype or grade). It is hypothesised in this study that in these dogs the lymphoma could have been primary in the eye and the enucleation could have been curative.

Histiocytic Sarcoma

Although it is a systemic tumour, it is not uncommon for it to initially appear in the eye, without other associated clinical signs. It is usually a unilateral tumour, which presents as a mass in the uvea, with uveitis and/or secondary glaucoma.

A very marked breed predisposition is observed: the three most frequently affected breeds are Rottweilers, Golden Retrievers and Labrador Retrievers. Much less frequently it is observed in Bernese Mountain Dogs (Figure 19). They are usually adult or elderly animals, without a sex predisposition.

Macroscopically, a solid whitish mass is observed that invades the uvea, although less discrete and infiltrative forms can also be observed, mostly in the anterior uvea.

Microscopically, neoplastic cells are round, with abundant eosinophilic cytoplasm (frequently vacuolised) and present prominent atypia, including karyomegaly and multinucleation. Immunohistochemically, neoplastic cells are positive for CD18, in addition to vimentin, and negative for Melan-A and other melanocytic markers.

Prognosis is poor and dogs show a very short survival time (between zero and six months after enucleation), since after diagnosis in the eye, masses are typically observed in other organs (Naranjo et al., 2007).

Schwannoma of Blue-eyed Dogs (Spindle Cell Tumour of Blue-eyed Dogs)

This is a rare tumour that occurs in dogs with blue eyes or a partially blue uvea (heterochromic). The first case of this neoplasm has recently been described in a dog with a completely brown iris (Marlo et al., 2018). It usually occurs in adult dogs (middle aged), and the breeds that appear to be most commonly affected are the Siberian Husky, Australian Shepherd and Catahoula.

In less than half of the cases, a tumour is suspected at the time of enucleation, since these tumours do not often form discrete masses, but instead invade the uvea in a diffuse and poorly delineated way, causing it to thicken, so that they can be confused with uveitis. The most frequent location is the iris, with invasion of the ciliary body, although occasionally they are exclusively observed in the choroid.

Histologically, they are spindle cell tumours forming bundles ranging from small and delicate cells, without anaplastic features, to plump spindle cells with marked karyomegaly and anaplasia. Antoni A and Antoni B type organisations can be seen, similar to what is seen in peripheral nerve sheath tumours.

The immunohistochemical staining pattern of these tumours is as follows: vimentin, S-100 and GFAP positive, whereas Melan-A is usually negative. Although GFAP is used to label astrocytes (central nervous system), Schwann cells from unmyelinated nerve fibres are GFAP-positive, suggesting that this tumour originates from these cells (Zarfoss et al., 2007).

They are locally infiltrative tumours, so that they can recur in the fibrous tunica after evisceration or in the orbit after enucleation, although metastases are considered rare, with only one case described so far (Duke et al., 2013), in which metastases were confirmed in the lung, liver and mesenteric lymph node. It was speculated that invasion of the sclera, which is not typical of these uveal schwannomas and was observed in this case, could be a predictor of poor prognosis.

Post-traumatic Sarcoma in the Cat

This is the third most frequent intraocular tumour in cats (the second if only primary ones are considered). Three histological variants of post-traumatic sarcoma are described.

Spindle Cell Variant

This is the most common variant, derived from lens epithelial cells, in approximately 70% of cases. It occurs in cats with a history of severe, chronic intraocular disease. Although the owner may not witness the traumatic episode, it usually occurs in outdoor cats or rescue cats in which "the eye was already affected". Furthermore, the latency period from the traumatic event to the development of the tumour can vary from two months to more than ten years, although longer periods are more frequent (mean of seven years). The initial trauma can even be from intraocular surgery or intraocular gentamicin injections (Duke et al., 2013).

Macroscopically, the tumour has a tendency to line the inner surfaces of the eyeball, invade the uvea, retina, and cornea and finally progresses to fill the eyeball, forming a solid mass (Figure 20), with possible extension beyond the fibrous tunic into the orbit, infiltration of the peripheral nerves and/or invasion of the optic nerve. In early cases, neoplastic cells are seen in the equatorial region of the lens.

Microscopically, spindle cells with marked pleomorphism and anaplasia are observed, with the presence of multinucleated cells on some occasions. Most cases show evidence of lens capsule rupture (Figure 21). PAS-positive basement membranes can be seen surrounding the neoplastic cells.

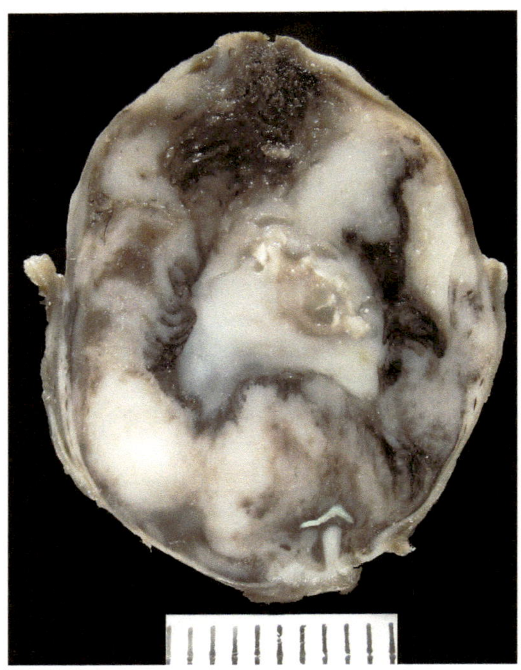

Figure 20. Post-traumatic sarcoma in a cat, spindle cell variant. The neoplasm fills all the cavities of the eyeball, destroying their structures. Remnants of the lens can be seen in the centre, embedded in the tumour.

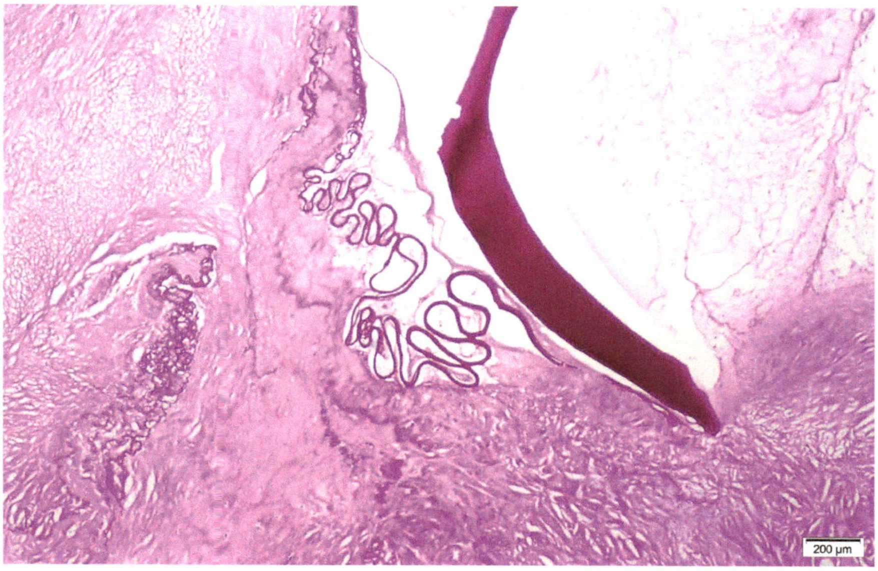

Figure 21. Post-traumatic sarcoma in a cat, spindle cell variant. Fragments of the lens capsule can be seen, which appears broken and wrinkled (magenta colour). PAS stain.

Immunohistochemically, these tumours are characterised by being vimentin positive and, in some cases, labelling with smooth muscle actin, cytokeratin, and α-crystallin is observed. This last protein is exclusive to lenticular fibres. PAS-positive membranes show type IV collagen labelling, the typical collagen from basement membranes.

Many of the **characteristics of this tumour** suggest that it originates from lenticular epithelial cells (Zeiss et al., 2003):

- lenticular capsule rupture in almost all cases;
- early tumours are seen around the lens;
- presence of basement membranes similar to the lenticular capsule around neoplastic cells; and
- α-crystallin labelling in approximately one third of tumours.

Although these tumours have sporadically been described in other species (rabbit, dog and bird), no neoplasms originating from the lens have been described in humans (Albert et al., 2015). These tumours are usually highly locally infiltrative, invading the orbit through the tunica fibrosa, so local recurrence is possible and frequent after enucleation. In addition, the tumour can invade the peripheral nerves and the optic nerve, ascending towards the optic chiasm and the brain. Distant metastases can occur, although the frequency is difficult to establish.

Round Cell Variant (Post-traumatic Lymphoma)

Approximately 24% of cases. It is a type of lymphoma, although with the typical distribution of post-traumatic sarcoma. It is also seen in animals with long-lasting intraocular disease.

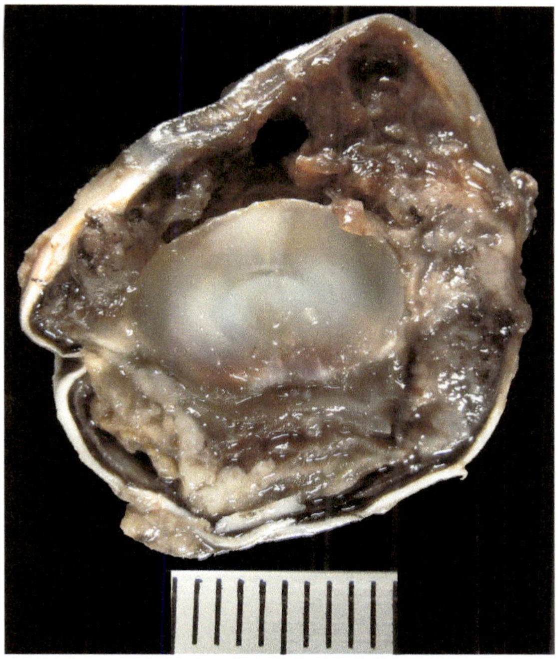

Figure 22. Post-traumatic sarcoma in a cat, round cell variant. The neoplasm appears poorly defined, lining the internal surfaces of the eyeball.

Macroscopically, the tumour has a tendency to fill the eyeball, destroying the uvea and other intraocular structures (Figure 22). It can end up spreading through the sclera or to the optic nerve.

Microscopically, it usually shows extensive areas of necrosis, with a tendency for neoplastic cells to survive around the blood vessels. The morphology of the cells is typical of a lymphoma, with monomorphic round cells, with little cytoplasm and abundant mitoses. Rupture of the lens capsule is usually seen, although not in all cases.

Immunohistochemically, these tumours are positive for B-cell markers (CD20), although a mixture with cells positive for T-cell markers (CD3) is usually seen. In the cases where clonality has been determined, the majority have been found to be of B-cell origin. The behaviour of this tumour is locally infiltrative and local recurrences and systemic involvement have been described, although it is difficult to determine if there are histological characteristics that help to predict this behaviour.

Osteosarcoma/ Chondrosarcoma Variant

This is the least frequent variant (6% of cases) and, therefore, the one where the least information is available.

Macroscopically, this tumour usually fills the eyeball, forming a solid mass, which is frequently mineralised.

Microscopically, areas of osteoid and/or chondroid matrix deposition and rupture of the lens capsule are observed in all cases. In some cases, characteristics can be detected that suggest that it may originate from the lenticular epithelium.

The behaviour of this tumour is difficult to predict since few cases have been described and not much information is currently available. A case has recently been published in which intrathoracic metastases were confirmed (lung, tracheobronchial and mediastinal lymph nodes, pericardium, parietal pleura; Moreira et al., 2018). Recently, what are presumably primary chondrosarcomas have been described in the eye of cats and are not associated with post-traumatic sarcoma (Beckwith-Cohen et al., 2014), which is why a good description of macro and microscopic features, as well as an exhaustive history and clinical examination are necessary to make one diagnosis or another since the prognosis is radically different (although rare and the numbers are low, enucleation is presumably curative in these presumed primary ocular chondrosarcomas in cats).

Metastatic Tumours (Cat and Dog)

These tumours have a different distribution pattern in the eye in dogs and cats. In dogs, the most common metastatic tumours are lymphoma and histiocytic sarcoma (in this order), followed by carcinoma, melanoma haemangiosarcoma, osteosarcoma, and many others. Among epithelial tumours, mammary carcinomas are the most frequently diagnosed.

The general characteristics are:

- metastases may be present unilaterally, but recurrence of the neoplasm in the contralateral eye is common;
- the anterior uvea is affected more often than the choroid;
- neoplastic cells are frequently identified within blood vessels; and
- two patterns of involvement are described:
  - formation of a discrete mass
  - diffuse infiltrates without forming a mass, in which neoplastic cells tend to line the inner surfaces of the eye.

It must be considered that extraskeletal osteosarcomas or chondrosarcomas are rarely described in the eye, so a thorough search for a primary tumour is essential and this differential must be ruled out before considering a primary extraskeletal neoplasm.

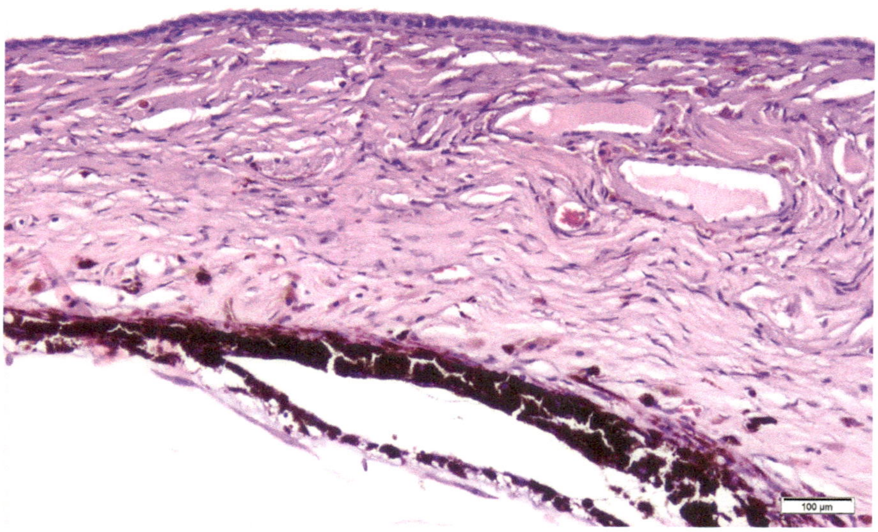

Figure 23. Metastatic carcinoma in the eye of a cat. One layer of cuboidal epithelial cells lines the anterior surface of the iris. The iris does not show an epithelial lining on its anterior surface normally. HE stain.

In **cats**, the most common metastatic tumours include lung carcinomas ("lung-eye syndrome"), squamous cell carcinomas, and fibrosarcomas. Key features include:

- uni- or bilateral ocular involvement;
- choroidal involvement more frequent than involvement of the anterior uvea;
- if the anterior uvea is affected, neoplastic tumour cells usually line the inner surface of the iris and the ciliary body (Figure 23);
- the blood vessels appear to be invaded extensively, which can cause infarcts in the choroid (wedge-shaped areas in which the tapetum appears discoloured and with vascular attenuation); and
- the orbit can be affected along with invasion of the posterior segment

Miscellaneous

Isolated cases of leiomyomas, leiomyosarcomas and primary extraskeletal osteosarcomas in the dog as well as primary extraskeletal chondrosarcomas in the cat (Beckwith-Cohen et al., 2014) have been described.

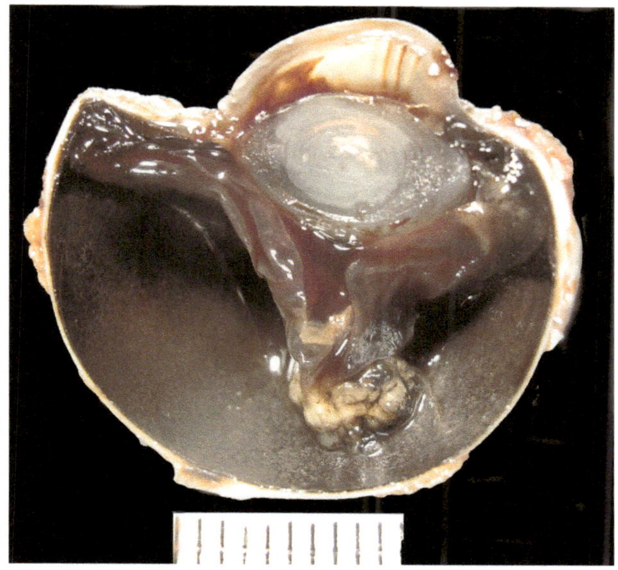

Figure 24. Retinal glioma in a dog. The subtle mass originates from the retina and causes complete detachment. Haemorrhage can be seen in the vitreous and anterior chamber.

Retina and Optic Nerve Tumours

Gliomas of the Retina and Optic Nerve in the Dog

Gliomas, most commonly astrocytomas, can occur in the retina and optic nerve. They are the most common primary tumour in the retina. In these cases, the central retina is most frequently affected, close to or contiguous with the optic nerve, and the tumour usually forms a discrete mass that protrudes into the vitreous humour (Figure 24). The tumour may also present with expansion of the optic nerve and may manifest as a protrusion of the papilla into the eyeball. Exophthalmia is rare.

Microscopically, a proliferation of spindle-shaped to stellate cells is usually observed, replacing the optic nerve neuropil, with characteristics similar to intracranial gliomas.

Immunohistochemically, these tumours are positive for glial markers (GFAP), which is consistent with an astrocytic origin. Less frequently, these tumours show differentiation towards oligodendroglioma, in which case they are GFAP-negative.

The prognosis is good if the surgical margins (optic nerve) appear free of neoplastic cells. In cases where the tumour extends to the surgical margins of the optic nerve, it usually recurs and ascends towards the optic chiasm and even the base of the brain. No metastases are reported (Naranjo et al., 2008).

Orbital Meningioma in Dogs

This tumour originates from released meningothelial cells of the arachnoid that surrounds the optic nerve.

Macroscopically, a mass is observed that surrounds and encompasses the optic nerve and extends to fill the orbit, conforming to the space, which is why most of the time the mass has a conical shape (Figure 25).

Microscopically, the tumour is composed of polygonal cells that form solid aggregates and nests and invade the orbital tissue. Foci of metaplastic bone, cartilage, or myxomatous matrix can be seen between neoplastic cells. Cell morphology corresponds to the histological subtype of meningotheliomatous meningioma. Less frequently, the cells have spindle-shaped morphology, similar to a transitional meningioma. The optic nerve appears compressed, and retinal ganglion cells may be lost from the retrograde degeneration that occurs.

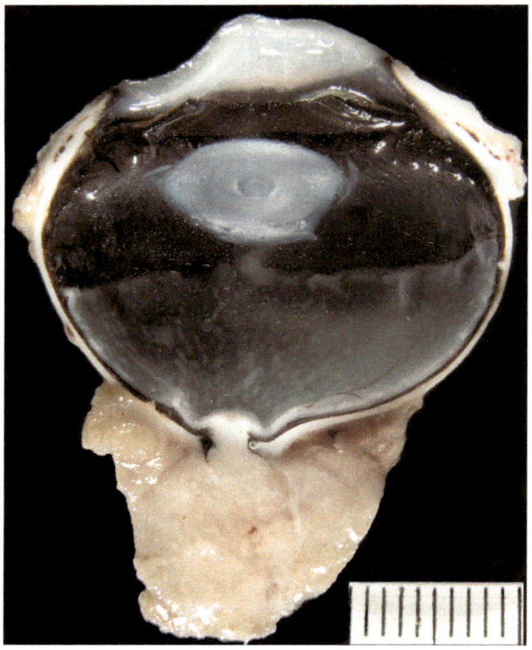

Figure 25. Orbital meningioma. The mass has a conical shape, as it eventually adapts to the shape of the orbit. The posterior sclera appears indented by the neoplasm.

Due to its microscopic appearance, it can be confused with an epithelial neoplasia (such as squamous cell carcinoma), but immunohistochemically meningiomas are positive for vimentin and NSE and are negative for cytokeratin (unlike most epithelial neoplasms).

The prognosis is guarded because, although the tumour is slow growing, complete resection is difficult and therefore local recurrences are frequent. They can ascend through the optic foramen into the calvarium, compressing or displacing the brain, or they can grow through the chiasm into the contralateral optic nerve (Mauldin et al., 2000). Metastases are reported very infrequently.

The extension of an intracranial meningioma from the calvarium into the optic nerve is much less frequently seen. In this case, the tumour remains within the dura, diffusely expands the thickness of the optic nerve, and the involvement is usually bilateral. In this case, any histological subtype of meningioma can occur.

Retinal Tumours with Neural Differentiation

PNET (primitive neuroectodermal tumours) is a generic name used to classify embryonal tumours that arise from the germinal neuroepithelium of the neural tube (neuroectoderm). They can include tumours such as neuroblastomas, ependymoblastomas, retinoblastomas, and medulloepitheliomas.

In the eye, PNETs usually occur in the peripheral retina or in the area adjacent to the ciliary body. Medulloepitheliomas originate in the ciliary body or optic nerve, although they are seen more rarely in the retina.

Cases of **retinoblastoma** in dogs found in the veterinary literature are rare and debatable. Although tumours with neural differentiation are seen, it is unusual for them to meet the histological features specified for human retinoblastomas.

PNET with characteristics similar to retinoblastomas (four cases) have recently been identified. Dogs with this type of tumour were less than two years old, had tumours in the retina or ciliary body and had histological characteristics similar to retinoblastomas in humans: rosettes and fleurettes composed of a single layer of cells, in contrast to medulloepitheliomas, that were detected in dogs older than seven years of age and in which true rosettes were not observed (Regan et al., 2013). Retinoblastoma-like tumours also showed immunohistochemical labelling with an antibody against IRBP, a protein that is only seen in retinal photoreceptors; medulloepitheliomas were negative for this marker.

Orbital Tumours

Orbital tumours can be very varied, due to the variety of tissues found in the orbit (fibroblasts, adipocytes, vessels, nerves, salivary and lacrimal glands, bone etc.). In the many published studies, **epithelial tumours** (carcinomas and adenocarcinomas) (Figure 26) are considered to be the **most frequently diagnosed in both dogs and cats**, followed by sarcomas (fibrosarcoma, osteosarcoma, multilobular osteochondrosarcoma). These tumours can also spread from adjacent structures (such as nasal and sinus carcinomas) or, less frequently, be metastatic. Orbital lymphoma is considered part of a systemic disease.

Most importantly, **most of these tumours are malignant**, so the prognosis is, at the very least, guarded.

Canine Orbital Multilobular Adenoma

This tumour presents as either a bulge in the conjunctiva or a mass-like lesion in the orbit (exophthalmia, periocular bulge). It is not clear which gland gives rise to this tumour since it can originate in different areas of the orbit (lacrimal or salivary glands).

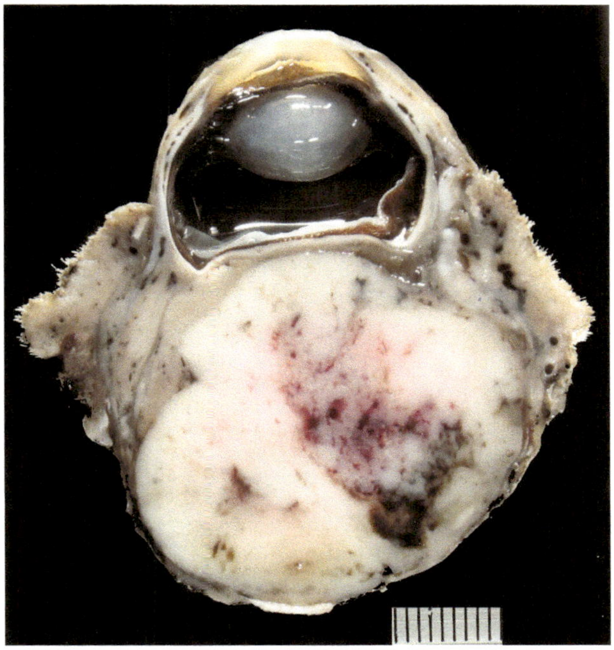

Figure 26. Orbital adenocarcinoma in a dog. These tumours can originate from the main lacrimal gland or from the zygomatic salivary gland.

Macroscopically, a soft, translucent, multilobulated tissue is observed, with a thin capsule surrounding each of the lobules, which appear loosely cohesive, and where tissue is very friable and falls apart quickly. For this reason, the tissue is difficult to grasp with forceps and it breaks easily and, therefore, it is easy for excision to be incomplete unless exenteration is performed.

Microscopically, well-differentiated glandular tissue without atypia is seen, although no ducts are observed between the acini. Secretory cells contain abundant, vacuolised, and granular cytoplasm. A PAS stain demonstrating mucopolysaccharides in the cytoplasm of these secretory cells can be performed.

They are benign tumours insofar as they do not metastasise, but they frequently recur in the orbit one or two years after diagnosis and are occasionally bilateral, so they often require exenteration (Headrick et al., 2004).

Canine Orbital Hibernoma

A benign neoplasm of brown adipose tissue that can arise in the orbit (Ravi et al., 2014), although it can spread to the subconjunctival tissue. They occur in adult to geriatric dogs and are rare.

Macroscopically, they are slightly lobulated whitish masses with a soft consistency, which are often well defined, and can cause exophthalmos or a mass effect in the periocular tissues.

Histologically, the masses appear lobulated and are composed of polygonal cells with finely vacuolated or granular cytoplasm (Figure 27).

These tumours must be differentiated from sebaceous neoplasms (sebaceous adenomas/adenocarcinomas), from white adipose tissue neoplasms (lipoma/liposarcoma), granular cell tumours, oncocytomas, and rhabdomyomas. Immunohistochemically, they are positive for the UCP-1 protein (uncoupling

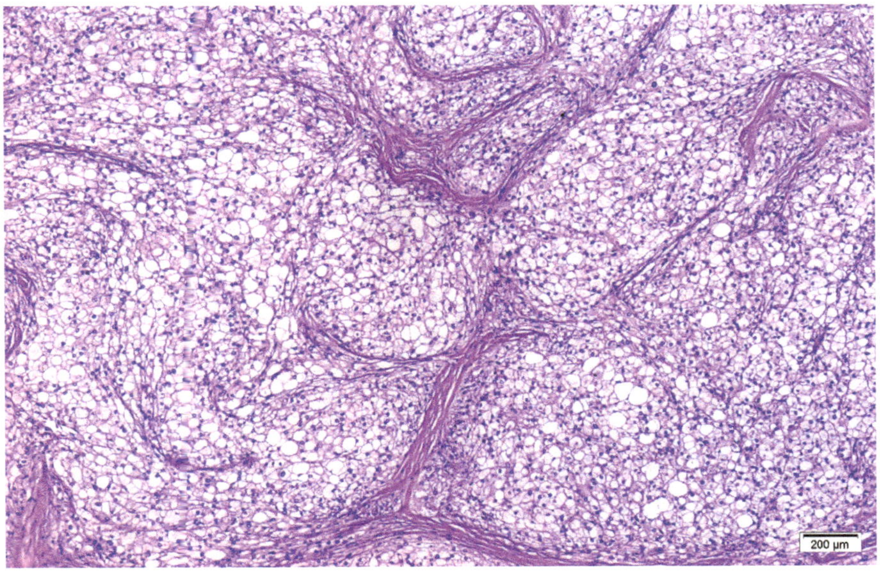

Figure 27. Orbital hibernoma in a dog. The neoplasm is multilobulated with polygonal cells which have a highly vacuolated cytoplasm. This tumour was positive for desmin, consistent with the description of canine hibernomas. HE stain.

protein I), which is consistent with differentiation towards brown fat; as this antibody has limited availability, muscle cell markers can be used to detect these tumours, mainly desmin, since a common progenitor is suggested for neoplastic cells of brown adipose tissue and skeletal myocytes.

These are benign neoplasms whose complete removal is considered curative.

Canine Orbital Rhabdomyosarcoma

Rhabdomyosarcomas are biologically very aggressive and are rare skeletal muscle neoplasms, although in the vicinity of the eyeball they usually occur relatively frequently in the orbit. They occur in young dogs, mainly in large or giant breeds, and the nasal and lower orbit seems to be the most affected area. Dogs present with orbital clinical signs (exophthalmia, deviation of the visual axis, resistance to retropulsion).

Macroscopically, they are poorly delineated tumours that are highly infiltrative towards the adjacent orbital tissues, including the possibility of infiltrating the adjacent bone. They are whitish tumours with haemorrhagic areas and a firm consistency.

Histologically, their microscopic appearance is consistent with embryonal rhabdomiosarcomas. They may show cells with a round to plump spindle to polygonal morphology, in some cases with multinucleated cells or the presence of striations in the cytoplasm (Figure 28).

Immunohistochemically, these tumours can be differentiated from other sarcomas or round cell tumours because they are positive for desmin and most for skeletal muscle actin as well.

In young dogs the prognosis is poor, with tumours that progress rapidly, recur frequently and develop metastatic disease, with a median survival time of six months. In older dogs, the prognosis is better, with no relapses or metastases reported after exenteration (Scott et al., 2016).

Feline Restrictive Orbital Myofibroblastic Sarcoma

This condition was known as "feline orbital pseudotumour", but the recent trend is to consider it as a neoplasm, due to its invasive behaviour. This tumour typically presents with reduced motility of the eyeball, which may show a fixed position, as well as secondary exposure keratitis or corneal ulceration/perforation. Furthermore, most cats present concurrent alterations in the contralateral eye and/or in the oral cavity. Recently, a subset of squamous cell carcinomas in the orbit and ocular adnexa that can present with similar clinical signs has been described, so a differential diagnosis between these two neoplasms must be established in cats that present with these clinical signs (Diehl et al., 2018).

Macroscopically, there are no discrete masses and, in addition to the clinical signs referred to, there is a thickening of the orbital structures, the eyelids and periocular structures, as well as the oral cavity.

Microscopically, a poorly delineated and infiltrative population of bland spindle cells is observed that invades the structures of the orbit, periocular skin and submucosa of the oral cavity, with associated collagen deposition. An associated lymphoplasmacytic infiltrate is usually seen. Due to the benign cytological appearance of the cells that compose it, this tumour can easily be confused with a reactive process (reactive fibroplasia or granulation tissue), so the history is crucial at the time of submission of the biopsy (Figure 29).

Immunohistochemically, spindle cells are positive for vimentin, S100 and smooth muscle actin.

The prognosis of this tumour is considered poor, since the spindle cells continue their progression and invade the contralateral orbit and periocular structures and the oral cavity, which is why euthanasia is elected in many of these cats. The average time for progression from one eye to the other or for the appearance of lesions in the oral cavity is four to five months. Survival time is described as being between three and fifteen months after enucleation of the first eye, although these cats are usually euthanised due to a reduced quality of life, since so far metastases have not been described (Bell et al., 2011).

Secondary/metastatic Tumours in the Orbit (Cat and Dog)

Adenocarcinomas can frequently infiltrate the orbit from the nasal cavity or paranasal sinuses, both in dogs and cats.

In cats, and less frequently in dogs, epithelial tumours (carcinomas) can metastasise to the orbit (and invade the eyeball.) Some of the more common primary sites include the lung, nasal cavity, middle ear, oral cavity, conjunctiva, and lacrimal gland.

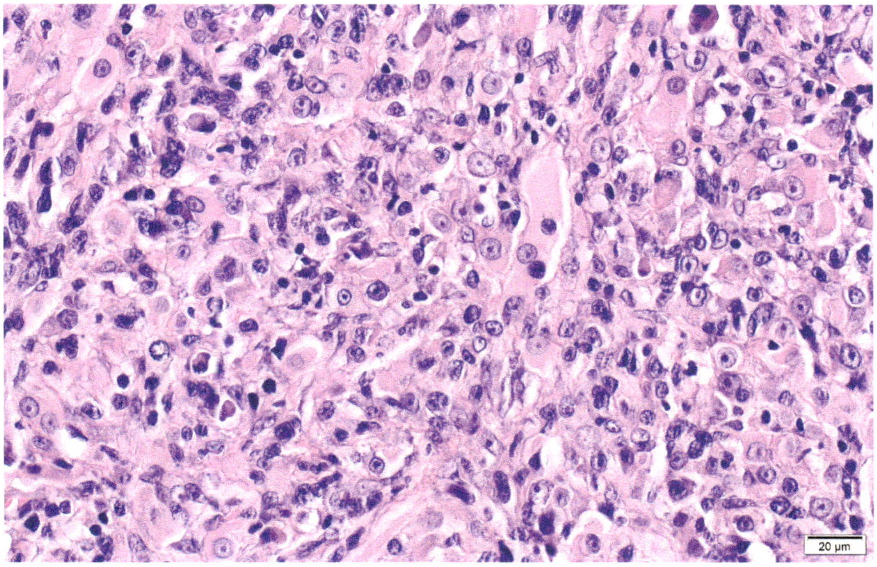

Figure 28. Rhabdomyosarcoma in the orbit of a dog. Neoplastic cells are highly pleomorphic, round and spindle shaped, and some are multinucleated. HE stain.

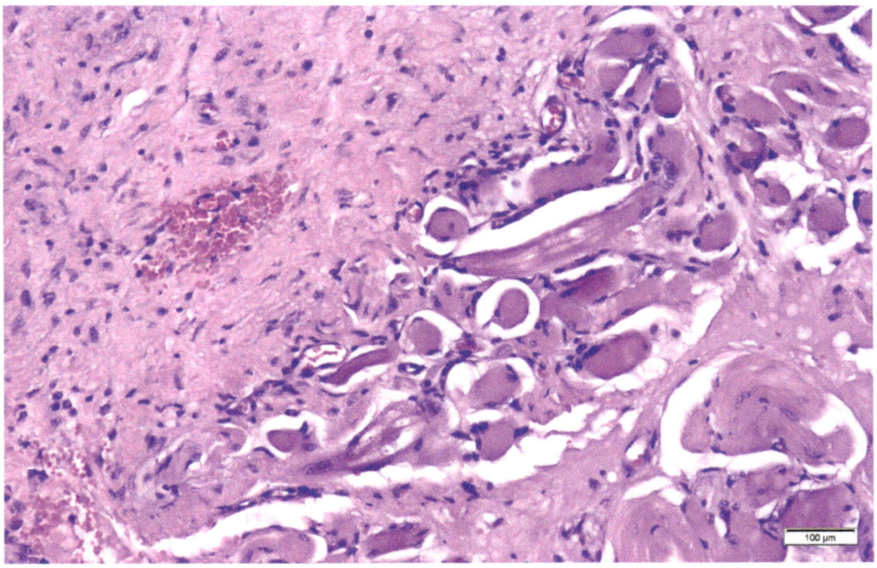

Figure 29. Restrictive orbital myofibroblastic sarcoma in a cat. In the upper left of the image spindle cells without cytological atypica can be seen separated by abundant collagen which infiltrate remains of extraocular muscle myocytes (bottom right). HE stain.

Bibliography

- Albert, D.M., Phelps, P.O., Surapaneni, K.R. et al. (2015) The significance of the discordant occurrence of lens tumors in humans versus other species. *Ophthalmology*, 122(122):1765–1770.
- Beckwith-Cohen, B., Teixeira, L.B., Dubielzig, R.R. (2014) Presumed primary intraocular chondrosarcoma in cats. *J Vet Diagn Invest*, 26(26):664–68.
- Beckwith-Cohen, B., Bentley, E., Dubielzig, R.R. (2015) Outcome of iridociliary epithelial tumor biopsies in dogs: a retrospective study. *Vet Rec*, 176(176):147.
- Beckwith-Cohen, B., Teixeira, L.B., Ramos-Vara, J.A. et al. (2015) Squamous papillomas of the conjunctiva in dogs: a condition not associated with papillomavirus infection. *Vet Pathol*, 52(52):676–680.
- Bell, C.M., Schwarz, T., Dubielzig, R.R. (2011) Diagnostic features of feline restrictive orbital myofibroblastic sarcoma. *Vet Pathol*, 48(48):742–750.
- Cantaloube, B., Raymond-Letron, I., Regnier, A. (2004) Multiple eyelid apocrina hidrocystomas in two Persian cats. *Vet Ophthalmol*, 7(7):121–155.
- Chaitman, J., van der Woerdt, A., Bartick, T.E. (1999) Multiple eyelid cysts resembling apocrine hidrocystomas in three Persian cats and one Himalayan cat. *Vet Pathol*, 36(36):474–476.
- Collins, B.K., Collier, L.L., Miller, M.A. et al. (1993) Biologic behavior and histologic characteristics of canine conjunctival melanoma. *Prog Vet Comp Ophthalmol*, 3(4): 135–140.
- Dees, D.D., Maclaren, N.E., Teixeira, L. et al. (2013) An unusual case of ocular melanosis and limbal melanocytoma with benign intraorbital extension in a dog. *Vet Ophthalmol*, 16(1):117–122.
- Dees, D.D., Schobert, C.S., Dubielzig, R.R. et al. (2016) Third eyelid gland neoplasms of dogs and cats: a retrospective histopathologic study of 145 cases. *Vet Ophthalmol*, 19(2):138–143.
- Diehl, K.A., Pryor, S.G., Teixeira, L.B.C. (2018) Orbital invasive squamous cell carcinoma with adnexal involvement clinically mimicking feline restrictive orbital myofibroblastic sarcoma: 19 cases (1990–2016). *Vet Ophthalmol*, 21(21):281–289.
- Dreyfus, J., Schobert, C.S., Dubielzig, R.R. (2011) Superficial corneal squamous cell carcinoma occurring in dogs with chronic keratitis. *Vet Ophthalmol*, 14(14):161–168.
- Dubielzig, R.R. (1984) Ocular sarcoma following trauma in three cats. *J Am Vet Med Assoc*, 184(184):578–581.
- Dubielzig, R.R., Everitt, J., Shadduck, J.A. et al. (1990) Clinical and morphologic features of post-traumatic ocular sarcomas in cats. *Vet Pathol*, 27(27):62–65.
- Dubielzig, R.R., Steinberg, H., Garvin, H. et al. (1998) Iridociliary tumors in 100 dogs and 17 cats: a morphological study. *Vet Ophthalmol*, 1: 223–231.
- Dubielzig, R.R., Ketring, K.L., MLellan, G.J. et al. (2010) *Veterinary Ocular Pathology: A Comparative Review.* Saunders Elsevier.
- Dubielzig, R.R. (2017) Tumors of the Eye. En: *Tumors in Domestic Animals* 5th edition (ed. Meuten DJ). Wiley Blackwell: Ames, IA, 892–922.
- Duke, F.D., Brudenall, D.K., Scott, E.M. et al. (2013) Metastatic uveal schwannoma of blue-eyed dogs. *Vet Ophthalmol*, 1:141–144.
- Duke, F.D., Strong, T.D., Bentley, E. et al. (2013) Canine ocular tumors following ciliary body ablation with intravitreal gentamicin. *Vet Ophthalmol*, 16(16):159–162.
- Duke, F.D., Strong, T.D., Bentley, E. et al. (2013) Feline ocular tumors following ciliary body ablation with intravitreal gentamicin. *Vet Ophthalmol*, 1:188–190.
- Duncan, D.E., Peiffer, R.L. (1991) Morphology and prognostic indicators of anterior uveal melanomas in cats. *Prog Vet Comp Ophthalmol*, 1(1): 25–32.
- Fife, M., Blocker, T., Fife, T. et al. (2011) Canine conjunctival mast cell tumors: a retrospective study. *Vet Ophthalmol*, 14(14):153–160.
- Finn, M., Krohne, S., Stiles, J. (2008) Ocular melanocytic neoplasia. *Compend Contin Educ Vet*, 30(1):19–25.
- Fragola, J.A., Dubielzig, R.R., Bentley, E. et al. (2018) Iridociliary cysts masquerading as neoplasia in cats: a morphologic review of 14 cases. *Vet Ophthalmol*, 21(2): 125–131.
- Giudice, C., Muscolo, M.C., Rondena, M. et al. (2009) Eyelid multiple cysts of the apocrine gland of Moll in Persian cats. *J Feline Med Surg*, 11(11):487–491.
- Headrick, J.F., Bentley, E., Dubielzig, R.R. (2004) Canine lobular orbital adenoma: a report of 15 cases with distinctive features. *Vet Ophthalmol*, 7(7):47–51.
- Hoffman, A., Blocker, T., Dubielzig, R. et al. (2005) Feline periocular peripheral nerve sheath tumor: a case series. *Vet Ophthalmol*, 8(3):153–158.
- Holt, E., Goldschmidt, M.H., Skorupski, K. (2006) Extranodal conjunctival Hodgkin's-like lymphoma in a cat. *Vet Ophthalmol*, 9(9):141–144.
- Hong, I.H., Bae, S.H., Lee, S.G. et al. (2011) Mucosa-associated lymphoid tissue lymphoma of the third eyelid conjunctiva in a dog. *Vet Ophthalmol*, 14(14):61–65.
- Kafarnik, C., Calvarese, S., Dubielzig, R.R. (2010) Canine mesenchymal hamartoma of the eyelid. *Vet Ophthalmol*, 13(13):94–98.
- Kalishman, J.B., Chappell, R., Flood, L.A. et al. (1998) A matched observational study of survival in cats with enucleation due to diffuse iris melanoma. *Vet Ophthalmol*, 1(1):25–29.
- Kiupel, M., Webster, J.D., Bailey, K.L. et al. (2011) Proposal of a 2-tier histologic grading system for canine cutaneous mast cell tumours to more accurately predict biological behavior. *Vet Pathol*, 48(48):147–155.
- Klosterman, E., Colitz, C.M., Chandler, H.L. et al. (2006) Immunohistochemical properties of ocular adenomas, adenocarcinomas and medulloepitheliomas. *Vet Ophthalmol*, 9(9):387–394.
- Komnenou, A.T., Thomas, A.L., Kyriazis, A.P. et al. (2015) Ocular manifestations of canine transmissible venereal tumor: a retrospective study of 25 cases in Greece. *Vet Rec*, 176(176):523.
- Krohne, S.G., Henderson, N.M., Richardson, R.C. et al. (1994) Prevalence of ocular involvement in dogs with multicentric lymphoma: prospective evaluation of 94 cases. *Vet Comp Ophthalmol*, 4(3): 127–135.

■ Labelle, A.L., Labelle, P. (2013) Canine ocular neoplasia: a review. *Vet Ophthalmol*, 1:3–14.
■ Lanza, M.R., Musciano, A.R., Dubielzig, R.D. et al. (2018) Clinical and pathological classification of canine intraocular lymphoma. *Vet Ophthalmol*, 21(21):167–173.
■ Malmberg, J.L., Garcia, T., Dubielzig, R.R. et al. (2017) Canine and feline retinal lymphoma: a retrospective review of 12 cases. *Vet Ophthalmol*, 20(20):73–78.
■ Marlo, T.L., Giuliano, E.A., Moore, C.P. et al. (2018) Uveal schwannoma in a brown-eyed dog. *Vet Ophthalmol*, 21(21):205–209.
■ Mauldin, E.A., Deehr, A.J., Hertzke, D. et al. (2000) Canine orbital meningiomas: a review of 22 cases. *Vet Ophthalmol*, 3(3):11–16.
■ McCowan, C., Malcolm, J., Hurn, S. et al. (2014) Conjunctival lymphoma: immunophenotype and outcome in five dogs and three cats. *Vet Ophthalmol*, 17(5):351–357.
■ McLaughlin, S.A., Whitley, R.D., Gilger, B.C. et al. (1988) Eyelid neoplasia in cats: a review of demographic data (1979–1989). *J Am Anim Hosp Assoc*, 29: 63–67.
■ Montgomery, K.W., van der Woerdt, A., Aquino, S.M. et al. (2010) Periocular cutaneous mast cell tumors in cats: evaluation of surgical excision (33 cases). *Vet Ophthalmol*, 13(13):26–30.
■ Moreira, M.V.L., de Andrade, M.C., Fulgencio, G.O. et al. (2018) Presumed post-traumatic ocular chondrosarcoma with intrathoracic metastases in a cat. *Vet Ophthalmol*, 21(21):535–538.
■ Naranjo, C., Dubielzig, R.R., Friedrichs, K.R. (2007) Canine ocular histiocytic sarcoma. *Vet Ophthalmol*, 10(10):179–185.
■ Naranjo, C., Schobert, C., Dubielzig, R. (2008) Canine ocular gliomas: a retrospective study. *Vet Ophthalmol*, 11(11):356–362.
■ Nerschbach, V., Eule, J.C., Eberle, N. et al. (2016) Ocular manifestation of lymphoma in newly diagnosed cats. *Vet Comp Oncol*, 14(14):58–66.
■ Newkirk, K.M., Rohrbach, B.W. (2009) A retrospective study of eyelid tumors from 43 cats. *Vet Pathol*, 46(46):916–927.
■ Olbertz, L., Lima, L., Langohr, I. et al. (2013) Supposed primary conjunctival lymphoma in a dog. *Vet Ophthalmol*, 1:100–104.
■ Ota-Kuroki, J., Ragsdale, J.M., Bawa, B. et al. (2014) Intraocular and periocular lymphoma in dogs and cats: a retrospective review of 21 cases (2001–2012). *Vet Ophthalmol*, 17(17):389–396.
■ Patnaik, A.K., Ehler, W.J., MacEwen, E.G. (1984) Canine cutaneous mast cell tumor: morphologic grading and survival time in 83 dogs. *Vet Pathol*, 21(21):469–474.
■ Patnaik, A.K., Mooney, S. (1988) Feline melanoma: a comparative study of ocular, oral, and dermal neoplasms. *Vet Pathol*, 25(25):105–112.
■ Pirie, C.G., Knollinger, A.M., Thomas, C.B. et al. (2006) Canine conjunctival hemangioma and hemangiosarcoma: a retrospective evaluation of 108 cases (1989–2004). *Vet Ophthalmol*, 9(9):215–226.
■ Pirie, C.G., Dubielzig, R.R. (2006) Feline conjunctival hemangioma and hemangiosarcoma: a retrospective evaluation of eight cases (1993–2004). *Vet Ophthalmol*, 9(9):227–231.
■ Planellas, M., Pastor, J., Torres, M.D. et al. (2010) Unusual presentation of a metastatic uveal melanoma in a cat. *Vet Ophthalmol*, 13(6):391–4.
■ Radi, Z.A., Miller, D.L., Hines, M.E. (2004) B-cell conjunctival lymphoma in a cat. *Vet Ophthalmol*, 7(7):413–415.
■ Ravi, M., Schobert, C.S., Kiupel, M. (2014) Clinical, morphologic, and immunohistochemical features of canine orbital hibernomas. *Vet Pathol*, 51(51):563–568.
■ Regan, D.P., Dubielzig, R.R., Zeiss, C.J. et al. (2013) Primary primitive neuroectodermal tumor of the retina and ciliary body in dogs. *Vet Ophthalmol*, 1:87–93.
■ Reilly, C.R., Dubielzig, R.R., Newman, S.J. et al. (2005) Features of canine conjunctival melanocytic tumors [abstract]. *Proc Am Coll Vet Ophthalmol*, 40.
■ Roberts, S.M., Severin, G.A., Lavach, J.D. (1986) Prevalence and treatment of palpebral neoplasms in the dog: 200 cases (1975–1983). *J Am Vet Med Assoc*, 189(10):1355–1359.
■ Schobert, C.S., Labelle, P., Dubielzig, R.R. (2010) Feline conjunctival melanoma: histopathological characteristics and clinical outcomes. *Vet Ophthalmol*, 13(1):43–46.
■ Scott, E.M., Teixeira, L.B., Flanders, D.J. et al. (2016) Canine orbital rhabdomyosarcoma: a report of 18 cases. *Vet Ophthalmol*, 19(2):137.
■ Vascellari, M., Multari, D., Mutinelli, F. (2005) Unicentric extranodal lymphoma of the upper eyelid conjunctiva in a dog. *Vet Ophthalmol*, 8(1):67–70.
■ Wang, A.L., Kern, T. (2015) Melanocytic ophthalmic neoplasms of the domestic veterinary species: a review. *Top Companion Anim Med*, 30(4):148–157.
■ Wiggans, K.T., Skorupski, K.A., Reilly, C.M. et al. (2014) Presumed solitary intraocular or conjunctival lymphoma in dogs and cats: 9 cases (1985–2013). *J Am Vet Med Assoc*, 244(4):460–470.
■ Wiggans, K.T., Reilly, C.M., Kass, P.H. et al. (2016) Histologic and immunohistochemical predictors of clinical behavior for feline diffuse iris melanoma. *Vet Ophthalmol*, 1:44–55.
■ Zarfoss, M.K., Dubielzig, R.R. (2007) Metastatic iridociliary adenocarcinoma in a Labrador retriever. *Vet Pathol*, 44(5):672–676.
■ Zarfoss, M.K., Klauss, G., Newkirk, K. et al. (2007) Uveal spindle cell tumor of blue-eyed dogs: an immunohistochemical study. *Vet Pathol*, 44(3):276–284.
■ Zeiss, C.J., Johnson, E.M., Dubielzig, R.R. (2003) Feline intraocular tumors may arise from transformation of lens epithelium. *Vet Pathol*, 40(4):355–362.

Test

Answers on Page 272

1. **Regarding eyelid neoplasms in domestic carnivores, which of the following statements is incorrect?**
   a. Most eyelid neoplasms in dogs are benign.
   b. In the dog, the upper eyelid is affected more frequently than the lower one.
   c. In dogs, mesenchymal tumours are more common than epithelial ones.
   d. In cats, the most common eyelid tumour is squamous cell carcinoma.

2. **Which of these statements about apocrine hydrocystomas in the cat is correct?**
   a. They are usually solitary neoplasms.
   b. Macroscopically, the main differential diagnosis is melanocytic neoplasms.
   c. They originate from the glands of Zeis.
   d. They are tumours that frequently recur and develop distant metastases.

3. **Point out the incorrect statement regarding squamous cell carcinomas on the margin of the eyelid of the cat:**
   a. The upper eyelid is affected more frequently than the lower one.
   b. They form poorly defined, ulcerated lesions.
   c. They can be multifocal tumours.
   d. They are more common than primary conjunctival squamous cell carcinomas.

4. **Which statement is incorrect regarding ocular and periocular melanocytic neoplasms in the dog:**
   a. Most melanocytic neoplasms on the cutaneous surface of the eyelid are benign.
   b. Most melanocytic neoplasms of the eyelid margin are benign.
   c. Most conjunctival melanocytic neoplasms are benign.
   d. Most uveal melanocytic neoplasms are benign.

5. **Regarding conjunctival mast cell tumours in the dog, which of the following statements is correct:**
   a. Most metastasise to regional lymph nodes.
   b. They are assessed using the same grading systems as cutaneous mast cell tumours.
   c. Most occur in the bulbar conjunctiva.
   d. They are rare tumours compared to the rest of conjunctival tumours.

6. **Regarding neoplasms of the nictitating membrane gland in domestic carnivores, point out which statement is incorrect:**
   a. Adenomas are only described in the dog.
   b. Most are squamous cell carcinomas.
   c. They can present with exophthalmia.
   d. Metastases are more common in cats than dogs.

7. **Indicate which answer is incorrect regarding purely corneal squamous cell carcinomas in the dog:**
   a. Exposure to ultraviolet radiation is the most important risk factor.
   b. Most occur in brachycephalic dog breeds.
   c. There is usually a history of chronic ocular surface disease.
   d. They are minimally invasive tumours, affecting at most the anterior third of the stroma.

8. **Which of these histological parameters is not associated with prognosis in diffuse iris melanoma in cats according to Wiggans et al., 2016?**
   a. Mitotic index greater than 7.
   b. Extrascleral extension.
   c. Necrosis within the tumour.
   d. Invasion of the scleral venous plexus vessels.

9. **Indicate the correct answer regarding iridociliary epithelial tumours in domestic carnivores:**
   a. They are the most common primary intraocular neoplasm in dogs.
   b. In cats, they are aggressive neoplasms which metastasise frequently.
   c. They are positive for vimentin in dogs and cats.
   d. Pigmented tumours are more common than non-pigmented ones in the dog.

10. **Regarding uveal lymphoma in domestic carnivores, indicate the correct answer:**
   a. In cats, they are associated with FeLV infection.
   b. The choroid is affected more often than the anterior uvea.
   c. In cats, it is the second most common intraocular neoplasm.
   d. In dogs, the phenotype is associated with the prognosis.

11. Indicate which answer is incorrect regarding schwannoma of blue-eyed dogs:

a. Huskies are one of the most frequently affected breeds.
b. Most present as discrete masses.
c. Metastases are rare.
d. It has been described in a dog with a brown iris.

12. Regarding post-traumatic sarcoma in the cat, indicate the correct answer:

a. No metastases have been described.
b. The round cell variant is the most common.
c. The round cell variant is a T-cell lymphoma.
d. The spindle cell variant originates from lens epithelial cells.

13. Identify which of the following answers is incorrect regarding metastatic neoplasms to the eye in dogs and cats:

a. Lung-eye syndrome is typical in dogs.
b. In dogs, the anterior uvea is more frequently affected than the posterior.
c. The presence of neoplastic cells lining the inner surface of the uvea is suggestive of metastatic neoplasia.
d. In cats, they can present as choroidal infarcts.

14. Regarding optic nerve tumours in the dog, indicate which is the correct answer:

a. Most gliomas are astrocytomas.
b. Metastasis of orbital meningiomas are not reported.
c. Most orbital meningiomas are of a transitional type.
d. Exophthalmia is the most common ocular sign for gliomas.

15. Indicate which of the following is incorrect regarding feline restrictive orbital myofibroblastic sarcoma:

a. Affected cats frequently present with corneal problems.
b. They do not usually form discrete masses.
c. The oral cavity can be affected.
d. Its spread is mainly by distant metastasis.

Clinical Case

Signalment: 15-year-old female entire Yorkshire Terrier.

Presenting complaint: blindness in the right eye.

Ophthalmological examination: exophthalmia and blindness in the right eye with retinal indentation. Retrobulbar mass.

- Menace response: negative in the right eye (OD) and positive in the left eye (OS).
- Slight exophthalmia with painless resistance to retropulsion. Mydriatic pupil not reactive to the chromatic and achromatic photomotor reflex. Immature cataracts. Intraocular pressure within normal range.
- Examination of the retina is made difficult by the presence of cataracts. Despite this, cupping and a marked increase in the size of the optic disc can be observed.
- Ocular ultrasound: an indentation of the eyeball is evidenced in the region adjacent to the papilla, which makes it appear cupped.

Physical examination: without other significant abnormalities.

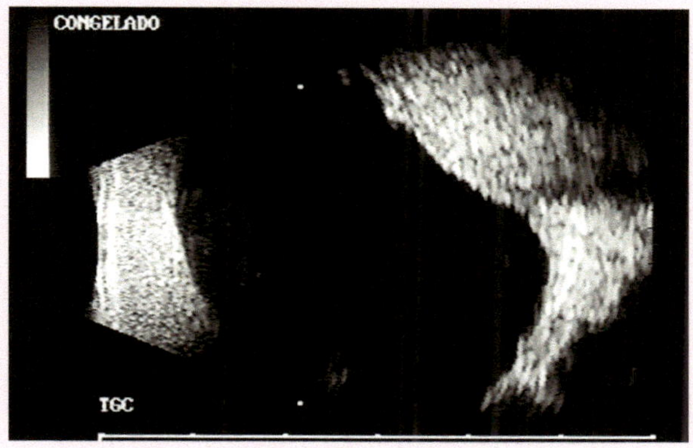

Ocular ultrasound (courtesy of Ocaña Veterinary Ophthalmology, Madrid.)

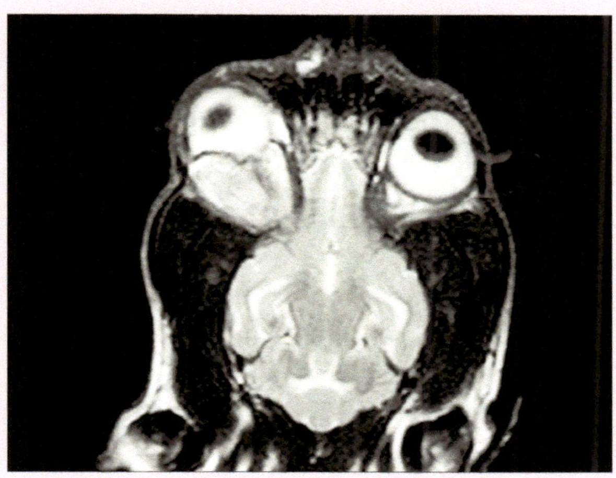

Magnetic resonance imaging (courtesy of Valentina Lorenzo, Veterinary Neurology, Getafe, Madrid.)

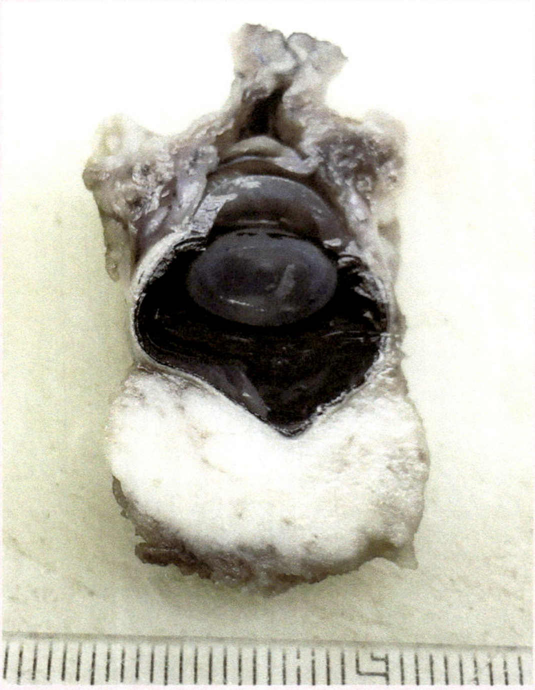

Gross image after fixation.

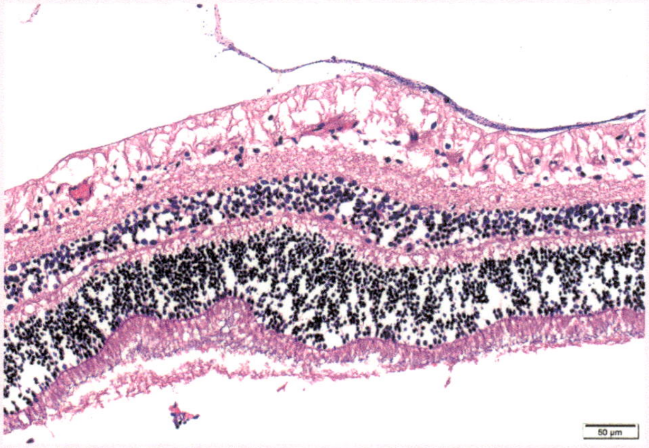

Microscopic image.

Questions:

1. **Based on the history and signalment, indicate the most likely cause of the clinical signs:**
   a. Orbital cellulitis due to a foreign body.
   b. Sialocele of the zygomatic gland.
   c. Retrobulbar neoplasm.
   d. Extraocular muscle myositis.

2. **Which of the following statements is most accurate regarding imaging studies?**
   a. Diffuse lesion of the right orbit that extends into the cranial vault.
   b. Mass lesion with scleral compression that displaces the eyeball outwards.
   c. Cavitary lesion with liquid material that compresses the eyeball.
   d. Hypermature cataract of the right eye.

3. **Considering the gross image, what would be the most likely diagnosis?**
   a. Orbital cellulitis.
   b. Sialocele of the zygomatic gland.
   c. Lacrimal gland adenocarcinoma.
   d. Orbital meningioma.

4. **What does the microscopic image of the retina show?**
   a. Ganglion cell loss.
   b. Loss of the inner nuclear layer.
   c. Loss of the outer nuclear layer.
   d. The retina is histologically normal.

5. **Which statement is most accurate regarding the prognosis?**
   a. Good after exenteration.
   b. Local recurrence is highly probable.
   c. Involvement of the orbit of the contralateral eye is very likely.
   d. Distant metastases are very likely.

Notes

Correct Answers:

Test

1. c
2. b
3. a
4. c
5. d
6. b
7. a
8. d
9. c
10. c
11. b
12. d
13. a
14. a
15. d

Clinical Case

1. c.
2. b.
3. d.
4. a.
5. b.

Notes

Gastrointestinal Neoplasms in Cats and Dogs

Pachi Clemente Vicario

Tumours of the Oral Cavity

Tumours of the oral cavity are **common in dogs** and constitute about 6–7% of tumours in this species. In general, about one third of the lesions in the mouth of dogs are malignant neoplasms of the gums, palate, or lips, one third are odontogenic tumours and the other third are inflammatory lesions. **In cats, inflammatory lesions are the most frequent**, representing half of the cases biopsied, and squamous cell carcinoma is the most common tumour, causing a third of oral lesions in the species. Regarding the tongue, half of the lesions that are biopsied are neoplasms, while in this location one in three tumours are benign.

Melanoma

Melanoma is the **most common malignant tumour in the dog's oral cavity**. Pigmented masses can be diagnosed with cytology, but unpigmented masses can be more difficult to identify as melanomas even with histopathology. Any mass diagnosed as an undifferentiated tumour in the oral cavity should include melanoma among its differentials and the use of immunohistochemistry may be necessary for a definitive diagnosis. The use of a panel of stains that includes PNL2, Melan-A, TRP-1 and TRP-2, has been proposed to increase sensitivity and specificity in the diagnosis.

Given the suspicion of oral melanoma, **establishing the clinical stage is essential** due to its importance in the prognosis and choice of treatment. Tumour size, lymph node evaluation and distant metastases (mainly in the lung) are the factors that affect the clinical stage.

To determine the true extent of the primary tumour, the use of **advanced imaging techniques** such as computed tomography is necessary. Studies with CT and contrast injected into the tumour have shown how oral melanoma can metastasise to different lymph nodes, both ipsilaterally and contralaterally, as well as submandibular and retropharyngeal. In more than a third of cases, all four lymph nodes are affected.

The size of the lymph node cannot be used to diagnose metastasis because **a normal size does not rule out the presence of tumour cells**. Cytology can be useful in clear cases in which melanocytes are recognised with characteristics of malignancy, which should not be confused with melanophages (Figure 1),

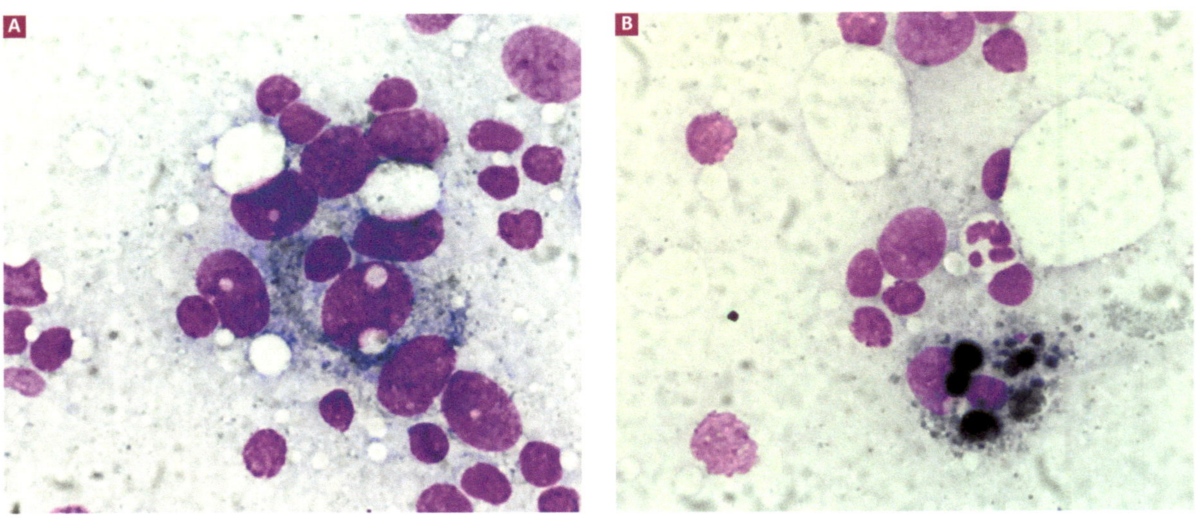

Figure 1. Cytological image of the mandibular lymph node of a dog with melanoma of the soft palate. The left image (**A**) shows a multinucleated melanocyte, with small, dark granules of dark pigment, which indicate lymphatic metastasis. In the image on the right hand side (**B**), of the same sample a melanophage can be seen. The granules are much larger in size. Melanophages can be observed after causing lesions in pigmented areas and this does not mean that there are metastasis.

although there is not a good correlation between cytology and histopathology and false negatives may occur.

In addition to the clinical stage, there are factors such as the location of the tumour that are important, since the prognosis is better in melanomas located on the lip or tongue compared to those located in the maxilla or palate when treated surgically.

In localised tumours, **surgery with curative intent (with wide margins)** can obtain particularly good results, especially in tumours smaller than 3 cm, with disease-free intervals of about fifteen months and an average survival time of two years (Figure 2). The use of adjuvant chemotherapy after surgery does not appear to offer any benefit. Median survivals with surgery are about two years for stages I and II, and about seven months for stage III.

In localised cases where surgery is not possible, **radiotherapy** can be used, with hypofractionated protocols (e.g. 4 x 8 Gy, administered once a week). Median survival times with radiotherapy depend on the clinical stage, but not on the location in the oral cavity, and are 25, 9, 5 and 2 months for clinical stages I, II, III, and IV, respectively.

For cases with distant metastasis, the treatment options are limited, since it is considered a **chemoresistant tumour** and only about a quarter of the tumours seem to respond to carboplatin, with only a partial response in most of the cases that respond.

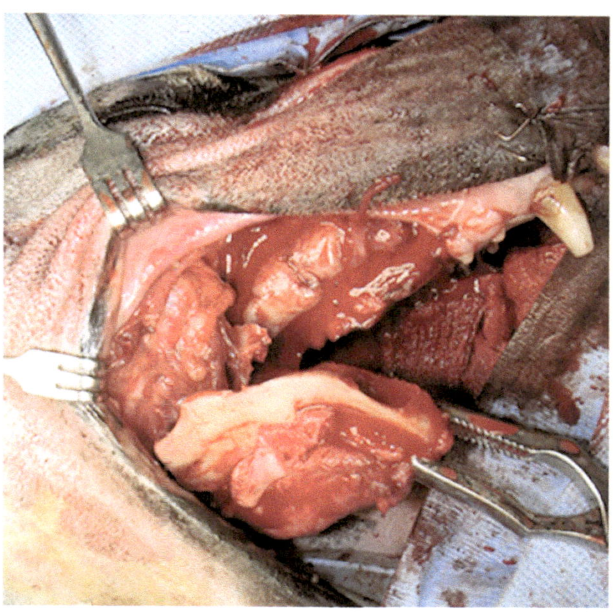

Figure 2. Surgery with curative intention: after performing studies with CT the tumour is removed with a margin of healthy tissue which includes bone from the maxilla. (Image courtesy of Judith Bertrán, DACVS fellowship Surgical Oncology).

Another therapeutic approach has included **immunotherapy**. A vaccine (Oncept Melanoma®) was developed against canine oral melanoma that uses a fragment of human DNA that encodes tyrosinase, a glycoprotein essential in the production of melanin and that is overexpressed in melanoma. By encoding human tyrosine, the canine immune system recognises it as foreign and produces a response against it (which also affects cells that express canine tyrosinase, which is similar).

In an initial study, when it was administered to dogs with clinical stage I to III (without distant metastases) and with good local control of the disease (after surgery and/or radiotherapy), a favourable response was observed, with survival in the group who received the vaccine for more than 1000 days versus 550 days for the group that did not receive it (using a historical control group). However, another study found no benefit in disease-free or survival time when the vaccinated and the non-vaccinated group were compared.

In summary, although it seems well tolerated, there is no clear evidence that its use represents a benefit in patient survival time, although, since these are patients who frequently receive multiple therapies, it is difficult to know the specific effects of each one. However, responses have been documented in some patients with gross disease treated with the vaccine alone.

Other approaches with immunotherapy, still under investigation, include the use of checkpoint inhibitors such as PD-L1 (Programmed Death Ligand 1).

Squamous Cell Carcinoma

This is the **second most frequent tumour type in the oral cavity of the dog and the first in cats. Diagnosis can be cytological**, and the samples contain basal and squamous cells, with angled edges and marked pleomorphism. Many of these squamous cells present an immature nucleus (compared to the mature, small, condensed, or absent nucleus of normal squamous cells), which represents a lack of synchronisation between nuclear and cytoplasmic maturation that is characteristic of this tumour. Sometimes they are accompanied by an inflammatory infiltrate that can make the cytological diagnosis between inflammation and dysplasia or neoplasia with secondary inflammation difficult. In these cases, a biopsy is necessary for diagnosis.

It is a **locally aggressive tumour and frequently invades the underlying bone**. In addition, in dogs there are lymph node **metastases** in a third of cases and distant ones in 5% although the rate of metastasis depends on the location of the tumour and is higher in caudal tumours and lower in rostral tumours. In cats, Soltero-Rivera et al. have shown that 30% of cases have regional lymph node metastases and 10% distant metastases. Thus, before making decisions about treatment, evaluation of the lymph nodes and the thorax is necessary, especially in cases of squamous cell carcinomas of the tonsils or base of the tongue, which are associated with a higher rate of metastasis.

For **canine tumours, aggressive surgery involving the underlying bone** is the treatment of choice when there is no metastasis. In dogs, mandibulectomy offers a median survival time of about two years and more than 90% of patients live for one year from diagnosis. The recurrence rate associated with mandibulectomy is 10%. However, with tumours originating in the maxilla, the prognosis is worse, and the recurrence rate is 29% and the median survival is only time 1–1.5 years, with 57% of dogs alive one year after diagnosis. For tumours treated with **surgery and radiation therapy** (for residual disease), the median survival time is more than two and a half years.

In cases treated with **radiotherapy**, the prognosis depends on the clinical stage, with a survival time of five years for tumours less than 2 cm, two years for tumours of 2–4 cm, and eight months for tumours greater than 4 cm. In patients with metastatic disease, **piroxicam** has a response rate of 17% and this increases to 56% if associated with cisplatin, although due to renal toxicity this combination is not recommended and a combination of piroxicam and carboplatin is used.

Recent studies confirm a good prognosis for squamous cell carcinoma treated with aggressive surgery, with long mean survival times (more than half of the cases were still alive and mean survival time could not be calculated) and differences depending on the location and size of the tumour. In cases with dirty margins, adjuvant radiation therapy helps control the disease. Preliminary data, to be confirmed with larger series of cases, indicate that in small tumours, less than 2 cm in size and not located in the tonsils, electrochemotherapy can achieve long-lasting complete remissions. Papillary squamous cell carcinoma in dogs appears to have a less aggressive clinical course and its immunohistochemical profile is well described.

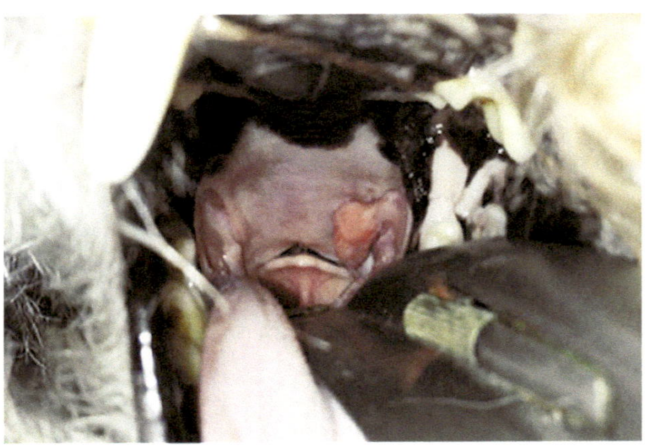

Figure 3. Abnormally large tonsil in a West Highland White Terrier who was brought for a consult due to a mass in the neck.

Squamous cell carcinoma is the **most common tumour in the tonsils**. Sometimes it can be diagnosed from an increase in their size (Figures 3 and 4), but in other cases the size can be normal and present marked metastatic lymphadenopathy. By location, tonsillar squamous cell carcinoma has the highest metastasis rate.

In the case of **feline squamous cell carcinoma**, the prognosis is worse, and the one-year survival rate is less than 10%. It is the most common tumour in the oral cavity in cats. One of the reasons for its poor prognosis is that it is considered a **chemoresistant** tumour. In fact, a study that tested nearly 2000 drugs in feline squamous carcinoma cell lines found only four that could potentially be effective, data that now need to be corroborated in vivo. The **results obtained with radiotherapy are also modest**, with progression-free intervals of about six months, but with marked toxicity associated with the treatment.

The use of **toceranib phosphate** (Palladia, Zoetis), associated with other therapies, with a mean treatment duration of two months, has also been investigated. In about half of the cases, progression or partial remission appears to stabilise, and these cases have longer survival times. However, overall, the median survival time for cats treated with toceranib is four months. If surgery is being considered for these tumours, it is necessary to inform owners of the need for oesophagostomy tubes, which in some cases may be required permanently.

Fibrosarcoma

Fibrosarcoma is the **third most common tumour in the oral cavity of dogs and the second most common in cats**. It is

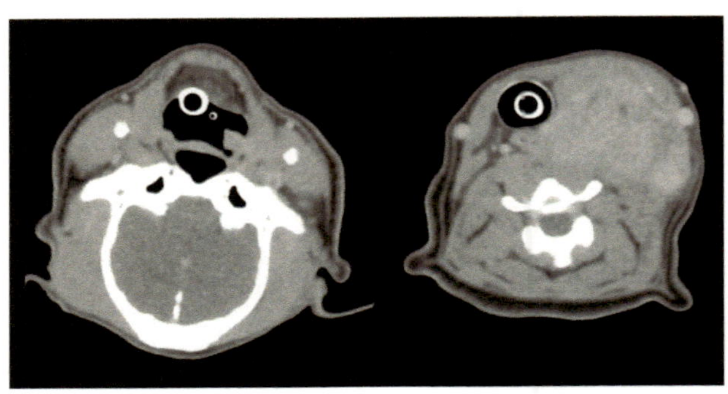

Figure 4. CT images of the case from Figure 3, where the enlarged tonsil and the large mass in the neck can be seen, result of lymphatic metastasis.

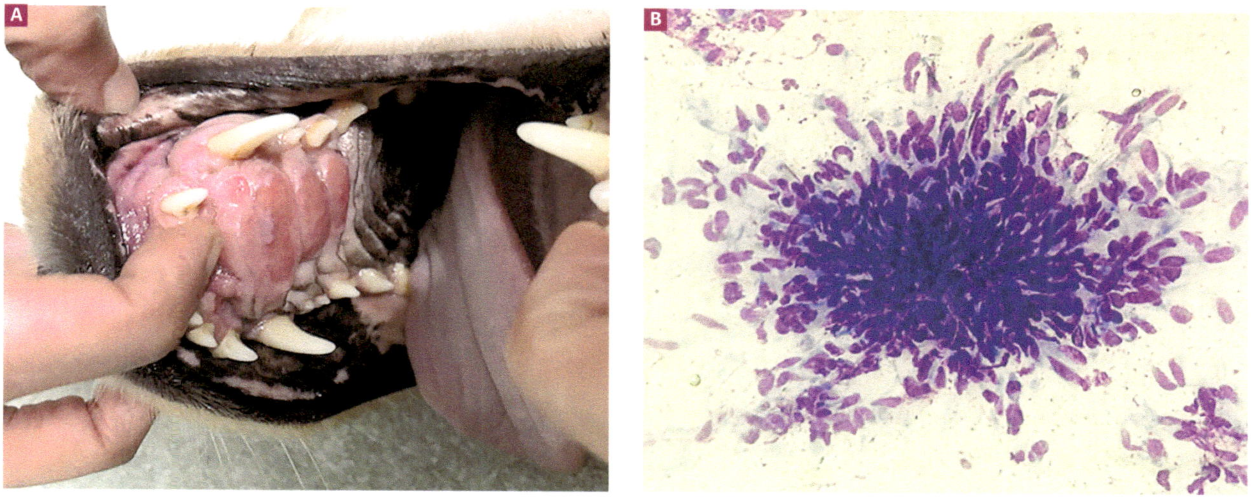

Figure 5. Macroscopic (**A**) and cytological (**B**) images of an oral fibrosarcoma in an 8-year-old Labrador Retriever. The cytology shows an abundant population of mesenchymal cells.

most often seen in large breed dogs (Labradors and Golden Retrievers, in particular) at 7–8 years of age (Figure 5).

The **cytological diagnosis** of sarcomas is based on the presence of spindle cells, with a moderate nucleus/cytoplasm ratio, basophilic cytoplasm, and an oval central nucleus with one or more nucleoli. However, cytology shows a well-differentiated population of fibroblasts in fibromas, well-differentiated fibrosarcoma's, or reactive fibroplasia, seen in granulation tissue or scars.

For a definitive diagnosis, a **biopsy is essential**, although it also has limitations from a prognostic point of view. A well-defined condition is low-grade, high-biological-grade fibrosarcoma, which appears histologically to be a low-grade process, but with a very aggressive biological behaviour that requires radical treatment. Furthermore, the histological grade of the pre-treatment biopsy does not coincide with the histological grade of the tumour after surgery in 40% of the cases: in 30% of the cases, it underestimates the grade and in 10% it indicates a grade higher than the real one. The owner should be informed of this possibility if the decision regarding treatment will be made based on the biopsy result.

Although fibrosarcoma is characterised by being locally aggressive and having a low rate of metastasis, the disease spreads to lymph nodes in about 20% of cases and to the lung in up to 27% so clinical staging should be performed in all cases before making therapeutic decisions.

The **prognosis is reserved** and, in general, local control is the greatest challenge, with a recurrence rate of 60% in mandibulectomies, 40% in maxillectomies, and a mean survival time of one year in both cases. Although they are considered resistant to radiotherapy (median survival time is seven months when treated with radiation alone), the use of **radiotherapy after surgery** reduces recurrence to 30% and increases median survival time to 18–26 months (with 75% of patients alive one year after diagnosis). Recent studies have found no benefit in irradiating cases of dirty margins, highlighting the importance of obtaining clean margins in surgery, due to the implication in the prognosis of the disease. In particular, the prognosis is better for smaller tumours (Table 1). In addition to the location (better in the maxilla), the clinical stage, the type of surgery (aggressive rather than conservative) and the histological grade (better in grade I than in II or III) are determining factors in the survival of the patient.

Regarding tumour recurrence, prognostic factors are the breed (worse prognosis in Golden Retrievers) and whether clean margins are achieved in surgery.

The prognosis has improved in recent years with longer survival times than in studies prior to 2000.

Table 1. Relationship between the size of fibrosarcoma's and the mean survival time of diagnosed patients.

Tumour size	Average survival time
<2 cm	45 months
2–4 cm	31 months
>4 cm	7 months

Odontogenic Tumours

Acanthomatous ameloblastoma occurs mainly in the rostral jaw and the Golden Retriever, Akita Inu and Cocker Spaniel are overrepresented breeds. Although it generally affects older dogs, it can also be seen in young dogs.

In advanced imaging studies (tomography) it can be seen that they affect multiple teeth with lysis of the alveolar bone and displacement of the tooth due to the mass effect.

Surgery is associated with a good prognosis with a very low recurrence rate. If surgery is not possible, the use of intratumoural chemotherapy may be considered (always using closed chemotherapy delivery systems to reduce environmental contamination).

Gastrointestinal Lymphoma

Gastrointestinal lymphoma can affect both dogs and cats, but while in the former it accounts for only 5–7% of cases of lymphoma, in cats the gastrointestinal form is the most frequent presentation of lymphoma at present. Since the feline leukaemia virus vaccine was marketed, there has been a decrease in lymphomas directly associated with the virus (mediastinal form, in young cats) and an increase in forms not associated with infection (mainly digestive, in older cats).

Lymphoma is the **most common gastrointestinal tumour in cats**. The clinical signs are non-specific and are associated with the digestive tract, with weight loss, vomiting or diarrhoea, and anorexia in most cases. It mainly affects 12–13-year-old cats and represents a variety of clinical presentations that include different immunophenotypes (B and T), grades (high and low), and anatomical locations. These factors are associated with different prognoses and treatments, so it is essential to have a complete diagnosis before making decisions regarding treatment.

High-grade Feline Gastrointestinal Lymphoma

Most of these cases can be diagnosed by **cytology** of digestive masses or enlarged lymph nodes, in which a homogeneous cell population of large lymphocytes is observed. Occasionally, digestive lymphoma is located only in the stomach, and in these cases, it is B-cell. In general, regardless of the location or the protocol used (COP type or CHOP type), the **most important prognostic factor is the response to treatment** (Table 2). Different studies show a response rate of around 50% for complete remission and an additional 20–25% for partial remission, with a mean survival time between ten and twenty months for complete remissions, although it is much lower in cases of stable or progressive disease.

Table 2. Treatment protocol commonly used by the author.

Week	Medication	Dose
1	Vincristine	0.5–0.7 mg/m² IV
2	Cyclophosphamide	50 mg/cat PO
3	Vincristine	0.5–0.7 mg/m² IV
4	Methotrexate	2.5 mg/cat PO

During the protocol, prednisone or prednisolone is administered at 1 mg/kg/day. This protocol is repeated weekly for six months, every two weeks for six more months, and every three weeks for six months (eighteen months total duration).

Feline Large Granular Lymphocyte Lymphoma

This subtype of large cell or high-grade lymphoma is **characterised by the presence of granules in the cytoplasm of large lymphocytes**. These granules may look different depending on the stain used. With Diff-Quick, the stain commonly used in most practices, they are eosinophilic in colour (Figure 6).

Lymphocyte lymphoma with granules in its cytoplasm has been associated with a **very poor prognosis** since it was first described, with average survival times of just a couple of weeks and a low response rate to treatment (less than 10%), data which is corroborated in a furthermore recent study of more than 100 cases (Finotello *et al.*, 2018). This latest study showed the difficulties in identifying these granules with haematoxylin-eosin, while with cytology they are more easily observed. Therefore, the author recommends performing an imprint cytology prior to specimen fixation when performing surgical or endoscopic biopsies.

Low-grade Feline Digestive Lymphoma

This is the **most common form of feline digestive lymphoma**, causing about 50–70% of cases. The clinical, analytical, and even histopathological presentation are similar in cases of

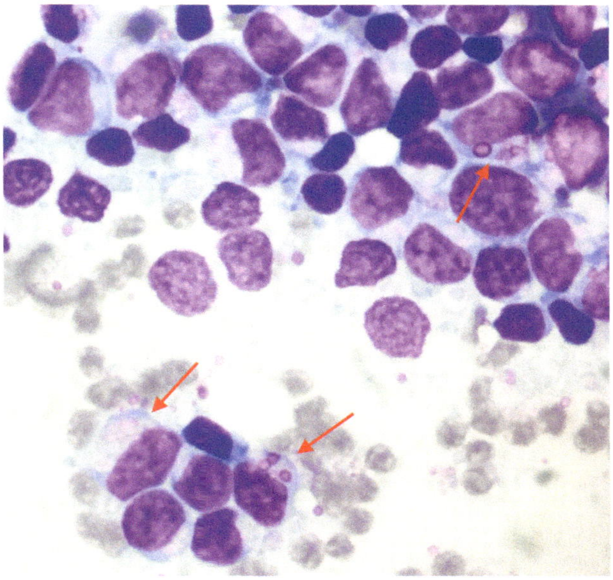

Figure 6. Cytological image of abdominal lymphadenopathy in a 6-year-old Common European cat. Eosinophilic granules can be seen in the cytoplasm of some lymphoblasts (arrows). The diagnosis is large granular lymphocyte lymphoma.

inflammatory bowel disease and low-grade feline lymphoma, and different studies show that different tests may be necessary to make a definitive diagnosis. By adding immunohistochemistry and clonality tests, many cases go from an initial diagnosis of inflammatory disease to that of lymphoma, increasing the percentage of lymphoma diagnoses from 20% (with biopsy) to 50% of cases (with biopsy, immunohistochemistry and clonality).

However, a study published in 2019 showed that more than half of healthy cats (12 out of 20), without digestive signs, had results compatible with the diagnosis of low-grade lymphoma when applying this diagnostic procedure (histopathology, immunohistochemistry and clonality test), although only two out of twenty developed clinical signs compatible with the disease months later. Therefore, a **clinical interpretation that combines the clinical signs with the findings of diagnostic tests** is necessary to assess when to start treatment, at least until there are more data on the necessary follow-up in these animals diagnosed before there are symptoms.

The cause of low-grade intestinal lymphoma is unknown. Some studies have shown that the microbiota present in cats with lymphoma and cats with inflammatory disease is different and a greater number of dendritic myeloid cells associated with these changes has been identified in cats with lymphoma. However, it is not known whether these changes are a cause or consequence of the disease and further studies are needed to determine this.

Small cell lymphoma is usually treated with **prednisone (or prednisolone) and chlorambucil**. The response rate is very high and the prognosis generally good, with a survival time of several years. However, it must be taken into account that it may take time to reach the maximum response and although only 25% of cases are in complete remission after one month of treatment, this increases to 50% after three months. Pope et al. propose that if there is complete remission one year after diagnosis, prednisone and chlorambucil therapy should be interrupted, to be reinstated when there is recurrence. This approach was more effective than maintaining prednisone/chlorambucil therapy indefinitely until relapse and administration of lomustine. In any case, if there is no response to prednisone/chlorambucil (after waiting the appropriate time), lomustine may be considered as a rescue option, which is associated with a response rate in about 50% of cases.

Digestive Lymphoma in Dogs

Gastrointestinal lymphoma in dogs is a **rare presentation** (about 5% of canine lymphomas). Prognosis depends on the grade (high or low) and location of the lesions. High-grade disease usually affects the entire digestive tract diffusely, with the lymph nodes and liver often also affected. Chemotherapy with CHOP-type protocols, in general, has not achieved good results and the prognosis is poor, with a mean survival time of two months. Although the difference is not significant, the cases treated with lomustine have a mean survival time of four months. However, these high-grade lymphomas that are located in the colon and rectum show a good response to chemotherapy with average survival times of 5–6 years.

Low-grade digestive lymphomas are less common. Two studies published in 2018 with a total of 37 cases showed the benefit of medical treatment, with a mean survival time of twenty months if they were treated, compared to nine months without treatment and eighteen months if remission was achieved (partial or total) compared to three months if they did not respond or were not treated. These cases can be difficult to differentiate from inflammatory bowel disease and molecular tests in addition to biopsy may be necessary, similar to what occurs in cats.

Gastric Carcinoma

This is a **rare tumour in dogs** (it represents less than 1% of tumours in this species) and is usually diagnosed in advanced stages with about 75% of cases with metastasis. Compared with chronic gastritis, dogs with carcinoma are usually older (nine years with carcinoma versus 6–7 in cases of gastritis) and present with worse body condition.

Ultrasound is useful to detect neoplasia in half of cases, while endoscopy is diagnostic in more than 90% of cases. The Belgian Tervuren Shepherd seems to be predisposed to this tumour, at least in northern Europe. The prognosis for this tumour is poor and survival times with surgery and/or chemotherapy do not usually exceed two months.

Many of these tumours overexpress HER-2, a tyrosine kinase receptor in the epidermal growth factor receptor (EGFR) family. Human tumours that overexpress this receptor can be treated with trastuzumab, an anti-HER-2 monoclonal antibody that has improved prognosis compared to conventional chemotherapy treatments. Although there is currently no monoclonal antibody against canine HER-2 the fact that this tumour expresses a large amount of this receptor opens the door to the option of immunotherapy.

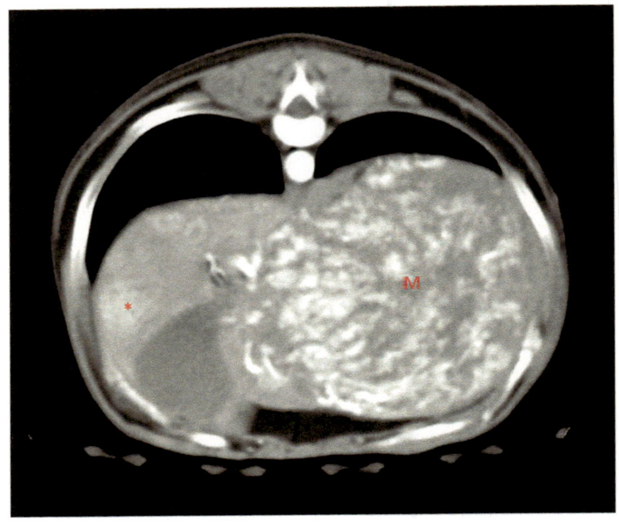

Figure 7. CT image of a massive hepatocellular carcinoma (M) on the left side which was surgically removed in its entirety. An area where contrast uptake can be seen in the right lobe (asterisk). The previous cytology of this area does not display signs of malignancy and the biopsy confirms hyperplasia.

Hepatic Tumours

Primary liver tumours are not common in dogs. However, **metastases** can present in the liver, from splenic, pancreatic, and digestive tumours from the portal venous system that drains these organs, or be affected by systemic conditions such as lymphoma, histiocytic tumours, or mast cell tumours. They can also present benign lesions such as nodular hyperplasia or extramedullary haematopoiesis. In cats, primary liver tumours are also less common than metastases.

The four **primary tumours** that affect dogs and cats are hepatocellular carcinoma, bile duct carcinoma, neuroendocrine tumours, and mesenchymal tumours (haemangiosarcoma, leiomyosarcoma, fibrosarcoma...). The malignant ones are more frequent in dogs and the benign ones more frequent in cats.

There are three types of tumour morphology:

- **massive**: single, large masses affecting a single lobe (Figure 7);
- **nodular**: multifocal tumours, affecting several liver lobes; and
- **diffuse**: multiple nodules, extending through all lobes and infiltrating most of the liver parenchyma. The prognosis depends on both the histological diagnosis and the morphological presentation, which is good for massive hepatocellular carcinoma and benign lesions and poor for nodular and diffuse lesions.

Imaging techniques are not sufficient to differentiate between the different histological types, although they have shown that size of the mass is related to different diagnoses: the smallest lesions (4 cm on average) are more frequently diagnosed as hyperplastic nodules, while lesions measuring 8 cm on average are usually diagnosed as adenomas and larger lesions measuring 10 cm on average as hepatocellular carcinomas.

However, **cytology or histology are necessary** for a definitive diagnosis. Cytology has different sensitivity and specificity for different types of tumours: it is more reliable for round cell tumours such as lymphoma and less reliable for hepatocellular carcinoma. This is because well-differentiated hepatocellular carcinomas (Figure 8) are cytologically similar to adenomas or hyperplastic nodules, making differentiation difficult. Although cytology (Figure 9) can be performed without complications, as long as there is an adequate number of platelets, biopsies are taken only after clotting tests are done.

The **treatment for massive hepatocellular carcinoma** (the most common presentation, forming more than half of the cases of hepatocellular carcinoma) is **surgical removal**. The technique has a mortality rate of 5% during surgery and a complication rate of around 30% with intrasurgical bleeding (which may require blood transfusion during or immediately after surgery) and hypoglycaemia, mainly. If it can be treated surgically, the prognosis is better (survival time greater than four years) than if not treated surgically (median survival time of nine months).

The location of the tumour in the liver is associated with different rates of complications: tumours on the right side present a greater risk of death during surgery (due to injuries to the

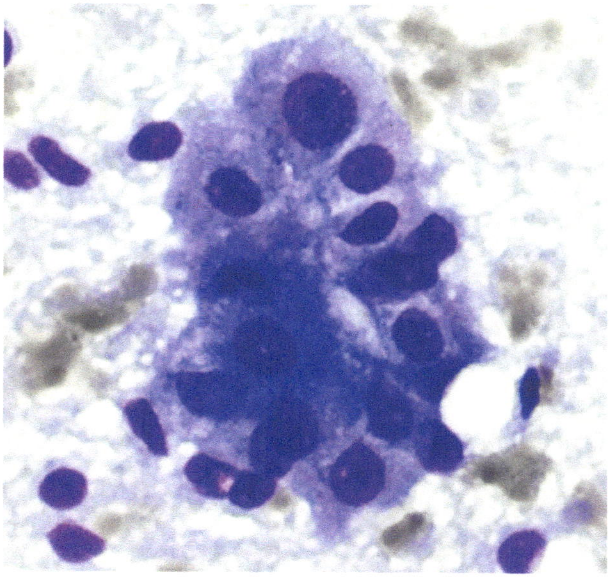

Figure 8. Cytology of the mass seen in Figure 7. The hepatocytes show marked anisocytosis and anisokaryosis. The histological diagnosis was hepatocellular carcinoma.

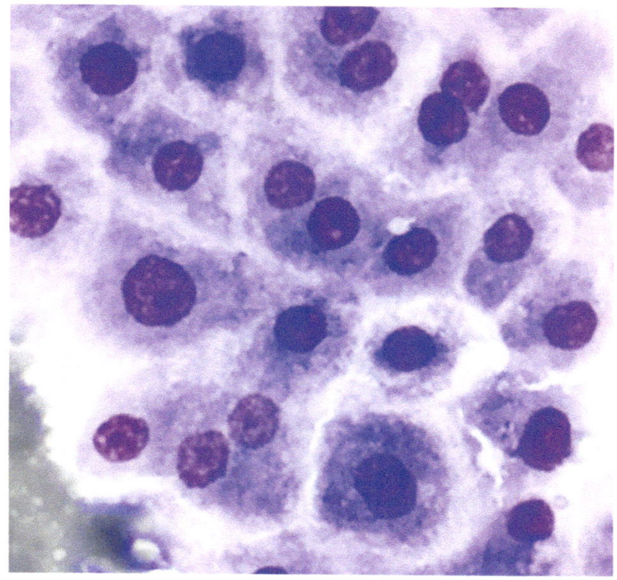

Figure 9. Cytology of the right liver lobe of the case seen in Figures 7 and 8. The cytology shows mild anisocytosis and anisokaryosis in some cells. It is difficult to differentiate between hyperplasia and well-differentiated carcinomas using cytology.

caudal vena cava). However, if the patient survives the procedure, the prognosis is similar to that of patients with tumours on the left side. Local recurrence is 0–13% and metastases are rare, although in postmortem studies they are present in up to 60%. Liver surgery should be performed by experienced surgeons and in hospitals with the capacity for intensive care if necessary.

The prognosis for nodular (30% of cases) and diffuse (10%) presentations of liver carcinoma is poor. Surgical resection is not possible and there are no good medical alternatives for this type of tumour. In addition, the metastasis rate is high (90% for the nodular form and 100% for the diffuse one).

In nonsurgical cases, the use of **radiofrequency or microwave ablation**, either guided by ultrasound or by laparotomy, may be considered. These techniques generate heat in the tumour tissue until it produces necrosis. Although there are a small series of cases, there are no data yet to provide information on response rate or survival. While more data is not available, **this should not replace surgery when performing it is possible**. Selective embolisation has also been investigated with promising results, although this is a technique that requires interventional radiology equipment. Partial remission of inoperable tumours has been documented in 50% of cases treated with toceranib phosphate (Palladia, Zoetis), which may be an option for cases where surgery is not possible.

Treatment for bile duct tumours is similar, with surgery for single lesions (or affecting up to two liver lobes). However, the prognosis is worse in the case of biliary carcinomas (compared to hepatocellular carcinoma) because the majority of cases present local recurrence or metastasis and have a median survival time of six months.

Intestinal Carcinoma

Carcinoma is the **second most common intestinal tumour in cats after digestive lymphoma**. Treatment with surgery improves the prognosis, with median survival times of less than one month when surgery is not performed versus one year when treated surgically. Initial studies have also shown the benefits of using adjuvant chemotherapy. The combination of surgery and chemotherapy (carboplatin) offers better results in cases without metastases to regional lymph nodes than in those with metastatic disease at diagnosis.

In **dogs**, surgical treatment of carcinomas is associated with a good prognosis and although a study showed that survival times after adding chemotherapy were increased by four months, the difference was not significant. The use of toceranib phosphate after surgery was associated with better survival times, of more than one year on average, than cases treated only with surgery, with a mean survival time of ten months. Excision at 3 cm from the palpable end of the intestinal mass was associated with complete excision in all cases.

Gastrointestinal Stromal Tumours

Different studies have found that **around half of tumours traditionally diagnosed as intestinal mesenchymal tumours** (mainly leiomyosarcomas) are intestinal stromal tumours. Gastrointestinal stromal tumours originate from cells of Cajal and are positive for KIT on immunohistochemistry.

In dogs, 3% of stromal tumours did not express KIT but did express DOG-1, a stain that can be used to confirm these cases. Gastrointestinal stromal tumours are also positive for vimentin. The distinction is important because biological behaviour and treatment are different. There are no characteristics that allow them to be distinguished sonographically and immunohistochemical tests are necessary.

A third of the cases present metastases (omentum, lymph nodes and liver, mainly) at the time of diagnosis. The prognosis is similar regardless of the location. Stromal tumours with a larger size and heterogeneous appearance on ultrasound (hypoechoic areas) are correlated with more aggressive tumours and an increased risk of metastasis.

The c-kit receptor has a mutation on exon 11 in about one third of gastrointestinal stromal tumour cases. With techniques such as reverse transcriptase PCR (RT-PCR), up to ten different mutations have been detected in almost 75% of tumours, although the presence or absence of mutations could not be correlated with different KIT staining patterns.

Complete remissions have been documented in metastatic cases treated with c-kit inhibitors, both with imatinib in the presence of a c-kit mutation, and with toceranib (Palladia®) in cases without a mutation. Recent studies with toceranib show a clinical benefit (complete or partial remission or stable disease) in 70% of cases, with a better prognosis in cases without metastases at diagnosis and with lower mitotic counts.

For the most part, leiomyosarcomas do not usually metastasise, although more advanced cases can affect all intestinal layers, reach the exterior and affect the omentum locally. Median survival times are 1 year and 8 months for stromal tumours and leiomyosarcomas, respectively. However, if those cases in which death occurs in the immediate postoperative period (perforations, peritonitis) are excluded, the median survival time for stromal tumours is 37 months, compared to 8 months for leiomyosarcomas.

Undifferentiated sarcomas are a group (12–25% of intestinal sarcomas) that cannot be classified as stromal tumours or leiomyosarcomas as they are negative for KIT and SMA but are positive for vimentin. Their behaviour is more aggressive, with an average survival time of about three months.

Perianal Tumours: Anal Sac Adenocarcinoma

The clinical signs associated with anal sac adenocarcinoma may be caused by the primary tumour (perianal inflammation or pain) or by metastatic disease in regional lymph nodes (tenesmus and constipation). In some cases, the animals have clinical signs secondary to paraneoplastic hypercalcaemia (polyuria, polydipsia, anorexia, vomiting, and lethargy). Up to 30% of cases are diagnosed after the incidental finding during a routine physical examination. If an anal sac tumour is suspected, diagnostic tests are necessary to confirm the diagnosis and determine the extent of the tumour.

The **initial diagnosis can be made by cytology** (Figure 10). Although it does not have a neuroendocrine origin, the cytological appearance is similar to these tumours. They are highly cellular samples with clusters of cells with poorly defined cytoplasmic margins and intercellular junctions. Cells are fragile and it is common to find numerous free, intact nuclei from ruptured cells, which are called bare nuclei in some texts. Criteria for malignancy are very subtle, and anisocytosis and anisokaryosis can be very mild. Despite the cytological appearance, the biological behaviour of the tumour is aggressive, and a complete clinical staging is necessary before making treatment decisions.

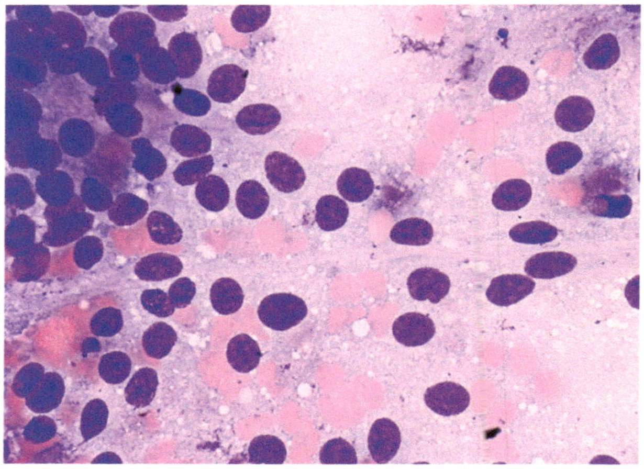

Figure 10. Cytological image of an anal sac carcinoma. There is very moderate anisokaryosis. The nucleoli can also be seen, but there are not marked features of malignancy even though the tumour had metastasised to lymph nodes at the time of diagnosis.

Radiographs or abdominal ultrasound may show marked regional lymphadenopathy, although the second method is superior to radiographs in detecting metastatic disease, not only in the appearance of the lymph nodes (cavitation or uniformity of the node parenchyma), but in the evaluation of lesions in other organs such as spleen or liver. However, **advanced imaging techniques such as tomography are more sensitive** in detecting lymphadenopathy. Pollard et al. identified sacral lymphadenopathy in fifteen cases using computed tomography, which was not identified in any of the cases using ultrasound.

The sacral lymph nodes, in addition to the iliac ones, are sentinel nodes for anal sac tumours, both ipsilateral and contralateral, so a thorough examination is necessary before offering the owner information on prognosis or treatment options. To rule out the presence of pulmonary metastases, three thoracic radiographs (right and left lateral, and ventrodorsal) should be performed.

The clinical stage is associated with differences in prognosis, with tumours smaller than 2 cm in diameter associated with tumour control for more than two years in 60% of cases. Similarly, in tumours less than 3 cm in diameter, without metastasis, surgery as the only treatment can achieve good long-term control with a median survival time of 4 years. However, 20% of the dogs had local recurrence (on average, one year after surgery) and 26% metastasis (18 months after surgery).

Up to 50% of cases have metastases at the time of diagnosis. Traditionally, removal of the primary tumour and lymph node metastases followed occasionally by chemotherapy has been recommended. When treated with surgery alone (by removing the primary tumour and metastases), the median survival time is about 10 months. The presence of lymphatic or vascular invasion is associated with a worse prognosis. The complication rate when removing iliac lymph nodes is low if the procedure is performed by an experienced surgeon, but it should always be carried out in centres that can provide intensive care and blood transfusions if necessary. The rate of local recurrence and recurrence of lymph node metastasis is 12 and 42% respectively.

In cases with lymph node metastases, **radiotherapy** with hypofractionated protocols (8 x 3.8 Gy over 2.5 weeks) obtain disease-free intervals (11 months) and survival times (15 months) which are longer than with surgery (5 and 6 months respectively). Symptoms secondary to the tumour, such as difficulty defaecating or hypercalcaemia, improved rapidly with the administration of radiotherapy.

The **benefit of chemotherapy is unclear**. Median survival times of 20 months (surgery and chemotherapy with melphalan), 17 months (surgery, chemotherapy with carboplatin and radiotherapy), or 31 months (surgery, radiotherapy and chemotherapy with mitoxantrone) have been reported, but the most effective treatment in each case is not clear, because there are no well-designed clinical trials and the data currently available come from series of cases treated very differently and with different clinical stages. Although some studies show poorer survival if chemotherapy is used, it may be because it is used in more advanced cases or with metastases, which may in themselves worsen the prognosis. It is the clinical stage (size of the primary tumour and presence of metastases) that affects the prognosis and not the use or not of adjuvant chemotherapy.

In cases of hypercalcaemia, this can be resolved if the primary tumour can be removed. A relapse of hypercalcaemia is usually associated with local recurrence or metastasis. However, due to the size of the published case series, the role of hypercalcaemia in the prognosis of the disease is unclear.

The use of **tyrosine kinase inhibitors** has shown efficacy in the management of metastatic disease. The mechanism by which they respond to toceranib is not completely clear, but it appears that it is not dependent on KIT or vascular endothelial growth factor receptor (VEGFR), but rather dependent on RET inhibition. About 20% of cases show partial remission and 50% stable disease, with prolonged survival. A study of 36 dogs (80% of them with lymph node metastases and 16% with lung metastases) had a mean survival time of 27 months, which was better in cases with a partial response (mean survival time of 34 months) than in those with stable disease (12 months) or progressive disease (2.5 months).

Bibliography

- Amory, J.T., Reetz, J.A., Sánchez, M.D. et al. (2014) Computed tomographic characteristics of odontogenic neoplasms in dogs. *Vet Radiol Ultrasound*, 55(2):147–158. doi:10.1111/vru.12101.
- Arteaga, T.A., McKnight, J., Bergman, P.J. (2012) A Review of 18 Cases of Feline Colonic Adenocarcinoma Treated with Subtotal Colectomies and Adjuvant Carboplatin. *Journal of the American Animal Hospital Association*, 48(6):399–404. doi:10.5326/JAAHA-MS-5807.
- Bahr, K.L., Sharkey. L.C., Murakami, T. et al. (2013) Accuracy of US-guided FNA of focal liver lesions in dogs: 140 cases (2005–2008). *Journal of the American Animal Hospital Association*, 49(3):190–196. doi:10.5326/JAAHA-MS-5851.
- Barnes, D.C., Demetriou, J.L. (2017) Surgical management of primary, metastatic, and recurrent anal sac adenocarcinoma in the dog: 52 cases. *Journal of Small Animal Practice*, 58(5):263–268. doi:10.1111/jsap.12633.
- Berger, E.P., Johannes, C.M., Jergens, A.E. et al. (2018) Retrospective evaluation of toceranib phosphate (Palladia®) use in the treatment of gastrointestinal stromal tumors of dogs. *J Vet Intern Med*, 50(1):412. doi:10.1111/jvim.15335.
- Boston, S.E., Lu, X., Culp, W.T.N. et al. (2014) Efficacy of systemic adjuvant therapies administered to dogs after excision of oral malignant melanomas: 151 cases (2001–2012). *J Am Vet Med Assoc*, 245(4):401–407. doi:10.2460/javma.245.4.401.
- Brockley, L.K., Cooper, M.A., Bennett, P.F. (2013) Malignant melanoma in 63 dogs (2001–2011): the effect of carboplatin chemotherapy on survival. *New Zealand Veterinary Journal*, 61(1):25–31. doi:10.1080/00480169.2012.699433.
- Candido, M.V., Syrjä, P., Kilpinen, S. et al. (2018) Canine breeds associated with gastric carcinoma, metaplasia and dysplasia diagnosed by histopathology of endoscopic biopsy samples. *Acta Veterinaria Scandinavica*, 60(1):37. doi:10.1186/s13028-018-0392-6.
- Carrasco, V., Rodriguez-Bertos, A., Rodriguez-Franco. F. et al. (2015) Distinguishing Intestinal Lymphoma From Inflammatory Bowel Disease in Canine Duodenal Endoscopic Biopsy Samples. *Veterinary Pathology*, 52(4):668–675. doi:10.1177/0300985814559398.
- Ciekot, P.A., Powers, B.E., Withrow, S.J. et al. (1994) Histologically low-grade, yet biologically high-grade, fibrosarcomas of the mandible and maxilla in dogs: 25 cases (1982–1991). *J Am Vet Med Assoc*, 204(4):610–615.
- Couto, K.M., Moore, P.F., Zwingenberger, A.L. et al. (2018) Clinical characteristics and outcome in dogs with small cell T-cell intestinal lymphoma. *Veterinary and Comparative Oncology*, 16(3):337–343. doi:10.1111/vco.12384.
- Dailey, D.D., Ehrhart, E.J., Duval, D.L. et al. (2015) DOG1 is a sensitive and specific immunohistochemical marker for diagnosis of canine gastrointestinal stromal tumors. *J Vet Diagn Invest*, 27(3):268–277. doi:10.1177/1040638715578878.
- Dennis, M.M., Ehrhart, N., Duncan, C.G. et al. (2006) Frequency of and risk factors associated with lingual lesions in dogs: 1,196 cases (1995–2004). *J Am Vet Med Assoc*, 228(10):1533–1537. doi:10.2460/javma.228.10.1533.
- Desmas, I., Burton, J.H., Post, G. et al. (2017) Clinical presentation, treatment, and outcome in 31 dogs with presumed primary colorectal lymphoma (2001–2013). *Veterinary and Comparative Oncology*, 15(2):504–517. doi:10.1111/vco.12194.
- Dutelle, A.L., Bulman-Fleming, J.C., Lewis, C.A. et al. (2012) Evaluation of lomustine as a rescue agent for cats with resistant lymphoma. *Journal of Feline Medicine and Surgery*, 14(10):694–700. doi:10.1177/1098612X12448017.
- Elliott, J.W., Swinbourne, F., Parry, A. et al. (2017) Successful treatment of a metastatic, gastrointestinal stromal tumour in a dog with toceranib phosphate (Palladia). *Journal of Small Animal Practice*, 58(7):416–418. doi:10.1111/jsap.12657.
- Fiani, N., Verstraete, F.J.M., Kass, P.H. et al. (2011) Clinicopathologic characterization of odontogenic tumors and focal fibrous hyperplasia in dogs: 152 cases (1995–2005). *J Am Vet Med Assoc*, 238(4):495–500. doi:10.2460/javma.238.4.495.
- Finotello, R., Vasconi, M.E., Sabattini, S. et al. (2018) Feline large granular lymphocyte lymphoma: An Italian Society of Veterinary Oncology (SIONCOV) retrospective study. *Veterinary and Comparative Oncology*, 16(1):159–166. doi:10.1111/vco.12325.
- Frazier, S.A., Johns, S.M., Ortega, J. et al. (2012) Outcome in dogs with surgically resected oral fibrosarcoma (1997–2008). *Veterinary and Comparative Oncology*, 10(1):33–43. doi:10.1111/j.1476–5829.2011.00272.x.
- Frost, D., Lasota, J., Miettinen, M. (2003) Gastrointestinal stromal tumors and leiomyomas in the dog: a histopathologic, immunohistochemical, and molecular genetic study of 50 cases. *Veterinary Pathology*, 40(1):42–54. doi:10.1354/vp.40-1-42.
- Fukushima, K., Kanemoto, H., Ohno, K. et al. (2012) Ct characteristics of primary hepatic mass lesions in dogs. *Veterinary Radiology & Ultrasound*, n/a–n/a. doi:10.1111/j.1740-8261.2011.01917.x.
- Gardner, H., Fidel, J., Haldorson, G. et al. (2015) Canine oral fibrosarcomas: a retrospective analysis of 65 cases (1998–2010). *Veterinary and Comparative Oncology*, 13(1):40–47. doi:10.1111/vco.12017.
- Garraway, K., Johannes, C.M., Bryan, A. et al. (2018) Relationship of the mucosal microbiota to gastrointestinal inflammation and small cell intestinal lymphoma in cats. *Journal of Veterinary Internal Medicine*, 32(5):1692–1702. doi:10.1111/jvim.15291.
- Goldschmidt, S.L., Bell, C.M., Hetzel, S. et al. (2017) Clinical Characterization of Canine Acanthomatous Ameloblastoma (CAA) in 263 dogs and the Influence of Postsurgical Histopathological Margin on Local Recurrence. *J Vet Dent*, 34(4):241–247. doi:10.1177/0898756417734312.
- Green, M.L., Smith, J.D., Kass, P.H. (2011) Surgical versus non-surgical treatment of feline small intestinal adenocarcinoma and the influence of metastasis on long-term survival in 18 cats (2000–2007). *Can Vet J*, 52(10):1101–1105.
- Gregory-Bryson, E., Bartlett, E., Kiupel, M. et al. (2010) Canine and human gastrointestinal stromal tumors display similar mutations in c-KIT exon 11. *BMC Cancer*, 10(1):559. doi:10.1186/1471-2407-10-559.

■ Grimes, J.A., Matz, B.M., Christopherson, P.W. et al. (2017) Agreement Between Cytology and Histopathology for Regional Lymph Node Metastasis in Dogs With Melanocytic Neoplasms. *Veterinary Pathology*, 54(4):579–587. doi:10.1177/0300985817698209.

■ Grimes, J.A., Mestrinho, L.A., Berg, J. et al. (2019) Histologic evaluation of mandibular and medial retropharyngeal lymph nodes during staging of oral malignant melanoma and squamous cell carcinoma in dogs. *J Am Vet Med Assoc*, 254(8):938–943. doi:10.2460/javma.254.8.938.

■ Grimes, J.A., Secrest, S.A., Northrup, N.C. et al. (2017) Indirect computed tomography lymphangiography with aqueous contrast for evaluation of sentinel lymph nodes in dogs with tumors of the head. *Vet Radiol Ultrasound*, 58(5):559–564. doi:10.1111/vru.12514.

■ Grosenbaugh, D.A., Leard, A.T., Bergman, P.J. et al. (2011) Safety and efficacy of a xenogeneic DNA vaccine encoding for human tyrosinase as adjunctive treatment for oral malignant melanoma in dogs following surgical excision of the primary tumor. *American Journal of veterinary research*, 72(12):1631–1638. doi:10.2460/ajvr.72.12.1631.

■ Gustafson, T.L., Villamil, A., Taylor, B.E. et al. (2014) A retrospective study of feline gastric lymphoma in 16 chemotherapy-treated cats. *Journal of the American Animal Hospital Association*, 50(1):46–52. doi:10.5326/JAAHA-MS-5989.

■ Hanazono, K., Fukumoto, S., Hirayama, K. et al. (2012) Predicting metastatic potential of gastrointestinal stromal tumors in dog by ultrasonography. *J Vet Med Sci*, 74(11):1477–1482.

■ Hayes, S., Yuzbasiyan-Gurkan, V., Gregory-Bryson, E. et al. (2013) Classification of Canine Nonangiogenic, Nonlymphogenic, Gastrointestinal Sarcomas Based on Microscopic, Immunohistochemical, and Molecular Characteristics. *Veterinary Pathology*, 50(5):779–788. doi:10.1177/0300985813478211.

■ Heaton, C.M., Fernandes, A.F.A., Jark, P.C. et al. (2020) Evaluation of toceranib for treatment of apocrine gland anal sac adenocarcinoma in dogs. *Journal of Veterinary Internal Medicine*, 9:2755. doi:10.1111/jvim.15706.

■ Heishima, K., Iwasaki, R., Kawabe, M. et al. (2018) Short-Term Administration of Single-Agent Toceranib in Six Cases of Inoperable Massive Canine Hepatocellular Carcinoma. *Journal of the American Animal Hospital Association*, JAAHA–MS–6788. doi:10.5326/JAAHA-MS-6788.

■ Hobbs, J., Sutherland-Smith, J., Penninck, D. et al. (2015) Ultrasonographic features of canine gastrointestinal stromal tumors compared to other gastrointestinal spindle cell tumors. *Vet Radiol Ultrasound*, 56(4):432–438. doi:10.1111/vru.12253.

■ Hugen, S., Thomas, R.E., German, A.J. et al. (2017) Gastric carcinoma in canines and humans, a review. *Veterinary and Comparative Oncology*, 15(3):692–705. doi:10.1111/vco.12249.

■ Irie, M., Takeuchi, Y., Ohtake, Y. et al. (2015) Imatinib mesylate treatment in a dog with gastrointestinal stromal tumors with a c-kit mutation. *J Vet Med Sci*, 77(11):1535–1539. doi:10.1292/jvms.15-0096.

■ Kawabe, M. Mori, T., Ito, Y. et al. (2015) Outcomes of dogs undergoing radiotherapy for treatment of oral malignant melanoma: 111 cases (2006–2012). *J Am Vet Med Assoc*, 247(10):1146–1153. doi:10.2460/javma.247.10.1146.

■ Kelly, J.M., Belding, B.A., Schaefer, A.K. (2010) Acanthomatous ameloblastoma in dogs treated with intralesional bleomycin. *Veterinary and Comparative Oncology*, 8(2):81–86. doi:10.1111/j.1476-5829.2010.00208.x.

■ Kiselow, M.A., Rassnick, K.M., McDonough, S.P. et al. (2008) Outcome of cats with low-grade lymphocytic lymphoma: 41 cases (1995–2005). *J Am Vet Med Assoc*, 232(3):405–410. doi:10.2460/javma.232.3.405.

■ Kiupel, M., Smedley, R.C., Pfent, C. et al. (2011) Diagnostic Algorithm to Differentiate Lymphoma From Inflammation in Feline Small Intestinal Biopsy Samples. *Veterinary Pathology*, 48(1):212–222. doi:10.1177/0300985810389479.

■ Krick, E.L., Little, L., Patel, R. et al. (2008) Description of clinical and pathological findings, treatment, and outcome of feline large granular lymphocyte lymphoma (1996–2004). *Veterinary and Comparative Oncology*, 6(2):102–110. doi:10.1111/j.1476-5829.2007.00146.x.

■ Lane, J., Price, J., Moore, A. et al. (2018) Low-grade gastrointestinal lymphoma in dogs: 20 cases (2010 to 2016). *Journal of Small Animal Practice*, 59(3):147–153. doi:10.1111/jsap.12769.

■ Lingard, A.E., Briscoe, K., Beatty, J.A. et al. (2009) Low-grade alimentary lymphoma: clinicopathological findings and response to treatment in 17 cases. *Journal of Feline Medicine and Surgery*, 11(8):692–700. doi:10.1016/j.jfms.2009.05.021.

■ Maekawa, N., Konnai, S., Takagi, S. et al. (2017) A canine chimeric monoclonal antibody targeting PD-L1 and its clinical efficacy in canine oral malignant melanoma or undifferentiated sarcoma. *Sci Rep*, 7(1):8951–12. doi:10.1038/s41598-017-09444-2.

■ Majeski, S.A., Steffey, M.A., Fuller, M. et al. (2017) Indirect computed tomographic lymphography for iliosacral lymphatic mapping in a cohort of dogs with anal sac gland adenocarcinoma: technique description. *Vet Radiol Ultrasound*, 58(3):295–303. doi:10.1111/vru.12482.

■ Marconato, L., Weyland, M., Tresch, N. (2019) Toxicity and outcome in cats with oral squamous cell carcinoma after accelerated hypofractionated radiotherapy and concurrent systemic treatment. *Veterinary and Comparative Oncology*, vco.12557. doi:10.1111/vco.12557.

■ Marolf, A.J., Bachand, A.M., Sharber, J. et al. (2015) Comparison of endoscopy and sonography findings in dogs and cats with histologically confirmed gastric neoplasia. *Journal of Small Animal Practice*, 56(5):339–344. doi:10.1111/jsap.12324.

■ Marsilio, S., Ackermann, M.R., Lidbury, J.A. et al. (2019) Results of histopathology, immunohistochemistry, and molecular clonality testing of small intestinal biopsy specimens from clinically healthy client-owned cats. *Journal of Veterinary Internal Medicine*, 138(Suppl 1):S1. doi:10.1111/jvim.15455.

■ Martano, M., Iussich, S., Morello, E. et al. (2018) Canine oral fibrosarcoma: Changes in prognosis over the last 30 years? *Vet J*, 241:1-7. doi:10.1016/j.tvjl.2018.09.005.

■ Masserdotti, C., Drigo, M. (2012) Retrospective study of cytologic features of well-differentiated hepatocellular carcinoma in dogs. *Vet Clin Pathol*, 41(3):382–390. doi:10.1111/j.1939-165X.2012.00436.x.

■ Meier, V., Polton, G., Cancedda, S. et al. (2017) Outcome in dogs with advanced (stage 3b) anal sac gland carcinoma treated with surgery or hypofractionated radiation therapy. *Veterinary and Comparative Oncology*, 15(3):1073–1086. doi:10.1111/vco.12248.

■ Mestrinho, L.A., Pissarra, H., Carvalho, S. et al. (2017) Comparison of Histological and Proliferation Features of Canine Oral Squamous Cell Carcinoma Based on Intraoral Location: 36 Cases. *J Vet Dent*, 34(2):92–99. doi:10.1177/0898756417713979.

■ Mikiewicz, M., Paździor-Czapula, K., Gesek, M. et al. (2019) Canine and Feline Oral Cavity Tumours and Tumour-like Lesions: a Retrospective Study of 486 Cases (2015–2017). *Journal of Comparative Pathology*, 172:80–87. doi:10.1016/j.jcpa.2019.09.007.

■ Morrice, M., Polton, G., Beck, S. (2019) Evaluation of the extent of neoplastic infiltration in small intestinal tumours in dogs. *Vet Med Sci*, 135:635. doi:10.1002/vms3.147.

■ Murphy, S., Hayes, A.M., Blackwood, L. et al. (2005) Oral malignant melanoma - the effect of coarse fractionation radiotherapy alone or with adjuvant carboplatin therapy. *Veterinary and Comparative Oncology*, 3(4):222–229. doi:10.1111/j.1476-5810.2005.00082.x.

■ Nemoto, Y., Shosu, K., Okuda, M. et al. (2018) Development and characterization of monoclonal antibodies against canine PD-1 and PD-L1. *Veterinary Immunology and Immunopathology*. 2018;198:19–25. doi:10.1016/j.vetimm.2018.02.007.

■ Oishi, Y., Tani, K., Taura, Y. (2018) Transcatheter arterial embolisation in four dogs with hepatocellular carcinoma. *Journal of Small Animal Practice*, 1:191. doi:10.1111/jsap.12944.

■ Olmsted, G.A., Farrelly, J., Post, G.S. et al. (2017) Tolerability of toceranib phosphate (Palladia) when used in conjunction with other therapies in 35 cats with feline oral squamous cell carcinoma: 2009-2013. *Journal of Feline Medicine and Surgery*, 19(6):568–575. doi:10.1177/1098612X16638118.

■ Ottnod, J.M., Smedley, R.C., Walshaw, R. et al. (2013) A retrospective analysis of the efficacy of Oncept vaccine for the adjunct treatment of canine oral malignant melanoma. *Veterinary and Comparative Oncology*, 11(3):219–229. doi:10.1111/vco.12057.

■ Paulin, M.V., Couronné, L., Beguin, J. et al. (2018) Feline low-grade alimentary lymphoma: an emerging entity and a potential animal model for human disease. *BMC Vet Res*, 14(1):306. doi:10.1186/s12917-018-1635-5.

■ Perry, J.A., Culp, W.T.N., Dailey, D.D. et al. (2014) Diagnostic accuracy of pre-treatment biopsy for grading soft tissue sarcomas in dogs. *Veterinary and Comparative Oncology*, 12(2):106–113. doi:10.1111/j.1476-5829.2012.00333.x.

■ Piegols, H.J., Takada, M., Parys, M. et al. (2018) Investigation of novel chemotherapeutics for feline oral squamous cell carcinoma. *Oncotarget*, 9(69):33098-33109. doi:10.18632/oncotarget.26006.

■ Pollard, R.E., Fuller, M.C., Steffey, M.A. (2017) Ultrasound and computed tomography of the iliosacral lymphatic centre in dogs with anal sac gland carcinoma. *Veterinary and Comparative Oncology*, 15(2):299–306. doi:10.1111/vco.12160.

■ Pope, K.V., Tun, A.E., McNeill, C.J. et al. (2015) Outcome and toxicity assessment of feline small cell lymphoma: 56 cases (2000–2010). *Vet Med Sci*, 1(2):51–62. doi:10.1002/vms3.9.

■ Potanas, C.P., Padgett, S., Gamblin, R.M. (2015) Surgical excision of anal sac apocrine gland adenocarcinomas with and without adjunctive chemotherapy in dogs: 42 cases (2005–2011). *J Am Vet Med Assoc*, 246(8):877–884. doi:10.2460/javma.246.8.877.

■ Pradel, J., Berlato, D., Dobromylskyj, M. et al. (2018) Prognostic significance of histopathology in canine anal sac gland adenocarcinomas: Preliminary results in a retrospective study of 39 cases. *Veterinary and Comparative Oncology*, 16(4):518–528. doi:10.1111/vco.12410.

■ Rassnick, K.M., Ruslander, D.M., Cotter, S.M. et al. (2001) Use of carboplatin for treatment of dogs with malignant melanoma: 27 cases (1989–2000). *J Am Vet Med Assoc*, 218(9):1444–1448. doi:10.2460/javma.2001.218.1444.

■ Riggs, J., Adams, V.J., Hermer, J.V. et al. (2018) Outcomes following surgical excision or surgical excision combined with adjunctive, hypofractionated radiotherapy in dogs with oral squamous cell carcinoma or fibrosarcoma. *J Am Vet Med Assoc*, 253(1):73–83. doi:10.2460/javma.253.1.73.

■ Russell, K.N., Mehler, S.J., Skorupski, K.A. et al. (2007) Clinical and immunohistochemical differentiation of gastrointestinal stromal tumors from leiomyosarcomas in dogs: 42 cases (1990–2003). *J Am Vet Med Assoc*, 230(9):1329–1333. doi:10.2460/javma.230.9.1329.

■ Sabattini, S., Bottero, E., Turba, M.E. et al. (2016) Differentiating feline inflammatory bowel disease from alimentary lymphoma in duodenal endoscopic biopsies. *Journal of Small Animal Practice*, 57(8):396–401. doi:10.1111/jsap.12494.

■ Seim-Wikse, T., Skancke, E., Nødtvedt, A. et al. (2019) Comparison of body condition score and other minimally invasive biomarkers between dogs with gastric carcinoma and dogs with chronic gastritis. *J Am Vet Med Assoc* 254(2):226–235. doi:10.2460/javma.254.2.226.

■ Selmic, L.E. (2017) Hepatobiliary Neoplasia. *Vet Clin North Am Small Anim Pract*, 47(3):725–735. doi:10.1016/j.cvsm.2016.11.016.

■ Shosu, K., Sakurai, M., Inoue, K. et al. (2016) Programmed Cell Death Ligand 1 Expression in Canine Cancer. *In Vivo*, 30(3):195–204.

■ Simčič, P., Lowe, R., Granziera, V. et al. (2019) Electrochemotherapy in treatment of canine oral non-tonsillar squamous cell carcinoma. A case series report. *Veterinary and Comparative Oncology*, 58(3):381. doi:10.1111/vco.12530.

■ Skinner, O.T., Boston, S.E., Souza, CH de M. (2017) Patterns of lymph node metastasis identified following bilateral mandibular and medial retropharyngeal lymphadenectomy in 31 dogs with malignancies of the head. *Veterinary and Comparative Oncology*, 15(3):881–889. doi:10.1111/vco.12229.

■ Skorupski, K.A., Alarcón, C.N., de Lorimier, L-P. et al. (2018) Outcome and clinical, pathological, and immunohistochemical factors associated with prognosis for dogs with early-stage anal sac adenocarcinoma treated with surgery alone: 34 cases (2002–2013). *J Am Vet Med Assoc*, 253(1):84–91. doi:10.2460/javma.253.1.84.

■ Slawienski, M.J., Mauldin, G.E., Mauldin, G.N. et al. (1997) Malignant colonic neoplasia in cats: 46 cases (1990–1996). *J Am Vet Med Assoc*, 211(7):878–881.

■ Smedley, R.C., Lamoureux, J., Sledge, D.G. et al. (2011) Immunohistochemical diagnosis of canine oral amelanotic melanocytic neoplasms. *Veterinary Pathology*, 48(1):32–40. doi:10.1177/0300985810387447.

■ Smith, A.A., Frimberger, A.E., Moore, A.S. (2019) Retrospective study of survival time and prognostic factors for dogs with small intestinal adenocarcinoma treated by tumor excision with or without adjuvant chemotherapy. *J Am Vet Med Assoc*, 254(2):243–250. doi:10.2460/javma.254.2.243.

■ Sogame, N., Risbon, R., Burgess, K.E. (2018) Intestinal lymphoma in dogs: 84 cases (1997–2012). *J Am Vet Med Assoc*, 252(4):440–447. doi:10.2460/javma.252.4.440.

■ Syrcle, J.A., Bonczynski, J.J., Monette, S. et al. (2008) Retrospective evaluation of lingual tumors in 42 dogs: 1999–2005. *Journal of the American Animal Hospital Association*, 44(6):308–319. doi:10.5326/0440308.

■ Takanosu, M., Amano, S., Kagawa, Y. (2016) Analysis of c-KIT exon 11 mutations in canine gastrointestinal stromal tumours. *Vet J*, 207:118–123. doi:10.1016/j.tvjl.2015.10.051.

■ Thaiwong, T., Sledge, D.G., Collins-Webb, A. et al. (2018) Immunohistochemical Characterization of Canine Oral Papillary Squamous Cell Carcinoma. *Veterinary Pathology*, 55(2):224–232. doi:10.1177/0300985817741732.

■ Thierry, F., Longo, M., Pecceu, E. et al. (2018) Computed tomographic appearance of canine tonsillar neoplasia: 14 cases. *Vet Radiol Ultrasound*, 59(1):54–63. doi:10.1111/vru.12561.

■ Tuohy, J.L., Selmic, L.E., Worley, D.R. et al. (2014) Outcome following curative-intent surgery for oral melanoma in dogs: 70 cases (1998–2011). *J Am Vet Med Assoc*, 245(11):1266–1273. doi:10.2460/javma.245.11.1266.

■ Ugrappa, S., Jain, A., Fuloria, N.K. et al. (2017) Acanthomatous ameloblastoma in anterior mandibular region of a young patient: A rare case report. *Ann Afr Med*, 16(2):85–89. doi:10.4103/aam.aam_51_16.

■ Urie, B.K., Russell, D.S., Kisseberth, W.C. et al. (2012) Evaluation of expression and function of vascular endothelial growth factor receptor 2, platelet derived growth factor receptors-alpha and -beta, KIT, and RET in canine apocrine gland anal sac adenocarcinoma and thyroid carcinoma. *BMC Vet Res*, 8(1):67. doi:10.1186/1746-6148-8-67.

■ Van den Steen, N., Berlato, D., Polton, G. et al. (2012) Rectal lymphoma in 11 dogs - a retrospective study. *Journal of Small Animal Practice*, 53(10):586–591. doi:10.1111/j.1748-5827.2012.01258.x.

■ Verganti, S., Berlato, D., Blackwood, L. et al. (2017) Use of Oncept melanoma vaccine in 69 canine oral malignant melanomas in the UK. *Journal of Small Animal Practice*, 58(1):10–16. doi:10.1111/jsap.12613.

■ Waite, A.H.K., Jackson, K., Gregor, T.P. et al. (2013) Lymphoma in cats treated with a weekly cyclophosphamide-vincristine-, and prednisone-based protocol: 114 cases (1998–2008). *J Am Vet Med Assoc*, 242(8):1104–1109. doi:10.2460/javma.242.8.1104.

■ Wiles, V., Hohenhaus, A., Lamb, K. et al. (2017) Retrospective evaluation of toceranib phosphate (Palladia) in cats with oral squamous cell carcinoma. *Journal of Feline Medicine and Surgery*, 19(2):185–193. doi:10.1177/1098612X15622237.

■ Wingo, K. (2018) Histopathologic Diagnoses from Biopsies of the Oral Cavity in 403 Dogs and 73 Cats. *J Vet Dent*, 35(1):7–17. doi:10.1177/0898756418759760.

■ Wouda, R.M., Borrego, J., Keuler, N.S. et al. (2016) Evaluation of adjuvant carboplatin chemotherapy in the management of surgically excised anal sac apocrine gland adenocarcinoma in dogs. *Veterinary and Comparative Oncology*, 14(1):67–80. doi:10.1111/vco.12068.

■ Yang, T., Case, J.B., Boston, S. et al. (2017) Microwave ablation for treatment of hepatic neoplasia in five dogs. *J Am Vet Med Assoc*, 250(1):79–85. doi:10.2460/javma.250.1.79.

Test

Answers on Page 290

1. **Regarding the frequency of appearance of oral tumours in dogs and cats, what is the correct answer?**
   a. Oral tumours account for 10–12% of all tumours in dogs.
   b. In dogs, the most common tumour is squamous cell carcinoma.
   c. Approximately half of tumours of the tongue that are biopsied in cats are neoplasms.
   d. About half of the lesions in the mouths of dogs are malignant neoplasms of the gums, palate, or lips.

2. **Concerning canine oral melanoma, which answer is incorrect?**
   a. Melanoma is the most common malignant tumour in the oral cavity of the dog.
   b. Factors that mainly affect the clinical stage of canine oral melanoma are the size of the tumour, the involvement of the local lymph nodes, and the presence or absence of distant metastases.
   c. Ultrasound is the technique of choice to assess the extent of canine oral melanoma.
   d. Median survival times with radiation therapy (without surgery) are 25, 9, 5 and 2 months for clinical stages I, II, III, and IV, respectively.

3. **What are the characteristics of oral squamous cell carcinoma?**
   a. It is the second most frequent tumour type in the oral cavity of the dog and the first in cats.
   b. Cytological diagnosis is quite simple and does not require biopsy to be effective.
   c. It is a tumour type with a very low rate of metastasis, present in less than 5% of cases.
   d. In the case of feline squamous cell carcinoma, the prognosis is better than in the dog, and survival at one year is usually greater than 40%.

4. **Gastrointestinal lymphoma affects both dogs and cats, what is the correct answer?**
   a. The different forms of gastrointestinal lymphoma are more common in dogs than cats.
   b. Feline gastrointestinal large granular lymphocyte lymphoma is characterised by the presence of double and triple nuclei in tumour cells.
   c. In the dog, gastrointestinal lymphoma occurs infrequently, constituting about 15% of canine lymphomas.
   d. Lymphoma is the most common gastrointestinal tumour in cats.

5. **Which answer is wrong when it comes to treating the different gastrointestinal lymphomas in dogs and cats?**
   a. In the treatment of high-grade feline gastrointestinal lymphoma, various studies show a response rate of around 50% for complete remissions.
   b. High-grade lymphomas located in the colon and rectum have a poor response to chemotherapy with mean survival times of less than one year.
   c. Lymphocyte lymphoma with granules in its cytoplasm has been associated with a very poor prognosis since it was first described, with average survival times of just a couple of weeks.
   d. Small cell lymphoma is usually treated with prednisone (or prednisolone) and chlorambucil.

6. **Which is the correct answer?**
   a. The cause of low-grade intestinal lymphoma is unknown.
   b. Gastric carcinoma is a rare tumour in dogs: it constitutes about 5% of tumours in this species.
   c. Carcinoma is the second most common intestinal tumour in dogs after digestive lymphoma.
   d. Primary liver tumours are common in the dog.

7. **Which answer is incorrect when it comes to treating liver tumours in dogs and cats?**
   a. The most widely used technique is selective embolisation, leaving the tumour without blood supply.
   b. A partial remission of inoperable tumours has been documented in 50% of the cases treated with toceranib phosphate.
   c. Surgical resection of liver carcinoma is not possible and there are no good medical alternatives to treat this tumour.
   d. Radiofrequency or microwave ablation, either guided by ultrasound or by laparotomy, may be a treatment system for liver tumours, although there are still few studies in this regard.

8. **Regarding gastrointestinal stromal tumours, what is the correct answer?**
   a. In dogs, 13% of stromal tumours did not express KIT but did express DOG-1.
   b. Gastrointestinal stromal tumours originate from Cajal cells and are positive for KIT on immunohistochemistry.
   c. 20% of cases present metastases (mainly omentum, lymph nodes and liver) at the time of diagnosis.
   d. Leiomyosarcomas usually metastasise, and more advanced cases can affect all layers of the intestine.

9. **How is an anal sac adenocarcinoma diagnosed?**
    a. Cytology is a good initial diagnostic method.
    b. The safest method is immunohistochemistry since all are KIT positive.
    c. Advanced imaging techniques, such as tomography, are not very sensitive in detecting lymphadenopathy and are rarely used.
    d. Radiography is the technique that provides the most information when diagnosing this type of tumour.

10. **In which gastrointestinal tract tumour have complete remissions been recorded in cases of metastasis after treatment with c-kit inhibitors?**
    a. Anal sac adenocarcinoma.
    b. Liver carcinoma, but only in cats.
    c. Gastrointestinal stromal tumours.
    d. High-grade feline gastrointestinal lymphoma.

Correct Answers:

1. c
2. c
3. a
4. d
5. b
6. a
7. a
8. b
9. a
10. c

Notes

Tumours of the Musculoskeletal System

Pachi Clemente Vicario

Osteosarcoma

Osteosarcoma is the **most common skeletal tumour in dogs** and accounts for 85% of bone tumours. It affects middle-aged dogs, with a peak in incidence between seven and ten years old. This is one of the few differences with the same cancer in people, which mainly affects young people between 10 and 20 years of age.

Generally diagnosed in large and giant breed dogs, with a minority of cases in dogs under 15 kilograms. Frequently diagnosed breeds include Rottweilers, but also Golden and Labrador Retrievers. In terms of groups, mastiff-type dogs and giant mountain breeds are the most frequently represented. Among the risk factors for developing osteosarcomas, in addition to body size, some genetic factors have been identified. The most constant genetic alterations in canine osteosarcoma are the mutations that affect the SETD2 gene.

Most osteosarcomas originate in the extremities, specifically in the metaphysis of long bones, being **twice as frequent in the forelimbs as in the hindlimbs**. Generally, it is located away from the elbow (proximal humerus and distal radius) and close to the knee (distal femur and proximal tibia). However, tumours in the distal tibia are more frequent in some cases. Those that originate in the axial skeleton can do so in the mandible, maxilla, spine, skull, ribs, nasal cavity, and pelvis (in this order from most to least common)

Clinical Signs and Lesions

The clinical signs are lameness and swelling at the primary site for tumours of the extremities and are location dependent for those of the axial skeleton. When a bone tumour is suspected, diagnostic tests include radiology and cytological or histological diagnosis.

Osteosarcoma can cause both **bone lysis and proliferation** and is often associated with a soft tissue component. The radiological characteristics of an aggressive lesion (non-pathognomonic for osteosarcoma) are cortical destruction, periosteal reaction, and a poorly defined separation between normal and abnormal bone (Figure 1). **Codman's triangle**, a lesion that occurs when the tumour invades the bony cortex and elevates the periosteum in the peripheral area of the tumour, can be seen in many cases.

It is extremely rare for an osteosarcoma to affect two different bones on both sides of the joint, with most lesions being monostotic. The radiological changes described can also be observed in other diseases such as osteomyelitis, especially the fungal type.

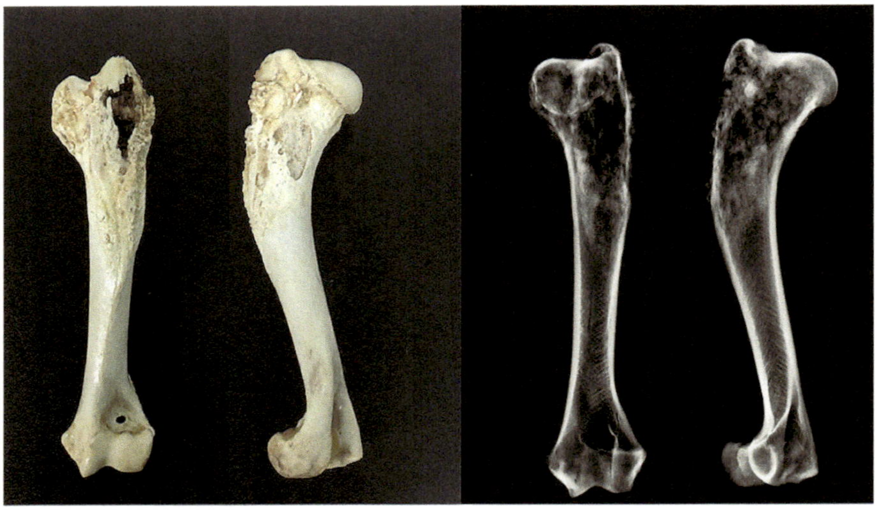

Figure 1. Macroscopic and radiographic image of an osteosarcoma. There is a lesion with destruction of the cortical area, periosteal reaction, and poorly defined margins between the pathological and normal areas.

Diagnosis

Based on the clinical history (including prevalence of fungal diseases), breed and age, and radiological changes, a presumptive diagnosis of osteosarcoma can be made. It is important to rule out other tumours that could produce bone metastases such as genitourinary carcinomas.

Osteosarcoma is a malignant bone tumour, and its **histological diagnosis is based on the identification of osteoid extracellular matrix**, which differentiates it from other tumours that can originate in bone.

Small or superficial biopsies can lead to misdiagnoses that can include other sarcomas such as chondrosarcoma, fibrosarcoma or haemangiosarcoma, and non-tumour lesions such as reactive bone. If a biopsy is to be taken, it is important to **use the proper needles and to take samples from the centre of the lesion**, piercing the cortex of the bone.

Cytology (Figure 2) can give a definitive diagnosis in most cases. Furthermore, in the case of suspected sarcoma, the **use of specific stains such as alkaline phosphatase** allows a definitive diagnosis with a specificity of 94%.

The author performs an ultrasound-guided aspiration biopsy in cases in which it is required to confirm suspicions after evaluating the case and consulting with a radiologist. If a biopsy is to be performed, it should be done by the surgeon treating the case, especially if limb-saving surgery is being considered. As mentioned, the risk of a bone biopsy is that it is not diagnostic (small or superficial sample) or provides an incorrect diagnosis. It must be considered that different diagnoses may imply a completely different prognosis and treatment from that of osteosarcoma.

If osteosarcoma is suspected or confirmed, **thoracic radiographs** (three views: right and left lateral, and ventrodorsal) and a complete orthopaedic and **physical examination should be performed**. Although most cases will not have visible metastases at diagnosis, 10–15% of cases may be positive and have a worse prognosis.

Before considering amputation, injuries that may be associated with bone metastases (localised pain in other bones) should be ruled out as well as neurological or orthopaedic abnormalities that could contraindicate removal of the limb. Although in most cases that have pulmonary metastases these can be seen both on good quality radiographs and computed tomography, different studies show that **tomography is superior for detection of small lung lesions**, especially in large breed dogs, and that a greater number of lesions are seen on tomography than on radiology.

Treatment

The standard treatment for osteosarcoma consists of **amputation of the affected limb and administration of adjuvant chemotherapy**. The amputation should be complete in the forelimb (including scapula) and with hip disarticulation in the hindlimb. In some cases, surgery can be performed without amputation (Figure 3), but provided the necessary criteria are met including that the tumour does not affect more than

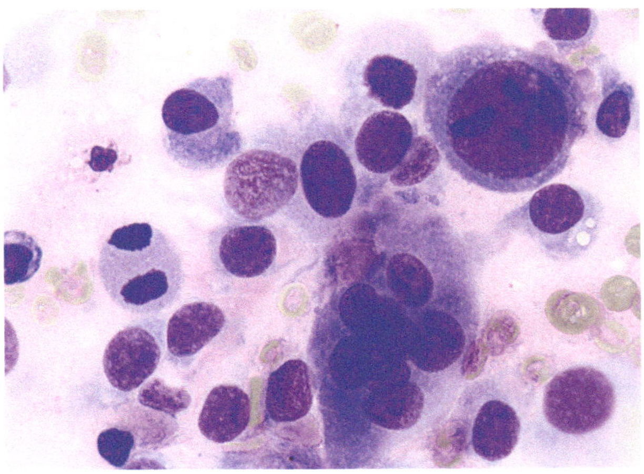

Figure 2. Cytology of an osseous lytic lesion which shows osteoblasts with anisocytosis and anisokaryosis, prominent nucleoli, mitosis, and different chromatin patterns. An osteoclast can be seen (multinucleated).

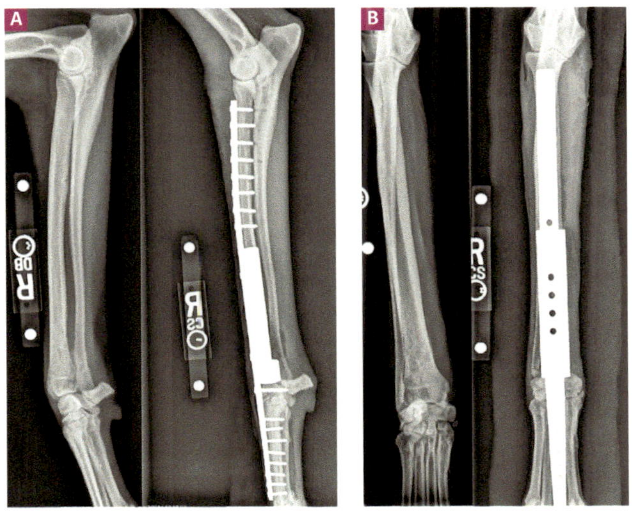

Figure 3. Lytic lesion from an osteosarcoma in lateral and cranial caudal views before (**A**) and after (**B**) the removal of the tumour to save the limb. The images show how an arthrodesis is performed using this technique.

50% of the bone, with soft tissue involvement that does not involve 360° and the absence of pathological fracture or of swollen lesions. When considering this type of surgery, it is important to perform advanced imaging tests such as CT (Figure 4) or MRI, because they offer better information about the actual size of the tumour lesion than radiographs. Osteosarcoma located in the distal radius offers the best prognosis in terms of limb functionality with this surgical technique. If cases in which the technique is indicated are carefully selected, the percentage of serious complications that may end up requiring amputation of the limb (severe infection of the surgical site or local recurrence of the tumour) is less than 20%.

Although amputation is the treatment of the primary tumour, **the main problem with osteosarcoma is metastatic disease**, and therefore the use of **systemic chemotherapy after amputation is recommended**.

The treatment which is currently recommended is **carboplatin** (300 mg/m^2 IV every three weeks, four treatments). None of the different combinations (simultaneous or alternate carboplatin and doxorubicin, or carboplatin and gemcitabine) achieve better survival times than carboplatin as a single agent. Nor does a greater number of doses offer better results than four treatments. A review of 470 cases treated with various protocols found none superior when assessing disease-free interval or survival. Between 50 and 70% of the animals developed metastases and the average survival time is one year, with 20% of cases surviving two years.

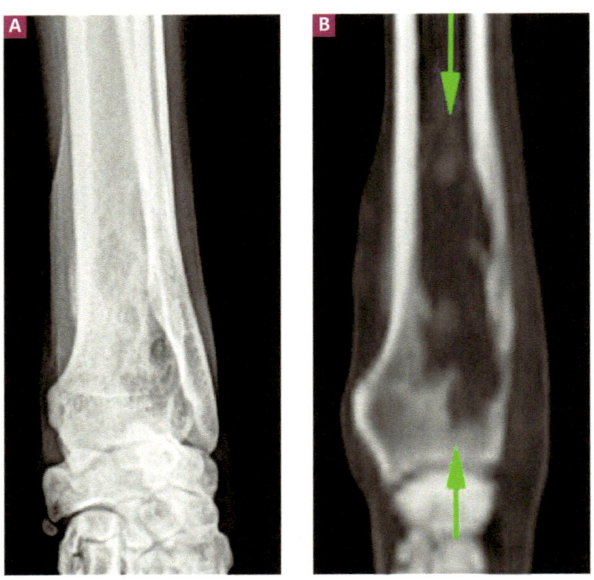

Figure 4. Comparison of radiographic (**A**) and CT (**B**) images from the same patient with osteosarcoma of the distal radius. On CT the lesion can be seen to be larger than when using radiography.

Elevation of alkaline phosphatase has been shown as a poor prognostic marker in some studies, while the histological grade of the tumour does not seem to affect prognosis. Infection of the surgical site in cases where surgery is performed to save the limb has been associated with a better prognosis.

Although chemotherapy is effective in delaying the development of metastases, treatments that allow better long-term control and prolong the survival of these animals are necessary. New approaches have used metronomic chemotherapy at the end of conventional chemotherapy. The authors data with Greyhounds (Clemente-Vicario and Couto, 2015 ACVIM Forum Research Abstract Program) show no benefit of using a combination of antiangiogenic drugs, including toceranib, when completing treatment with doxorubicin versus animals who were treated with doxorubicin alone. These data were confirmed by another study that did not show any benefit when using metronomic chemotherapy (with or without toceranib) after completing conventional chemotherapy. Not only were the disease-free interval and survival time similar, but there were more side effects (diarrhoea, weight loss) when toceranib was used. The simultaneous administration of metronomic and conventional chemotherapy (at maximum tolerated doses) was associated with an increase in toxicity; however, the mean survival time was not superior to historical data. These data show that **metronomic chemotherapy does not represent any benefit in the management of cases of canine osteosarcoma**.

Alternatively, a prospective clinical trial evaluated the response rate of osteosarcoma metastases to toceranib. In this case, instead of trying to delay the appearance of these metastases by using it to complete conventional chemotherapy, the animals were treated with toceranib once the appearance of metastases was documented. Twenty-two dogs were included in the trial, nine of which left the study within 8 weeks due to disease progression or adverse effects. At 8 weeks, only 17% of the cases achieved stable disease, while the rest had progressive disease. The results of the study **do not justify the recommendation of the use of toceranib for the treatment of metastatic osteosarcoma**.

Osteosarcoma is considered an immunogenic tumour, so **immunotherapy could offer an improvement in the prognosis of this disease**. The epidermal growth factor receptor (EGFR) is considered a therapeutic target and antibodies have been developed to stimulate an immune response that recognises and attacks tumour cells. A clinical trial using *Listeria* to induce an immune response to HER-2 has shown promising results in dogs, with a mean disease-free interval of 615 days and a mean survival time of 956 days. The survival rates at one, two and three years were 77.67 and 56% respectively, much higher than that obtained with conventional chemotherapy. However, the documentation of cases of listeriosis in dogs treated with the vaccine and the zoonotic risk led to the discontinuation of the trial.

Prognosis

Without the most aggressive treatment, the prognosis for dogs with osteosarcoma is **very poor**, with most animals requiring euthanasia due to pain associated with the primary tumour.

If a pathological fracture occurs, the only option at that time is amputation or euthanasia. Among the different palliative treatments studied, **radiotherapy seems the most effective in terms of local pain control**. However, a frequent complication in the cases treated with palliative radiotherapy is the risk of pathological fractures. These fractures can occur within a few weeks of treatment and owners should be informed of this complication. Other palliative treatments, such as the use of bisphosphonates (pamidronate) are not effective at controlling pain. Although in initial studies a good response was observed, with 28% of the animals demonstrating less pain, there were no differences when comparing pamidronate with a placebo.

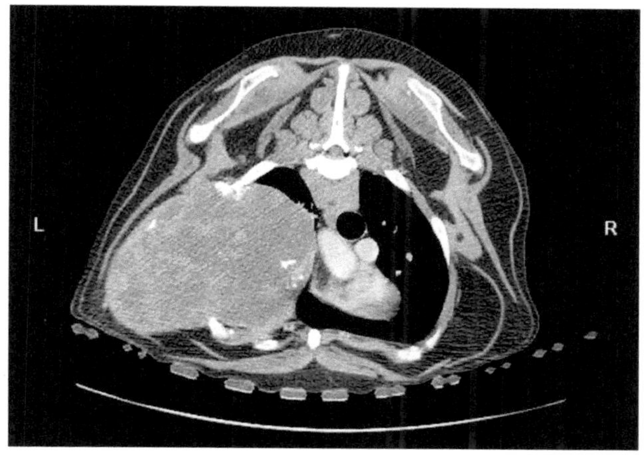

Figure 5. Costal chondrosarcoma. These lesions can become large but aggressive surgery without adjuvant therapy is associated with a good prognosis.

Other Tumours of the Bone and Musculoskeletal System

Chondrosarcoma, haemangiosarcoma, fibrosarcoma, lymphoma, and plasma cell tumour can appear in bone as the primary site. Other tumours, such as carcinomas, can affect the bone as metastatic disease.

Chondrosarcoma

It is the **second most common bone tumour** and accounts for about 10% of primary bone tumours. Its diagnosis is based on the presence of cartilaginous extracellular matrix, without the presence of osteoid matrix. 90% of cases in dogs are in flat bones such as the ribs, nasal cavity, or pelvis. Despite being a malignant tumour, it is considered a local disease and **aggressive surgery is associated with good survival** even without adjuvant treatments. In costal chondrosarcoma (Figure 5), median survival times after resection of the affected rib along with the immediately caudal and proximal rib are almost 4 years, compared with a median survival of 10 months in cases of costal osteosarcoma.

It is important to remember that a complete tumour analysis is necessary for a definitive diagnosis since some parts of a rib osteosarcoma (with a much worse prognosis than chondrosarcomas) may have areas with cartilage production. If this part is biopsied, a misdiagnosis of chondrosarcoma could be made.

Fibrosarcoma

A **rare tumour as a primary bone tumour** (about 5% of primary bone tumours) and can be difficult to distinguish from a fibroblastic osteosarcoma if the sample is small. The recommended treatment is aggressive surgery, although this does not rule out the appearance of metastases.

Haemangiosarcoma

Haemangiosarcoma (HSA) **can present with the primary lesion in both bone and muscle** (in addition to the most frequent locations, such as spleen, heart, or subcutaneous tissue, among others). In bone, it accounts primarily for less than 1% of bone tumours. It can also develop metastatic lesions in the muscle from primary lesions in other locations.

The lesions are irregular, ill-defined, and hypoechoic on ultrasound. On CT, they are heterogeneous, invasive of adjacent tissues, with heterogeneous contrast uptake. Haemangiosarcoma can be difficult to differentiate from the telangiectatic presentation of osteosarcoma (Figure 6), and the use of immunohistochemistry changes the diagnosis in up to 20% of cases.

Unlike chondrosarcoma, **HSA has a high rate of metastasis**, and most cases will develop metastatic disease in the months following diagnosis. Before performing any treatment, it is essential to perform clinical staging Median survival time for intramuscular haemangiosarcomas is about 9 months when treated with doxorubicin.

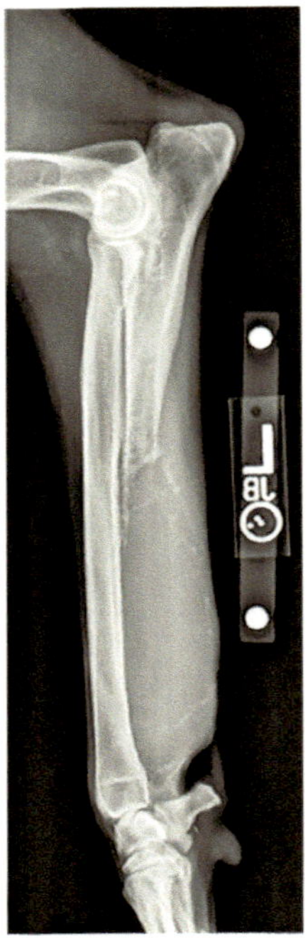

Figure 6. Lytic osseous lesion of the ulna. The histological diagnosis was of telangiectatic haemangiosarcoma.

The presence of metastases at the time of haemangiosarcoma diagnosis does not seem to worsen the prognosis if they are treated with chemotherapy protocols such as VAC (vincristine, actinomycin D and cyclophosphamide), since there is a high response rate although it may not be very long lived.

Multilobular Bone Tumour

A **rare** tumour of the skull that affects dogs. It has also been called chondroma rodens and multilobular osteoma. It has a typical radiological appearance (popcorn image). The bone structure is replaced by a mass with soft tissue density (Figure 7) with multifocal calcification.

Complete surgical resection can be complicated (but possible), and tumour recurrence occurs in about half of the cases, even in cases with clean margins at surgery. Recurrence generally occurs within a year after surgery and cases that recur have a higher risk of developing metastases, usually pulmonary ones. Due to the slow growth of metastatic lesions, their surgical removal (metastasectomy) may be indicated in some cases. The role of chemotherapy in these slow-growing tumours is unclear.

Histological grade and complete resection are important for prognosis. Due to the surgical complication (due to the location and the need for clean margins), it should only be performed by surgeons with experience with this type of tumours.

Secondary Bone Tumours

Among secondary bone tumours, **carcinomas are the most common**, especially genitourinary, mammary (Figure 8) and prostate, but metastases from **squamous cell carcinomas** (**Figure 9**) **are also frequently seen**, which usually present lesions in different bones, including the vertebrae in many cases.

A particular presentation that is seen with relative frequency is the so-called "lung-digit syndrome" in cats, where metastases develop in the phalanges of one or more digits from a primary lung tumour. Although they are treated for the injury of the toes, a study of these cases shows that they usually present metastases in multiple sites including muscle, eyes, or large vessels such as the aorta.

Multiple Myeloma

Multiple myeloma, a plasma cell tumour in the bone marrow, can also **produce numerous lytic lesions in different bones** (Figure 10), but it is considered a primary bone tumour.

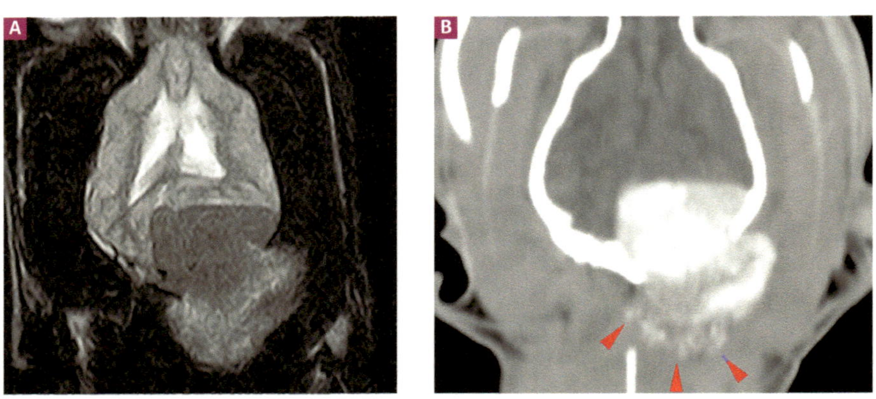

Figure 7. MRI (**A**) and CT (**B**) images of a multilobular osseous tumour. The tumour can be seen invading the cranial cavity.

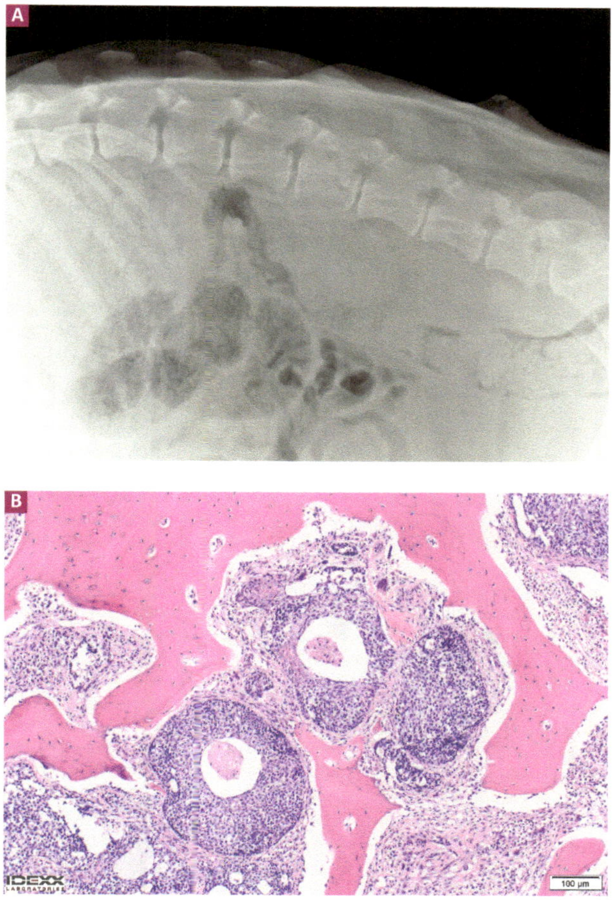

Figure 8. Lateral radiograph of the abdomen of a female German Shepherd dog with mammary carcinoma which shows lysis of the L4 vertebral body (**A**). Microscopic image which shows tumour proliferation between the vertebral bone (**B**). (Courtesy of Carolina Naranjo, DACVP).

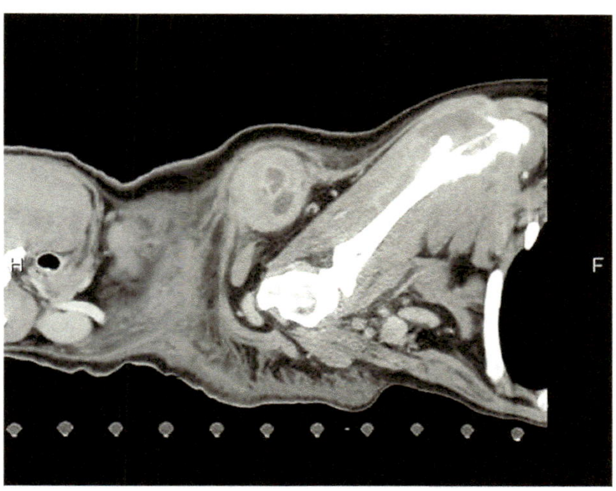

Figure 9. CT image in a soft tissue window, where a mass level with the cervical musculature and a lesion in the dorsal area of the scapula can be seen. Both lesions were metastasis from a pulmonary squamous cell carcinoma.

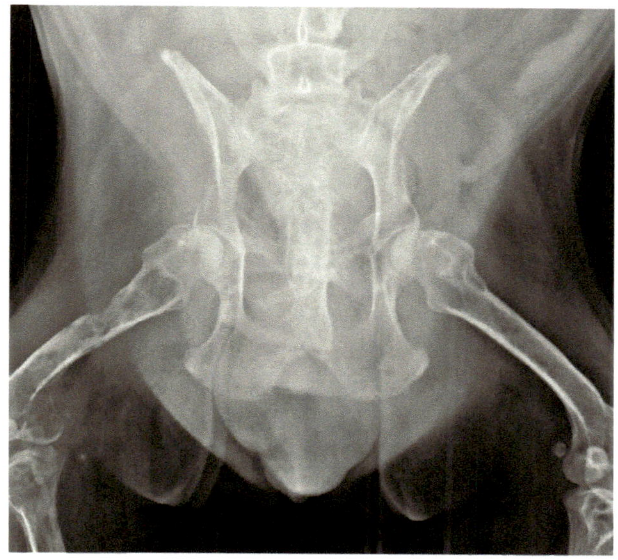

Figure 10. Lytic lesions in femurs and tibias in a dog with multiple myeloma.

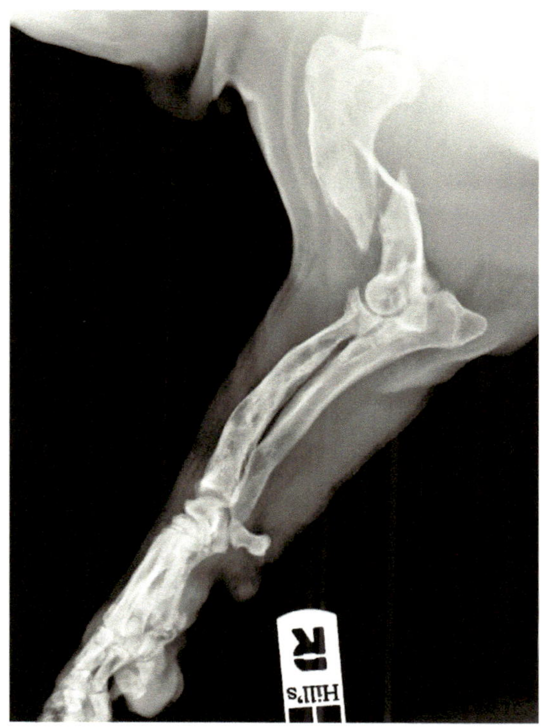

Figure 11. Pathological fracture in a dog with multiple myeloma. Multiple lesions can be seen in the ulna, radius, and femur.

These cases also usually present hyperproteinaemia, with monoclonal gammopathies, and are diagnosed with cytology of the bone marrow. When lytic lesions are extensive, there is a risk of pathological fractures (Figure 11).

Joint Tumours

Synovial sarcoma is the tumour that has traditionally been considered the most common in dogs' joints, although with the routine use of immunohistochemistry, **histiocytic tumours are now considered the most common**. In fact, it is currently unclear whether synovial sarcoma actually exists in dogs.

In people, synovial sarcoma is caused by a chromosomal translocation that has later been observed in sarcomas located primarily in locations other than the joint, so that it is considered a soft-tissue sarcoma that sometimes affects the synovial membrane rather than a sarcoma originating in the joint. These tumours that originate from stem cells, which explains why they are sometimes positive for cytokeratin, while normal synoviocytes are not.

Similar genetic studies have not been carried out in dogs to establish whether the same occurs in this species, but the current recommendation is not to use this nomenclature until there is a way to identify the synovial origin of these sarcomas and **it is not really known if the synovial sarcoma exists in dogs or whether it is a form of soft-tissue sarcoma**, as can occur in other parts of the body.

Thus, the **most common joint tumour is now histiocytic sarcoma**, which originates from A synoviocytes. In immunohistochemistry they are vimentin and CD18 positive. Other markers that show positivity are CD1 and CD11c, but these can only be studied in frozen samples and not after being fixed with formalin, so they are less useful. The Golden Retriever, Labrador Retriever, Rottweiler, and Flat-Coated Retriever are the breeds that most frequently suffer from periarticular histiocytic sarcoma.

Most dogs suffering from this tumour have a previous history of trauma to the same joint. The usual clinical signs are lameness and inflammation and, on radiological study, most cases present lysis and bone proliferation.

Although histiocytic tumours generally have a poor prognosis, joint or periarticular tumours have a more favourable course, with a median survival time of just over one year after surgery compared to four months for non-joint tumours. Among the periarticular histiocytic tumours, those that do not present with metastases at diagnosis have a better prognosis, with a median survival time greater than 2.5 years, while for those with metastases it is only 8 months.

Due to the importance of metastases in prognosis, before advising amputation, a complete clinical study should be performed (Figure 12). The presence of periarticular lesions is frequent in the disseminated form of the disease, which again highlights the importance of conducting a complete clinical examination. On the other hand, cases with disseminated histiocytic sarcoma, which is associated with a worse prognosis, usually present with systemic clinical signs (such as anorexia, weight loss, and lethargy). Thus, a thorough clinical history and physical examination are important when distinguishing between both presentations since the histopathology of the tumour is the same in both cases.

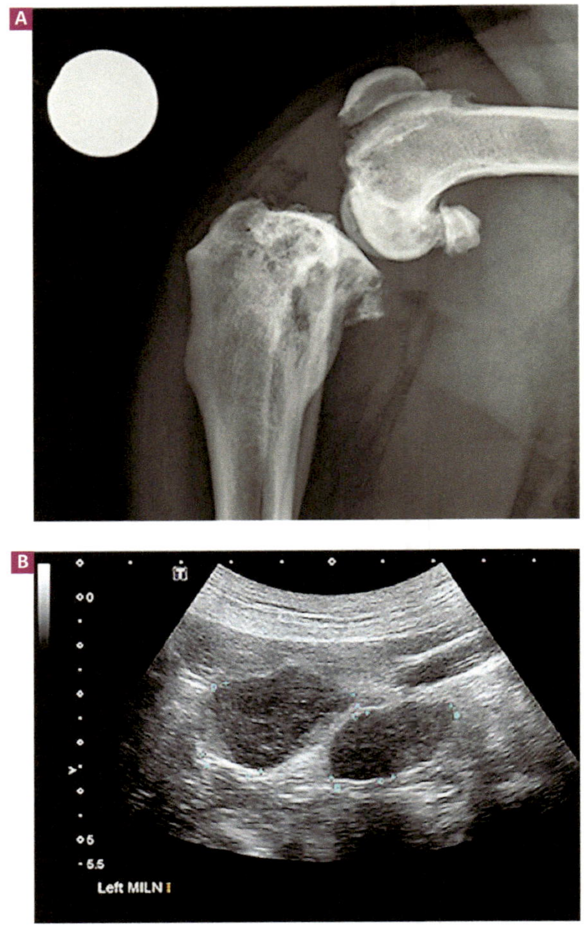

Figure 12. Joint lesion in a dog with histiocytic sarcoma presenting with lameness (**A**). The abdominal ultrasound showed lymphadenopathy (**B**) and cytology confirmed iliac lymphatic metastasis.

In the joint, **benign tumours and non-neoplastic lesions can also develop**.

The most common benign tumour in the joint is the **synovial myxoma**, which mainly affects large breed dogs (Labrador and Dobermann), and adult dogs (8 years old on average, although it can be diagnosed between 2 and 14 years of age). It is characterised by the presence of abundant myxoid matrix, but neither cytology nor radiology provides a diagnosis, so histopathology is necessary. The abundance of myxoid matrix may indicate an origin in B synoviocytes (producers of synovial fluid), but this origin has not been demonstrated as there is no specific marker for these cells.

At a cytological level, the findings are similar to inflamed synovial fluid, while on radiology there are changes similar to those observed in malignant tumours. It is a benign tumour because it does not metastasise, and the prognosis is good. Cases without bone involvement or extension outside the capsule can be treated with removal of the capsule with 10% local recurrence. More advanced cases can be treated with radiotherapy or amputation.

Synovial chondromatosis is a pathology that appears neoplastic since masses form in the joint. It can appear primarily or secondary to degenerative joint disease, and multiple nodules (1–10 mm) of cartilaginous metaplasia occur that can become ossified.

Some dogs may recover after removal of the synovium, but in other cases they may require arthrodesis or amputation. Very rarely, they can progress to chondrosarcomas.

Bibliography

- Alvarez, F.J., Hosoya, K., Lara-Garcia, A. et al. (2013) VAC Protocol for Treatment of Dogs with Stage III Hemangiosarcoma. *Journal of the American Animal Hospital Association*, 49(6):370–377. doi:10.5326/JAAHA-MS-5954.
- Armbrust, L.J., Biller, D.S., Bamford, A. et al. (2012) Comparison of three-view thoracic radiography and computed tomography for detection of pulmonary nodules in dogs with neoplasia. *J Am Vet Med Assoc*, 240(9):1088–1094. doi:10.2460/javma.240.9.1088.
- Boerman, I., Selvarajah, G.T., Nielen, M. et al. (2012) Prognostic factors in canine appendicular osteosarcoma - a meta-analysis. *BMC Vet Res*, 8(1):56. doi:10.1186/1746-6148-8-56.
- Bracha, S., Walshaw, R., Danton, T. et al. (2014) Evaluation of toxicities from combined metronomic and maximal-tolerated dose chemotherapy in dogs with osteosarcoma. *Journal of Small Animal Practice*, 55(7):369–374. doi:10.1111/jsap.12228.
- Britt, T., Clifford, C., Barger, A. et al. (2007) Diagnosing appendicular osteosarcoma with ultrasound-guided fine-needle aspiration: 36 cases. *J Small Anim Pract*, 48(3):145–150. doi:10.1111/j.1748-5827.2006.00243.x.
- Bulakowski, E.J., Philibert, J.C., Siegel, S. et al. (2008) Evaluation of outcome associated with subcutaneous and intramuscular hemangiosarcoma treated with adjuvant doxorubicin in dogs: 21 cases (2001–2006). *J Am Vet Med Assoc*, 233(1):122–128. doi:10.2460/javma.233.1.122.
- Culp, W.T.N., Olea-Popelka, F., Sefton, J. et al. (2014) Evaluation of outcome and prognostic factors for dogs living greater than one year after diagnosis of osteosarcoma: 90 cases (1997–2008). *J Am Vet Med Assoc*, 245(10):1141-1146. doi:10.2460/javma.245.10.1141.
- Davis, G.J., Kapatkin, A.S., Craig, L.E. et al. (2002) Comparison of radiography, computed tomography, and magnetic resonance imaging for evaluation of appendicular osteosarcoma in dogs. *J Am Vet Med Assoc*, 220(8):1171–1176. doi:10.2460/javma.2002.220.1171.
- Eberle, N., Fork, M., Babo von, V. et al. (2011) Comparison of examination of thoracic radiographs and thoracic computed tomography in dogs with appendicular osteosarcoma. *Veterinary and Comparative Oncology*, 9(2):131–140. doi:10.1111/j.1476-5829.2010.00241.x.
- Fabbi, M., Di Palma, S., Manfredi, S. et al. (2017) Imaging diagnosis-ultrasonographic appearance of skeletal muscle metastases in a dog with hemangiosarcoma. *Vet Radiol Ultrasound*, 58(6):E64–E67. doi:10.1111/vru.12432.
- Fan, T.M., Charney, S.C., de Lorimier, L.P. et al. (2009) Double-Blind Placebo-Controlled Trial of Adjuvant Pamidronate with Palliative Radiotherapy and Intravenous Doxorubicin for Canine Appendicular Osteosarcoma Bone Pain. *Journal of Veterinary Internal Medicine*, 23(1):152–160. doi:10.1111/j.1939-1676.2008.0221.x.
- Fan, T.M., de Lorimier, L-P., O'Dell-Anderson, K. et al. (2007) Single-agent pamidronate for palliative therapy of canine appendicular osteosarcoma bone pain. *J Vet Intern Med*, 21(3):431–439. doi:10.1892/0891-6640(2007)21[431:spfpto]2.0.co;2.
- Fukuda, S., Kobayashi, T., Robertson, I.D. et al. (2014) Computed tomographic features of canine nonparenchymal hemangiosarcoma. *Vet Radiol Ultrasound*, 55(4):374–379. doi:10.1111/vru.12136.
- Gardner, H.L., Sivaprakasam, K., Briones, N. et al. (2019) Canine osteosarcoma genome sequencing identifies recurrent mutations in DMD and the histone methyltransferase gene SETD2. *Commun Biol*, 2(1):266–13. doi:10.1038/s42003-019-0487-2.
- Giuffrida, M.A., Bacon, N.J., Kamstock, D.A. (2017) Use of routine histopathology and factor VIII-related antigen/von Willebrand factor immunohistochemistry to differentiate primary hemangiosarcoma of bone from telangiectatic osteosarcoma in 54 dogs. *Veterinary and Comparative Oncology*, 15(4):1232–1239. doi:10.1111/vco.12259.
- Goldfinch, N., Argyle, D.J. (2012) Feline lung-digit syndrome: unusual metastatic patterns of primary lung tumours in cats. *Journal of Feline Medicine and Surgery*, 14(3):202–208. doi:10.1177/1098612X12439267.
- Klahn, S.L., Kitchell, B.E., Dervisis, N.G. (2011) Evaluation and comparison of outcomes in dogs with periarticular and nonperiarticular histiocytic sarcoma. *J Am Vet Med Assoc*, 239(1):90–96. doi:10.2460/javma.239.1.90.
- Laver, T., London, C.A., Vail, D.M. et al. (2018) Prospective evaluation of toceranib phosphate in metastatic canine osteosarcoma. *Veterinary and Comparative Oncology*, 16(1):E23–E29. doi:10.1111/vco.12328.
- Liptak, J.M., Kamstock, D.A., Dernell, W.S. et al. (2008) Oncologic Outcome after Curative-Intent Treatment in 39 Dogs with Primary Chest Wall Tumors (19922005). *Veterinary Surgery*, 37(5):488–496. doi:10.1111/j.1532-950X.2008.00415.x.
- London, C.A., Gardner, H.L., Mathie, T. et al. (2015) Impact of Toceranib/Piroxicam/Cyclophosphamide Maintenance Therapy on Outcome of Dogs with Appendicular Osteosarcoma following Amputation and Carboplatin Chemotherapy: A Multi-Institutional Study. *PLoS ONE*, 10(4):e0124889. doi:10.1371/journal.pone.0124889.
- Makielski, K.M., Mills, L.J., Sarver, A.L. et al. (2019) Risk Factors for Development of Canine and Human Osteosarcoma: A Comparative Review. *Veterinary Sciences*, 6(2):48. doi:10.3390/vetsci6020048.
- Manor, E.K., Craig, L.E., Sun, X. et al. (2018) Prior joint disease is associated with increased risk of periarticular histiocytic sarcoma in dogs. *Veterinary and Comparative Oncology*, 16(1):E83–E88. doi:10.1111/vco.12338.
- Mason, N.J., Gnanandarajah, J.S., Engiles, J.B. et al. (2016) Immunotherapy with a HER2-Targeting Listeria Induces HER2-Specific Immunity and Demonstrates Potential Therapeutic Effects in a Phase I Trial in Canine Osteosarcoma. *Clin Cancer Res*, 22(17):4380–4390. doi:10.1158/1078-0432.CCR-16-0088.
- Meuten, D.J. (2016) *Tumors in Domestic Animals*. John Wiley & Sons.
- Musser, M.L., Berger, E.P., Parsons, C. et al. (2019) Vaccine strain Listeria monocytogenes abscess in a dog: a case report. *BMC Vet Res*, 15(1):467–4. doi:10.1186/s12917-019-2216-y.

■ Pagano, C., Boudreaux, B., Shiomitsu, K. (2016) Safety and toxicity of an accelerated coarsely fractionated radiation protocol for treatment of appendicular osteosarcoma in 14 dogs: 10 GY × 2 Fractions. *Vet Radiol Ultrasound*, 57(5):551–556. doi:10.1111/vru.12389.

■ Ryseff, J.K., Bohn, A.A. (2012) Detection of alkaline phosphatase in canine cells previously stained with Wright-Giemsa and its utility in differentiating osteosarcoma from other mesenchymal tumors. *Vet Clin Pathol*, 41(3):391–395. doi:10.1111/j.1939-165X.2012.00445.x.

■ Sakthikumar, S., Elvers, I., Kim, J. et al. (2018) SETD2 Is Recurrently Mutated in Whole-Exome Sequenced Canine Osteosarcoma. *Cancer Res*, 78(13):3421–3431. doi:10.1158/0008-5472.CAN-17-3558.

■ Schmidt, A.F., Nielen, M., Klungel, O.H. et al. (2013) Prognostic factors of early metastasis and mortality in dogs with appendicular osteosarcoma after receiving surgery: an individual patient data meta-analysis. *Prev Vet Med*, 112(3–4):414–422. doi:10.1016/j.prevetmed.2013.08.011.

■ Schott, C.R., Tatiersky, L.J., Foster, R.A. et al. (2018) Histologic Grade Does Not Predict Outcome in Dogs with Appendicular Osteosarcoma Receiving the Standard of Care. *Veterinary Pathology*, 55(2):202-211. doi:10.1177/0300985817747329.

■ Selmic, L.E., Burton, J.H., Thamm, D.H. et al. (2014) Comparison of Carboplatin and Doxorubicin-Based Chemotherapy Protocols in 470 Dogs after Amputation for Treatment of Appendicular Osteosarcoma. *Journal of veterinary internal medicine*, (28):554–563. doi:10.1111/jvim.12313.

■ Singer, J., Fazekas, J., Wang, W. et al. (2014) Generation of a Canine Anti-EGFR (ErbB-1) Antibody for Passive Immunotherapy in Dog Cancer Patients. *Molecular Cancer Therapeutics*, 13(7):1777–1790. doi:10.1158/1535-7163.MCT-13-0288.

■ Thrift, E., Greenwell, C., Turner, A-L. et al. (2017) Metastatic pulmonary carcinomas in cats ("feline lung-digit syndrome"): further variations on a theme. *JFMS Open Rep*, 3(1):2055116917691069. doi:10.1177/2055116917691069.

■ Tuohy, J.L., Shaevitz, M.H., Garrett, L.D. et al. (2019) Demographic characteristics, site, and phylogenetic distribution of dogs with appendicular osteosarcoma: 744 dogs (2000–2015). *Heymann D, ed. PLoS ONE*, 14(12):e0223243. doi:10.1371/journal.pone.0223243.

■ Wustefeld-Janssens, B.G., Seguin, B., Ehrhart, N.P. et al. (2020) Analysis of outcome in dogs that undergo secondary amputation as an end-point for managing complications related to limb salvage surgery for treatment of appendicular osteosarcoma. *Veterinary and Comparative Oncology*, 18(1):84–91. doi:10.1111/vco.12513.

■ Wycislo, K.L., Fan, T.M. (2015) The immunotherapy of canine osteosarcoma: a historical and systematic review. *J Vet Intern Med*, 29(3):759–769. doi:10.1111/jvim.12603.

Test

Answers on Page 304

1. **Osteosarcoma is the most common skeletal tumour in the dog. What percentage of all bone tumours are osteosarcomas in the canine species?**
   a. 75%.
   b. 80%.
   c. 85%.
   d. 90%.

2. **Most osteosarcomas originate in the extremities, specifically in the metaphysis of long bones. Which of the following are risk factors for the development of sarcomas in the dog?**
   a. That the dog is a mastiff type breed.
   b. That the animal is a giant mountain type breed.
   c. Genetic alterations such as mutations that affect the SETD2 gene.
   d. All of the above answers are correct.

3. **When talking about diagnosis of canine osteosarcoma, which of the following answers is incorrect?**
   a. It is important to rule out whether the tumour in question is a metastasis from another tumour which has not been located.
   b. Biopsies which are too small or superficial can lead to erroneous diagnoses.
   c. Cytology almost never gives a definitive diagnosis, more tests are needed.
   d. For biopsies, it is important to take samples from the centre of the lesion.

4. **Regarding the treatment of canine osteosarcoma, which answer is the correct one?**
   a. Recent studies show that when a tumour is located in a limb, traditional amputation of the limb should be avoided, and less aggressive treatments should be carried out.
   b. The chemotherapy treatment which is currently recommended is based on carboplatin.
   c. The latest studies recommend replacing carboplatin with toceranib, especially when it comes to metastatic osteosarcoma.
   d. If the affected limb is amputated, other treatments can be dispensed with because the tumour, which has minimal capacity to metastasise, has already been removed.

5. **Regarding the prognosis of different tumours that affect the musculoskeletal system, what is the wrong answer?**
   a. Osteosarcoma has a moderately good prognosis if the affected limb is amputated.
   b. Aggressive surgery is associated with good survival rate with chondrosarcoma.
   c. Primary haemangiosarcoma in bone or muscle has a high rate of metastasis.
   d. Multilobular bone tumours recur in half of cases, even though clean margins have been achieved during surgery.

6. **What are the most common secondary bone tumours?**
   a. Squamous cell tumours.
   b. Multiple myeloma.
   c. Leiomyomas.
   d. Carcinomas.

7. **What is the most common malignant tumour that affects joints?**
   a. Synovial sarcoma.
   b. Histiocytic sarcoma.
   c. Synovial myxoma.
   d. Chondrosarcoma.

8. **What is synovial chondromatosis?**
   a. A malignant tumour originating in synoviocytes.
   b. A pathology that appears neoplastic, since masses are formed in the joint, but it is not.
   c. One of the most common joint tumours in dogs.
   d. It has a very characteristic radiological appearance, shaped like popcorn.

Notes

Correct Answers:

1. c
2. d
3. c
4. b
5. a
6. d
7. b
8. b

Notes

Tumours of the Nasal Cavity and Pulmonary Tumours

Pachi Clemente Vicario

Nasal Tumours

Nasal Plane

The most frequent tumour of the nasal plane is **squamous cell carcinoma**, which is common in cats (with an unpigmented nasal plane and in areas exposed to sunlight) and rare in dogs. Other tumours that can be seen in this location are mast cell tumours or fibrosarcomas (Figure 1), but they are rarely diagnosed.

Cytology from a fine needle aspirate can help to make a diagnosis in cases of mast cell tumours or fibrosarcomas. In the case of squamous cell carcinomas, there is often a lot of inflammation and secondary infection in the most superficial part, so instead of taking impression smears, obtaining deeper samples by aspiration is recommended (Figure 2).

Squamous cell carcinoma is an epithelial tumour that can develop in different anatomical locations. Aspects related only to the nasal plane are briefly described here. In cats, it affects older outdoor cats, where the area is depigmented, since **exposure to ultraviolet light is a predisposing factor**.

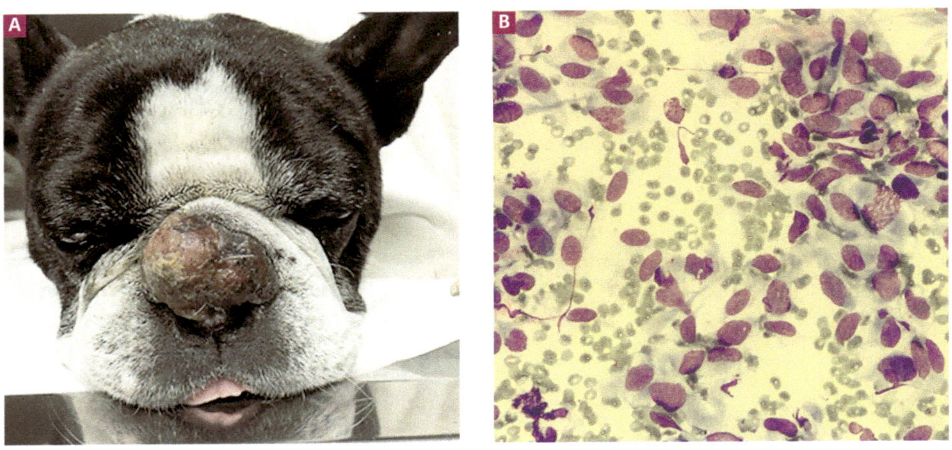

Figure 1. Macroscopic lesion of the nasal plane in a French Bulldog (**A**). Cytology from the lesion showed moderate cellularity, without signs of secondary inflammation, with a homogenous population of mesenchymal cells, elongated, with little cytoplasm, oval nuclei, and the presence of minimal extracellular matrix (top right corner of the image), compatible with soft-tissue sarcoma (**B**).

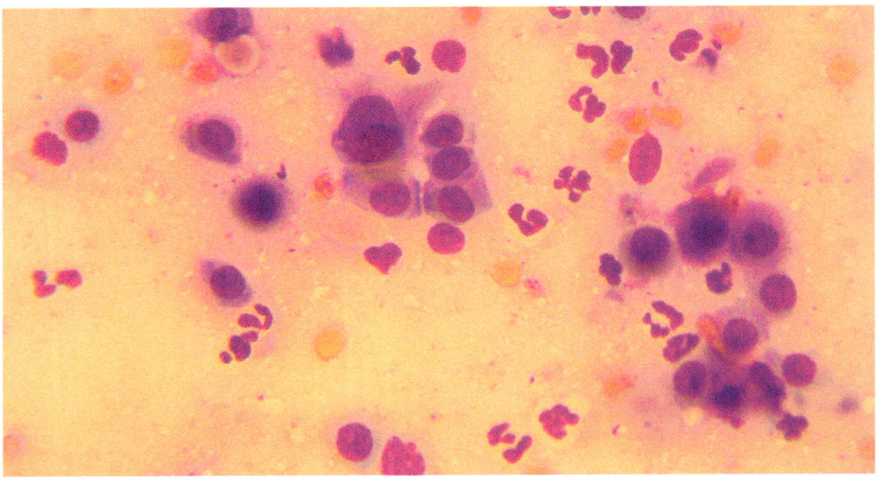

Figure 2. Cytology from an aspiration of an ulcerated lesion on the nasal plane of a Pug, which shows a population of squamous cells, with cytoplasm with angulated edges, a high nucleus/cytoplasm ratio, anisocytosis, anisokaryosis and occasional binucleated cells. There are also abundant neutrophils. The biopsy confirmed the presence of a squamous cell carcinoma.

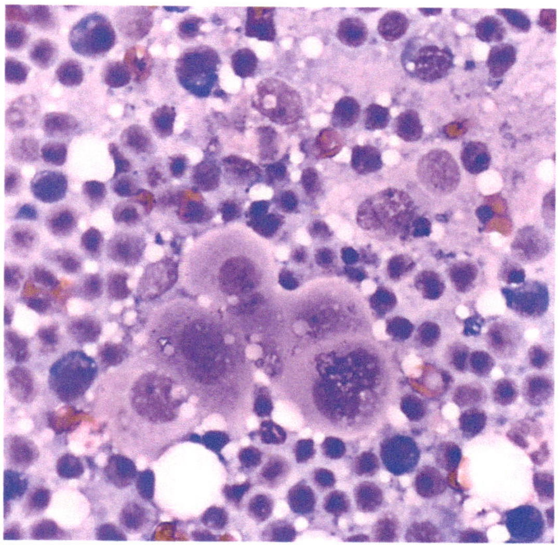

Figure 3. Cluster of normal sized epithelial cells from the submandibular lymph nodes of a dog with squamous cell carcinoma of the nasal plane.

The lesion initially appears traumatic but progresses as an ulcer with tissue destruction. Although the rate of metastasis to regional lymph nodes is low, evaluation using cytology it is always recommended (Figure 3) before offering local treatment such as surgery or electrochemotherapy.

In cats, electrochemotherapy combining intravenous bleomycin and local electrical pulses offers good results (Figure 4) in squamous cell carcinomas of the nasal plane.

In dogs it can be treated surgically if there are no lymph node metastases. Only the nasal plane can be removed, or the maxillary bone can be included in tumours that require wider margins.

The result from a cosmetic point of view is acceptable and the functional result is very good, but informing the owner regarding the results is essential before surgery. Showing them images of similar cases, which have undergone surgery, so they are aware of the cosmetic result before making the decision whether to intervene on their pet.

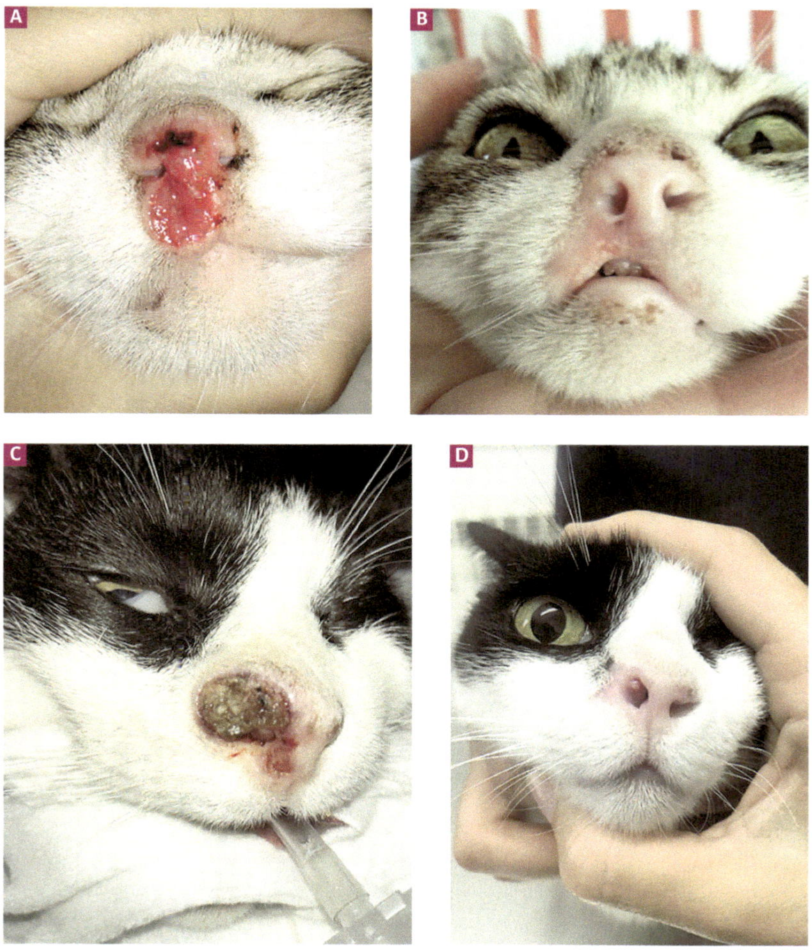

Figure 4. Examples of squamous cell carcinomas before (**A** and **C**) and after (**B** and **D**) electrochemotherapy treatment.

The prognosis is good for tumours that can be completely removed, but the risk of local recurrence is high if clean margins are not achieved, so prior to this it is important to have advanced imaging studies (CT or MRI) to help plan the surgical procedure.

Nasal Cavity

Tumours of the nasal cavity and paranasal sinuses constitute **about 1% of tumours in dogs** and affect older animals (10 years old on average). They can be both **carcinomas** (adenocarcinomas, squamous cell carcinoma and undifferentiated carcinomas) as well as **sarcomas** (fibrosarcomas, chondrosarcomas, osteosarcomas, and undifferentiated sarcomas). About two thirds of the cases are carcinomas and one third are sarcomas. In both cases, it is considered a locally aggressive tumour with a low metastasis rate at the time of diagnosis, but which can be 40–50% at the time of death of the animal. Other tumours, such as round cell tumours, can occasionally be found in dogs.

They share **clinical signs** with other nasal diseases, but a history of epistaxis or mucopurulent discharge, unilateral (initially), in older dogs (8–10 years of age on average), should mean this neoplasm is included on the list of differentials. These clinical signs may be present several months prior to consultation, and nasal neoplasia is the most common cause of chronic nasal discharge or epistaxis. In most cases there are no systemic clinical signs. It is important to bear in mind that an improvement after treatment with antibiotics or anti-inflammatory drugs does not rule out tumoural origin of the disease.

If there is facial deformation, the most likely diagnosis is cancer. If the tumour affects the caudal portion of the nasal cavity, some neurological signs may be present, although the absence of these does not rule out the spread of the tumour caudal to the cribriform plate.

From the clinical signs and imaging tests, a presumptive diagnosis of a nasal tumour can be made, but the **definitive diagnosis is by histopathology**.

CT or MRI are the preferred imaging modalities because they are superior to radiographs. CT is also more reliable than rhinoscopy in detecting nasal masses and may be considered the first option when nasal tumours are suspected. Under the same anaesthesia, and after visualising the tumour, a biopsy sample must be taken. Even in "blind" samples a diagnosis can be obtained, although it is often necessary to repeat the sampling.

One study showed no difference between the probability of making a diagnosis with samples obtained blindly, using advanced image-guided or rhinoscopy. The first sample was diagnostic in about half of cases, but at least three or four samples should be taken for a diagnosis, since due to the rhinitis present in many tumours secondary to the caudal location of some tumours in the nasal cavity or a poor-quality biopsy, false negatives are common. **A special precaution when taking the biopsy is not to advance caudally to the cribriform plate** (if the biopsy is taken from the nostril, this should not go further caudally than the medial canthus of the eye).

As part of the clinical staging (Table 1), lymph nodes must be aspirated (positive in 10–24% of cases) and thoracic radiographs taken (three views: right and left lateral and ventrodorsal). Most cases do not have metastases at the time of diagnosis, but it is essential to rule them out before starting treatment, especially if a local treatment such as radiotherapy is to be recommended.

Table 1. The modified Adams classification is generally used to determine the clinical stage of the tumour.

Stage	Description
I	Unilateral. No bone involvement beyond the turbinates
II	Bone involvement (in addition to the turbinates), but without involvement of the orbit, subcutaneous tissue, or submucosa
III	Affected orbit or subcutaneous, submucosal, or nasopharyngeal mass
IV	Cribriform plate lysis

With the result of the biopsy and the CT images (Figure 5), the owner can be provided with prognostic information. Of the tumours that receive radiotherapy, in those that are poorly differentiated or anaplastic this provides a median survival time of 4.4 months, while patients with differentiated sarcomas and carcinomas live on average 10.6 months. Regarding CT images, unilateral tumours that do not destroy the nasal turbinates have a median survival time of 24 months, compared to those that penetrate the cribriform plate that live on average 6 months. When comparing MRI and CT to perform clinical staging, the tumour volume is greater (18%) with MRI compared with CT. Visualisation of the CNS is also better with MRI than with CT, but for most cases the information was similar with both techniques.

Nasal cavity tumours are **usually treated with radiotherapy**, while surgery has generally been limited to benign lesions or surgery adjunctive to radiation therapy. Median survival times with radiotherapy range from 11 to 19 months, with survival rates at one year of 43–68% and 11–44% at two years. In more detail, the prognosis depends on the clinical stage and the histological type. Median survival times are two years

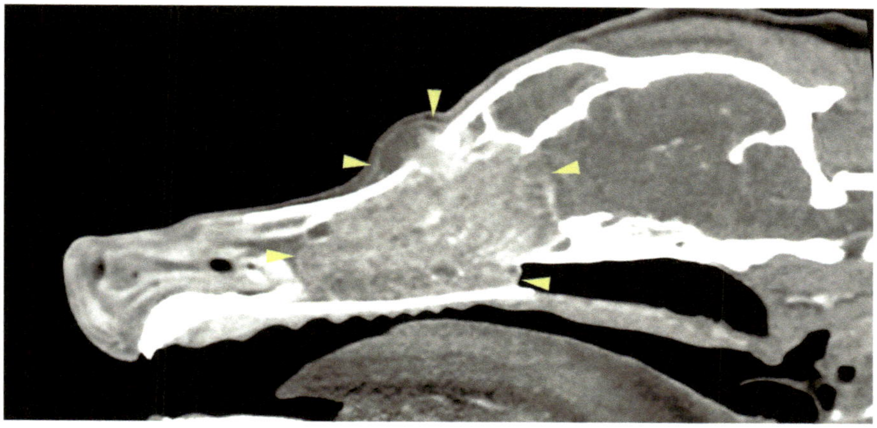

Figure 5. CT section where facial deformation can be seen in addition to how the mass has gone through the cribriform plate and invaded the cranial cavity (stage IV).

for stage I, fifteen months for stages II and III, and about six months for stage IV

In sarcomas treated with radiation, the median survival for fibrosarcomas and chondrosarcomas is one year, while osteosarcomas have median survival times of 1.7 years or undifferentiated sarcomas 11 months. This same study showed better results in definitive protocols (with daily treatments) than with those that were reduced to three weekly treatments or palliative protocols.

The experience of the veterinary team that performs the treatment is extremely important because notable differences have been documented when delimiting the tumour tissue and separating it from normal structures that should not be irradiated.

It is crucial to inform the owner that **radiotherapy helps control the tumour, but cure is unlikely**, especially in advanced stages, since what radiation achieves is a significant reduction in tumour volume, of around 60% in carcinomas, but only 20% in sarcomas.

Protocols that include fewer treatments are possible with some linear accelerators. An example of these protocols, called stereotactic radiation, would be only three treatments administered in 3–5 days, with a radiation dose of 10 Gy per fraction, which has been associated with average survival times of 18 months and one and two year survival rate of 50% and 40% respectively, similar to other protocols that require more treatments (with the corresponding anaesthesia).

In **stage IV tumours the prognosis is poor**, and they are often treated with palliative protocols, trying to control symptoms and improve quality of life. The median survival time for these cases is about four months. The presence of midline deviation of the frontal or olfactory lobe is associated with a worse prognosis and in one study the animals that presented it had a mean survival time of 2 months while those that did not present it had a mean survival time of 7 months.

When radiotherapy is not an option, medical treatment may be considered. There is **little information on the role of chemotherapy in the management of nasal tumours in dogs**. The use of alternating carboplatin and doxorubicin (three doses of each, administered every three weeks) achieved median survival times of 9 months in carcinomas and 15 months in sarcomas. When carcinomas were separated by clinical stage, the mean survival times were 10 months in stages I and II, 5 months in stage III, and only 1 month in stage IV.

In 2011 an article was published on the use of toceranib phosphate in solid tumours. Among the tumours in which a response was observed were nasal carcinomas. Although 70% of the cases showed clinical benefit (which includes complete remission, partial remission, and stable disease), the majority had stable disease. Toceranib phosphate is an inhibitor of different tyrosine kinases, such as c-Kit, the vascular endothelial growth factor receptor (VEGFR) or the platelet-derived growth factor receptor (PDGFR). Nasal carcinomas mostly express receptors that can be blocked with toceranib such as VEGFR and PDGFR-α, as evidenced in a group of more than 180 samples of these tumours. However, a second study found that, even though these receptors were expressed in all cases, they were not phosphorylated.

Protein phosphorylation is used as an indicator of activity in cell signalling and therefore it is considered that proteins that are active (phosphorylated) may be more relevant in cell proliferation compared to those that are present, but not active. The antiangiogenic effect of toceranib (by inhibiting receptors present on vascular endothelial cells) does not seem to explain the response either.

Changes in contrast uptake on tomography are used as an indicator of antiangiogenic effect. One study showed that although 83% of dogs with nasal carcinoma treated with toceranib showed decreased contrast uptake, this did not correlate with the partial remission observed in 22% or stable disease in 61% of cases treated. More studies are needed to understand the mechanism responsible for the cell proliferation of these tumours and their response to toceranib.

In **cats, lymphoma is the most common tumour in the nasal cavity**, although rhinitis is more common. In a study comparing response to radiation therapy, chemotherapy, or a combination of both, no differences were seen between the three groups, with 44% of cats living for more than two years. There was a response to radiotherapy in 93% of the cases. Similarly, when treated with chemotherapy, 93% of them went into remission (73% complete remission and 20% partial remission), with a median survival time of 2 years for those who showed complete remission and about 2 months for those who showed partial remission. When treated with hypofractionated protocols, 86% of cats show an improvement in symptoms, the mean time until the tumour progresses after treatment is about 7 months, and the mean survival time is 1 year. However, it is important to bear in mind that, despite being initially located in the nasal cavity, the lymphoma can progress to other locations and there is a 20% relapse rate in different locations when treated with localised therapies such as radiotherapy.

Carcinomas of the nasal cavity in cats can also be treated with radiotherapy with a median survival time of 15 months and survival rates of 57% at a year and 27% at 2 years using protocols of ten fractions of 4.2 Gy. Palliative protocols achieve lower survival rates, especially in cats with stage IV (modified Adams classification) or with facial deformation.

Pulmonary Tumours

Pulmonary tumours are **much less common in dogs than in people**. In human patients, it is the cancer that causes the most deaths per year, with more deaths than breast, colon and prostate tumours combined, with tobacco as the main risk factor. However, in dogs no relationship has been found between exposure to smoke (dogs in homes of smokers) and an increased risk of lung cancer.

It affects older animals, with an average age of 11 years old, although less differentiated forms, such as anaplastic carcinoma, affect younger animals (7.5 years old on average). Genetic studies with canine lung carcinoma cell lines show alterations in the number of copies (with a lower number) in the CDKN2A/B/B-AS1 gene, a gene that participates in the control of the cell cycle and is considered a tumour suppressor. In people with lung adenocarcinoma, the lack of this gene is also common.

The most comprehensive genetic study of canine lung carcinomas analysed samples from eighty-eight tumours. Almost 70% of the total diagnosed cases were between 10 and 13 years of age and the most frequent breed diagnosed was the Labrador Retriever (21% of the cases). The study confirmed fewer copies of CDKN2A/B/B-AS1 in 40% of the samples analysed and also showed that more than a third of canine lung carcinomas have the V659E mutation in the HER2 gene. This gene encodes the HER2 receptor (Human Epidermal growth factor Receptor type 2) which is related to cell growth and proliferation, and which remains constantly active with this mutation, thus contributing to tumour growth.

Histologically, **lung tumours can derive from the epithelium of the airways**, in which case the masses are observed near the pulmonary hilum, or the **lung parenchyma**, when they are in the lung periphery, but classification of tumours is based on histological type and not on location. About 85% of primary lung tumours are bronchoalveolar carcinomas, while the remaining 15% are made up of adenocarcinomas and squamous cell carcinomas. Small cell carcinoma, which affects 25% of human lung cancer patients, is rare in dogs.

Lung tumours **have a strong tendency to metastasise**. In fact, in people, the tumour is only located in the lung at the time of diagnosis in 15% of cases, with more than 50% of cases with distant metastases. In dogs, 23% of cases have distant metastases when diagnosed, but about 70% show evidence of vascular or lymphatic invasion (an indicator of a high risk of metastasis). In the case of more aggressive carcinomas, such as squamous cell or anaplastic types, the rate of metastasis at diagnosis exceeds 50 and 90% respectively. 25% of cases are diagnosed incidentally on thoracic radiographs of asymptomatic animals (for example, during preanaesthetic check-ups in geriatric animals). When they present with clinical signs, cough is the most frequent and is present in half of cases, but dyspnoea (25%) or systemic signs such as lethargy, anorexia or weight loss may also be present. Occasionally, the reason for consultation may be lameness secondary to hypertrophic osteopathy in dogs or digital metastasis in cats (Figure 6). In a series of thirty-six cats with digital metastases from a primary lung tumour, none of them had respiratory symptoms. In addition to the toes, they can have metastases in other locations including the eye or muscles. The use of term MODAL (Muscle/Ocular/Digit/Aorta/Lung) syndrome has been proposed because it at least affects these organs.

On radiographs, half of the cases have lesions that affect a single lung lobe. In a review of seventy-four cases, the radiological characteristics were described according to the tumour (confirmed with histopathology in all cases). Histiocytic sarcomas

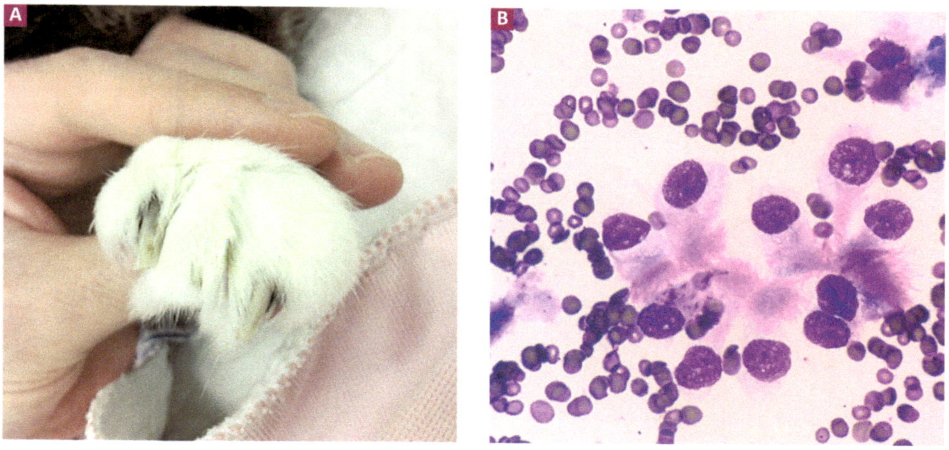

Figure 6. Inflammation in the digit of a cat with pulmonary carcinoma (**A**) and cytology from the lesion where well-differentiated respiratory epithelial cells can be seen (**B**). Generally, cytology shows epithelial cells with malignancy criteria in which specific characteristics of respiratory cells cannot normally be recognised.

were tumours of greater volume (271 cm³), with bronchograms in half of cases, and were more frequently located in the left and right middle cranial lobes, while adenocarcinomas were frequently located in the left caudal lobe. However, these descriptions refer to most cases of each tumour, but do not allow a final diagnosis simply based on location.

In most of the cases treated by the author, an **ultrasound-guided fine needle aspiration was attempted first if the tumour was close to the thoracic wall to make a diagnosis**. Sensitivity is 77–90% and correlates well (over 80%) with histopathology. For tumours located outside ultrasound range, sometimes a CT-guided biopsy can be performed, but in many of these cases the diagnosis is made after surgical removal of the mass. **Tomography is superior to radiography for evaluation of the tracheobronchial nodes** (whose status is important for the prognosis, since patients in whom lymphadenopathy is detected have a mean survival time of 2 months, compared to 10 months in those without lymphadenopathy). In human patients, non-operable tumours are biopsied because the treatment depends not only on the histological type, but also on the presence of certain molecular alterations (for example, the mutation in the epithelial growth factor receptor, EGFR). If surgery is to be performed prior to the definitive diagnosis, it is important to inform the owner that the prognosis depends on the histological type. As mentioned, some canine lung carcinomas have a HER2 mutation. In about a third of these cases, the mutation could be found in the plasma of these animals, which opens the door to non-invasive genetic diagnosis (liquid biopsy).

The prognosis for cases in which the tumour can be completely removed with surgery is better (one year) than in those in which macroscopic disease remains (one month) after the procedure. Thus, before operating, assessing whether all the visible disease can be removed is necessary. The **prognosis depends on the clinical stage and the histological type and grade**. Median survival time for solitary tumours (treated with surgery) is 26 months, compared to 7 months for multiple lesions or 3 months for lesions invading adjacent tissues. Cases with lymph node metastases had a shorter survival time (1 month) than those without metastases (15 months).

The histological type is also important, with a survival time for squamous carcinomas of 8 months, compared to 19 months for adenocarcinomas, as well as the histological grade, with a better prognosis for grade I carcinomas (26 months on average) than for grade II (8 months) or III (only a few days). Finally, the combination of both factors; clinical stage and histological type, has also shown its prognostic value, with papillary adenocarcinomas with clinical stage T1N0M0, with a mean survival time of 555 days, and other histological types with a more advanced clinical stage, of only 72 days.

Information on the role of chemotherapy is scarce. In people, platinum derivatives and vinorelbine are used for cases that do not present molecular alterations that can be treated with targeted therapies. Studies with cell lines show inhibitory concentrations 50% below therapeutic levels of carboplatin, although there are no clinical data to confirm this potential benefit. Vinorelbine has also been used in canine lung carcinoma with no clear benefit from its adjuvant use, although there may be partial remissions when surgery is not possible. In advanced cases (T3, N1 or M1), the use of protocols that include thalidomide seems to slightly improve mean survival time (4 months), compared to surgery (3 months) or palliative treatment (2 months).

In 2020 an update of the clinical stage system for canine lung tumours was proposed (Table 2), adapted from the classification used in human medicine, compared to the one which has been in use since the 80's.

Table 2. Update of the clinical staging system for canine lung tumours (Lee et al., 2020).

Stage	Size	Solitary vs. multiple	Organ invasion
		T	
T1	< 3 cm	Solitary	No
T2	3–5 cm	Solitary	Visceral pleura, main bronchus (not carina)
T3	>5–7 cm	Nodules in the same lung lobe	Costal wall, pericardium, phrenic nerve
T4	> 7 cm	Nodules in ipsilateral lobes	Mediastinum, diaphragm, heart, great vessels, recurrent laryngeal nerve, carina, trachea, oesophagus, spine
		N	
N0	No lymph node metastasis		
N1	Ipsilateral tracheobronchial lymph node		
N2	Distant lymph node metastasis		
		M	
M0	Distant metastases		
M1	Malignant effusion, extrathoracic metastasis or in contralateral lung		
		Clinical stage	
Clinical stage I	T1, N0, M0		
Clinical stage II	T2–3, N0, M0; T1–2, N1, M0		
Clinical stage III	T4, N0, M0; T3–4, N1, M0; T1–2, N2, M0		
Clinical stage IV	M1		

The study shows how in a group of 71 dogs treated with surgery, those diagnosed in the early stages of the disease (clinical stages I–II) had a much better prognosis with a mean survival time of 25 months, compared to those with more advanced disease (stages III–IV) who lived an average of 5 months. In cases that received adjuvant chemotherapy no benefit was seen in either group (early or advanced disease) when compared with those that were treated with surgery alone.

The survival rates associated with each clinical stage are shown in Table 3.

Better understanding of the disease at a molecular and genetic level could lead to more effective treatments. Analysis of the expression of receptor tyrosine kinase in canine lung carcinoma shows a high expression of PDGRF-α and its phosphoprotein (which would indicate the activation of this receptor). In veterinary medicine, toceranib phosphate has been used with some reported cases of stable disease. The author has treated cases with multiple nodules, achieving survival rates of more than one year with a particularly good quality of life (Figure 7).

Table 3. Survival times associated with clinical stage.

Clinical stage	n	TNM (n)	Average tumour associated survival time* in days (95% interval)	Average survival time in days (95% interval)
Stage I	7	T1, N0, M0 (7)	No reached	925 (211–1693)
Stage II	32	T2, N0, M0 (13) T3, N0, M0 (19)	731 (621–841)	658 (392–924)
Stage III	24	T4, N0, M0 (15) T3–4, N1–2, M0 (9)	158 (115–201)	158 (115–201)
Stage IV	8	M1 (8)	52 (2–102)	52 (2–102)

*Time from surgery until death due to the tumour.

Analysis of the receptors also showed that 100% of lung carcinomas expressed the HER2 receptor and, subsequently, the same group has described the presence of a mutation in this gene in a third of the tumours and has shown that lung carcinoma cell lines with the mutation are sensitive to neratinib (a HER2 inhibitor), whereas those without the mutation are unresponsive to this drug.

Histiocytic Sarcoma

In addition to primary lung tumours, **histiocytic sarcoma is frequently diagnosed primarily in the lung**. It mainly affects the Golden Retriever and Bernese Mountain dog, but the Miniature Schnauzer and the Pembroke Welsh Corgi have recently been recognised as other at-risk breeds. In general, the animals present systemic clinical signs (weight loss, fever, anorexia, lethargy) and clinicopathological alterations such as anaemia, thrombocytopaenia and hypoalbuminaemia (more marked if they have haemophagocytic syndrome).

Histiocytic sarcoma can present in **two clinical forms, localised, or disseminated** (in the second case it affects the lymph nodes, liver, spleen, or joints). When it is located only in the lung, the right middle lobe is usually most affected. Although the prognosis is worse than for primary tumours, it depends on the clinical form. Patients with localised disease have a better prognosis (up to a year and a half if treated with surgery and lomustine chemotherapy).

Lung Tumours in Cats

In cats, lung tumours **have a more aggressive clinical course** with the development of metastases in up to 80% of cases, including involvement of tracheobronchial lymph nodes, intrathoracic metastases or in different extrathoracic structures.

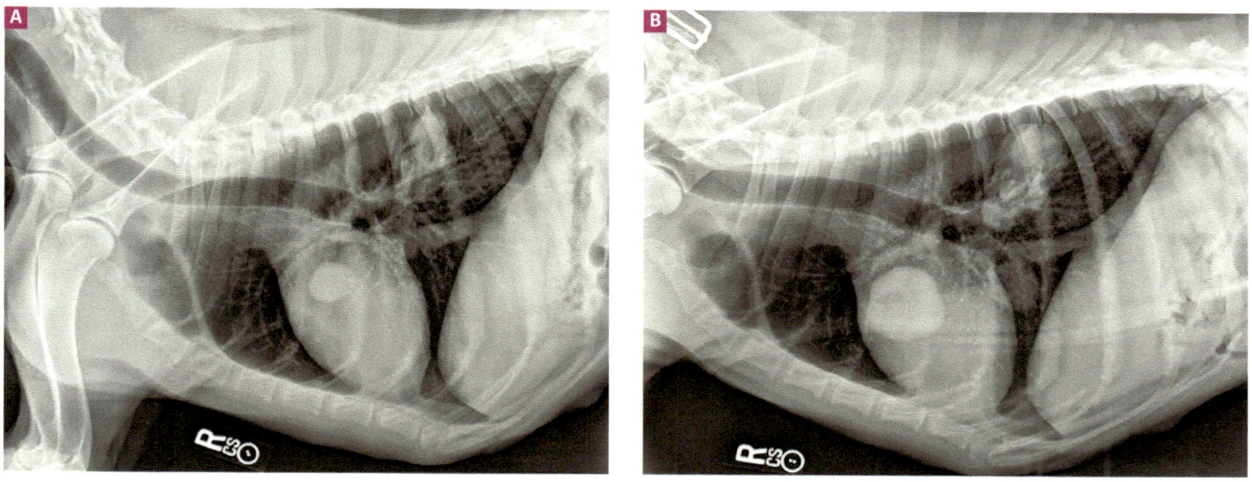

Figure 7. Radiographs of a pulmonary carcinoma with multiple nodules which were treated with toceranib phosphate. The image to the right (**B**), which shows progressive disease was taken 13 months after the one on the left (**A**). This patient lived for another 2 years, during which she was treated with toceranib.

Bibliography

■ Adams, W.M., Kleiter, M.M., Thrall, D.E. et al. (2009) Prognostic significance of tumor histology and computed tomographic staging for radiation treatment response of canine nasal tumors. *Veterinary Radiology & Ultrasound*. 50(50):330–335. doi:10.1111/j.1740-8261.2009.01545.x.

■ Barrett, L.E., Pollard, R.E., Zwingenberger, A. et al. (2014) Radiographic characterization of primary lung tumors in 74 dogs. *Veterinary Radiology & Ultrasound*. 55(55):480–487. doi:10.1111/vru.12154.

■ Cemazar, M., Tamzali, Y., Sersa, G. et al. (2008). Electrochemotherapy in veterinary oncology. *J Vet Intern Med*. 22(22):826–831. doi:10.1111/j.1939-1676.2008.0117.x.

■ Christensen, N.I., Forrest, L.J., White, P.J. et al. (2016) Single institution variability in intensity modulated radiation target delineation for canine nasal neoplasia. *Vet Radiol Ultrasound*. 57(57):639–645. doi:10.1111/vru.12398.

■ Clemente-Vicario, F., Alvarez, C.E., Rowell, J.L. et al. (2015) Human Genetic Relevance and Potent Antitumor Activity of Heat Shock Protein 90 Inhibition in Canine Lung Adenocarcinoma Cell Lines. Multhoff G, ed. *PLoS ONE*. 10(11):e0142007-e0142025. doi:10.1371/journal.pone.0142007.

■ Cohn, L.A. (2020) Canine Nasal Disease: An Update. *Vet Clin North Am Small Anim Pract*. 50(50):359–374. doi:10.1016/j.cvsm.2019.11.002.

■ Ferguson, S., Smith, K.C., Welsh, C.E. et al. (2019) A retrospective study of more than 400 feline nasal biopsy samples in the UK (2006–2013). *Journal of Feline Medicine and Surgery*. 1098612X19881847. doi:10.1177/1098612X19881847.

■ Finck, M., Ponce, F., Guilbaud, L. et al. (2015) Computed tomography or rhinoscopy as the first-line procedure for suspected nasal tumor: a pilot study. *Can Vet J*. 56(56):185–192.

■ Fox-Alvarez, S., Shiomitsu, K., Lejeune, A.T. et al. (2020) Outcome of intensity-modulated radiation therapy-based stereotactic radiation therapy for treatment of canine nasal carcinomas. *Vet Radiol Ultrasound*. 170:45. doi:10.1111/vru.12854.

■ Fujiwara-Igarashi, A., Fujimori, T., Oka, M. et al. (2014) Evaluation of outcomes and radiation complications in 65 cats with nasal tumours treated with palliative hypofractionated radiotherapy. *Vet J*. 202(202):455–461. doi:10.1016/j.tvjl.2014.09.016.

■ Gieger, T.L., Nolan, M.W. (2018) Linac-based stereotactic radiation therapy for canine non-lymphomatous nasal tumours: 29 cases (2013–2016). *Veterinary and Comparative Oncology*. 16(1):E68–E75. doi:10.1111/vco.12334.

■ Giuliano, A., Dobson, J. (2020) Clinical response and survival time of cats with carcinoma of the nasal cavity treated with palliative coarse fractionated radiotherapy. *Journal of Feline Medicine and Surgery*. 204:1098612X19893445. doi:10.1177/1098612X19893445.

■ Gottfried, S.D., Popovitch, C.A., Goldschmidt, M.H. et al. (2000) Metastatic digital carcinoma in the cat: a retrospective study of 36 cats (1992–1998). *Journal of the American Animal Hospital Association*. 36(36):501–509. doi:10.5326/15473317-36-6-501.

■ Gramer, I., Killick, D., Scase, T. et al. (2017) Expression of VEGFR and PDGFR-α/-β in 187 canine nasal carcinomas. *Veterinary and Comparative Oncology*. 15(15):1041–1050. doi:10.1111/vco.12245.

■ Haney, S.M., Beaver, L., Turrel, J. et al. (2009) Survival analysis of 97 cats with nasal lymphoma: a multi-institutional retrospective study (1986–2006). *J Vet Intern Med*. 23(23):287-294. doi:10.1111/j.1939-1676.2008.0243.x.

■ Harris, B.J., Lourenço, B.N., Dobson, J.M. et al. (2014) Diagnostic accuracy of three biopsy techniques in 117 dogs with intra-nasal neoplasia. *Journal of Small Animal Practice*. 55(55):219–224. doi:10.1111/jsap.12187.

■ Hocker, S.E., Higginbotham, M.L., Schermerhorn, T. et al. (2017) Receptor tyrosine kinase expression and phosphorylation in canine nasal carcinoma. *Res Vet Sci*. 115:484–489. doi:10.1016/j.rvsc.2017.07.030.

■ Impellizeri, J., Aurisicchio, L., Forde, P. et al. (2016) Electroporation in veterinary oncology. *Vet J*. 217:18–25. doi:10.1016/j.tvjl.2016.05.015.

■ Kagawa, Y., Nakano, Y., Kobayashi, T. et al. (2016) Localized pulmonary histiocytic sarcomas in Pembroke Welsh Corgi. *J Vet Med Sci*. 77(77):1659–1661. doi:10.1292/jvms.15-0284.

■ Lee, B.M., Clarke, D., Watson, M. et al. (2020) Retrospective evaluation of a modified human lung cancer stage classification in dogs with surgically excised primary pulmonary carcinomas. *Veterinary and Comparative Oncology*. 211(211):432. doi:10.1111/vco.12582.

■ Lenz, J.A., Furrow, E., Craig, L.E. et al. (2017) Histiocytic sarcoma in 14 miniature schnauzers – a new breed predisposition? *Journal of Small Animal Practice*. 58(58):461–467. doi:10.1111/jsap.12688.

■ London, C.A., Hannah, A.L., Zadovoskaya, R. et al. (2003) Phase I dose-escalating study of SU11654, a small molecule receptor tyrosine kinase inhibitor, in dogs with spontaneous malignancies. *Clin Cancer Res*. 2755–2768.

■ Lorch, G., Sivaprakasam, K., Zismann, V. et al. (2019) Identification of Recurrent Activating HER2 Mutations in Primary Canine Pulmonary Adenocarcinoma. *Clin Cancer Res*. 25(25):5866–5877. doi:10.1158/1078-0432.CCR-19-1145.

■ Lux, C.N., Culp, W.T.N., Johnson, L.R. et al. (2017) Prospective comparison of tumor staging using computed tomography versus magnetic resonance imaging findings in dogs with nasal neoplasia: a pilot study. *Vet Radiol Ultrasound*. 58(58):315–325. doi:10.1111/vru.12486.

■ Mariotti, E.T., Premanandan, C., Lorch, G. (2014) Canine pulmonary adenocarcinoma tyrosine kinase receptor expression and phosphorylation. *BMC Vet Res*. 10(1):19–13. doi:10.1186/1746-6148-10-19.

■ Marlowe, K.W., Robat, C.S., Clarke, D.M. et al. (2018) Primary pulmonary histiocytic sarcoma in dogs: A retrospective analysis of 37 cases (2000–2015). *Veterinary and Comparative Oncology*. 16(16):658–663. doi:10.1111/vco.12437.

■ Meier, V.S., Beatrice, L., Turek, M. et al. (2019) Outcome and failure patterns of localized sinonasal lymphoma in cats treated with first-line single-modality radiation therapy: A retrospective study. *Veterinary and Comparative Oncology*. 1(1):51. doi:10.1111/vco.12517.

■ Meuten, D.J. (2016) *Tumors in Domestic Animals*. John Wiley & Sons.

■ Morgan. M.J., Lurie. D.M., Villamil, A.J. (2018) Evaluation of tumor volume reduction of nasal carcinomas versus sarcomas in dogs treated with definitive fractionated megavoltage radiation: 15 cases (2010–2016). *BMC Res Notes*. 11(11):70–76. doi:10.1186/s13104-018-3190-3.

■ Polton, G., Finotello, R., Sabattini, S. et al. (2018) Survival analysis of dogs with advanced primary lung carcinoma treated by metronomic cyclophosphamide, piroxicam and thalidomide. *Veterinary and Comparative Oncology*. 16(16):399–408. doi:10.1111/vco.12393.

■ Savas, P., Hughes, B., Solomon, B. (2013) Targeted therapy in lung cancer: IPASS and beyond, keeping abreast of the explosion of targeted therapies for lung cancer. *Journal of thoracic disease*. 5 Suppl 5(5):S579–S592. doi:10.3978/j.issn.2072-1439.2013.08.52.

■ Stiborova, K., Meier, V.S., Takada, M., et al. (2020) Definitive-intent radiotherapy for sinonasal carcinoma in cats: A multicenter retrospective assessment. *Veterinary and Comparative Oncology*. vco.12583. doi:10.1111/vco.12583.

■ Takagi, S., Yamazaki, H., Izumi, Y., et al. (2020) Assessment of tumor enhancement by contrast-enhanced CT in solid tumor-bearing dogs treated with toceranib phosphate. *Vet Radiol Ultrasound*. vru.12856. doi:10.1111/vru.12856.

■ Taylor, S.S., Goodfellow, M.R., Browne, W.J. et al. (2009) Feline extranodal lymphoma: response to chemotherapy and survival in 110 cats. *Journal of Small Animal Practice*. 50(50):584–592. doi:10.1111/j.1743-5827.2009.00813.x.

■ Thrift, E., Greenwell, C., Turner, A-L. et al. (2017) Metastatic pulmonary carcinomas in cats ("feline lung-digit syndrome"): further variations on a theme. *JFMS Open Rep*. 3(3):2055116917691069. doi:10.1177/2055116917691069.

■ Tozon, N., Pavlin, D., Sersa, G. et al. (2014) Electrochemotherapy with intravenous bleomycin injection: an observational study in superficial squamous cell carcinoma in cats. *Journal of Feline Medicine and Surgery*. 16(16):291–299. doi:10.1177/1098612X13507071.

■ Valenciano, A.C., Cowell, R.L. (2019) *Cowell and Tyler's Diagnostic Cytology and Hematology of the Dog and Cat* - E-Book. Elsevier Health Sciences.

■ Wada, Y., Noguchi, S., Sasaki, H. et al. (2018) Prognostic significance of midline shift of the olfactory or frontal lobes of the brain in canine nasal carcinomas treated by palliative radiotherapy: a pilot study. *J Vet Med Sci*. 80(80):1724–1727. doi:10.1292/jvms.18-0347.

■ Weeden, A.M., Degner, D.A. (2016) Surgical Approaches to the Nasal Cavity and Sinuses. *Vet Clin North Am Small Anim Pract*. 46(46):719–733. doi:10.1016/j.cvsm.2016.02.004.

■ Woodruff, M.J., Heading, K.L., Bennett, P. (2019) Canine intranasal tumours treated with alternating carboplatin and doxorubin in conjunction with oral piroxicam: 29 cases. *Veterinary and Comparative Oncology*. 17(17):42–48. doi:10.1111/vco.12443.

■ Wouda, R.M., Miller, M.E., Chon, E. et al. (2015) Clinical effects of vinorelbine administration in the management of various malignant tumor types in dogs: 58 cases (1997–2012). *J Am Vet Med Assoc*. 246(246):1230–1237. doi:10.2460/javma.246.11.1230.

■ Zierenberg-Ripoll, A., Pollard, R.E., Stewart, S.L. et al. (2018) Association between environmental factors including second-hand smoke and primary lung cancer in dogs. *Journal of Small Animal Practice*. 59(59):343–349. doi:10.1111/jsap.12778.

Test

Answers on Page 318

Answers on page 318

1. **The most common tumour of the nasal plane is squamous cell carcinoma, in which species is it most common?**
   a. It is more common in cats than in dogs.
   b. It is more common in dogs than in cats.
   c. The occurrence is similar in dogs and cats.
   d. It is a tumour which occurs exclusively in cats with a light coat colour.

2. **Squamous cell carcinoma is an epithelial tumour which can develop in different anatomical locations. Which is the correct answer regarding nasal plane tumours.**
   a. Electrochemotherapy treatment has been studied in cats, but with poor results.
   b. Usually cats which are affected are older, with a loss of pigmentation in the area and outdoor access, as exposure to UV light is a predisposing factor.
   c. The rate of metastasis to regional lymph nodes is high and they should therefore be biopsied in all patients to rule this out.
   d. Surgical treatment is not effective, as recurrence occurs in 100% of cases.

3. **Nasal cavity tumours:**
   a. Are always carcinomas.
   b. Make up about 10% of the nasal tumours in dogs.
   c. Can be both carcinomas and sarcomas.
   d. The absence of neurological signs in tumours which are positioned more caudally assures that there is no involvement of the cribriform plate.

4. **According to the modified Adams classification, a grade III nasal tumour has the following characteristics:**
   a. Osseous involvement (in addition to the turbinates), but does not affect the orbit, subcutaneous tissue, or submucosa.
   b. The orbit is affected or there is a subcutaneous, submucosal, or nasopharyngeal mass.
   c. Lysis of the cribriform plate.
   d. Unilateral. Without osseous involvement of anything else apart from the turbinates.

5. **Which answer is correct when referring to treatment of nasal cavity tumours in dogs and cats?**
   a. Nasal cavity tumours are usually treated using radiotherapy.
   b. Surgery is always the first step in treating the tumour.
   c. COP or CHOP protocols provide the best results.
   d. Tumours of the nasal cavity are usually treated with radiotherapy, although complete cure is unlikely.

6. **Which answer is incorrect regarding pulmonary tumours?**
   a. Histologically, pulmonary tumours can be derived from respiratory epithelium or pulmonary parenchyma.
   b. Pulmonary tumours frequently metastasise.
   c. 35% of cases are diagnosed incidentally.
   d. They are usually diagnosed in older animals, although undifferentiated forms, such as anaplastic carcinoma can affect younger animals.

7. **In the update to the clinical staging system for canine pulmonary tumours published in 2020 by Lee et al.:**
   a. N2 means that there is malignant effusion and extrathoracic or contralateral pulmonary involvement.
   b. T3 means there is invasion of the mediastinum, diaphragm, heart, large vessels, recurrent laryngeal nerve, carina, trachea, oesophagus and/or spine.
   c. N1 means that there is metastasis to distant lymph nodes.
   d. N1 means there is involvement of the ipsilateral tracheobronchial lymph node.

8. **Which answer is incorrect?**
   a. Histiocytic sarcoma is frequently diagnosed in its primary form in the lung.
   b. A study has documented that 100% of pulmonary carcinomas express the HER2 receptor.
   c. Pulmonary tumours have a more aggressive clinical course in cats than in dogs.
   d. Histiocytic sarcoma always presents with diffuse signs and is difficult to treat.

9. The presence of a pulmonary tumour can be suspected due to:

a. Secondary lameness and hypertrophic osteopathy in dogs.
b. Secondary lameness and digital metastasis in cats.
c. The presence of coughing, which affects around 50% of cases.
d. The three previous responses are correct.

10. For diagnosis of nasal plane tumours:

a. CT or MRI are the preferred imaging modalities as they are better than radiographs.
b. Radiography is the preferred imaging modality.
c. Histology is not necessary in most cases if a good staging is performed.
d. Biopsies do not provide conclusive results in most cases.

Correct Answers:

1. a
2. b
3. c
4. b
5. d
6. c
7. d
8. d
9. d
10. a

Notes

Practical Principles of Oncology Surgery

Judith Bertrán

Principles of Surgical Oncology of the Respiratory System

Nasal Tumours

The nasal cavity can be approached dorsally, ventrally, or laterally using rhinotomy. Even so, for tumours of the nasal cavity, **surgical techniques are rarely used via rhinotomy** since biopsies are usually acquired either blind or with rhinoscopy.

Nasal tumours are **rare in dogs and cats**, constituting 1–2% of tumours in these animals. The vast majority are malignant (80%) and 75% are of epithelial origin, with carcinoma and adenocarcinoma being the most common. Squamous cell carcinoma and undifferentiated carcinoma are other types of tumours affecting the nasal cavity, along with chondrosarcoma, osteosarcoma, or other mesenchymal tumours. Lymphoma is the most common nasal tumour in cats. Normally, these tumours affect dolichocephalic and mesocephalic dogs, are locally invasive and do not tend to metastasise at the time of diagnosis, although metastases can develop in about 50% of patients during the progression of the disease. Thus, treatment is aimed at the primary lesion. Dogs with untreated nasal tumours have a life expectancy of 3 months. **Medical only treatment with corticosteroids or COX-2 inhibitors does not improve the prognosis**.

The treatment par excellence for these nasal tumours is radiation therapy. The median survival time of dogs with nasal adenocarcinoma treated with radiotherapy is 14–21 months (depending on clinical stage), which is significantly longer than dogs treated with surgery alone (126 days). Mesenchymal tumours, such as chondrosarcomas, do not respond as well as epithelial tumours, although surgery can alleviate clinical signs. In cats with nasal lymphoma, radiation therapy with or without adjuvant chemotherapy can achieve long survival times and is a better tolerated therapeutic combination than surgery with chemotherapy.

Diagnosis and Clinical Staging

Diagnosis of nasal tumours can be performed by combining clinical findings with imaging techniques and biopsy results. The most frequent clinical sign is unilateral epistaxis, although it can occur bilaterally once the tumour has invaded the other nasal cavity. Other signs include excessive nasal or ocular discharge, intermittent sneezing, nasal cavity occlusion, facial deformation, and exophthalmos.

Clinical suspicions should be confirmed with imaging and biopsy of the lesion. There are different biopsy techniques for the nasal cavity. **Biopsies can be obtained with a rigid endoscope** to locate the lesion(s) and then with biopsy forceps, which can give a false negative result due to the size of the biopsy and severe inflammation of the nasal cavity in pathological conditions (e.g. inflammatory rhinitis). The results can be optimised with a large calibre cannula or with the tube technique, although these techniques can only be used in medium to large sized dogs. In these cases, it is important to make sure that the endotracheal tube cuff is inflated to protect the respiratory tract from aspiration due to nasal bleeding.

To avoid penetrating the cribriform plate and causing iatrogenic damage to the brain, the distance from the tip of the nose to the medial rim of the eye is measured with the instrument used for the biopsy. The instrument is marked at the aforementioned length and inserted into the nasal cavity for biopsies. During these procedures bleeding can be significant, so these patients should be tested for clotting and a platelet count performed (usually, these tests have already been performed to rule out epistaxis due to problems with haemostasis). If the bleeding is profuse, a gauze pad with diluted epinephrine (1:100,000) can be introduced into the nostril or 0.05% oxymetazoline applied to the nasal cavity.

Scrape cytology only achieves a diagnosis in 50% of cases, so it is not a technique which is recommended.

All **imaging techniques** should be performed before the biopsy is taken to prevent bleeding from making images difficult to interpret. Radiographs of the head can help with diagnosis: osteolysis, bone proliferation, increases in soft tissue opacity, or even the presence of radiopaque foreign bodies can be seen. The best projections are the ventrodorsal view with the mouth open and intraoral dorsoventral view.

Although radiographs may show radiographic signs suggestive of neoplasia, they are not pathognomonic since fungal infections or inflammatory diseases may have similar radiographic appearances. Thoracic radiography with three views completes the staging of the tumour, as far as imaging is concerned.

CT scanning is superior to radiography in that it allows for a much more thorough assessment of tumour extent (including assessment of the cribriform plate, assessment of the caudal extent of the tumour and invasion of adjacent structures) and is more sensitive for early stages (Figure 1). CT is also an imaging technique that is necessary in order to plan radiation therapy correctly and accurately. It is currently the technique used for the diagnosis and treatment approach to nasal tumours.

Rhinoscopy allows direct visualisation of the nasal cavities and is usually performed with a combined approach, such as rostral and/or caudal. The caudal approach is usually performed first with a flexible endoscope inserted through the oral cavity. If a tumour is present at this level, biopsy forceps are inserted into the endoscope to acquire a sample. Rostral rhinoscopy is performed using a rigid rhinoscope through the nostril and provides images of the nasal meatus, ventral turbinate, alar cartilage, and common ventral passages (Figure 2). Biopsies are taken at the end when the endoscopic examination is finished.

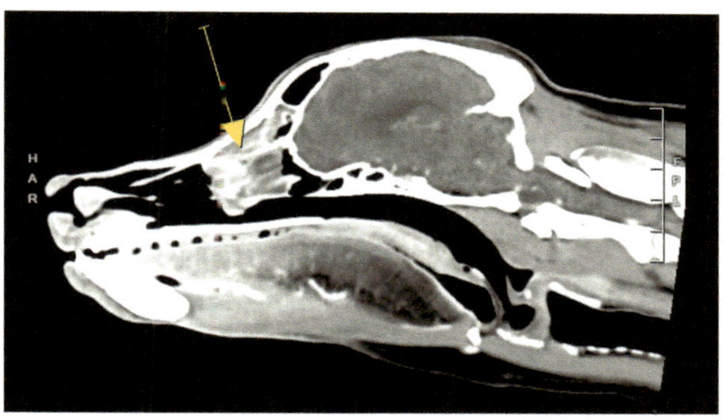

Figure 1. Sagittal section from a CT of the head and neck in a dog with stage 1 nasal adenocarcinoma (arrow). There is no nasal or cribriform plate osteolysis present.

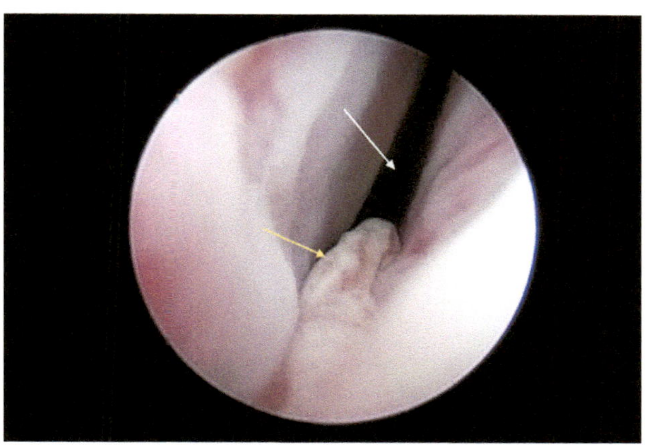

Figure 2. Rostral endoscopic image from the same patient shown in Figure 1. The nasal adenocarcinoma (orange arrow) can be visualised obstructing part of the nasal passage (white arrow).

General Surgical Considerations

Dorsal (Figure 3) or **ventral rhinotomy** is indicated for biopsies of pathologies in the nasal cavity when other techniques have failed to obtain diagnostic samples and for cytoreductive surgeries.

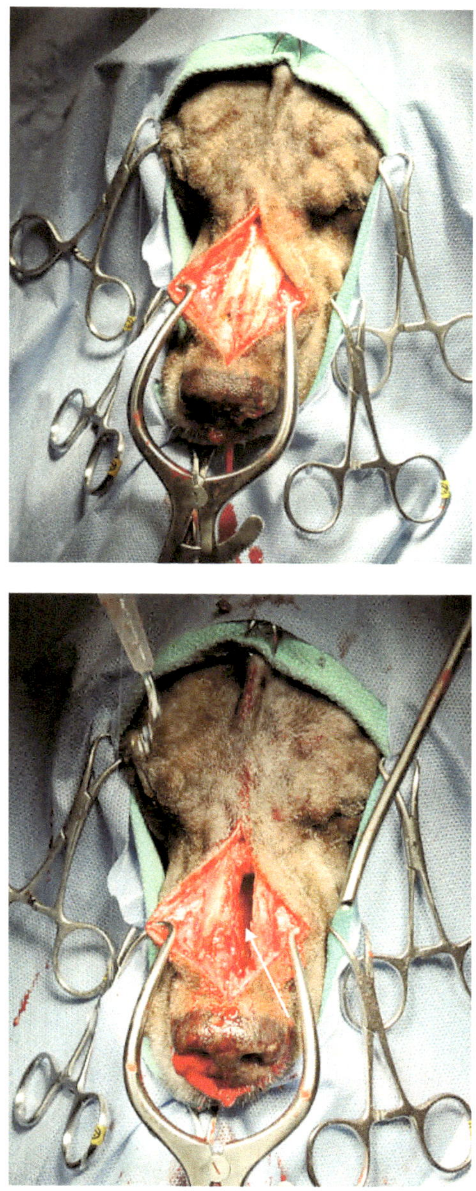

Figure 3. Dorsal approach for rhinotomy (**A**) and dorsal rhinotomy of the left nasal fossa (arrow) (**B**).

Surgery for nasal tumours on its own is not curative and should always be combined with other treatment protocols, including both neoadjuvant and adjuvant. In all procedures, after the patient has been anaesthetised and intubated, the larynx is stuffed with gauze to prevent aspiration of blood or other secretions during surgery. When the patient is extubated, the cuff is left inflated to remove any secretions which have accumulated at this level.

For **maxillofacial surgery**, a temporary carotid artery occlusion may be performed. This procedure does not have any sequelae in dogs, since they have collateral cerebral perfusion that comes from the vertebral arteries. In cats, the serious risk of cerebral hypoperfusion, even with temporary occlusion, means this procedure is contraindicated in this species. The occlusion can be temporary or permanent, depending on the surgical procedure or the proposed treatment. Normally, during release of the temporary occlusion, bleeding from the nose is not usually profuse after taking biopsies by rhinotomy.

Tumours of the Larynx

In cats, the most common tumours of the larynx are lymphoma and squamous cell carcinoma. In dogs, different types of tumours have been reported, such as rhabdomyosarcoma and rhabdomyoma. Other tumours reported in dogs are carcinoma, squamous cell carcinoma, mastocytomas, osteosarcoma, melanoma, lipomas, adenocarcinoma, chondrosarcoma, leiomyoma, fibropapilloma, fibrosarcoma, myxochondroma, invasive thyroid carcinoma, granular cell tumour and plasmacytoma.

Laryngeal lymphoma in cats is not a surgical disease and should be treated with a combination of chemotherapy with or without radiation therapy. Radiation therapy is not normally used in laryngeal tumours, although it should be considered as an option in cases of incomplete surgeries or when surgery is not an option. In the latter, permanent tracheostomy can alleviate clinical signs of upper airway obstruction.

Diagnosis and Clinical Staging

If there is any suspicion of a laryngeal mass, the next step for diagnosis is **general anaesthesia with intubation and direct examination of the oral cavity and larynx**. Patients usually present with some degree of dyspnoea and, if the obstruction is severe, passing an endotracheal tube may be difficult or impossible. In this case, the patient should be prepared for a tracheostomy (usually not needed), and it should be ensured that instruments (independent of those used for the biopsy) are available. Depending on the time it takes to perform a direct examination, it can be done under the effects of injectable anaesthetics, although intubation of the patient is recommended for obtaining biopsies.

The **biopsy** should be incisional for histopathology. Access to the laryngeal mass may be intraoral (with excision of a wedge from the mass), maintaining haemostasis by applying direct pressure to the biopsy area.

Cytology is not indicated for laryngeal masses since a diagnosis is often not obtained due to lack of cellularity. In cats, cytology may be beneficial in distinguishing between lymphoma and squamous cell carcinoma, although a more definitive diagnosis should be made before treatment begins.

The medial submandibular and retropharyngeal lymph nodes are responsible for draining the larynx. Although they have not been studied, deeper lymph nodes, such as the medial retropharyngeal or parotid, may also drain areas of the larynx and should be evaluated with cytology and/or biopsy (removal of the lymph nodes) to determine the presence of metastases. Evaluation of all lymph nodes in the head and neck can be performed using advanced imaging.

Radiographs can help localise the disease by showing a soft tissue opacity in the lumen of the larynx. **Ultrasound** is mostly used in patients where sedation and changes in position can produce respiratory stress although it can also be used to help diagnose laryngeal tumours. Ultrasound can also assist fine needle aspiration of lesions for cytology For the diagnosis of lung metastases or aspiration pneumonia, three thoracic radiographic views or chest CT scans are the most commonly used techniques. For cases where tumour resection or, alternatively, radiation therapy is taken into consideration, CT scans help to determine the extent of the tumour and the feasibility of surgery. Ideally, CT scans are performed before the biopsy is taken to prevent inflammation or bleeding secondary to the biopsy affecting interpretation.

General Surgical Considerations

Laryngeal tumours that are relatively confined to the larynx and do not invade the pharynx or oesophagus are candidates for possible surgery. Surgical techniques for the excision of laryngeal tumours depend on their location and extent, their behaviour and also on the curative or palliative objective of the surgical procedure (previously agreed and discussed with the owner).

Surgical techniques for the larynx include:

- **cordectomy**, excision of small tumours in the vocal folds
- **hemilaryngectomy**, excision of part of the larynx, including the cartilage
- **epiglotectomy**, excision of the epiglotis
- **total laryngectomy**, complete excision of the larynx and creation of a permanent tracheostomy.

Patients undergoing laryngeal surgeries should be monitored closely to detect complications as soon as possible. An intensive care unit with 24-hour monitoring and ability to provide oxygen therapy is needed. Tracheostomy tubes should be changed or cleaned every 24 hours and can usually be removed 3–4 days after surgery. Because of the risk of laryngeal oedema after a cordectomy or hemilaryngectomy, patients should receive intravenous corticosteroids in the perioperative and postoperative periods.

Surgical complications in these patients are the formation of scar tissue, laryngeal stenosis, incomplete margins of tumour excision and pneumonia due to aspiration of blood (in the immediate postoperative period) or food (during the postoperative period, due to laryngeal dysfunction).

In general, there is little information regarding the results after partial or total hemilaryngectomies and results in human medicine are used as a reference. In a study that analysed the performance of hemilaryngectomies in two cases for the treatment of laryngeal mastocytomas, the two recurred locally, in most likelihood due to the difficulty in excising complete margins in an area as critical as the larynx.

Tumours of the Trachea

Tumours of the trachea are **rare**. In dogs, the most common types are osteochondroma, chondroma, osteosarcoma, chondrosarcoma, adenocarcinoma, carcinoma, leiomyoma, mastocytoma, plasmacytoma, fibrosarcoma, and rhabdomyosarcoma. Osteochondromas are benign tumours that occur in young dogs and can be successfully treated with surgical resection. In cats, the most common tumours are lymphoma, adenocarcinoma, disseminated histiocytic sarcoma, inflammatory polyp, and carcinoma.

The distinction between lymphoma and other tumours is very important, since the treatment for lymphoma is not surgical, as for other tumours. For resection of benign tumours, such as an inflammatory polyp, surgical margins are more conservative.

Diagnostic Imaging and Clinical Staging

Tracheoscopy is a very important step in the diagnosis and treatment of tracheal masses. This technique allows visualisation of the mass and evaluation of the rest of the trachea to rule out other possible lesions. Normally, when clinical signs are present, the tumour is large in size, so it can prevent the use of an endotracheal tube or a bronchoscope caudal to the tumour. Tracheoscopy also allows biopsies of the tumour to be taken before definitive surgery.

Intratracheal masses can normally be diagnosed by **normal radiographs**, as the air within the trachea allows for contrast differences with soft tissues (Figure 4). Lateral projections are usually best for identifying tracheal masses. The most common radiographic signs are a soft tissue opacity in the tracheal lumen or stenosis. Generally, these tumours are not mineralised, except for osteochondromas.

For diagnosis in patients with dyspnoea, three thoracic projections are necessary, as well as for part of the staging of patients with tracheal masses. **CT is a very useful diagnostic tool** to evaluate the size, location, and extent of the tumour, propose surgical treatment and evaluate lung regions and lymph nodes (Figure 5).

General Surgical Considerations

The most commonly used treatment for tracheal tumours is **tracheal resection and anastomosis**, except for lymphomas.

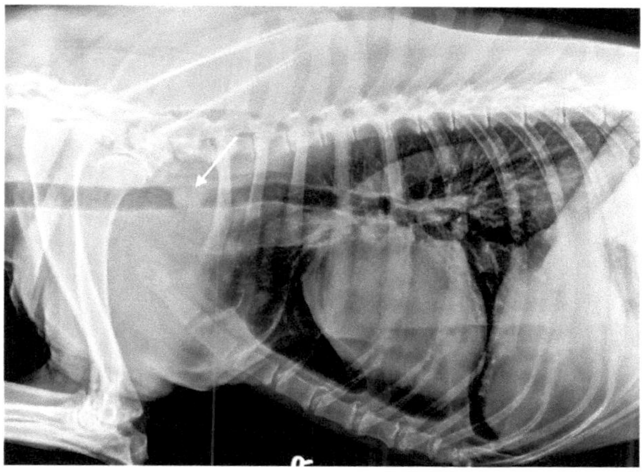

Figure 4. Right lateral radiograph of a canine patient with a carcinoma in the thoracic trachea (arrow).

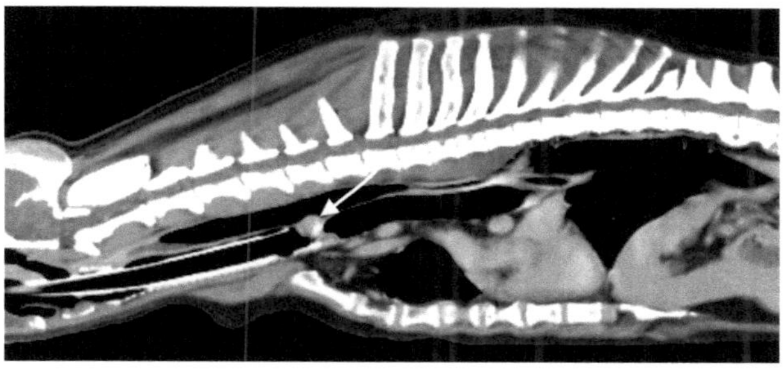

Figure 5. Sagittal postcontrast CT image with a soft tissue window in the same patient as in Figure 4. The tumour in the cervical trachea (arrow) shows contrast enhancement and the regional lymph nodes are of normal size with normal contrast.

The surgical approach depends on the location and extension of the tumour, so it is essential to have a good diagnosis before deciding on the approach.

For tracheal surgery it is important to note that this organ is wrapped in **adventitia with lateral pedicles** containing segmental vascularisation (branches of the cranial and caudal thyroid vein and artery, bronchoesophageal veins and arteries and internal jugular vein). Recurrent laryngeal nerves are also found within these lateral pedicles and should be protected during dissection and resection. This resection requires airway preservation at all times and good communication with the anaesthesiologist.

There are **two options for maintaining airway access during resection**:

- the endotracheal tube can be retracted cranially so that it is not right in the resection zone, using previously placed traction sutures (Figure 6) that serve to quickly join the two segments of trachea and allow the endotracheal tube to be advanced; and
- the second method uses a sterile endotracheal tube that

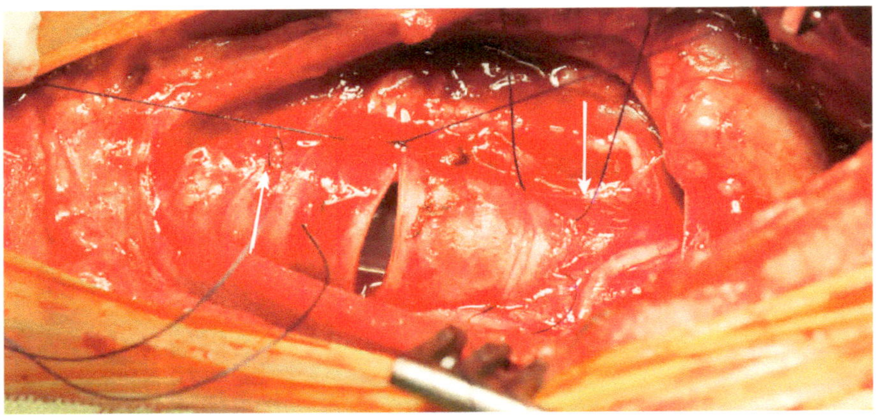

Figure 6. Traction sutures are positioned (arrows) in the trachea to ensure gentle handling of this structure.

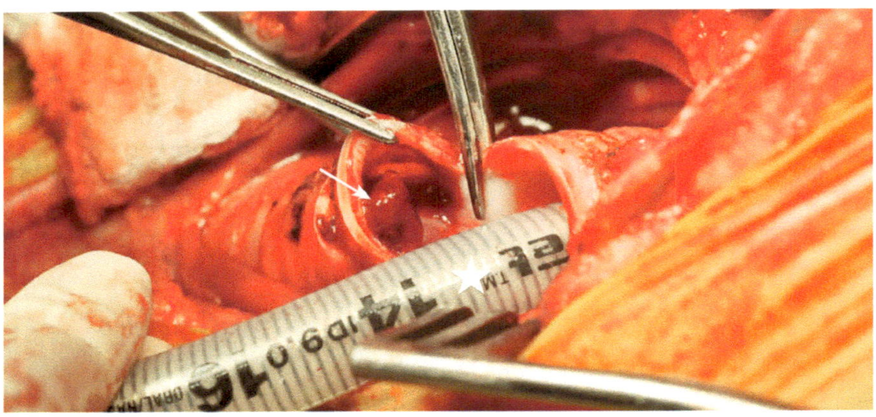

Figure 7. Ventral approach to the cervical trachea. In this case the marginal excision of the tracheal tumour (arrow) is performed whilst ventilating the patient with a sterile endotracheal tube (asterisk) in the distal trachea. In this case the technique used is cartilage division.

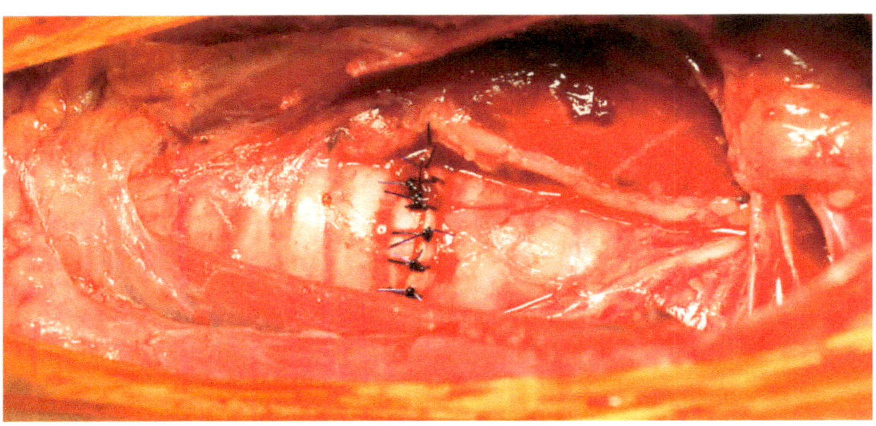

Figure 8. Anastomosis of the cervical trachea using simple interrupted sutures.

is inserted into the distal segment of the trachea after making an incision at the distal point of the resection (Figure 7). The cranial endotracheal tube is retracted cranially, but the patient is not extubated. Resection of the tumour containing segment is continued and the two tracheal segments are approximated to advance the cranial endotracheal tube (removing the caudal endotracheal tube).

Regardless of the method used, a sterile endotracheal tube should always be available for the surgeon to use if needed.

The inner surface of the trachea is a clean/contaminated surface, so there is likely contamination with manipulation of the intraoral endotracheal tube. After resection, the surgical field should be washed, a culture sample taken, and broad-spectrum antibiotics used. The two main objectives of anastomosis are that there is a perfect apposition of the tissues and that there is no tension. The presence of tension at the anastomosis site, although minimal, can create a tracheal stenosis.

The two methods for performing a tracheal resection and anastomosis are:

- the **cartilage division technique** (Figure 7), in which the proximal and distal incisions are made in the middle of the tracheal cartilage (just in the middle of the width of the tracheal cartilage) so that, when anastomosed, the two portions of the resected rings are aligned; and
- the **annular ligament technique**, in which tracheal incisions are made in the annular ligament, between two cartilaginous rings.

The **first technique is preferred**, because anatomically the apposition is better to achieve a first intention closure. It is recommended that the traction sutures be placed prior to resection, so that the tracheal segments do not retract, especially in cases of resection of the caudal cervical trachea, where it can retract towards the entrance to the thorax.

Suture patterns for anastomosis are a matter of debate, but the interrupted simple pattern tends to further aid anatomical and histological apposition of tracheal tissues (Figure 8). This anastomosis can be reinforced with mattress sutures using tracheal rings farther from the anastomosis line, especially when there is tension. All suture knots should be placed extraluminally and sutures in the dorsal trachea should be placed first. To reduce tension in the anastomosis area, a thorough knowledge of the different techniques for relieving tension in the trachea is of vital importance. However, this chapter will not go into detail regarding the different techniques.

The **approach to the intrathoracic trachea is done with an intercostal thoracotomy** from intercostal spaces three to five on the right side. The approach to the **cervical trachea is through the ventral midline**.

The use of **tracheal stents** that preserve the lumen of the trachea is an alternative when there are tumours that are not good candidates for surgical excision or to relieve signs of airway obstruction caused by stenosis secondary to surgery. The most commonly used stents are metal self-expanding stents, which must be introduced under fluoroscopy in the same way as for a tracheal collapse.

These patients, like all patients undergoing airway surgeries, should be monitored 24 hours a day and kept in an intensive care unit for prompt intervention if necessary. Harnesses should be used to walk them, and excessive pressure and tension avoided at the anastomosis site. Cough suppressants may be used if the patient continues to cough a week after surgery or to prevent excessive tension if the cough after surgery is severe. Postsurgical tracheostomy is a useful tool for monitoring lesions, alleviating the appearance of stenosis, and evaluating the healing of the anastomosis.

The complications that can occur with this type of surgery have already been discussed, but the most common and important is stenosis, probably due to excessive tension in the anastomosis area (which causes healing by second intention) or due to poor surgical apposition during anastomosis.

Recommendations on the maximum length of an uncomplicated tracheal resection are based on human literature. The most commonly reported veterinary recommendations are 25% in puppies and 20 to 60% in adult dogs.

Pulmonary Tumours

Surgical procedures performed on the lungs for oncology problems in dogs and cats include taking biopsies to diagnose local or diffuse disease and surgical treatment for primary (or metastatic) lung tumours.

Primary tumours are not common in dogs or cats, although their **prevalence seems to be increasing**. This trend is likely due to pets living longer, the development of more accurate diagnostic tools and more biopsies being taken. Primary lung tumours are described by their place of origin (bronchial, bronchoalveolar or alveolar) or by their histopathology (adenocarcinoma, squamous cell carcinoma, histiocytic sarcoma etc.). Adenocarcinomas are the most common primary lung tumours in companion animals; squamous cell carcinomas, anaplastic carcinomas, and other types of carcinomas are less common.

Benign lung tumours such as pulmonary adenomas and primary mesenchymal tumours (osteosarcoma, haemangiosarcoma, and fibrosarcoma) are rare. A more common lung disease is eosinophilic granuloma, with pulmonary consolidation, tracheobronchial lymphadenopathy, leucocytosis and basophilia. **Metastatic tumours** are **more frequent** lung lesions compared to primary pulmonary tumours. The lungs are a target organ for many tumours, such as sarcomas and carcinomas. The distinction between primary and secondary tumours is complicated, so a complete staging is essential.

Primary lung tumours are aggressive and tend to metastasise to pulmonary and regional lymph nodes (most commonly), the pleural space, skeletal muscle, bone, heart, liver, kidney, etc.

Patients with primary lung tumours may be asymptomatic (30% of cases) or have a chronic cough and/or other clinical signs (dyspnoea, decreased exercise tolerance, etc.). In cats, clinical signs related to the respiratory tract are less frequent. Most of the time, the identification of a lung tumour is incidental, when thoracic radiographs are taken for another reason, as the symptomatology may be non-specific to lung disease.

Paraneoplastic syndromes are not usually associated with lung tumours, although there are two very clearly identifiable syndromes: **hypertrophic osteopathy** (in dogs) (Figure 9) and **lung digit syndrome** (in cats) (Figure 10). Other paraneoplastic syndromes secondary to lung tumours are hypercalcaemia, fever, and adrenocorticotropic hormone secretion induced by the lung tumour.

The **most significant prognostic factors** in primary lung tumours (in dogs) are:

- clinical stage
- histological grade of the tumour (well-differentiated tumours have a better prognosis)
- presence of clinical signs (worse prognosis in dogs with clinical signs, as this is usually due to the disease being more advanced)
- tumour size (tumours of less than 5 cm have a better prognosis)
- tumour type (lung carcinoma has a better prognosis than histiocytic sarcoma)
- presence of pleural effusion.

The prognosis is usually worse in cats than in dogs, as the disease is usually more advanced when they begin to show non-tumour specific clinical signs. In domestic felines, the degree of tumour differentiation and regional metastases to the lymph nodes are of prognostic value.

Diagnosis and Clinical Staging

Definitive diagnosis of lung lesions is made by **cytology or histopathology**. Cytology is the most commonly used technique prior to surgery, as many primary lung malignancies can be diagnosed by combining cytology and advanced imaging. Cytology is obtained with a fine needle transthoracic biopsy guided by ultrasound, fluoroscopy, or CT. The author does not recommend blind fine needle biopsy, as it may lead to further complications (puncture of contaminated structures, such as the stomach, or of delicate structures, such as blood vessels or heart).

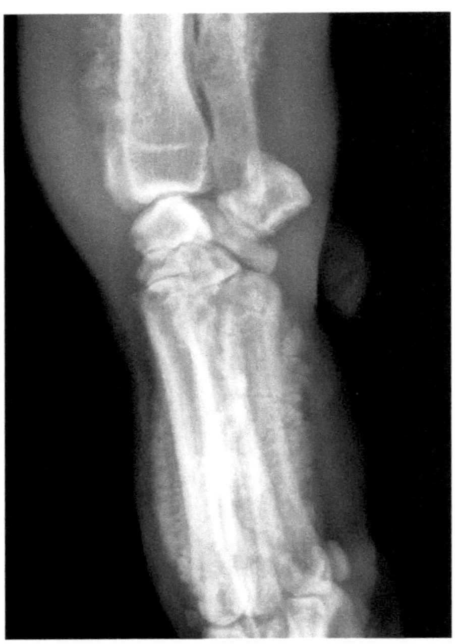

Figure 9. Mediolateral projection of the forelimb showing a periosteal reaction in the metacarpals, radius and ulnar in a patient with a pulmonary tumour.

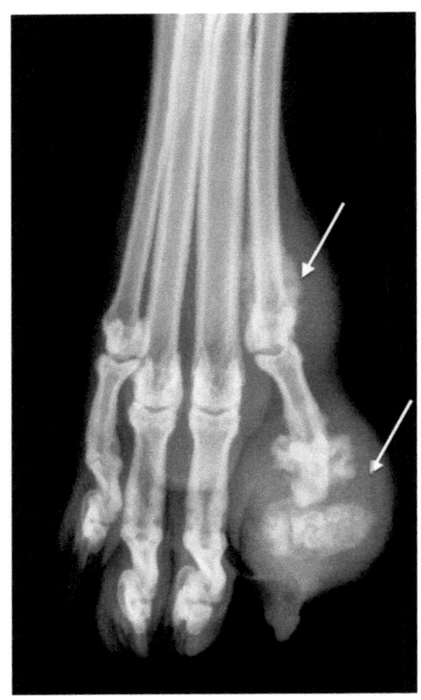

Figure 10. Craniocaudal projection of the tarsus of a cat with pulmonary carcinoma. The arrows show the metastases from the carcinoma to the phalanges and the metatarsus of the second digit.

The technique depends on the accessibility to the injury. Diagnoses obtained by cytopathology are correct in 82% of cases, with higher numbers (up to 91%) if an imaging tool is used to guide the puncture. Although complications associated with these procedures can be as high as 43% (pneumothorax and/or haemorrhage), these patients do not usually experience clinical signs, so they do not need treatment. Lung tumours may have a necrotic and/or purulent focal centre that sometimes confuses the diagnosis, therefore some clinicians recommend surgical excision without a presurgical diagnosis. This decision may also be conditioned by the location and size of the nodule on CT, by evidence of other lung nodules that may suggest metastasis or fungal infection, and by the clinical status of the patient and discussion with the owner.

Tracheal or bronchoalveolar lavage has little sensitivity for diagnosing lung cancer unless the tumour invades the bronchial tree. These techniques are best for cases where there is interstitial or alveolar disease rather than focal disease.

Obtaining cytology samples from pulmonary effusions in cases of lung tumour is debatable. In one study, cytology in cats with pleural effusion due to a lung neoplasm was diagnostic in twelve out of thirteen cats, while other studies have not shown such accuracy.

The methods for the biopsy of intrathoracic structures are multiple: Tru-Cut® biopsy, thoracoscopy or thoracotomy (intercostal or sternotomy).

For thoracic imaging, **radiography is key** to getting started with the diagnosis of lung tumours. Obtaining left, right and ventrodorsal projections is recommended. The radiographic appearance of lung tumours is variable, from a single nodule to multiple and/or diffuse lesions. Occasionally, pneumothorax or pleural effusions secondary to pulmonary neoplasia may be seen. However, thoracic radiographs still have several limitations, including poor accuracy in identifying lung metastases, pulmonary carcinosis, and tracheobronchial lymphadenopathy. CT has been identified as a more accurate diagnostic tool than conventional radiographs for the detection of lung metastases, showing lesions as small as 1 mm, while radiographs are not reliable until lesions measure up to 7–9 mm.

The high sensitivity of CT and its low specificity may result in the diagnosis of false positives. The use of automatic computerised schemes can mitigate the problem of detecting false positive nodules.

Distinguishing poorly differentiated primary lung tumours from metastatic carcinoma can sometimes be a diagnostic challenge. Immunohistochemistry using antibodies directed against thyroid transcription factor 1, cytokeratin or vimentin may be useful for differentiating primary lung tumours from metastatic disease. Antibodies against CD18 may also be useful for differentiating lung tumours of histiocytic origin.

General Surgical Considerations

For pulmonary surgery, the surgeon should be well familiarised with thoracic anatomy as well as **have surgical skills in a moving surgical field** (heart and lungs maintain constant movement).

Other essential requirements to ensure optimal results are:

- to have the hospitalisation capacity and medical equipment necessary to keep these patients monitored 24 hours a day; and
- to have surgical tools (and knowledge of their operation and applications) to make surgery safer and faster. Essential surgical instruments are automatic staplers, a bipolar sealing instrument or bipolar electric scalpel, and automatic ventilation equipment for anaesthesia.

The approach to the chest cavity can be performed using different routes. The **intercostal approach is the most widely used for lung surgery**. It is essential to know which intercostal space should be used, as dissection and removal of a lung from a more cranial or caudal intercostal space can complicate surgery and increase patient morbidity. For the identification of the intercostal space, the surgeon must have knowledge of the pulmonary lobe and structures to be addressed and also of the individual anatomy of the patient (CT images are also useful for the surgical approach).

Medium ventral sternotomy is an approach that allows bilateral exploration of the thorax and allows biopsies to be obtained, as well as allowing pulmonary lobectomies to be carried out. One of the significant limitations of this approach is the difficulty of accessing dorsal structures such as the root of the lung or dorsal lung lesions, so it is not used for the excision of solitary lung tumours. During the excision of lung tumours, the tracheobronchial lymph nodes should be palpated and excised and/or biopsied if they become enlarged.

Pneumonectomy is the complete excision of all lung lobes of a hemithorax (left or right). It can be performed in both dogs and cats. Acute excision of more than 50% of lung volume can have fatal consequences, so exceeding this lung volume is not recommended. It is important to know that the total lung volume of the left lung is 48% and that of the right lung is 52% so dogs and cats tolerate a left lung excision as long as the right lung is healthy (Figure 11). This technique is indicated for neoplasms that affect all ipsilateral lung lobes or the main bronchus of a lung. The mortality associated with this procedure is 6% in dogs and 20% in cats.

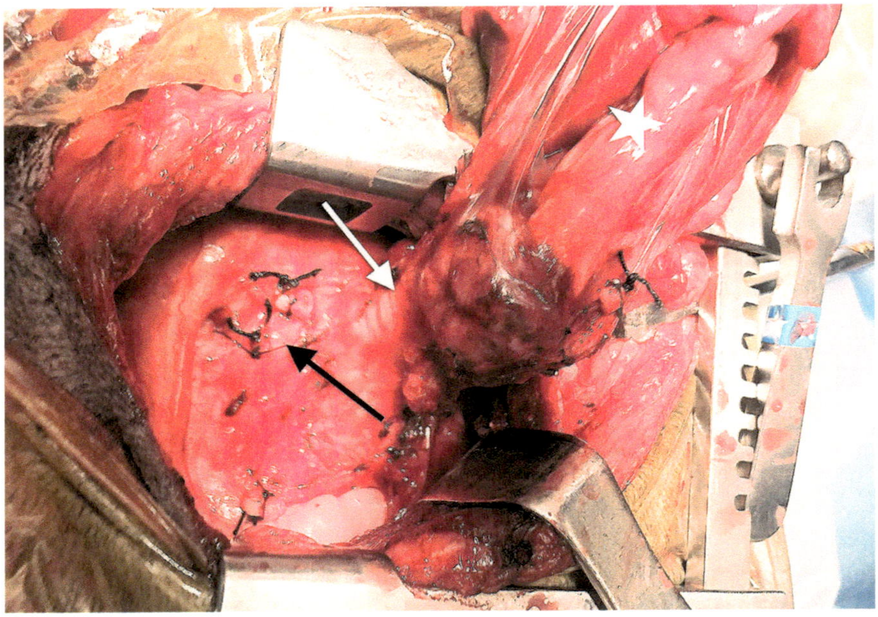

Figure 11. Left pneumonectomy in a patient with bronchial carcinoma. The left lung (asterisk) has been removed after dissection of the pulmonary ligament, ligation and resection of the pulmonary artery and vein (black arrow). The main left bronchus (white arrow) is the only anatomical structure which joins the left lung to the trachea and will be ligated and sectioned with a mechanical stapler.

Metastasectomy is an option for patients with metastases who meet specific requirements. In dogs and cats, metastasectomies may be indicated for metastatic lesions of sarcomas.

Even after permanent local monitoring and adjuvant chemotherapy, the metastatic rate varies depending on tumour type, clinical stage, location, species, and histological grade. The most common example is osteosarcoma, with a metastatic rate of 90% (while soft-tissue sarcomas have rates of 25%). Although metastases are usually biologically very heterogeneous and can progress rapidly, there are occasionally cases where metastasectomy may make sense. The biology of metastasis is complex but can be understood with the seed (tumour cell) and soil (site of metastasis) theory.

Simply put, **many sarcomas metastasise to the lung haematogenously and then to lymph nodes and bone**. With this in mind, routine follow-up for these patients should consist of a conventional physical examination and thoracic radiographs every three months for the first year after diagnosis, with fewer intervals during the second and subsequent year. Once metastases are identified, a complete clinical staging should be performed: thoracic and/or abdominal CT, abdominal ultrasound, and a full bone scintigraphy. As pulmonary metastasis of osteosarcoma is the most common and the most predictable, the requirements for metastasectomy are detailed based on this tumour type (Box 1).

Postoperative care for these patients includes monitoring in an intensive care unit. Oxygen therapy can help maintain a better oxygenation of the patient during the first few hours after surgery, providing an extra source of oxygen, although they do not normally need it.

These patients may suffer from hypoventilation and hypoxia due to several factors:

- narcotics, as opioids that are administered for postoperative analgesia can cause respiratory depression;
- the pain caused by moving the chest wall to breathe after surgery;
- lung lobe atelectasis due to positioning during surgery and anaesthesia; and
- pleural disease (pneumothorax or postoperative pleural effusion).

Although these patients usually recover very well, the first few hours after surgery are critical for good clinical progression. A **thoracic drainage tube is essential** after thoracic surgery, to allow the evacuation of air or fluids that accumulate in the pleural space after surgery. Unless the patient is suffering from hypoventilation or a respiratory crisis, serial drains are performed at 6–8 hour intervals, noting the volume of fluid and air being drawn. The thoracic drainage tube is removed when there is a negative pressure (no pneumothorax), the fluid volume decreases and/or the fluid volume is 2 ml/kg/day.

These are guidelines that normally allow the drainage tube to be removed within 24–48 hours after surgery unless there is a malignant pleural effusion, hypoalbuminaemia, iatrogenic pneumothorax, or a pyothorax.

> **Box 1. General considerations for performing a pulmonary metastasectomy**
>
> 1. **Detection time**: the longer the interval from primary tumour control to metastasis detection, the better, with 300 days suggested as the point from early onset versus late onset.
> 2. **Number of lesions**: biologically, the fewer apparent metastases there are, the greater the possibility that surgery can positively affect average survival. In general, surgery is indicated in cases where three or fewer metastases are found. CT scanning can help identify more metastases, so if two or more lesions are seen on conventional radiographs (three projections), a CT scan is recommended to identify the total number (although some nodules may be non-tumour, such as granulomas or osteomas) and the location of these metastases.
> 3. **Duplication time**: once one or two nodules are noted on thoracic radiographs, repeating radiographs within thirty days to determine the growth rate and possible clinical detection of new lesions is generally recommended that would make surgical intervention more problematic. In general, it is considered that the patients most likely to be good candidates for metastasectomy will still be good candidates in thirty days. It is not clear that the use of chemotherapy during this period has advantages.
> 4. **Technique**: open thoracotomies are usually recommended over thoracoscopies since they allow the direct palpation of potentially hidden lesions on the pleural surface. Most lesions are peripheral, discrete and subpleural, and can be excised with a partial lobectomy. Approach via intercostal thoracotomy or ventral sternotomy depends on the location and number of metastases the patient has.

Principles of Oncological Surgery of the Digestive System

Oral Tumours

Oral tumours are **common in dogs and cats (3–12% and 6% of all tumours, respectively)**. These tumours can affect any tissue of the oral cavity, but normally affect the mandible, maxilla, tongue, and palate. Because most tumours of the oral cavity require surgical treatment, the surgeon has a very important role in the diagnosis, staging, and treatment of these tumours. For example, an incisional biopsy is usually required to obtain the definitive diagnosis of an oral tumour, and this must be planned so that the biopsy tract does not have a negative impact on the surgical treatment plan with curative intent. In addition, clinical staging requires excision of regional lymph nodes, which is important in determining postoperative treatment and prognosis.

Diagnosis and Clinical Staging

Most dogs and cats affected by a tumour of the oral cavity end up seeing a veterinarian because the owner has detected a nodule. Even so, **there are tumours in the caudal area of the oral cavity that are imperceptible to owners**, such as cancer of the pharynx or soft palate.

Some of the most common clinical signs of oral tumours are hypersalivation, exophthalmos, facial inflammation, epistaxis, weight loss, halitosis, oral haemorrhage, dysphagia, or pain when opening the mouth, and occasionally cervical lymphadenopathy. Moving teeth, especially in animals with good dentition, should raise suspicions of a neoplastic process with secondary bone lysis. Performing a complete oropharyngeal examination (with the animal sedated or anaesthetised) is recommended, taking photographs or detailed notes about the tumour (appearance, measurement, 3D location) that are recorded in the patient file.

Diagnosis and clinical staging of animals with oral tumours is imperative prior to definitive surgical excision. A generous sized biopsy is required for definitive diagnosis, since fine needle aspiration and cytology usually gives little information in this type of tumour (haemodilution, excessive inflammation, false diagnosis) and requires sedation due to the location of the tumour. Regional lymph nodes and lungs are the most common sites of metastasis in animals with oral tumours.

Normally, oral tumours are necrotic or infected/inflamed, so it is very important to obtain a large biopsy sample. The use of an electric scalpel is not recommended, as it can affect the quality of the sample and diagnostic quality, so it should only be used after taking a biopsy with a scalpel or punch. Although large tumour samples increase the likelihood of diagnosis, peripheral samples that may contaminate normal tissue should be avoided.

In the oral cavity it should be noted that tissues for excision and reconstruction are limited, so contamination of tissues peripheral to the tumour should be completely avoided to **minimise the need to increase surgical margins**. Therefore, biopsies of oral tumours should always be taken with an intraoral approach, to avoid the seeding of cancer cells in other areas of the oral cavity. For small lesions, where taking a large sample involves an excisional biopsy, a photograph of the tumour with intraoral references is taken to record the details of its measurement and location in case a second surgery with wide margins for definitive treatment is required. Tumours that are attached to or come from the bones of the mandible, maxilla, or palate should be imaged under anaesthesia to determine the presence of bone lysis and the extent of local disease. Osteolysis is not detectable on a simple radiograph until 40% of the cortex has been destroyed by local disease, so skull **radiographs are not a good technique for detecting bone invasion by the tumour**. Currently, advanced imaging modalities are available in many veterinary centres and are highly recommended for imaging oral tumours,

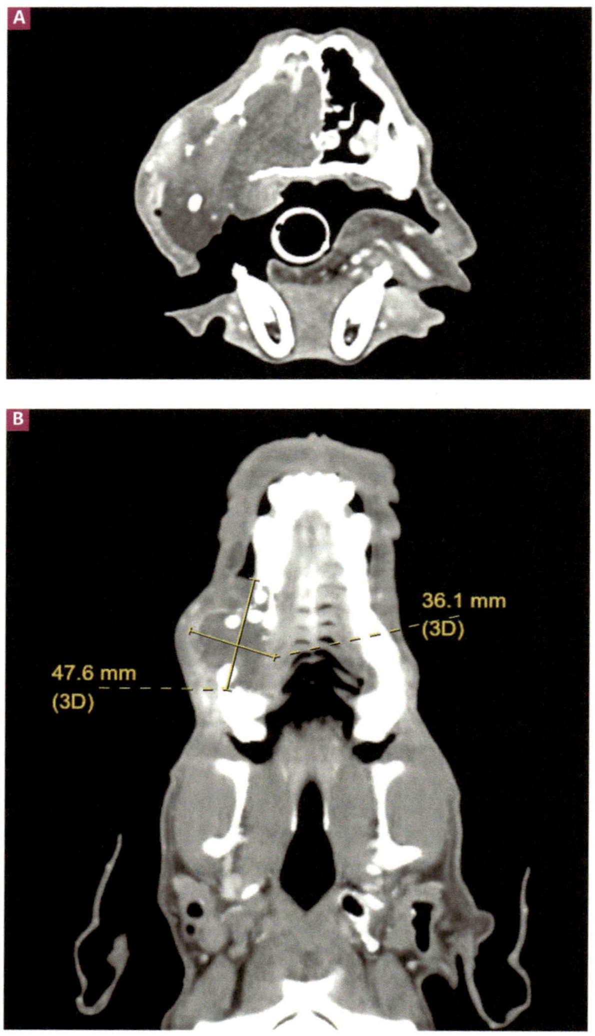

Figure 12. Transverse plane in a dog with a maxillary sarcoma which is invading the nasal cavity (**A**). Dorsal plane in the same patient which shows the size of the tumour and evidence of osteolysis of the maxillary bone (**B**).

particularly tumours originating in the maxilla, palate, and caudal mandible.

Generally, computed tomography (CT) is the preferred technique (Figure 12), rather than magnetic resonance imaging (MRI), since bone detail is superior in the former. This information is important for planning the definitive surgical procedure or, if indicated, radiation therapy.

Regional lymph nodes should be carefully palpated to determine if they are enlarged, asymmetrical, or harder than normal. Likewise, the clinical diagnosis cannot be based only on the size of the lymph node, which alone is not an accurate predictor of metastasis. In a study involving 100 dogs with oral melanoma, 40% with normal sized lymph nodes had metastases and 49% with enlarged lymph nodes had no metastases. In addition, regional lymph nodes include the mandibular, parotid, and middle retropharyngeal lymph nodes. Only 55% of the animals with metastases had affected mandibular lymph nodes, which are the only palpable ones in the head and neck region.

Detailed assessment of lymph nodes prior to surgery is recommended as part of clinical staging. Fine needle aspiration of lymph nodes is recommended regardless of their size or how firm they are. Currently, sentinel lymph node mapping is emerging as a technique and in the near future will be more widely accepted for lymph node evaluation.

The final step for staging is the **evaluation of distant metastases in the thoracic cavity**, particularly in the lungs. Thoracic radiography with three projections is the general recommendation. CT is more sensitive in detecting lung metastases when compared to standard radiography. Even so, for future staging in patients who are monitored for cancer, standard thoracic radiographs are typically cheaper, faster, less invasive, and can be compared over time. The author recommends a thoracic CT scan in patients undergoing a skull CT scan for surgical planning or in patients affected by oral tumours with high metastatic potential (e.g. malignant oral melanoma).

General Surgical Considerations

The surgical approach depends on the type of tumour and its location. Except for peripheral odontogenic fibroma, **most oral tumours have some bone involvement** and surgical resection of these tumours should include resection of the attached bone to ensure complete excision.

Radical surgeries such as mandibulectomy or maxillectomy are well tolerated in small animals. The minimum margins for malignant tumours are 2 cm, but the recommendation to increase the likelihood of a complete excision is 3 cm. Feline squamous cell carcinoma should be treated with a 2 cm margin

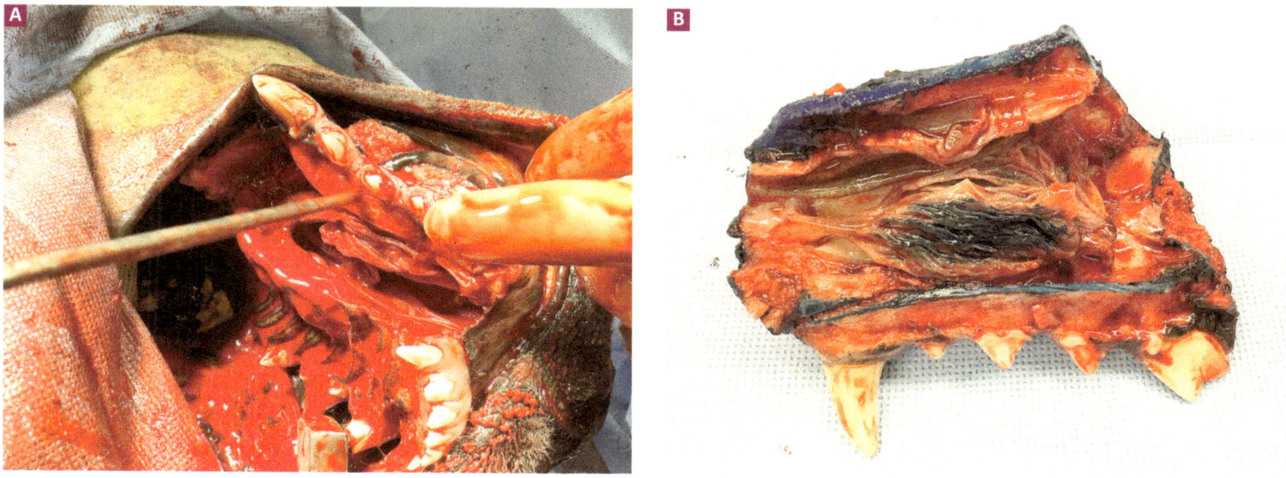

Figure 13. Left hemimaxillectomy for treatment of a maxillary osteosarcoma (**A**). Tumour excised with wide margins (**B**) on which the margins have been marked for pathological evaluation.

due to the high percentage of recurrence, although these margins are not always possible without increasing patient morbidity. Even so, in some studies it has been found that in cases where 2–3 cm margins are impossible (due to the extension of the tumour or its location), 1 cm margins for malignant tumours and 0.5 cm margins for benign tumours are acceptable with complete excisions.

Extensive resections, such as hemimandibulectomies, hemimaxilectomies (Figure 13), orbitectomies, and radical maxilectomies, are necessary to treat highly aggressive tumours, especially fibrosarcoma. Reconstruction of the bone in this type of surgery is not necessary, due to good function and postoperative cosmesis. It is important to have a detailed knowledge of regional anatomy prior to surgery and study the surgical area with CT or MRI to plan surgical approach, degree of resection and reconstruction.

The use of models of dog and cat skulls within the operating room facilitates the orientation of the surgeon and the approach to surgery.

In general, intraoperative administration of antibiotics in oral surgeries is not necessary since the risk of infection is minimal due to short surgical times and excellent vascularisation. Even so, the author uses prophylactic antibiotics in maxillary surgeries and in extensive caudal oral cavity surgeries due to the risk of acute bleeding (maxillary artery), to avoid intestinal bacterial translocation secondary to hypotension.

Multimodal perioperative analgesia is very important for this type of surgery. Combinations of regional anaesthetic nerve blocks, anti-inflammatories and narcotics are recommended to minimise morbidity and improve perioperative comfort.

In general, cats are more sensitive to oral interventions, especially aggressive surgeries. Mandibulectomy in cats is more complicated due to the small size of the jaw relative to tumours, so achieving surgical margins of 2–3 cm can be difficult. Therefore, the most commonly used procedures for the management of mandibular tumours in cats are usually subtotal or total mandibulectomies. The surgical technique is the same as in the dog, although adding oesophageal or gastric feeding tubes to facilitate nutrition after surgery is recommended. Eating difficulties have been reported in 44% of dogs and 73% of cats after a mandibulectomy.

Lingual tumours are not common in cats and dogs. Most of these tumours are located in the dorsal area of the tongue, but they are distributed equally between the tip, body and caudal areas. It has been found that 16% of dogs with lingual tumours have a second primary tumour, so performing a clinical staging and a thorough physical examination are very important.

Oesophageal Tumours

Oesophageal neoplasia can occur as a primary, secondary, or metastatic tumour, invasion by a tumour that comes from tissues adjacent to the oesophagus or by a tumour that occurs in conjunction with a *Spirocerca lupi* infection. Primary tumours reported in the oesophagus of small animals are osteosarcoma, fibrosarcoma, undifferentiated sarcoma, squamous cell carcinoma, undifferentiated carcinoma, adenocarcinoma, leiomyoma, leiomyosarcoma, plasmacytoma and adenomatous polyp. Thyroid tumours are most likely to invade the oesophagus, although respiratory neoplasms and stomach tumours have also been reported.

Dogs are the definitive host of *Spirocerca lupi*, a nematode that can migrate from the stomach to the thoracic aorta after ingestion. Once located in the thoracic aorta, these nematodes can penetrate the oesophageal wall causing nodules that can later transform into malignant nodules forming a sarcoma.

The prognosis in dogs and cats with oesophageal tumours depends on the nature of the tumour. In general, healing can be achieved for benign tumours (leiomyoma or plasmacytoma) that are surgically resected aggressively and early. Although the ability to diagnose oesophageal tumours is improving with the use of CT and oesophagoscopy, the rapid progression of malignant tumours, high metastatic index, and surgical challenges limit treatment success and prognosis. The use of adjuvant treatment is not well described, although chemotherapy and/or radiotherapy are considered treatments for oesophageal tumours.

Diagnosis and Clinical Staging

Obtaining cervical and thoracic radiographs of any patient presenting with clinical signs consistent with oesophageal pathology is essential. These radiographic projections allow soft tissue opacity nodules in the oesophageal area, a mass effect or lung metastases to be observed. If a mass effect is observed in the caudodorsal area of the mediastinum by means of a thoracic radiograph, it is most likely that the cause of the problem is an oesophageal pathology. Caudal mediastinal nodules are more easily diagnosed with dorsoventral or ventrodorsal radiographic views than with lateral views. On the other hand, positive contrast radiographs can help diagnose oesophageal tumours with radiographic signs such as an irregular surface of the mucosa, a decrease in the size of the oesophageal lumen, or the inability of the contrast to reach the stomach.

Ultrasound of the cervical oesophagus is easier and more accessible than that of the thoracic oesophagus. The use of ultrasound can help guide fine needle aspiration.

CT is an excellent imaging tool for intrathoracic structures. Although there is little information available on oesophageal tumours detected by CT, this technique provides added information about the size and shape of the tumour, if there are changes in organs peripheral to it and if there are lung or lymph node metastases.

Oesophagoscopy is excellent for evaluating oesophageal neoplasia. This technique allows the veterinarian to assess surgical resectability and obtain biopsies. It should be noted if there is any evidence of oesophageal perforation on thoracic radiographs prior to oesophagotomy, to avoid formation of a tension pneumothorax due to insufflation.

Oesophageal neoplasms are rare in dogs and cats. Oesophageal surgery is technically complicated and is generally considered difficult. For the treatment of oesophageal tumours, resection and anastomosis are recommended when possible. In rare cases of small benign tumours of the oesophagus (adenomatous polyps) resection via oesophagotomy may be considered.

Oesophageal tumours can be diagnosed by **fine needle aspiration or with a biopsy**. These techniques can be performed percutaneously, guided by ultrasound or CT. When the nodule is located in the cervical area, ultrasound is a very valuable tool, although its use is limited when the tumour is located in the thoracic oesophagus. Biopsies taken oesophagoscopically can be frustrating, as the results are usually non-diagnostic and tumours do not penetrate the mucosa. Open, ventral approaches to the cervical oesophagus and lateral intercostal approaches to the intrathoracic oesophagus may also be used for biopsy.

General Surgical Considerations

Surgical approaches to the oesophagus depend on the location of the lesion:

- the **cervical oesophagus** can be approached from the ventral midline with the patient in a dorsal position. In this area, neurovascular structures such as the carotid sheath, recurrent laryngeal nerves, thyroid glands, and parathyroid glands must be respected; and
- for the **thoracic oesophagus**, approaches vary depending on the location of the tumour: cranial (third or fourth left or right intercostal space) and caudal oesophagus (seventh, eighth or ninth left intercostal space). Regional anatomy should be well understood to avoid damaging the vagus nerve or thoracic blood vessels.

The **basic principles for oesophageal surgery** are to avoid contamination of the surrounding tissues, to try to achieve margins of non-neoplastic tissue, to include the submucosa in the closure and to use an apposition pattern, to treat the tissues with extreme delicacy (since the oesophagus has a segmental vascularisation), to omentalise the incision/anastomosis and to position a gastrostomy tube.

Oesophageal surgery has been associated with a considerable number of complications due to different factors. The oesophagus has no serosa, so an immediate seal with fibrin after a surgical incision does not form, increasing the risk of leakage of contents and contamination. After a tumour resection, the oesophagus is subjected to continuous and greater tension than other areas of the gastrointestinal tract due to the constant movement of breathing (contraction of the diaphragm). Finally, segmental vascularisation of the oesophagus means the surgeon must pay great attention to preserving the vascularisation of the cervical and thoracic area to avoid necrosis of the organ. Other factors that alter the healing of the oesophagus are the absence of omentum, peristaltic contractions, and the continuous passage of boluses of food, water, and saliva.

Tumours of the Stomach

Gastric neoplasia is not common in dogs, accounting for less than 1% of all canine tumours, with adenocarcinoma (AC) being the most common type of gastric tumour. Lymphoma is the most common gastric tumour in cats. Currently, the incidence of leukaemia virus related lymphoma has decreased due to virus control, but non-virus-related food tract lymphoma has increased. Other gastric tumours include leiomyoma, leiomyosarcoma, fibrosarcoma, extramedullary plasmacytoma, mastocytoma, and stromal tumours (GIST).

The **treatment indicated for AC is complete surgical resection**. Because the clinical signs are usually non-specific (intermittent vomiting, weight loss, decreased appetite etc.), diagnosis of this disease usually occurs late when the pathology is already advanced.

Diagnostic Imaging and Clinical Staging

Radiographs usually have limitations, but they can be useful for detecting obvious abnormalities within the stomach, lymphadenopathy, or ascites. **Positive contrast radiography** is the most sensitive modality for identifying stomach wall abnormalities. Despite the relatively low incidence of thoracic metastases secondary to gastric neoplasia, three radiographic views of the chest are recommended before proceeding with more invasive diagnostic techniques.

Abdominal ultrasound allows visualisation of changes associated with the gastric wall, as well as detecting metastatic tumours in the abdominal cavity. Ideally, gastric ultrasound should be performed on an empty stomach, with only water. In one study, common features between tumours regarding their shape, number of affected gastric layers and presence or absence of serous infiltration predicted histopathological type in more than 80% of cases. In that same study, the presence of a focal nodule, thickening of the stomach muscle layer, and abnormalities in the pyloric antrum were more consistent with the diagnosis of leiomyoma or leiomyosarcoma, while evidence of spread of pathology to the gastric serosa was suggestive of a carcinoma.

Ultrasound-guided aspiration is used as a first-line diagnostic tool and is a minimally invasive technique that is useful in animals that are weak, which rules out anaesthesia for surgery or endoscopy. Even so, 50% of samples may be non-diagnostic, as tumour inflammation and/or ulceration influences the accuracy of cytology on diagnosis. Despite poor accuracy, there are neoplasms that can be diagnosed or ruled out with fine needle aspiration and cytology, such as gastric lymphoma. The use of advanced imaging techniques has not yet been consolidated as a diagnostic tool.

Samples taken endoscopically are the mainstay for the diagnosis of gastric neoplasms. Endoscopy allows minimally invasive tissue visualisation and is particularly useful in defining the extent of disease. Endoscopy has limitations when the tumour does not infiltrate the gastric mucosa or because of the quality of the sample (size, percentage of necrosis etc.).

Laparoscopic techniques are gaining interest and use in veterinary medicine, as laparoscopic examination can be useful in defining the extent of the disease while it can also be used to obtain biopsies. For the stomach, laparoscopy is typically used to assist in the biopsy technique, taken outside the animal's abdomen via a minimally invasive approach.

General Surgical Considerations

During gastric tumour excision surgeries, diagnostic and therapeutic dilemmas are often encountered when the orientation or extent of the gastric mass is different from that anticipated according to preoperative staging. When, during an exploratory laparotomy, a gastric tumour is found unexpectedly, a decision must be taken regarding the technique necessary for the diagnosis of this nodule. Excisional biopsy is usually the most commonly used technique unless it interferes with the final or subsequent resection, once the diagnosis is obtained. Fine needle aspiration and intraoperative cytology are useful when gastric lesions are found accidentally; however, they are usually not possible unless there is a pathologist working at the practice.

There are some anatomical structures that should be considered when stomach surgery is recommended, such as the bile duct, pancreatic duct, hepatic artery, and portal vein. These structures should be protected when performing any surgical procedure on the pylorus area. The function, vascularisation and innervation of the stomach should be taken into account when performing surgery on this organ. Although the stomach receives a lot of collateral vascularisation from the celiac plexus, its location near the celiac artery and the cranial mesenteric artery should be taken into account when extensive resections are performed.

The general surgical principles applied in gastrointestinal surgery should also be applied in stomach surgery: gentle handling of tissues, ensuring these remain humid to minimise adhesion formation, simple continuous or interrupted patterns of a long-lasting monofilament absorbable suture, minimising contamination of the abdominal cavity and avoiding the use of an electric scalpel. The application of two layers of closure is acceptable, but not recommended in areas where the lumen of the stomach is limited, as it can cause an obstruction in cases of more complex gastric reconstructions.

Surgical techniques applied to the stomach include:

- resection of the submucosa
- partial gastrectomy
- Billroth I (pylorectomy and gastroduodenostomy)
- Billroth II (gastrojejunostomy) or complete gastrectomy (Figure 14).

In people with gastric neoplasia, the clinical stage of the disease has been shown to be of prognostic importance. In veterinary medicine, this information has not yet been demonstrated, so prognostic factors related to gastric lymph nodes have not been established.

Postsurgical enteral nutrition is extremely important in patients which have undergone gastric resections. Most patients have suffered some degree of malnutrition or nutritional deficiency prior to surgery due to gastric disease. In humans, preoperative malnutrition and weight loss have been linked to an increase in postoperative complications. For these patients, nutrition, and the placement of feeding tubes (nasogastric, oesophageal, jejunal or gastrojejunal) should be considered. Feeding should usually be started as soon as possible (12–24 hours after the procedure) with easy to digest, low fat, high carbohydrate diets. Early, aggressive enteral nutritional supplementation preserves the barrier function of the gastrointestinal mucosa, increases immune defence mechanisms, and decreases rates of bacterial translocation infection.

As with any procedure involving the gastrointestinal tract, postoperative analgesia is based on injectable opioids (intermittent injections or constant infusions). Multimodal analgesia is the most effective method of pain control, so that the

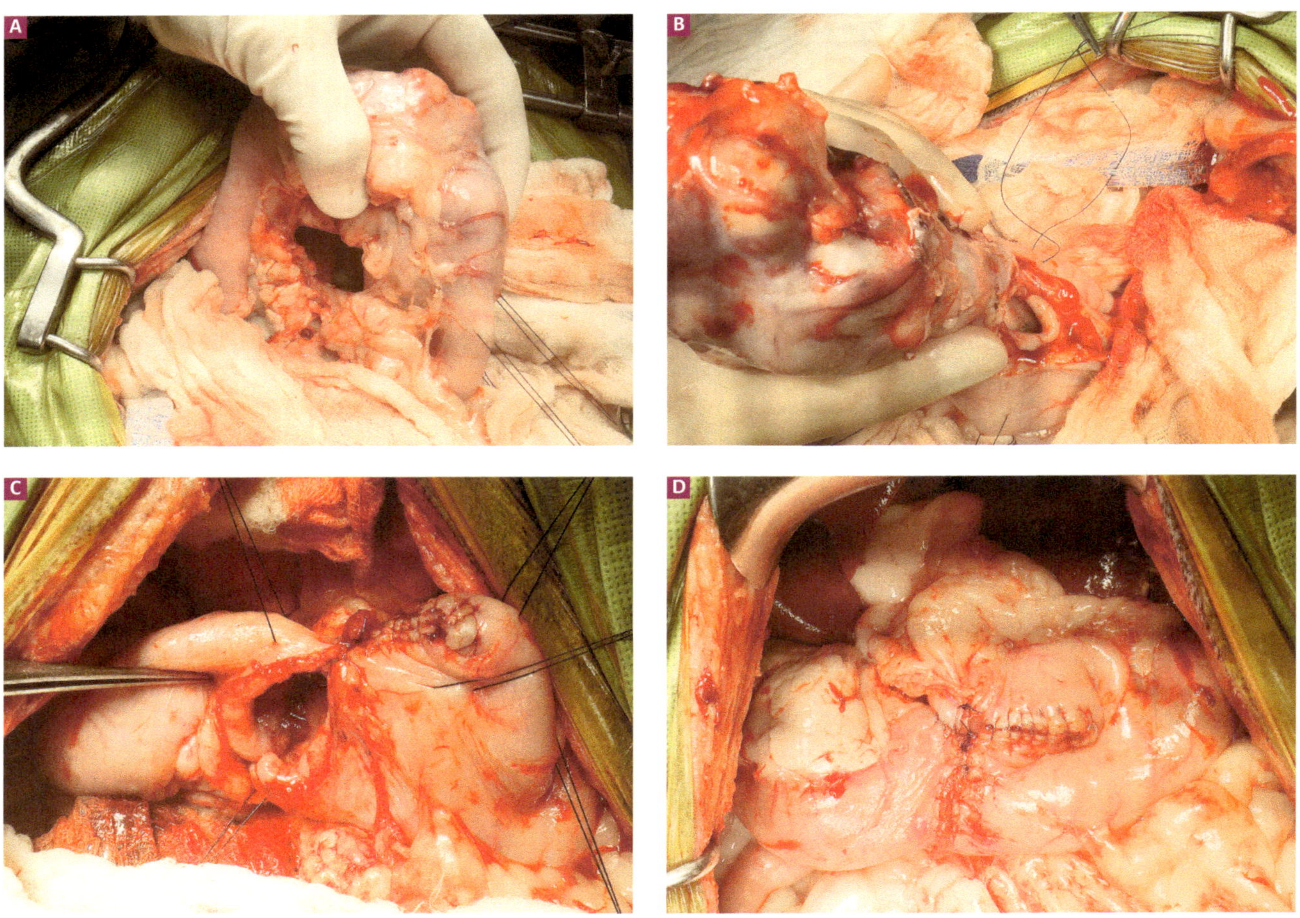

Figure 14. (**A**) Pyloric adenocarcinoma in a dog with obstruction syndrome of the gastric outflow tract. Traction sutures are used on the stomach and the area to be resected is dissected freeing it of omentum. (**B**) The marginal excision starts proximally, in the stomach area. Using the traction sutures and aspiration avoids contamination of the surgical field with gastric contents. (**C**) Once the tumour is excised distally (duodenum) gastroduodenal reconstruction is started. (**D**) The anastomosis is completed.

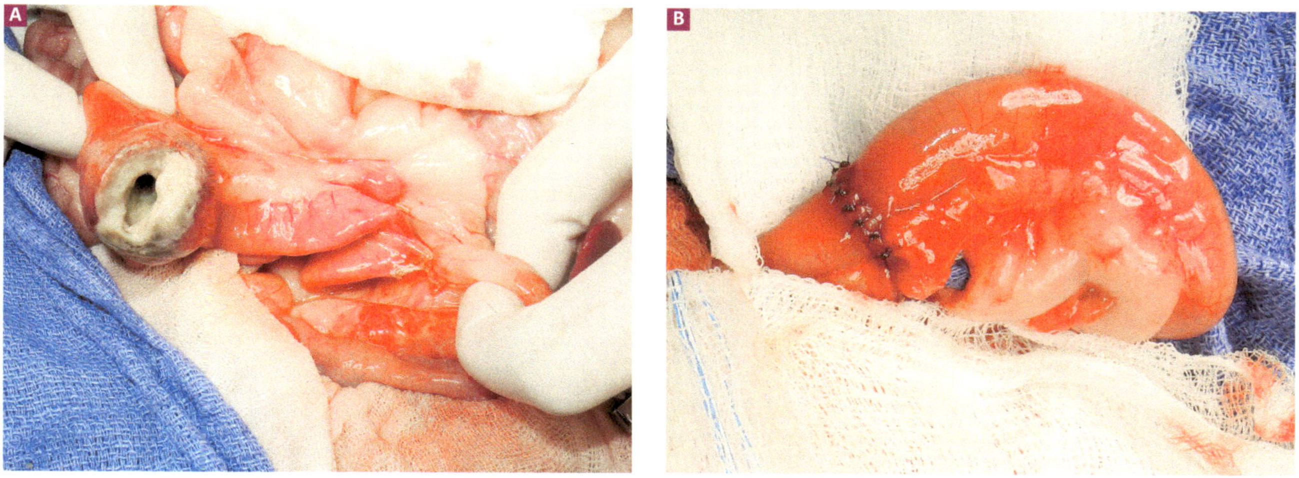

Figure 15. Feline intestinal lymphoma with perforation (**A**). Intestinal mass resection and anastomosis (**B**).

side effects of the analgesics used separately are limited due to the decrease in the doses needed when combining different medications. These advantages are of greater importance in the gastrointestinal tract, as several factors related to opioids and analgesia can complicate postoperative recovery. Negative factors include paralytic ileus and gastrointestinal dilation due to opioids, postsurgical pain, peritoneal inflammation, and segmental disruption of gastrointestinal innervation due to surgery. The **consequences of paralytic ileus can be extremely negative** if not treated quickly and aggressively.

Chronic regurgitation and vomiting can cause chronic oesophagitis and subsequent oesophageal stenosis, aspiration pneumonia, and chronic intestinal dilation. It is important to implement rapid, aggressive treatment so that these pathological processes do not continue as a vicious circle and/or end in sequelae. In a retrospective study of canine gastric carcinoma, major postsurgical complications occurred in eight out of forty dogs, including septic peritonitis in four of them.

The **prognosis in these patients depends on the type of tumour, its location, and postsurgical complications**. For example, dogs with gastric adenocarcinoma have an average survival time of three months without treatment or less than eight months with surgical treatment and chemotherapy. In a more recent article, the reported median survival time is 178 days in dogs with surgically resected gastric carcinoma. Chemotherapy has been used as a single agent or adjuvant with surgery. Unfortunately, the studies available in veterinary medicine looking at gastric tumours are limited to small groups of patients, so the effectiveness of chemotherapy regimens has not been established. However, it appears that the administration of adjuvant chemotherapy is correlated with improved survival times.

Tumours of the Intestine

There are four categories of tumours that occur in the small intestine of small animals:

- epithelial tumours (carcinomas)
- smooth muscle tumours (leiomyosarcomas)
- neuroendocrine tumours
- round cell neoplasms.

Lymphoma is the most common intestinal neoplasm of the small intestine, constituting 30% of all tumours in cats and 6% in dogs. Non-obstructive intestinal lymphomatous disease is usually treated medically, and treatment and prognosis depend on the tumour subtype. Although contradictory, solitary, obstructive lymphomatous lesions can be treated with a combination of surgery and medical treatment (Figure 15). In cases of large intestinal lymphoma tumours, medical treatment with chemotherapy can help reduce tumour size, although owners should be warned of the risk of intestinal perforation in case of positive tumour response. The prognosis for dogs affected by intestinal lymphoma that are treated medically with different chemotherapy protocols is an average survival time of 62 days.

Adenocarcinoma (AC) is the second most common intestinal tumour in dogs and cats. Approximately 40% of ACs have metastasised at the time of exploratory surgery, usually to regional lymph nodes, although the liver, peritoneum, mesentery, and omentum are also areas affected by adenocarcinoma metastases. In dogs, the prognosis for AC treated by surgical resection is 7–15 months survival time, if localised disease is present, or 3 months, if metastatic disease is present. Taking samples of regional lymph nodes (even if they appear normal) is advisable when performing exploratory laparotomy, as the prognosis varies significantly with the presence of metastasis. In cats with intestinal AC, the median survival time is 15 months.

Mesenchymal tumours of the gastrointestinal tract have been divided into gastrointestinal stromal tumours (GIST) and leiomyosarcomas (GILM). GISTs are found more often in the caecum and large intestine, while GILMs occur more commonly in the stomach and small intestine.

Diagnosis and Clinical Staging

Radiography with or without contrast and ultrasonography are the most widely used imaging modalities for the diagnosis and staging of animals with intestinal neoplasia. Due to the high incidence of systemic metastasis in these patients, thoracic radiography (three views) is indicated. The radiographic signs which can be identified in two abdominal views include aboral gas secondary to an obstructive intestinal mass and/or the presence of free air in the abdomen secondary to intestinal perforation due to a neoplastic process. Contrast radiography may be contraindicated in animals with suspected intestinal perforation.

Abdominal ultrasound has been described as the most effective and least invasive diagnostic technique for the detection of gastrointestinal tumours. Loss of identifiable intestinal layers on abdominal ultrasound is a predictive factor for intestinal tumours in dogs. Ultrasound also facilitates sampling via fine needle aspiration and evaluation of the entire abdomen to identify locoregional metastases.

For minimally invasive sampling of the gastrointestinal tract there are three methods before abdominal examination using laparotomy:

- **fine needle aspiration**, which requires ultrasound guidance. It has a specificity of 95% and a sensitivity of 70% for the diagnosis of intestinal lesions, compared to histopathology;
- **endoscopic biopsy** of the gastrointestinal mucosa (limited to the duodenum); and
- **laparoscopically assisted biopsies**.

Intraoperative cytological imprints can help guide surgical actions, although they do not typically provide a definitive diagnosis.

Endoscopy is an important diagnostic tool for staging in the animal with suspected intestinal neoplasia. Even so, the limitations of this modality must be taken into account, in terms of technique, instrumentation and variability in the histopathological interpretation of samples. The range of non-diagnostic or non-interpretable samples is 19–46% in dogs and 21–50% in cats. Therefore, and as a general rule, acquiring at least eight individual samples is recommended. Differentiation between intestinal lymphoma and inflammatory bowel disease is essential before establishing a treatment plan for these animals. Endoscopic biopsies have limitations for differentiation between these two pathologies, especially in cats. Since most cases of feline gastrointestinal lymphoma are associated with the small intestine (jejunum and ileum), obtaining full thickness biopsies via laparoscopy or exploratory laparotomy is recommended. No difference has been noted in the quality of the samples taken via laparotomy or laparoscopically.

General Surgical Considerations

At an anatomical level, the vascularisation, and anatomical limitations of areas of the small intestine must be understood by the surgeon.

The **jejunum** is a very mobile part of the small intestine, and this allows surgical interventions to occur outside the abdomen, thus decreasing possible peritoneal contamination.

In contrast, the **duodenum** has different constrictions (such as the duodenal colic ligament and mesoduodenum) that can complicate associated surgical procedures in this part of the small intestine. Surgical resections associated with the proximal duodenum are especially difficult due to the proximity of the entrance to the duodenum of the pancreatic and bile ducts. In cats, the pancreatic duct enters through the major duodenal papilla, and is the sole source of drainage for pancreatic secretions in 80% of feline patients. Therefore, preventing obstruction of pancreatic drainage due to surgical procedures in these patients is essential. In dogs, the lesser duodenal papilla is the primary entry for pancreatic secretions to the duodenum, and is more distal, so the greater duodenal papilla can be excised thus maintaining pancreatic secretion. The proximity of the right pancreas to the duodenum, within the mesoduodenum, also complicates resection in this area due to shared vascularisation between these two anatomical structures.

Vascularisation of the small intestine comes from the branches of the cranial mesenteric artery. The branches of this artery anastomose with branches of the caudal coeliac and mesenteric arteries, forming a redundant vascularisation loop for irrigation of the intestine. The venous return of the intestines comes from the cranial mesenteric, splenic, caudal mesenteric and gastroduodenal veins, which form the portal vein.

For any surgical procedure in the gastrointestinal tract, **Halsted's surgical principles** must be followed:

- minimisation of tension
- maintenance of vascularisation
- minimisation of contamination
- delicate tissue management.

Postoperative management varies for each patient, depending on the preoperative and intraoperative state. For example, a patient who has septic peritonitis secondary to an intestinal mass that has perforated the intestine will need to be treated differently to a more stable patient.

As discussed in the section on stomach tumours, **perioperative nutrition** is essential, especially in cases with septic peritonitis or tumours that cause gastrointestinal bleeding. For cases of extreme intestinal resection, the most efficient feeding tubes are gastrojejunal, as they provide the advantage of a double lumen (stomach and intestine) and decreased morbidity with a single incision in the stomach. Due to the common gastroparesis or paralytic ileus experienced by the gastrointestinal system, early gastric decompression is necessary to decrease the risk of nausea and vomiting, which can lead to aspiration pneumonia in debilitated animals. If gastrointestinal motility is severely decreased, the gastrojejunal feeding tube may serve to ensure nutrition, via the jejunal component, and aspirate residual gastric contents, via the gastric component of the tube. Motility can be managed with medication and residual volume calculations to modify therapy and nutrition.

Monitoring biochemical parameters is an objective way to monitor patient recovery. Typically, animals presented for elective surgical treatment of an intestinal tumour recover readily with supportive treatment and analgesia. Conversely, weakened animals with postsurgical complications, septic peritonitis, or clinical signs of intestinal obstruction need more intensive monitoring. Daily assessment of electrolytes and kidney parameters serve to make changes to treatment and assess patient hydration. Assessment of albumin and total protein levels are necessary to assess the need for colloids or transfusions. The most efficient transfusion to increase albumin levels is a human or canine albumin transfusion which, although a potential to cause hypersensitivity has been identified, is normally safe for healthy and hypoalbuminaemic dogs. Alternatively, some clinicians use plasma to combat hypoperfusion and hypoalbuminaemia, although it is much less efficient as 22.5 ml/kg is needed to increase blood albumin levels by 0.5 g/dl.

Antibiotic therapy is used in the perioperative period, but its postoperative use is controversial. Typically, it is prescribed thirty minutes before the operation and first- or second-generation enhanced penicillins or cephalosporins are used in the perioperative period. For the postoperative period, antibiotics are not indicated unless there is an active infection during the surgical procedure.

Daily monitoring of glucose levels is important, as hypoglycaemia can indicate intestinal dehiscence and sepsis. Body temperature, degree of abdominal pain and volume of intra-abdominal fluid are parameters indicative of complications related to intestinal surgery.

Postsurgical intestinal dehiscence is the most significant complication and usually occurs within 3–5 days after surgery, although it may occur later. This is due to the gastrointestinal tract healing process, in which there is a latency phase where the strength of the anastomosis is at its weakest. Dehiscence rates after intestinal surgery are between 7% and 16% and reach 12% when intestinal surgery is performed due to the presence of a tumour.

Short-bowel syndrome can occur with aggressive intestinal resection (>75% of bowel length, although it usually depends on the areas resected). Resection of the jejunum is tolerated better than resection of the duodenum or ileum/colon. Clinical signs include diarrhoea, steatorrhoea, malnutrition and weight loss. Over time, the intestinal mucosa adapts, and this causes an increase in the number and size of enterocytes, with an increase in the number of intestinal villi and crypts, which increases the total intestinal absorption surface. It appears that maintenance of the ileocolic valve is essential to limit the development of short-bowel syndrome. Although this problem may occur, 80% of animals that undergo aggressive bowel resection have a good long-term prognosis.

Colorectal Tumours

During a complete physical examination, **abdominal palpation** and **rectal examination should be performed**. During rectal examination, it is important to identify the location of the tumour with respect to the length of the rectum, the location of the tumour with respect to the gastrointestinal layer (mucosa versus other deeper layers), the extent of the tumour (focal or circumferential), and whether there are multiple or solitary lesions. Tumours are normally palpable between 3–8 cm aboral in dogs. If the tumour is circumferential, a stenosis may be noted on rectal palpation, but it is important to identify infiltrative tumours during palpation. Normally the rectum moves freely during intrarectal palpation, but in the case of full thickness tumour infiltration of the rectal layers or surrounding tissues it feels fixed and immobile. Conversely, the rectum may be invaded (less likely) by tumours of the pelvic cavity, usually prostate carcinoma. During rectal palpation, the sublumbar lymph nodes are also palpated, where colorectal tumours can metastasise locoregionally, in addition to the colic lymph nodes (in the mesocolon). Depending on the characteristics identified on rectal examination, the most appropriate type of diagnostic imaging is chosen.

The term "sublumbar" refers to a chain of lymph nodes that are located in the sublumbar area: the iliosacral lymphatic centre (which includes the middle iliac, hypogastric, and sacral nodes) and the iliofemoral lymph node. The hypogastric lymph nodes (which drain the anus, rectum, and colon) are located ventral to the 6th and 7th lumbar vertebrae and adjacent to the external and internal iliac arteries. The middle iliac lymph nodes are ventral to the 5th and 6th lumbar vertebrae between the deep circumflex and the external iliac lymph nodes. If these lymph nodes are swollen, they can be palpated variably by rectal examination and cytology of these lymph nodes can be taken transrectally or percutaneously or using imaging guidance. For staging of these lymph nodes, they can be felt and/or visualised with abdominal ultrasound in small dogs, but a CT scan of the abdomen and pelvis with contrast is recommended for visualisation of lymphatic structures within the pelvic canal.

Diagnosis and Clinical Staging

Any of these techniques can be used to **take biopsies** of lesions in the colorectal area, depending on the type of tumour and its location.

- Biopsies can be taken directly without the need for anaesthesia if the nodule prolapses through the anus. Despite this, this technique is not recommended as only superficial samples can be taken and bleeding can be significant.
- Using a Tru-Cut® needle or incisional wedge biopsy, transanal samples can be taken after causing eversion of the rectum with traction sutures. These traction sutures are placed in a cranial position to the anorectal line to successively expose the mucosa of the rectum.
- Proctocolonoscopy is a widely used technique to visualise the large intestine and rectum. Preparation for endoscopy typically requires a combination of fasting (24 hours before surgery) and enemas with warm water (10–20 ml/kg every 12 hours). This can also be combined with an osmotic laxative that is administered orally prior to the procedure. Proctocolonoscopy is necessary to characterise colorectal tumours: focal or multiple, location, measurements, length, if there is circumferential extension and to take biopsies. Biopsies taken through an endoscope are small and superficial, so they may be inadequate. Complications associated with this type of procedure are minimal and are usually related to colonic perforation and severe bleeding after the biopsy.
- Although colotomy is another technique for accessing the colonic lumen, it is rarely used to take biopsies.

For staging with imaging techniques, **abdominal ultrasound and/or abdominal and pelvic CT with contrast are the most efficient and widely used**. Abdominal ultrasound should be performed for colorectal tumours, although the pubic bone may prevent imaging of the rectum and other structures of the pelvic canal. Ultrasound is superior to CT for diagnosis of thickening of the intestinal wall (more than 4 mm) with loss of delineation of the normal intestinal layers. Abdominal ultrasound also allows fine needle aspirations to be taken directly for cytology.

Abdominal CT, as already discussed, is used to detect infiltration and for localisation of rectal tumours and/or intrapelvic lymph nodes (Figure 16). Thoracic evaluation can be performed with a simple radiograph (three views) or with a thoracic CT scan.

General Surgical Considerations

Recommendations for decreasing the risk of intraoperative contamination vary depending on the surgeon, but generally include a **low fibre diet** (for a week) and **not giving any laxatives or enema**, as liquid faecal matter is more difficult to control during standard surgery. In case of obstruction or perforation, attempts are made to avoid enemas. In patients who are debilitated due to disease, treatment with enteral or parenteral nutrition, plasma, or blood transfusions should be considered.

Preoperative antibiotic therapy is controversial, but since the risk of infection in colorectal surgeries is high antibiotics should be used against anaerobic and Gram-negative microorganisms (third generation cephalosporins, neomycin, metronidazole, erythromycin). Typically, the first dose is administered during the patient's anaesthetic induction and is repeated every two hours during surgery.

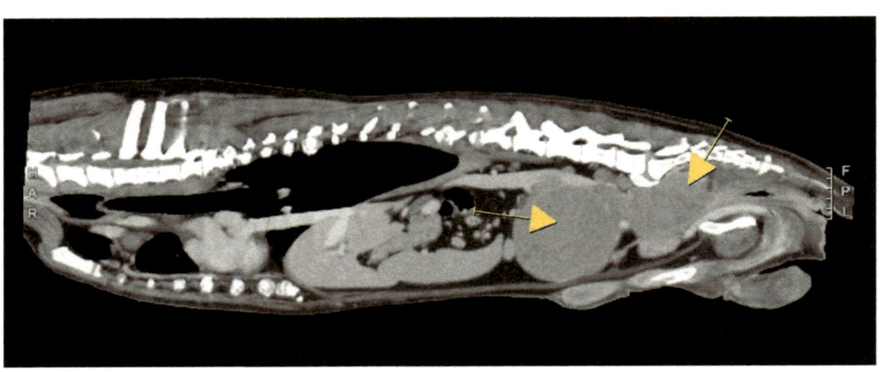

Figure 16. Sagittal thoracic and abdominal CT sections postcontrast. This patient had locoregional metastases in the sacral and iliac lymph nodes (arrows).

Serious complications of these surgeries are **dehiscence and infection**, since the bacterial load of the digestive tract, especially distally, is extremely high and harmful. These complications are usually the result of improper surgical technique and/or inappropriate suture material. Excision of the ileocolic junction in cats and dogs may result in clinical signs such as increased frequency of defaecation or softer stools over a variable time (weeks to months). These complications should be discussed with owners prior to surgery.

Colon resection or colectomy may be subtotal or total. Subtotal colectomy refers to the excision of a part of the colon without resecting the ileocaecal colic junction and leaving 3–5 cm of ascending colon from the caecum to obtain a tension free anastomosis.

The colon is externalised and isolated as far as possible from the abdomen and stools are massaged cranial or caudally to the portion of the colon to be resected. During preparation for resection of part of the colon, its vascularisation should be taken into account. Straight vessels, which are blood vessels perpendicular to the colon, come from the cranial ileocolic artery (branch of the cranial mesenteric artery) and the caudal mesenteric artery caudally. These blood vessels are ligated as distally as possible (near the colon).

The rectum has multiple sources of vascularisation from three main branches: the cranial rectal artery (branch of the caudal mesenteric artery), the middle and the caudal rectal arteries (branch of the internal pudendal artery). Most vascularisation of the rectum comes from the cranial rectal artery, so if this artery is ligated, most of the distal colon and proximal rectum must be excised to avoid necrosis of this area.

The positioning of the patient during the procedure depends on the type of surgery to be performed. For surgeries of the perineal area (rectal, anal, or perianal sacs), the patient is positioned in ventral recumbency with the tail retracted cranially and the perineal area elevated.

For **rectal surgery**, complications that may occur are short lived rectal bleeding, soft stools, rectal stenosis (may require a second surgery if it causes pain or obstruction), possible loss of storage capacity (faecal incontinence), dehiscence, and peritonitis. While cats are more tolerant of colon excision (90–95% colon), dogs appear to be less tolerant, although more than 70% of the colon has been excised without long term sequelae.

In one study, after subtotal colectomy in dogs, the elimination of liquid faeces was observed to be 10–12 times per day, normalising in 8–10 weeks, without tenesmus.

Resections of rectal or colic masses depend on the origin and behaviour of the tumour, its size and location. In general, malignant tumours are operated on with a wide margin resection, while benign masses are marginally resected. There are some tumours, such as carcinoma of the apocrine glands of the anal sacs, which although they are malignant with aggressive behaviour cannot be excised with wide margins due to their location. On the other hand, resection of locally aggressive tumours that infiltrate perirectal tissues is problematic or even contraindicated.

In general, approaches to the rectal area can be performed without having to access the pelvic canal via symphysiotomy of the pubis. Most surgeries can be undertaken with a caudal laparotomy approach (masses in the colon or proximal rectum and excision of sublumbar lymph nodes) (Figure 17) or by using a rectal mucosal eversion technique (masses located in the distal rectum). This chapter will not detail the approaches and type of surgery indicated for each type of colorectal tumour.

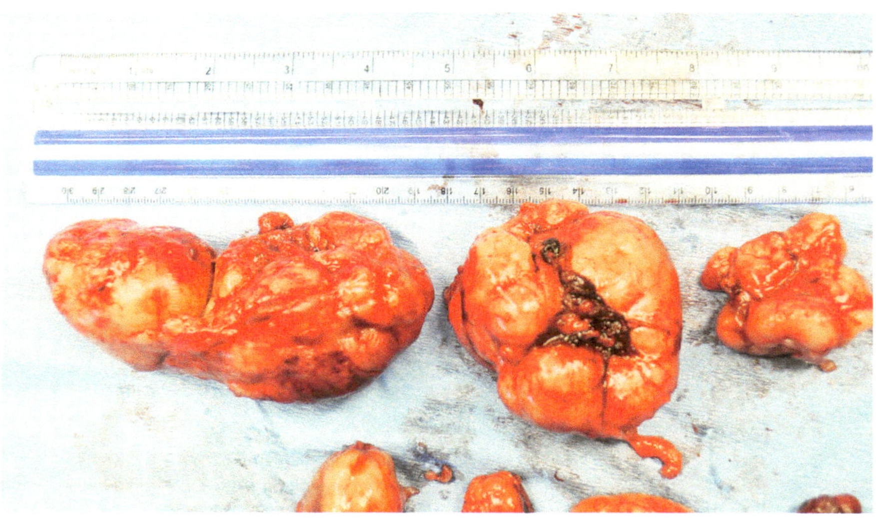

Figure 17. Excision of sublumbar lymph nodes in a patient with adenocarcinoma of the apocrine glands of the anal glands.

Principles of Oncological Skin Surgery

Prevalence

In dogs, 30% of neoplasms come from the skin. In a study evaluating 11,740 skin tumours in dogs, the most common tumours were mastocytomas (16.35%), lipomas (12.47%), hair follicle tumours (12.34%), histiocytomas (12.1%), soft-tissue sarcomas (10.86%), and melanocytic tumours (8.63%). Other skin and subcutaneous tissue tumours are basal cell tumours, sebaceous gland adenoma, sebaceous gland hyperplasia, hepatoid gland adenoma, apocrine adenocarcinoma, and fibroid.

These tumours are distributed over the trunk (30.08%), head and neck (20.9%), extremities (19.14%), anal and perianal areas (8.59%) and tail (3.91%). Other studies have shown similar percentages, as well as comparable distributions and percentages.

Classification

Skin tumours include skin and subcutaneous tissue. The World Health Organization (WHO) classifies epithelial and mesenchymal tumours histologically. Cutaneous tumours can be classified histologically by the type of tissue where the tumour originates from into epithelial, adnexal, mesenchymal, round cell, or melanocytic.

- **Epithelial**: these include basal cell tumours, papillomas, squamous cell carcinomas, and subungual tumours.
- **Adnexal**: originate from the adnexal structures of the skin, including sebaceous gland tumours (adenoma, adenocarcinoma), ceruminous gland adenoma, perianal tumours (adenoma, adenocarcinoma), anal gland apocrine gland adenocarcinoma, sweat gland tumours, hair follicle tumours (trichoepithelioma), pilomatrixoma, meibomian gland adenoma, and cornified intracutaneous epithelioma.
- **Mesenchymal**: originate in connective tissue and are normally located in subcutaneous tissue and/or invade the skin. Soft-tissue sarcomas are malignant mesenchymal tumours. Mesenchymal skin tumours include lipomas or liposarcomas, fibroids or fibrosarcomas, haemangiomas or haemangiosarcomas, myxomas or myxosarcomas, and peripheral nerve sheath tumours. Injection induced haemangiopericytomas and soft-tissue sarcomas are also included in this group, as their biological behaviour is identical to that of soft-tissue sarcomas.
- **Round cells**: include tumours from the population of round cells that reside in the skin. For example, mastocytomas, histiocytomas, melanocytic nevus, plasmacytoma, lymphoma, and transmissible venereal tumour.
- **Melanocytic**: most melanocytic tumours are benign (melanocytic nevus). The most common anatomical sites at which they occur are the eyelashes, face, trunk, and extremities. The biological behaviour of melanocytic tumours varies depending on anatomical location. Tumours located at the mucocutaneous junction or in the subungual area tend to be malignant and are associated with a worse prognosis. Tumours smaller than 1 cm in diameter are usually benign and those larger than 2.5 cm are usually malignant. Malignant melanoma metastasises to the regional lymph nodes and lungs via haematogenous and lymphatic pathways.

Diagnostic Approach and Staging

Presurgical Evaluation

Collecting information about the **clinical history of the skin tumour** is essential, which should include how long the tumour has been present, its growth rate, and whether there has been any change in that rate of growth. Knowledge of previous cytologies, biopsies and/or histologies performed on the tumour or other nodules in the patient is important as it can influence treatment decisions and prognosis. Details of any other clinical signs in the patient are also important, as they could indicate a paraneoplastic syndrome associated with a skin tumour (e.g. gastrointestinal ulcerations associated with mastocytomas).

A **thorough physical examination** should be part of the patient's routine clinical examination. Blood tests including complete blood count, biochemistry, and urinalysis can help investigate other subclinical diseases in middle aged or geriatric patients presenting with skin tumours, while providing general information about the patient's health for general anaesthesia.

Tumour Staging

Determining the **type of tumour, its histological grade and carrying out clinical staging with the TNM classification (tumour, lymph node, metastasis)** before the surgical intervention to plan an optimal treatment protocol and offer the client a rational prognosis is important. This information can be obtained with a good physical examination of the patient and tumour, fine needle aspiration, cytology, incisional (rather than excisional) nodule biopsy, regional lymph node cytology, and diagnostic imaging for distant metastases.

For evaluation of the skin nodule, the anatomical location must be described and measured in 3D to determine the tumour volume. This information should be documented on a patient map in the clinical records. Skin nodules should be palpated carefully to determine consistency, degree of attachment to surrounding tissues, and whether they appear ulcerated or painful.

Sampling Using Fine Needle Aspiration

Samples obtained using fine needle aspiration should be taken from **all skin nodules and subcutaneous tissue** as part of the diagnostic process prior to surgery. Most skin nodules are easily accessible for puncture, so this diagnostic technique is simple, low cost, is associated with minimal pain for the patient, does not need sedation and can provide a quick diagnosis.

Tumour cytology **provides information on tumour type** (e.g. round cells versus epithelial cells), but typically the specific cell type of origin or tumour grade cannot be determined, as it is not possible to observe tumour cytomorphology and architecture with this technique.

Round cell and epithelial tumours tend to exfoliate better and are more likely to offer a diagnostic sample when compared to mesenchymal tumours.

For the diagnosis of skin neoplasia, puncture cytology has a sensitivity of 89.3% and a specificity of 97.9%.

Tumour Biopsy for Histopathological Diagnosis

If cytology does not provide information about the type of tumour or if the cytological diagnosis does not correlate with the clinical diagnosis, an incisional biopsy is indicated to obtain sufficient tissue for histopathology and for determination of treatment options.

Before definitive treatment, **a biopsy is indicated when**:

- the type of treatment will be altered with knowledge of the type of tumour. For example, cutaneous lymphoma (chemotherapy) versus fibrosarcoma (surgery);
- surgery for definitive treatment may be altered with knowledge of the type and grade of the tumour. For example, a grade III soft-tissue sarcoma is more aggressive than a grade I soft-tissue sarcoma. Even so, this aspect should be studied with caution, since the tumour grade obtained by an incisional biopsy is not indicative of the grade of the tumour in its entirety;
- the tumour is located in an anatomical area with limited reconstruction possibilities; and
- knowledge of the type of tumour and/or its grade affects the owner's decision regarding treatment, depending on the prognosis.

Determination of Tumour Stage

Staging determines the extent of the primary tumour and the presence of local or distant metastases. Results of accurate staging with cytology and/or tumour biopsy will indicate the need for additional clinical staging and development of a treatment plan, providing a more realistic expectation of prognosis. This is more important for skin tumours that have high metastatic potential.

Tests for clinical staging typically include assessment of regional lymph nodes, thoracic radiographs (three views), abdominal ultrasound, and possibly advanced imaging to assess for the presence of metastases.

Options for Treatment of Skin Tumours

Appropriate treatment options in individual cases are based on the type of tumour, the degree of local disease, the results of staging tests, the presence or absence of metastases, and the condition of the patient.

Most solid skin tumours can be treated successfully with surgical resection. Surgery may be used as a single treatment or in combination with chemotherapy, radiation therapy, or other adjuvant therapies. Tumours that are sensitive to radiation therapy are squamous cell carcinoma, basal cell carcinoma, cutaneous lymphoma, and mast cell carcinomas.

Principles of Surgical Excision

The objective of surgical excision of malignant tumours of the skin is to obtain a **block excision with wide surgical margins free of tumour cells**, with a normal tissue margin in all three dimensions. The extent of the surgical margins depends on the type of tumour and the location.

Resection requires the excision of any tissue that is in contact with the tumour, including fascia, muscle, subcutaneous fat, or even bone. The first surgery usually provides the best opportunity to achieve local tumour control.

Excision of the skin tumour must be done following **basic surgical principles**: an aseptic surgical technique, with absolute care of the tissues, maintaining vascularisation and minimising dead space and skin tension. Any previously performed biopsy tract should be excised *en bloc* with the tumour and relevant margins. Ideally, a surgical excision (of wide or marginal margins) should not penetrate the tumour capsule and will prevent seeding and contamination of tumour cells to local or distant tissues.

Veins should be ligated before arteries to prevent tumour manipulation from shedding neoplastic cells that can access systemic vascularisation and haematogenous dissemination.

Instruments, gloves, and surgical drapes should be changed immediately after tumour excision. The **use of postoperative drains should be avoided**, as when introduced they can contaminate healthy tissues which they pass through with tumour cells. However, the use of drains may be considered if the surgery results in a large dead space area or is located in an anatomical area with a lot of movement, which predisposes to the formation of a seroma. Still, many seromas can be managed conservatively and disappear spontaneously.

Surgical Margins

Guidelines for surgical margins depend on the type of tumour, suspected biological behaviour, tumour grade, anatomical location, and normal tissues adjacent to the tumour.

Margin resection (surgical doses) for skin tumours may be:

- **intracapsular** or cytoreductive resection, which clinically leaves macroscopic tumour tissue in the patient. Therefore, by applying this surgical dose to a malignant tumour local recurrence is assured unless a local adjuvant treatment (radiation, electrochemotherapy) is added to the tumour site. These surgeries are usually performed to alleviate the clinical signs caused by the tumour (Figure 18);
- **marginal excision**: is the resection of the tumour immediately outside the pseudocapsule, thus leaving microscopic tumour tissue in the patient in cases of malignant invasive tumours. Local recurrence is quite common unless a second surgery with wide margins is performed, or local adjuvant therapy is applied. An example for this type of surgical dose is to resect soft-tissue sarcomas

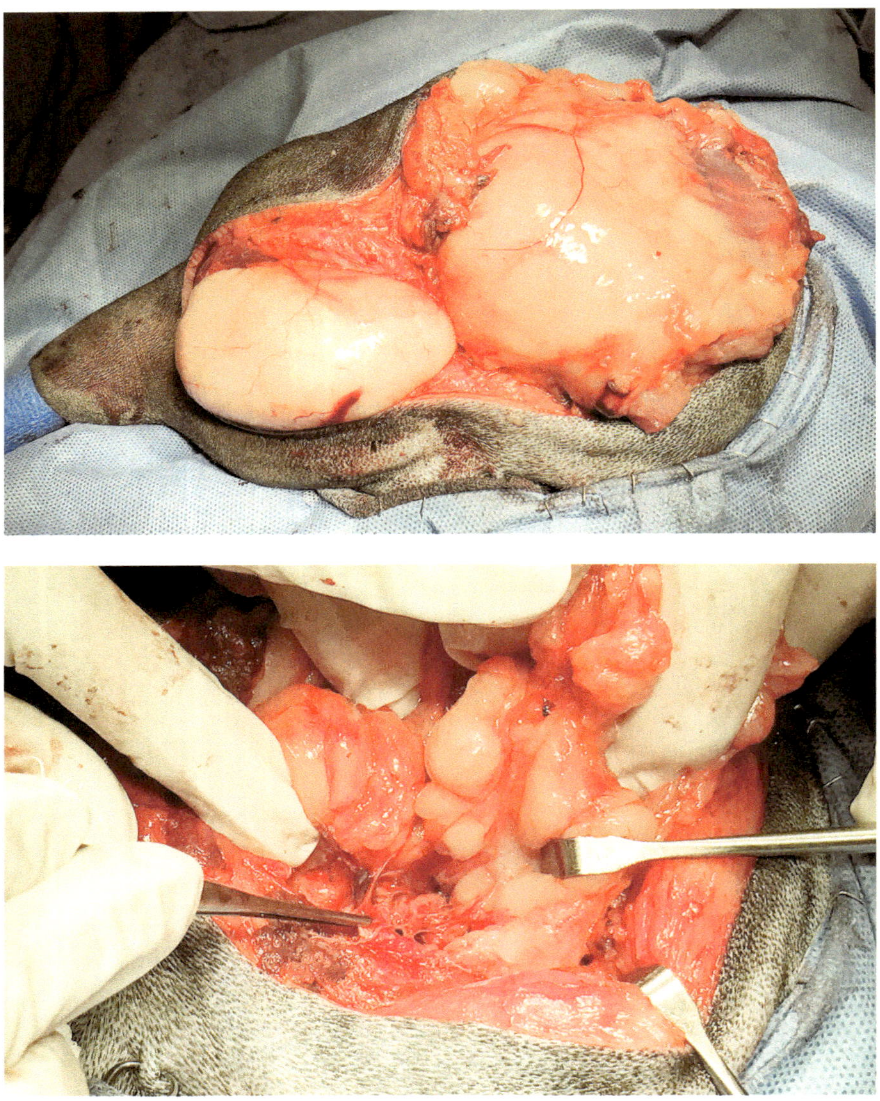

Figure 18. Intracapsular excision of an infiltrative lipoma on the left hindlimb of a dog.

that appear well encapsulated, but in fact are removed just around the pseudocapsule (composed of compressed tumour cells) thus leaving microscopic tissue and cancer cell projections on the surgical periphery (Figure 19);

- **wide margin resection** is the excision of the tumour with non-carcinogenic tissue margins in all three dimensions. Local recurrence is unlikely. An example of wide margin resection for skin tumours are mast cell tumours of the trunk, which are excised with 2–3 cm lateral margins and a deep fascial plane (Figure 20); and
- **radical resection**: refers to the resection of the entire anatomical part containing the tumour. Local recurrence

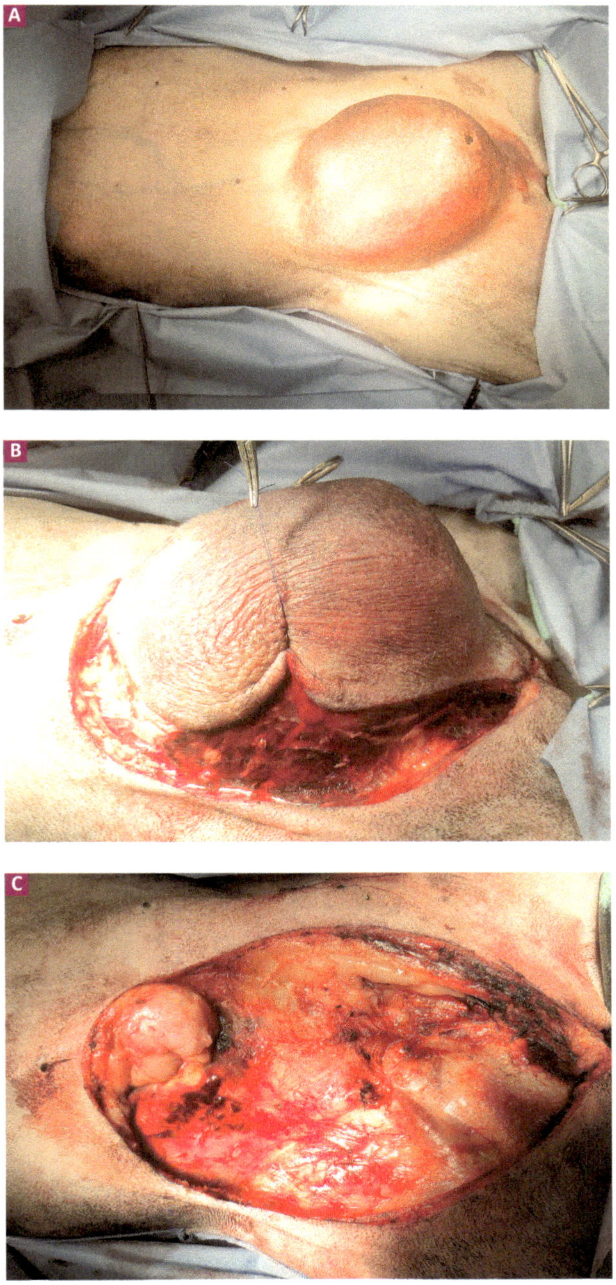

Figure 19. Inguinal grade III mastocytoma (**A**). Marginal excision of the tumour, without extra margins of the apparently normal tissue (**B**). Tissue bed after marginal excision (**C**). This patient received definitive adjuvant radiotherapy two weeks after surgery.

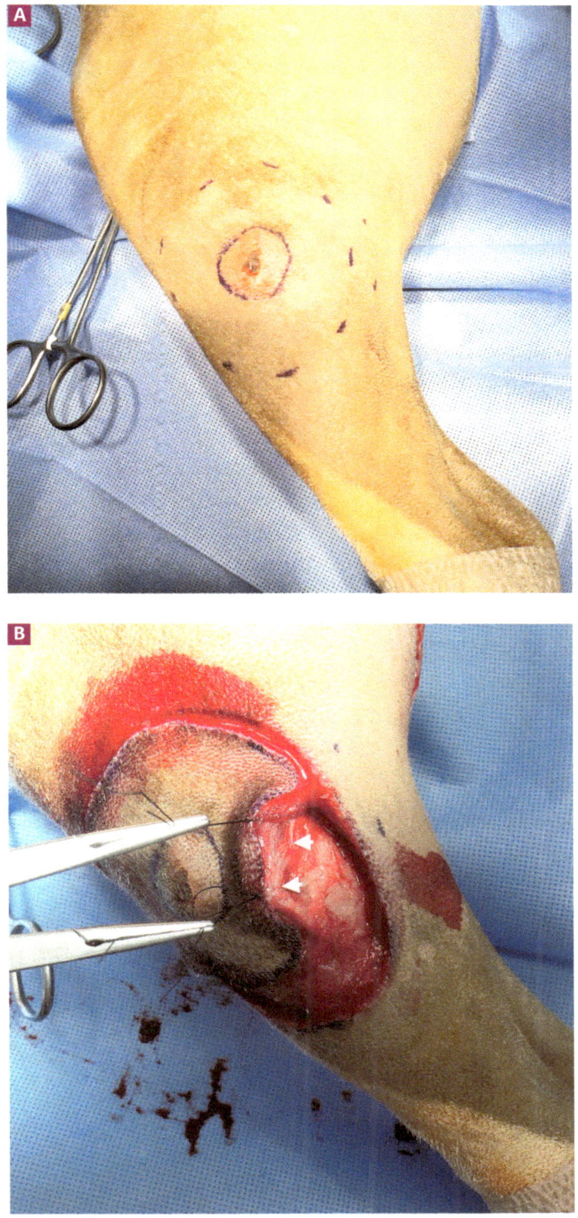

Figure 20. Surgical approach to a grade II soft-tissue sarcoma distal to the left stifle. The tumour is marked using a sterile marker and 3 cm lateral to this is measured. Whether the excision is feasible is checked (**A**). The excision is started in the skin and subcutaneously until the fascia is reached, dissecting below the fascia to remove the tumour block (**B**).

is unlikely. An appropriate example of radical resection for skin tumours is limb amputation due to grade III soft-tissue sarcoma. Radical resection requires extensive knowledge of regional anatomy as well as postoperative strategies, side effects of more extreme surgery, and knowledge of reconstructive surgery (Figure 21).

As a general principle, all tissues which the tumour comes into contact with or invades must be resected with a margin of normal tissue. Adipose tissue is a poor biological barrier in terms of protection for tumour invasion, so using subcutaneous fat as a deep margin barrier in skin tumours is not advisable. Muscle fascia and bone are the most effective barriers to tumour growth, so the recommendation is to use these tissues as a deep margin. When possible, dissection should be performed through non-tumour tissue (normal tissue) and a block excision. Higher grade tumours usually require more aggressive resection, with wider surgical margins.

Surgical margins should be determined taking the closure of the surgical wound into account, in addition to the complete resection of the tumour. The quality and quantity of surgical margins should not be compromised to facilitate surgical closure. From an oncological and surgical perspective, **it is preferable to have to deal with a large surgical wound rather than a resection of a malignant tumour with incomplete margins**.

There are a variety of surgical options for reconstruction, such as using flaps or skin grafts or even allowing the wound to close by second intention, and these should be used appropriately for different situations. Mohs micrographic surgery technique has been described in a pilot study for the total evaluation of surgical margins for skin tumours in veterinary oncology.

Evaluation of Surgical Margins

After local resection of a tumour, the surgeon plays an important role in communicating with the pathologist. This communication is essential for the identification of the sample and its margins. Detailed information of the procedure and surgical margins can be provided in the histopathology application document, including the clinical history, by attempting to maintain normal tissue architecture and by drawing the surgical margins (lateral and deep) with tissue ink.

The surgeon is responsible for interpreting the pathology report in the context of the surgery performed. The pathology report should contain three important points that help the surgeon decide on the need for adjuvant therapy to surgery: histological diagnosis, tumour grade, and quality of surgical margins.

If the surgical margins are incomplete, the entire wound is assumed to be contaminated with tumour cells, so a more aggressive surgical resection or other adjuvant treatment modality is indicated (Figure 22).

Surgical Reconstruction Procedures

Reconstruction procedures are indicated after tumour resection for reconstruction of skin defects. These procedures may

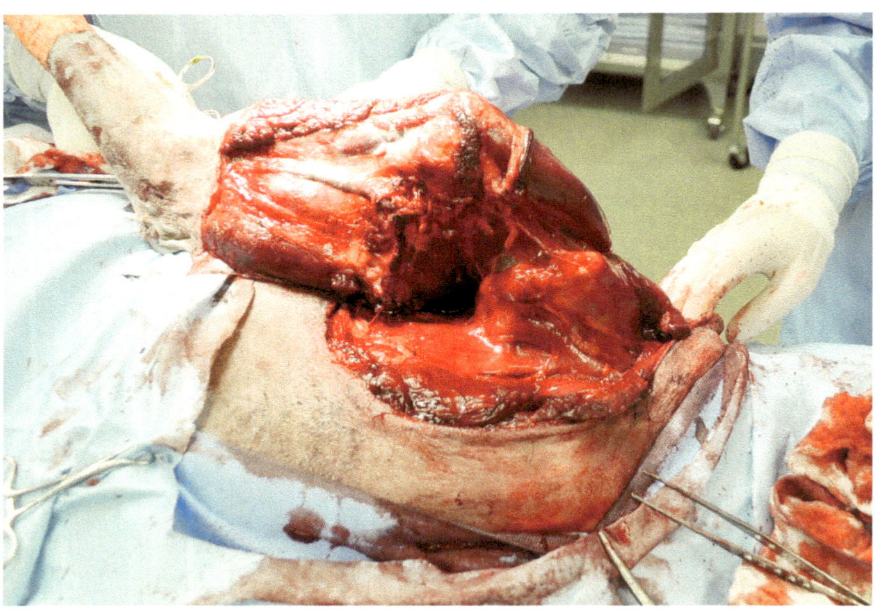

Figure 21. Radical excision (amputation of the right forelimb) due to an osteosarcoma.

include local or pedicle flaps, delayed or secondary primary closure, skin free grafting, or myocutaneous flaps.

The surgeon should plan the reconstructive procedure prior to excision of the tumour, marking its margins, surgical margins, and the proposed site for the flap with a sterile marker pen.

Each situation should be considered individually, with the degree of resection necessary for each type of tumour and location. For example, a low-grade mastocytoma located on the limb can be appropriately treated with a more conservative wide margin resection (1 cm lateral margin and a deep fascial plane), a high-grade mastocytoma ulcerated with regional lymph node metastasis can be treated with a palliative marginal resection, while a grade II (intermediate) mastocytoma in the pelvic area requires a broad excision with a reconstructive skin flap.

If a flap or graft is used for reconstruction, the donor and recipient surgical fields should be treated with different instruments and gloves to avoid cross contamination of tumour cells.

Adjuvant Therapies for Skin Tumours

Adjuvant therapies are those that complement the definitive primary therapy. Radiation or chemotherapy are the main adjuvant treatments to surgery for skin tumours. These therapies can be used palliatively or curatively. Indications for the need for adjuvant therapy are based on specific tumour type, tumour biology, histological grade, clinical stage, and quality of surgical margins. Other less common but emerging adjuvant therapies are immunotherapy, photodynamic therapy, ablative radiofrequency, and cryotherapy.

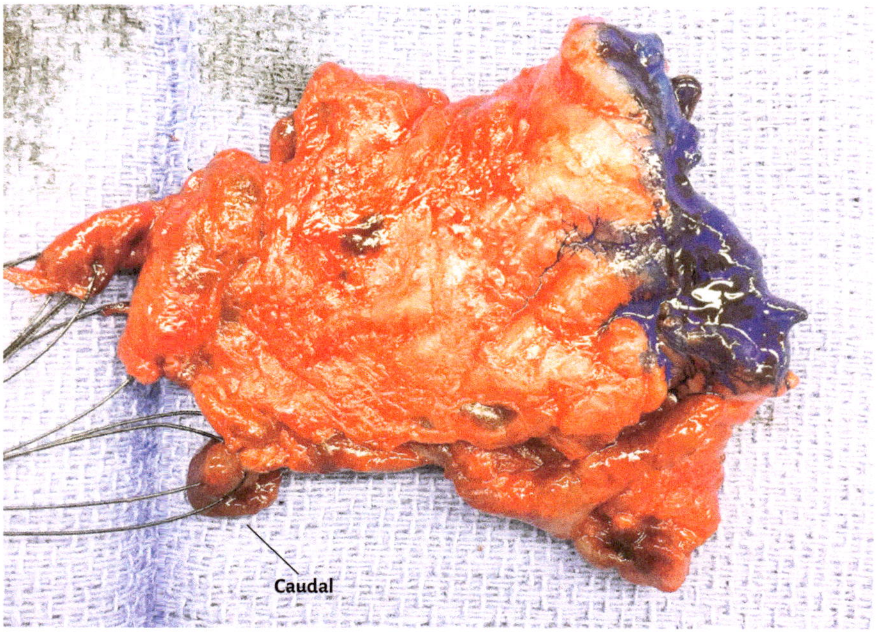

Figure 22. Marking of margins with surgical tissue ink (or equivalent) to communicate the margins which need to be identified to the pathologist. Communication with the pathologist is extremely important and this photo should be included for the benefit of the pathology department.

Bibliography

- Abrams, B., Wavreille, V.A., Husbands, B.D. et al. (2019) Perioperative complications and outcome after surgery for treatment of gastric carcinoma in dogs: A Veterinary Society of Surgical Oncology retrospective study of 40 cases (2004–2018). *Vet Surg.* 48(6):923–932.
- Aitken, M.L., Patnaik, A.K. (2000) Comparison of needle-core (Tru-Cut®) biopsy and surgical biopsy for the diagnosis of cutaneous and subcutaneous masses: a prospective study of 51 cases (November 1997-August 1998). *J Am Anim Hosp Assoc.* 36(2):153–7.
- Bernstein, J.A., Hodgin E.C., Holloway H.W. et al. (2006) Mohs micrographic surgery: a technique for total margin assessment in veterinary cutaneous oncologic surgery. *Vet Comp Oncol.* 4(3):151–60.
- Bonfanti, U., Bertazzolo, W., Bottero, E. et al. (2006) Diagnostic value of cytologic examination of gastrointestinal tract tumors in dogs and cats: 83 cases (2001–2004). *J Am Vet Med Assoc.* 229(7):1130–3.
- Bray, J.P., Polton, G.A., McSporran, K.D. et al. (2014) Canine soft tissue sarcoma managed in first opinion practice: outcome in 350 cases. *Vet Surg.* 43(7):774–82.
- Dvorak, L.D., Beaver, D.P., Ellison, G.W. et al. (2004) Major glossectomy in dogs: a case series and proposed classification system. *J Am Anim Hosp Assoc.* 40(4):331–7.
- Freeman, L.J. (2009) Gastrointestinal laparoscopy in small animals. *Vet Clin North Am Small Anim Pract.* 39(5):903–24.
- Ghisleni, G., Roccabianca, P., Ceruti, R. et al. (2006) Correlation between fine-needle aspiration cytology and histopathology in the evaluation of cutaneous and subcutaneous masses from dogs and cats. *Vet Clin Pathol.* 35(1):24–30.
- Graf, R., Pospischil, A., Guscetti, F. et al. (2018) Cutaneous Tumors in Swiss Dogs: Retrospective Data From the Swiss Canine Cancer Registry, 2008–2013. *Vet Pathol.* 55(6):809–820.
- Herring, E.S., Smith, M.M., Robertson J.L. (2002) Lymph node staging of oral and maxillofacial neoplasms in 31 dogs and cats. *J Vet Dent.* 19(3):122–6.
- Jakubiak, M.J., Siedlecki, C.T., Zenger, E. et al. (2005) Laryngeal, laryngotracheal, and tracheal masses in cats: 27 cases (1998–2003). *J Am Anim Hosp Assoc.* 41(5):310–6.
- Kok, M.K., Chambers, J.K., Tsuboi, M. et al. (2019) Retrospective study of canine cutaneous tumors in Japan, 2008–2017. *J Vet Med Sci.* 28.
- Lamb, C.R., Grierson, J. (1999) Ultrasonographic appearance of primary gastric neoplasia in 21 dogs. *J Small Anim Pract.* 40(5):211–5.
- Nemeth, T., Solymosi, N., Balka, G. (2008) Long-term results of subtotal colectomy for acquired hypertrophic megacolon in eight dogs. *J Small Anim Pract.* 49(12):618–24.
- Northrup, N.C., Selting, K.A., Rassnick, K.M. et al. (2006) Outcomes of cats with oral tumors treated with mandibulectomy: 42 cases. *J Am Anim Hosp Assoc.* 42(5):350–60.
- Paoloni, M.C., Penninck, D.G., Moore A.S. (2002) Ultrasonographic and clinicopathologic findings in 21 dogs with intestinal adenocarcinoma. *Vet Radiol Ultrasound.* 43(6):562–7.
- Penninck, D., Smyers, B., Webster, C.R. et al. (2003) Diagnostic value of ultrasonography in differentiating enteritis from intestinal neoplasia in dogs. *Vet Radiol Ultrasound.* 44(5):570–5.
- Sogame, N., Risbon R., Burgess K.E. (2018) Intestinal lymphoma in dogs: 84 cases (1997–2012). *J Am Vet Med Assoc.* 252(4):440–447.
- Syrcle, J.A., Bonczynski, J.J., Monette, S. et al. (2008) Retrospective evaluation of lingual tumors in 42 dogs: 1999–2005. *J Am Anim Hosp Assoc.* 44(6):308–19.
- Willard, M.D., Lovering, S.L., Cohen, N.D. et al. (2001) Quality of tissue specimens obtained endoscopically from the duodenum of dogs and cats. *J Am Vet Med Assoc* 219(4):474–9.
- Williams, L.E., Packer R.A. (2003) Association between lymph node size and metastasis in dogs with oral malignant melanoma: 100 cases (1987–2001). *J Am Vet Med Assoc.* 222(9):1234–6.

Test

Answers on Page 350

Answers on page 350

1. **Which of the following are recognised as negative prognostic factors for lung tumours?**
    a. Tumour type, clinical stage, pleural effusion, presence of clinical signs, tumour size.
    b. Tumour type, time the tumour has been present, patient breed, affected lung lobe, pleural effusion.
    c. Clinical signs, tumour size, patient activity, time the tumour has been present, tumour type.
    d. Tumour size, patient activity, presence of clinical signs and clinical stage.

2. **Regarding detection of metastatic lung disease, which of the following statements is true?**
    a. Conventional radiography is a very sensitive imaging test.
    b. If metastases are detected with radiography, the next step should be a thoracic MRI.
    c. CT can detect lung lesions as small as 1 mm in diameter.
    d. Radiographs can only detect lesions which are 20 mm in diameter.

3. **A 16-year-old cat is brought into the practice with multiple nodules on the digits and anorexia. Cytology is performed on one of the digital nodules and pneumocytes are observed in the sample. What is the most likely diagnosis and what should the next step be?**
    a. Polydactyly – analgesia and rest.
    b. Multiple mast cell tumours – amputate affected digits.
    c. Digital abscesses, as it is an outdoor cat – antibiotics.
    d. Pulmonary digital syndrome - thoracic radiographs (three projections).

4. **A 12-year-old male neutered Labrador Retriever is brought into the practice with severe lameness and painful swelling of the front legs. When radiographs are performed on the right carpus, a transarticular periosteal reaction with soft tissue swelling, but no arthropathy is seen. What should the next step be?**
    a. Arthrocentesis of the affected joints, the transarticular swelling may be rheumatoid arthritis.
    b. Abdominal ultrasound, as polyarthropathy can be seen with gastrointestinal diseases.
    c. Analgesia and prednisone.
    d. Thoracic radiographs (three projections).

5. **A 9-year-old male neutered Labrador presents for voice changes and inspiratory dyspnoea. Laryngeal paralysis is suspected, but on physical examination an asymmetry in the area of the larynx is palpated. The owners have limited financial resources but want to know what the dog is suffering from and the prognosis. What would the best course of action be to help meet the owners' expectations?**
    a. Thoracic radiography (three projections) to rule out tracheal mass and lung metastases.
    b. Oral examination with sedation.
    c. CT of the head and neck, with cytology if there is a laryngeal mass.
    d. Oral examination with anaesthesia and intubation and incisional biopsy if there is a laryngeal mass.

6. **What type of biopsy is best for diagnosing oral tumours?**
    a. Incisional biopsy.
    b. Excisional biopsy.
    c. Needle biopsy.
    d. No biopsy is needed, as cytology is highly sensitive.

7. **For the staging of oral malignant melanoma, which of the following is true?**
    a. The most common sites of metastasis are the liver and spleen.
    b. Palpation of enlarged regional lymph nodes is predictive of metastasis to these lymph nodes.
    c. Regional lymph node cytology is essential to diagnose metastasis in these lymph nodes.
    d. It does not usually metastasise to the lungs.

8. **Which of these parasites has been identified with oesophageal sarcomas?**
    a. *Anaplasma platys.*
    b. *Dirofilaria immitis.*
    c. A tumour has not been identified as being associated with a parasite.
    d. *Spirocerca lupi.*

9. **Ideally, what surgical treatment (surgical dose) is needed to treat an intestinal AC?**
    a. Marginal excision.
    b. Cytoreduction.
    c. Excision with wide 10 cm margins, if it is in the small intestine and 2 cm if it is in the large intestine.
    d. Excision with wide 3–5 cm margins.

10. A 10-year-old Rottweiler presents with a mass in the proximal jejunum, diagnosed by cytology as an intestinal AC. After resection and anastomosis, the patient continues to vomit profusely and has cranial abdominal distension, despite intravenous antiemetics (maropitant, ondansetron and metoclopramide). Which pathology is most likely and which treatment method is most suitable for these clinical signs?

a. They are probably caused by abdominal pain, the opioid dose should be increased.
b. Fluid and peritoneal gas are present on abdominal radiographs, surgery should be performed as soon as possible to treat septic peritonitis.
c. On a FAST ultrasound the stomach is found to be dilated. The cause is probably gastroparesis, and a nasogastric tube is needed to empty the stomach.
d. It is advisable to wait for a day for the antiemetics to take effect.

11. What is the most common malignant skin tumour in dogs?

a. Mast cell tumour.
b. Soft-tissue sarcoma.
c. Melanoma.
d. Squamous cell carcinoma.

12. For staging of a soft-tissue sarcoma in the left hindlimb, which imaging modality would be most appropriate?

a. Ultrasound of the regional lymph node.
b. Abdominal ultrasound.
c. Thoracic radiographs (three projections).
d. Soft-tissue sarcomas are locally invasive, but do not metastasise.

13. What surgical dose is recommended for the excision of a subcutaneous soft-tissue sarcoma in the lateral thorax?

a. A marginal excision, since there is excess skin in this area, if it is of a high-grade it can be excised again later.
b. Excision with wide 3 cm margins.
c. Excisional biopsy to remove the tumour.
d. Excision with wide 3 cm margins and a deep fascial plane.

14. A 5-year-old male castrated Boxer is brought to the practice with a dermal nodule of 3 cm in diameter on the lateral area of the left thigh that has been present for 3 months with some variation in size. The owner just wants to remove it, what would the best recommendation be?

a. Remove the tumour with an excisional biopsy and send it a pathologist.
b. Remove the tumour during the next prophylactic dental and there is no need to send it to the pathologist.
c. As it almost certainly a lipoma, there is no need for surgical treatment, only monitoring.
d. Perform a fine needle aspiration for cytology and have it checked by a pathologist.

15. A 3-year-old Pit Bull is brought to the practice for an annual check-up. On the physical examination a skin nodule of 1.5 cm in diameter that moves in the skin of the left thigh is seen. A fine needle aspiration is performed, and the cytology results are shown here:

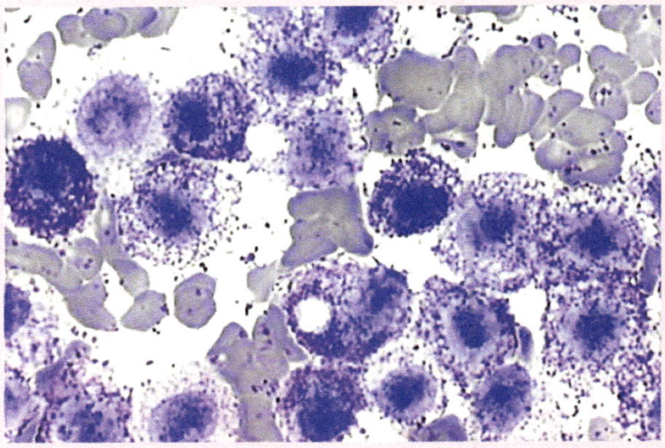

Which diagnostic tests necessary for staging should be recommended to the owners?

a. Thoracic radiographs.
b. Thoracic radiographs, abdominal ultrasound, bone marrow aspiration.
c. Locoregional lymph node puncture, abdominal ultrasound with liver and spleen puncture and cytology.
d. CT scan of the thorax and abdomen.

Notes

Correct Answers:

1. a
2. c
3. d
4. d
5. d
6. a
7. c
8. d
9. d
10. c
11. a
12. c
13. d
14. d
15. c

Notes

Urogenital System and Mammary Tumours

Juan Francisco Borrego

Kidneys

In dogs, **primary renal neoplasms are rare**, making up an estimated 0.3 to 1.5% of all canine neoplasms.

Epithelial tumours, and in particular **renal carcinoma, is the most common primary renal tumour in dogs** and should be distinguished from other primary epithelial neoplasms, including renal adenomas and oncocytomas, nephroblastomas, transitional cell carcinomas, and sarcomas. The mean age of dogs which are diagnosed with renal tumours is about nine years old and males are usually predisposed with a male/female ratio of 1.6/1 to 1.2/1. German Shepherd dogs may suffer from an unusual syndrome that includes the presence of cystadenocarcinomas with concurrent nodular dermatofibrosis, as well as uterine tumours.

The **most common kidney tumour in cats is lymphoma**. In contrast to older studies where most cats were feline leukaemia virus (FeLV) positive, this location it is not usually associated with the virus and the average age of onset is nine years old, with no breed or sex predisposition. In cats other primary tumours affecting the kidneys include adenoma, adenocarcinoma, transitional cell carcinoma, haemangiosarcoma, nephroblastoma, and squamous cell carcinoma.

Diagnosis

Patients may present with any combination of non-specific signs such as lack of appetite, weight loss, lethargy, vomiting, and haematuria. Physical examination may detect uni- or bilateral renomegaly, including pain on abdominal palpation. In German Shepherds renal cystadenocarcinoma may be associated with firm nodular skin lesions and benign uterine tumours.

Histopathological examination is required to reach a diagnosis, although ultrasound-guided cytology can be diagnostic in most cases of lymphoma and be helpful in a high percentage of epithelial neoplasms. Biopsies may be obtained percutaneously under ultrasound guidance or surgically. Patient staging should include complete blood count, biochemistry, and urinalysis, which may show anaemia or polycythaemia secondary to decreased or increased erythropoietin production. Non-specific changes such as azotaemia or hypoalbuminaemia, as well as paraneoplastic syndrome associated with some renal tumours, such as neutrophilic leucocytosis, may also be detected.

Thoracic radiographs should also form part of staging, as dogs and cats with epithelial renal tumours can present lung metastases in almost half of the cases. More up to date studies of renal carcinomas show a lower rate of lung metastasis (11–18%), which can probably be attributed to earlier clinical detection of the disease in recent years.

Although locoregional lymphadenopathies and other intra-abdominal structures can be detected on abdominal radiographs, **abdominal ultrasound is the imaging technique of choice**, as well as for guiding fine needle aspirates (FNA) of these organs. The combination of renomegaly, hypoechoic focal lesions, and bilateral involvement appear to be amongst the most common ultrasound features in canine lymphoma. Bilateral involvement is common in lymphoma, but rarely occurs in patients with renal carcinoma. Lymphoma in cats is usually bilateral (>80%), with irregular renomegaly with hypoechoic subcapsular thickening (detected on ultrasound) (Figure 1) and involvement of other organs.

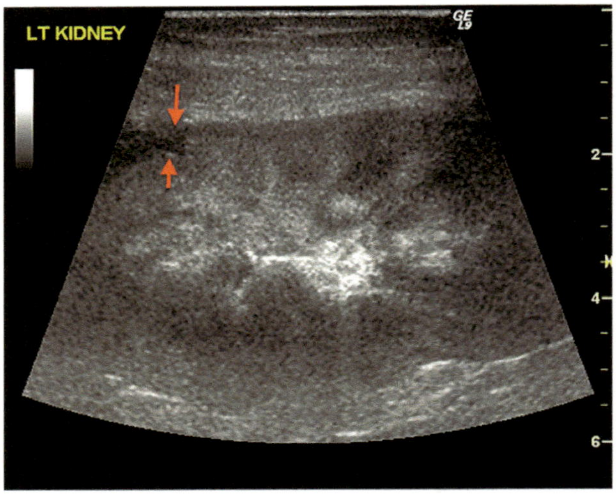

Figure 1. Ultrasound image of a feline patient with lymphoma where a subcapsular hypoechoic area typical in these patients can be seen.

Treatment

During surgical planning assessing renal function is vitally important: some of the tests available for this purpose include excretory urography, CT, and evaluation of glomerular filtration rate (GFR) using scintigraphy. Invasion of the vena cava by renal carcinoma is a rare finding, but should be assessed using ultrasound or CT.

Nephrectomy (Figure 2) is the most effective treatment for dogs with unilateral tumours, with a median survival time of 16 to 24 months for carcinomas, 9 months for haemangiosarcomas and 6 months for nephroblastomas. A mitotic index >30 appears to be associated with a worse prognosis in renal carcinomas after surgery.

The **role of adjuvant therapy in canine renal tumours is unclear**, as published studies do not demonstrate increased survival. Treatment with chemotherapy is indicated for cats and dogs with renal lymphoma. In addition to being bilateral, it is considered to be part of a systemic disease and is rarely the primary tumour. Extension to the central nervous system (CNS) is frequent, affecting up to 40–50% of cats. Multidrug protocols (COP/CHOP) are used most often with the addition of drugs that cross the blood brain barrier and reach the central nervous system (e.g. cytarabine). With treatment, the median survival time is 3–6 months. Surgery is the treatment of choice for cats with other kidney tumours. Renal cystadenocarcinomas in German Shepherds, although malignant and metastatic, progress more slowly than other renal neoplasms and survival times may be longer.

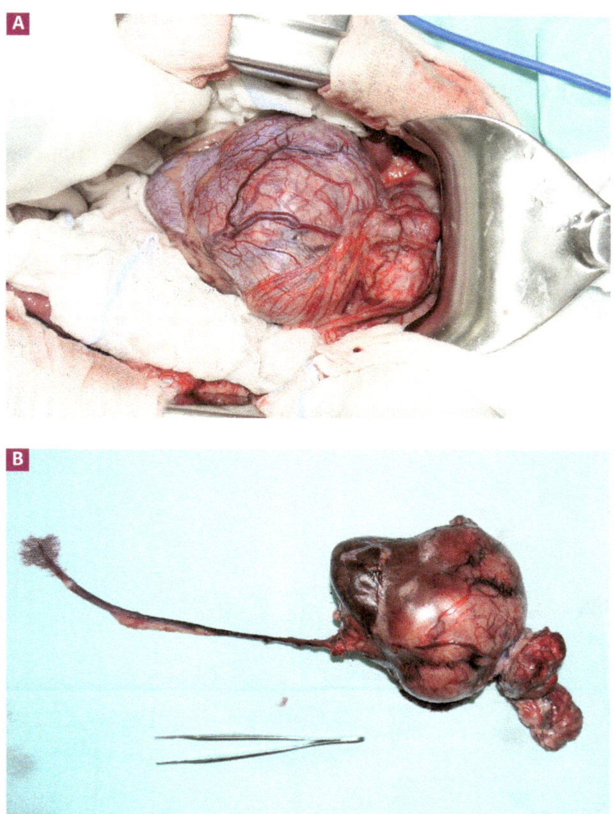

Figure 2. Intraoperative image of a renal carcinoma (**A**) in situ, and after a nephrectomy which included removal of the ureter (**B**). (Images courtesy of Manuel Jiménez Peláez).

Bladder and Urethra

Urinary bladder tumours are **common in dogs and uncommon in cats**. Most tumours affecting the bladder and urethra are malignant, epithelial tumours. The most common diagnosis affecting the urinary tract in both dogs and cats is intermediate to high-grade invasive transitional cell carcinoma (TCC). Other differentials include squamous cell carcinoma, adenocarcinoma, rhabdomyosarcoma, lymphoma, and other mesenchymal tumours. Urethral and prostate involvement is common with these types of tumours. As the clinical signs of these tumours are similar to those of bacterial cystitis and urolithiasis, both pathologies should be ruled out. Another important differential diagnosis for masses found in the urinary bladder, although rare, are benign polyps of the urinary bladder.

Feline TCC is a disease that affects geriatric cats, there does not appear to be any breed predisposition, and it is more common in male cats, without any known predisposing factors. Older bitches (9–11 years of age) appear to be predisposed and multiple risk factors have been described. Small breeds such as the Scottish Terrier are up to twenty times more likely to suffer from this type of tumour and others such as the West Highland White Terrier, Shetland Sheepdog, Beagle, and Fox Terrier are 3–5 times more likely to be affected compared to mixed breed dogs.

Other aetiologies described in dogs include obesity, sex (females are predisposed), castration, prior treatment with cyclophosphamide or exposure to insecticides (usually a consideration for older products, such as amitraz baths). The consumption of vegetables (mainly broccoli) seems to reduce the risk of suffering the disease in Scottish Terriers, a breed which is already predisposed.

Diagnosis

Clinical signs such as stranguria, pollakiuria, haematuria, dysuria, urinary incontinence, or any recurrent combination of these signs in a geriatric dog and, in particular, in the breeds described above, should lead to suspicions of the presence of a bladder mass and diagnostic tests should be performed. In cases where the disease is already more advanced, a mass in the caudal abdomen can sometimes be palpated, as well as abnormalities on rectal examination, such as a swollen urethra or enlarged intrapelvic/sublumbar lymph nodes.

Although less frequent TCCs can also metastasise to the inguinal lymph nodes and patients may also present with hindlimb lameness due to distant bone metastases (Figure 3) or hot, swollen, and painful limbs due to paraneoplastic hypertrophic osteopathy.

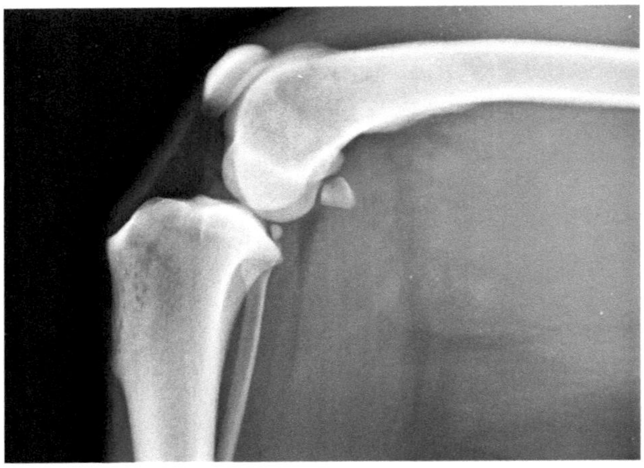

Figure 3. Aggressive lesion in the proximal tibia, showing a metastatic focus from a transitional cell carcinoma of the bladder. Although the rate of metastasis is low at diagnosis (<20%), transitional cell carcinomas can metastasise to the bones.

The **diagnostic work up** in any animal with the above clinical signs should begin with careful abdominal palpation and rectal examination. Complete blood count and biochemistry are usually normal, although in some cases azotaemia may be detected. Urine sediment, which can sometimes reveal the presence of cells with criteria of malignancy, does not provide a definitive diagnosis because any inflammatory process can cause dysplastic changes in cells which may resemble a carcinogenic process.

When a bladder tumour is suspected, urine should be obtained for analysis by catheterisation or ultrasound-guided cystocentesis to prevent the needle from penetrating the bladder through the tumour mass. A urine culture and antibiogram should be performed to rule out lower urinary tract infection, which is extremely common in these types of tumours (up to one third or more of patients). Unless the lesion is mineralised, **tumours are not usually detected on abdominal radiographs**, but sublumbar lymphadenopathy or bone metastases may be visible (Figure 4).

Although contrast radiology techniques can be used, **ultrasound is usually preferred** because of its ease of use and precision when detecting the presence of these masses. Ultrasound is an excellent technique for locating and defining the extent of the disease (Figure 5) and, to a lesser extent, for monitoring the response to therapy.

Cytology of cells from the urine pellet or those obtained by traumatic catheterisation can help in the presumptive diagnosis, with the characteristic intracytoplasmic pink bodies seen in transitional cells, although in most cases a biopsy (traumatic, surgical or via cystoscopic catheterisation) is required.

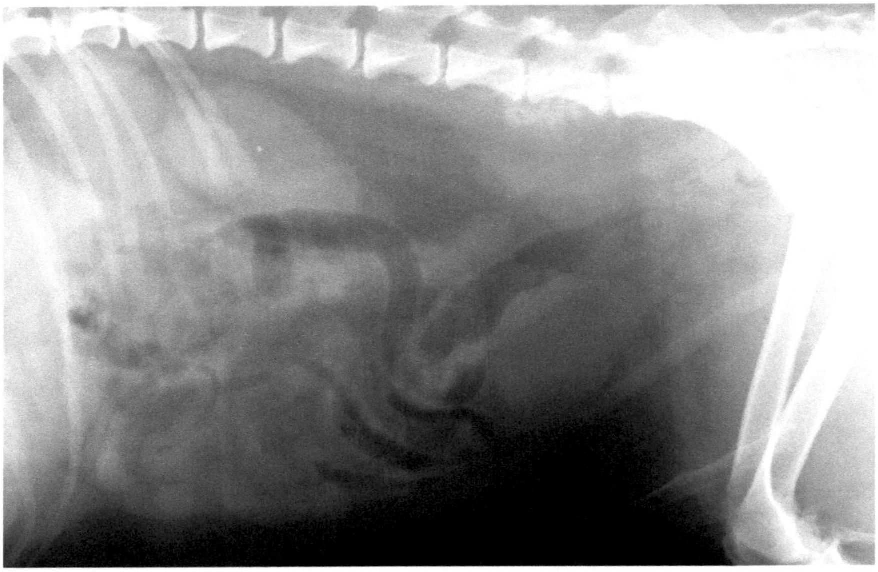

Figure 4. Aggressive osseous lesion between L5–L6 vertebrae with bone proliferation and marked sublumbar lymphadenopathy, showing a metastatic focus in a patient with transitional cell carcinoma of the bladder.

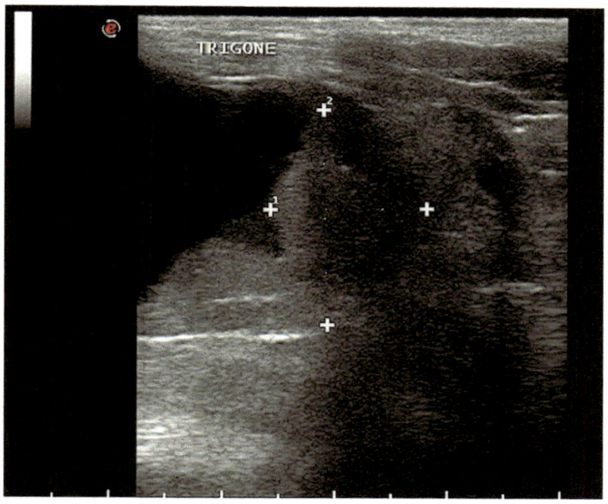

Figure 5. Ultrasound image which shows the presence of a mass in the urinary bladder trigone region, the most common location for transitional cell carcinomas located in the bladder.

Ultrasound-guided FNA is not recommended because of the risk of tumour spread through the needle tract. Obtaining a cystoscopic biopsy is the preferred technique for tumours in the urethra and bladder. A diagnostic quality sample acquired using cystoscopy is more likely to be obtained in females than in males. The sample is diagnostic in 65% of males and 96% of females.

TCC is uncommon in cats and most cases do not affect the bladder trigone. In addition, the presence of metastatic disease at the time of diagnosis is rare. In dogs, TCC usually affects the trigone. Obstruction of the ureters and urethra and invasion and involvement of the urethral sphincter are frequent.

Metastatic disease is detected at the time of clinical diagnosis in 10–20% of dogs and in up to 50% on postmortem.

The most common locations for metastases include the lymph nodes, lungs, bones, and skin. TCCs have also been described in the abdominal wall, most likely due to their highly exfoliative nature and implantation or dissemination during procedures such as biopsy surgery, tumour removal, tumour cytoreduction, placement of a cystotomy tube, FNA or mass cystocentesis (Figure 6).

Treatment

TCCs found in the abdominal wall present a much worse prognosis than those located in the bladder, so caution is recommended to avoid seeding the tumour in the abdomen or in the surgical area during the procedures mentioned in the previous section, and especially during surgery. Instruments and gloves used for tumour removal should be replaced and a different instrument should be used to close the abdomen.

Most dogs with TCC are managed with medical therapy or, less frequently, radiation therapy or surgery. Surgery should only be considered in tumours located cranially in the bladder, although it is unclear whether the prognosis is better than with the administration of medical treatment alone (Figure 7). Although very advanced surgical techniques have been described, it is rare that complete resection can be achieved with acceptable postoperative functionality for tumours located in the trigone region (most frequent). Radiation therapy is increasingly used in protocols combined with medical therapy, as new approaches to administering radiation

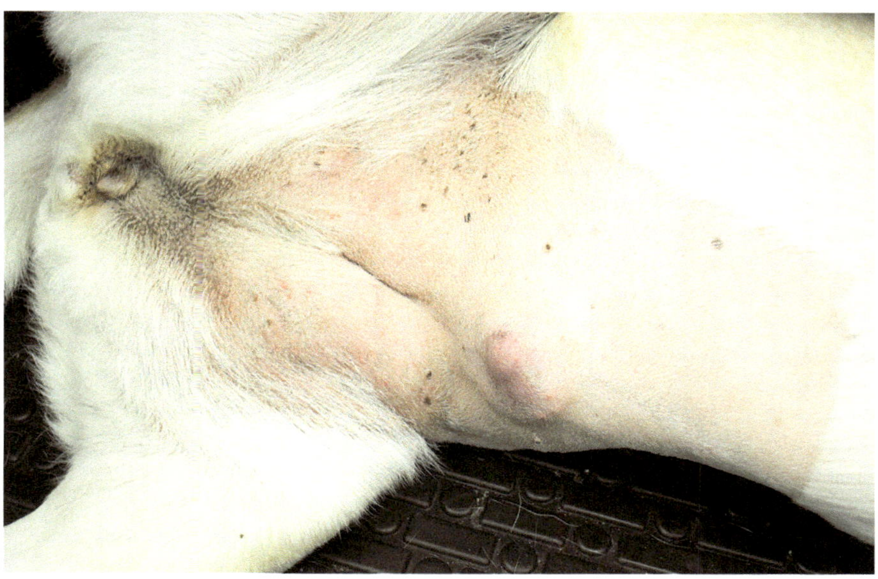

Figure 6. Patient with a mass in the abdominal wall as a result of the dissemination of a transitional cell carcinoma where fine needle aspiration and cytology were performed.

therapy are much better tolerated than they were in the past when the first treatments in this area were administered.

Chemotherapy, cyclooxygenase (COX) inhibitors, and combinations with other antineoplastic agents are the basis of TCC treatment in dogs. Remission rates are typically less than 20% with single drug treatment (NSAIDs or chemotherapy) and 35 to 50% with chemotherapy combined with a COX inhibitor. Platinum derived agents appear to be the most active in dogs with TCC, especially when combined with a COX inhibitor, although combinations of cisplatin and piroxicam should be avoided due to a high rate of renal failure. Some of the other chemotherapy medications most commonly used as single agents include mitoxantrone, chlorambucil, doxorubicin, and vinblastine.

Median survival time in dogs with TCC is 130 to 195 days after treatment with a single agent and more than 250 days with combination treatment. Current recommendations for treatments with single agents consist of a non-selective COX inhibitor such as piroxicam (0.3 mg/kg PO once daily) or a more selective COX-2 inhibitor such as deracoxib or firocoxib. In the case of combination therapy with a COX inhibitor and a chemotherapeutic, the response should be evaluated to determine whether treatment should be continued.

In feline patients, surgery should be considered, because the masses are usually located in the cranial bladder. The use of COX inhibitors (piroxicam and meloxicam), alone or in combination with chemotherapy, may play a role in the palliative treatment of bladder TCCs in cats. The survival times described range from 261 to 311 days.

In vitro studies suggest that radiation therapy protocols using higher doses of radiation with reduced fractionation may be more effective for the treatment of TCCs. **Stereotactic radiosurgery (SRS)**, which consists of the administration of a very high dose to clearly delimit the tissue to be irradiated, has led to the possibility of treating TCC with curative intent, with a very low risk of damaging the normal surrounding tissues. The advantage of this technique is that it is non-invasive, urinary continence is

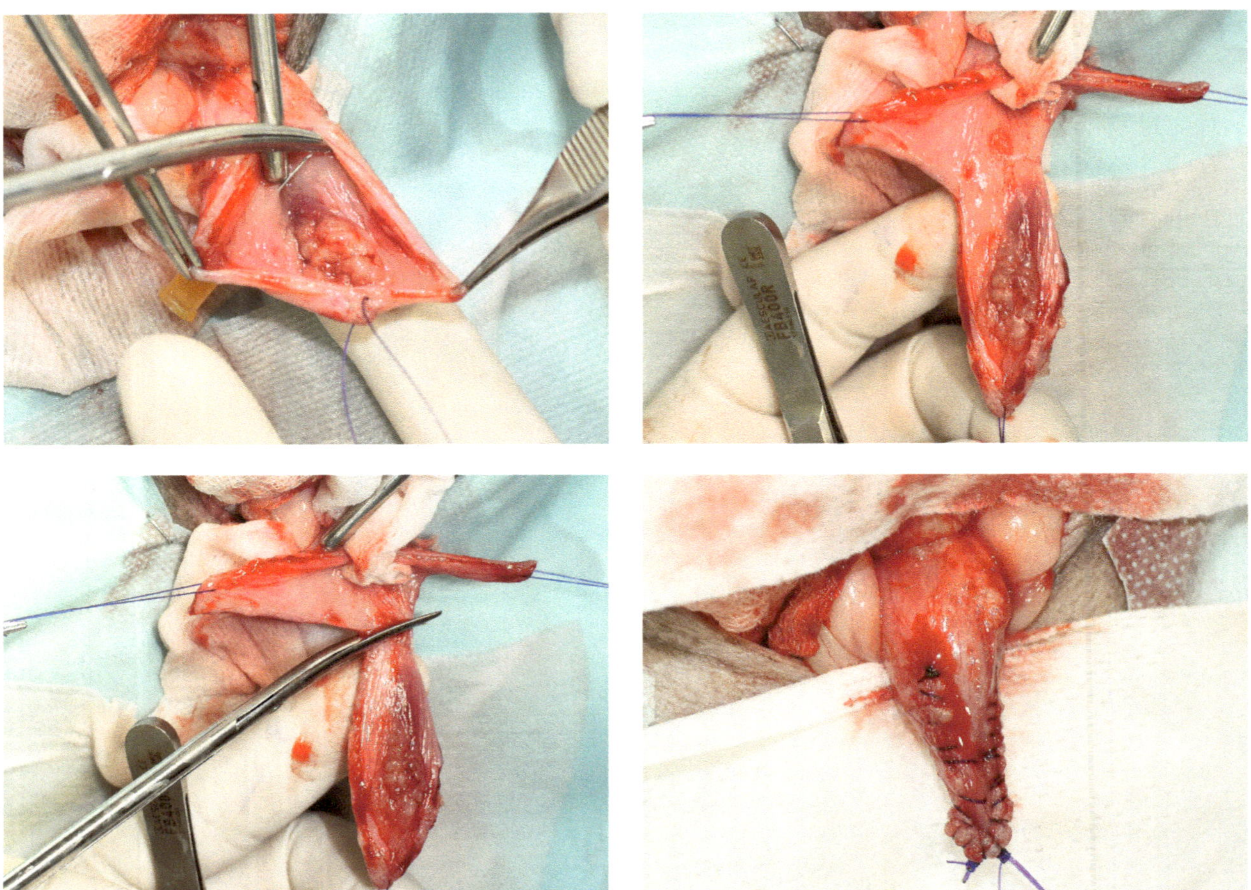

Figure 7. Surgery of bladder tumours is usually reserved for cases where the mass is located cranially, as shown in the image, and is tolerated quite well with mild transitory postsurgical incontinence. (Images courtesy of Manuel Jiménez Peláez).

usually maintained, and local tumour control is excellent. Disadvantages are related to the cost and availability of radiation facilities that are capable of administering SRS (Figure 8).

Most dogs with TCC die from obstructive disease and secondary complications before the development of metastatic disease. Several surgical techniques have been described in order to alleviate the symptoms caused by these obstructions. Ureterocolonic anastomosis is not recommended, as it is associated with neurological disorders and gastrointestinal complications secondary to hyperammonaemia, metabolic acidosis, uraemia, and chronic pyelonephritis. Other techniques have shown better results, including total cystectomy, in which the bladder neck and trigone are removed.

In cases of neoplasms limited to the urethra, vaginourethroplasty and/or transurethral resection may be performed. Cystostomy tubes also serve to relieve obstructions and are usually better tolerated; they allow an average survival time of three months from the time of obstruction. The techniques described for placement of the tubes are a traditional open technique or a minimally invasive approach to the abdomen, using laparoscopy or fluoroscopy. Another palliative option is the placement of a urethral stent using interventional radiology, although this can lead to urinary incontinence, which affects 26% of dogs. Despite this, urethral stents are well tolerated and resolve urinary tract obstructions in 97% of cases. Despite the good short term resolution rate of obstruction (97%), this technique is still considered palliative with short survival times if not combined with other therapies. Another option that may play a role in the palliative treatment of urinary tract obstructions is endoscopic ultrasound-guided carbon dioxide laser ablation, which is performed to reduce the volume of and potentially eliminate obstructive TCC lesions.

PROSTATE

Prostate tumours are **rare in cats and uncommon in dogs, with a prevalence of less than 1%**. The mean age at diagnosis is ten years old, with an increased risk in neutered dogs and certain breeds (Shetland Sheepdog and Scottish Terrier). Other prostate conditions that should be included in possible differential diagnoses include chronic prostatitis, prostatic abscesses, benign prostatic hyperplasia (BPH), and prostatic cysts, which are all more common in entire male dogs.

Due to rapid growth and high metastatic potential (up to 80% in postmortem studies) dogs may initially present due to clinical signs caused by the presence of metastases (weight loss, hindlimb lameness, pain, or neurological signs) rather than those of a primary urogenital disease (stranguria, haematuria, pollakiuria). Bone metastases occur in up to 40% of patients and can cause clinical signs such as pain, gait disturbances, or limping. Other clinical signs include those related to local obstruction due to an enlarged prostate or locoregional lymph nodes (dyschezia, tenesmus, constipation, flat shaped stools).

Diagnosis

The initial diagnostic evaluation should **begin with a rectal exam**. A neoplastic prostate is usually asymmetrical, fixed, firm in consistency, and can be painful. Careful rectal palpation is needed to detect lymphadenopathy of the nodes in the sacral region.

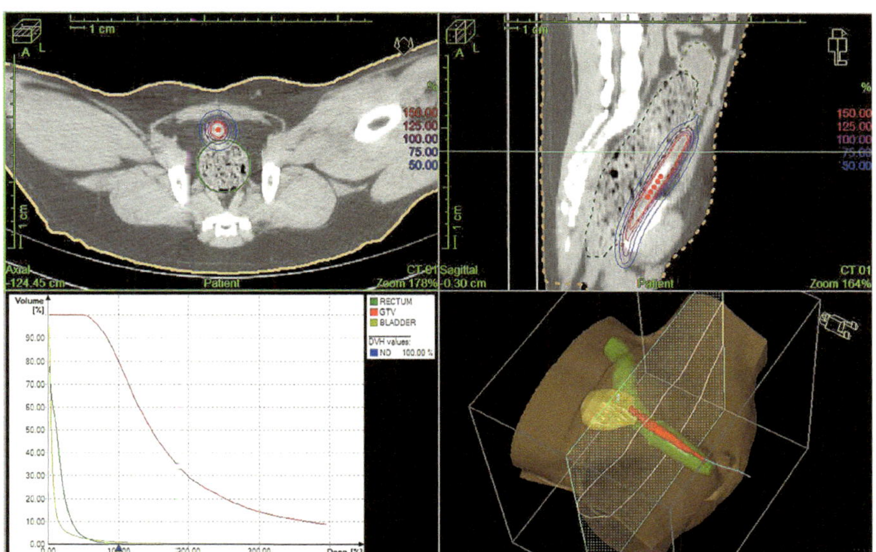

Figure 8. Images of a patient with transitional cell carcinoma treated with radiotherapy. The red colour (GTV) indicates the tumoural area of the urethra irradiated with the highest dose. The areas marked in green and yellow receive a lower dose as they are anatomically healthy areas. Radiotherapy has become an indispensable part of the treatment of this disease and that which offers the most promising future.

Complete blood count and biochemistry may show regenerative anaemia, leucocytosis, azotaemia due to potential obstructive disease, and hypercalcaemia. Urinalysis usually detects bacteriuria due to the high rate of secondary bacterial infections in these patients. Neoplastic cells can be seen in the urine sediment, although differentiation between reactive and neoplastic epithelial cells may not be possible.

Due to the high percentage of cases with distant metastases at diagnosis, **three radiographic views are recommended. Ultrasound is preferred over abdominal radiography** to determine the presence of locoregional metastasis in the lymph nodes (sublumbar), bladder/ureteral involvement, as well as involvement of other intra-abdominal organs. The finding of prostate mineralisation on abdominal radiographs or ultrasound is not pathognomonic of prostate carcinoma, since other benign processes can present in a similar way, however this finding in neutered male dogs is highly suggestive of neoplasia.

Bone metastasis can occur in any bone, although the lumbar vertebrae are most often affected, followed by the pelvis and femur. In radiographs, lesions have a lytic appearance and present as proliferative or mixed lesions. Performing more advanced imaging tests such as CT can help in the early detection of metastatic lesions due to this pathology.

Histological examination remains the definitive technique for the diagnosis of the disease, but a definitive diagnosis of prostate neoplasm can sometimes be made from cytology samples. Samples for cytological examination are usually obtained by traumatic catheterisation, cytological analysis of prostate washes, or ultrasound-guided puncture. Cytological sampling or histopathological analysis of any other lesions suspected of being metastases (lymph nodes or bone) may aid in diagnosis and staging of the disease. Ultrasound-guided aspirates or biopsies should be performed with caution due to the possibility of spreading the tumour with these procedures, although this has only been described in one case within the literature consulted (Figure 9).

Although secondary infections and inflammation are common, the diagnostic correlation between cytology and histopathology is very high in these cases. Adenocarcinoma is the most common type of tumour, followed by TCC. Immunohistochemistry can be performed to define the source cell more accurately. However, canine prostate carcinomas express markers of both urothelial and ductal origin, so differentiation between adenocarcinoma and TCC is complicated. Several histological subtypes have been described without appearing to be associated with prognosis.

Treatment

Overall prognosis is poor because most dogs with prostate cancer are diagnosed with advanced disease. Therapy is largely considered palliative and focuses on the control of local and remote metastatic disease.

Several surgical techniques have been described to try to achieve local control, although all have historically been associated with high morbidity and poor results (less than 3–4 months survival time), except in cases where the masses are relatively well defined and there are no metastases present, in which case total prostatectomies can be attempted.

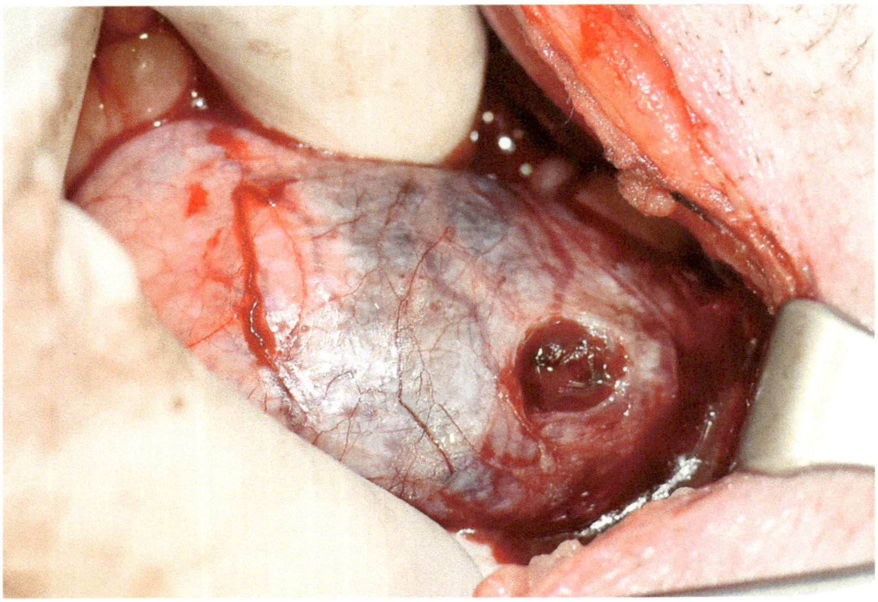

Figure 9. Image of a prostatic tumour where a sample has been taken via incisional biopsy during an exploratory laparotomy.

In dogs with early-stage disease subtotal intracapsular prostatectomy is an option which can lead to immediate relief of local clinical signs and is associated with a lower rate of postoperative complications than total prostatectomy.

Urethral obstructions can be managed as previously described, using palliative stents that relieve obstruction, with incontinence as one of the major complications. The best results with stent placement have been seen in obstructions of the prostatic urethra.

There is no consensus on the choice of medical therapy for prostate carcinomas although most include a COX-2 inhibitor in the combination used since studies have found the use of piroxicam or carprofen increased survival in a population of patients treated with and without chemotherapy, such as with mitoxantrone, providing several months of survival. The first results of radiation therapy in the treatment of prostate cancer seem promising, but the actual impact on the survival of these patients is unknown. In general, the prognosis of patients with prostate neoplasia is reserved to poor.

Penile, Scrotum, and Prepuce Tumours

Most penile tumours are of soft tissue origin and do not originate in the os penis, as is the case of transmissible venereal tumour (TVT), which is the most common presentation especially in countries with warm climates and stray dogs. There are tumours that occasionally originate in the os penis, such as ossifying fibroids, chondrosarcomas, osteosarcomas, or multilobular osteochondrosarcomas. The prepuce and scrotum can be affected by any skin tumour that affects the skin, such as mast cell tumours, squamous cell carcinoma etc.

Diagnosis and Treatment

The initial set of tests before surgery should include a complete blood count, biochemistry, and urinalysis, as well as evaluation of regional lymph nodes (palpation, FNA, or biopsy, and ultrasound).

General recommendations for the treatment of penile tumours depend on the location of the tumour and may require partial penile amputation or complete ablation of the external genitalia with scrotal urethrostomy.

Scrotal and preputial mast cell tumours are associated with a worse prognosis compared to other locations and require a multimodal approach including local (surgery/radiation therapy) and systemic (chemotherapy/tyrosine kinase inhibitors) treatment.

TVTs rarely metastasise and are easily diagnosed by cytology. They are curable with vincristine (0.5–0.7 mg/m^2 weekly IV) and the reduction of lesions is gradual with complete remission in 90% of treated cases, with administration between 2 to 8 doses. Treatment should be continued for 1 to 2 doses beyond the complete visible resolution of the lesion. Vincristine resistant lesions can be successfully treated with doxorubicin and radiation therapy.

Testicles

Testicular tumours (Figure 10) are the **second most frequent type of tumour in the uncastrated male dog** and mainly affect middle to old aged dogs (ten years old on average). The three major histological types include interstitial cell tumour, also called Leydig cell tumour, seminoma, and Sertoli cell tumour.

Historically, the rate of occurrence had been considered to be similar among the three histological types, although more recent studies show a lower prevalence of Sertoli cell tumours. Cryptorchid dogs have an increased risk of developing Sertoli cell tumours or seminomas, but not interstitial cell tumours. Cryptorchid patients tend to develop tumours in the right testicle, and this is more common in inguinal cryptorchid patients, compared to those with testicles in an abdominal location, as well as being younger than non-cryptorchid patients affected by the same tumour type. Approximately 25 to 50% of Sertoli cell tumours are functional and can cause hyperoestrogenaemia. Sertoli cell tumours are also the most likely type to metastasise, usually to regional lymph nodes, although this is relatively uncommon, at a rate of around 2 to 14%.

Diagnosis

Although the **majority of testicular tumours are found coincidentally on physical examination**, clinical signs may include decreased libido, signs of prostatomegaly (stranguria, tenesmus), and lack of appetite and/or weakness secondary to anaemia. Asymmetrical testicles, scrotal or inguinal swelling may be noted on palpation as well as signs of prostatomegaly, or signs of hyperoestrogenism including alopecia, gynecomastia, prepucial sagging, and poor coat quality.

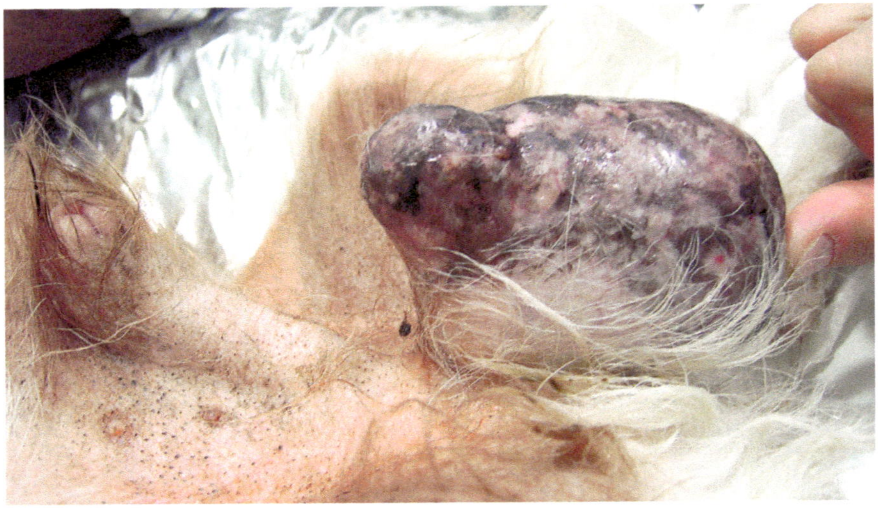

Figure 10. Macroscopic image of a testicular tumour.

Both testicles should be palpated simultaneously to compare size, shape, and firmness. Up to 20% of patients may have more than one type of testicular tumour. A rectal examination should be performed in these dogs, as prostatomegaly secondary to oestrogen induced squamous metaplasia is common.

Previous testing in these patients should include a complete blood count, abdominal ultrasound to assess regional lymphadenopathies and to detect or locate the cryptorchid testicle, as well as thoracic radiographs.

Histopathology is necessary for a final diagnosis, although a diagnosis may be obtained in some cases prior to surgery through FNA and cytology. In addition, testicular ultrasound and the vascularisation characteristics of these tumours can help to indicate the histological type.

Bone marrow suppression is a rare but well documented complication in cases of hyperoestrogenism. This syndrome is initially characterised by thrombocytopaenia and neutrophilic leucocytosis, which ultimately progresses to pancytopaenia.

Treatment

Bilateral orchiectomy with scrotal ablation is the surgical technique of choice and is curative in most cases in which there is only localised disease. If lymph node metastasis is suspected, an excisional biopsy of the enlarged nodes should be performed for confirmation.

Cisplatin has shown relative efficacy in a small number of dogs with metastatic disease. Radiation therapy has also been used to treat metastasis in the sublumbar lymph nodes in dogs with seminomas, which are tumours that overexpress KIT and VEGF receptors both in human and in veterinary medicine, so they are considered a model for comparative oncology.

Tumour response has been described in cases in human medicine, as well as in some isolated cases in veterinary medicine with the use of tyrosine kinase inhibitors such as toceranib phosphate, results that need to be supported in studies with a greater number of cases.

If oestrogen induced myelosuppression has occurred, the prognosis is reserved as aggressive supportive therapy is needed to treat marrow disorders for months with antibiotics, among other drugs.

Vagina and Vulva

Vaginal and vulvar tumours most commonly affect **entire geriatric nulliparous** bitches and are a **rare finding in felines**.

Most are benign smooth muscle tumours and leiomyoma is the predominant histological type. Polyps or fibroids are also relatively common in histopathological reports. Other benign tumours have been described in this area including lipomas and haemangiomas, some of which may be associated with vaginal bleeding. **The most common malignant tumour is leiomyosarcoma**, but other malignant tumours that originate in the lips of the vulva (melanoma, TVT, mast cell tumour) have been described. Other less common tumours in the area are adenocarcinoma that affects the clitoris or the extension of urethral tumours to the urethral papilla.

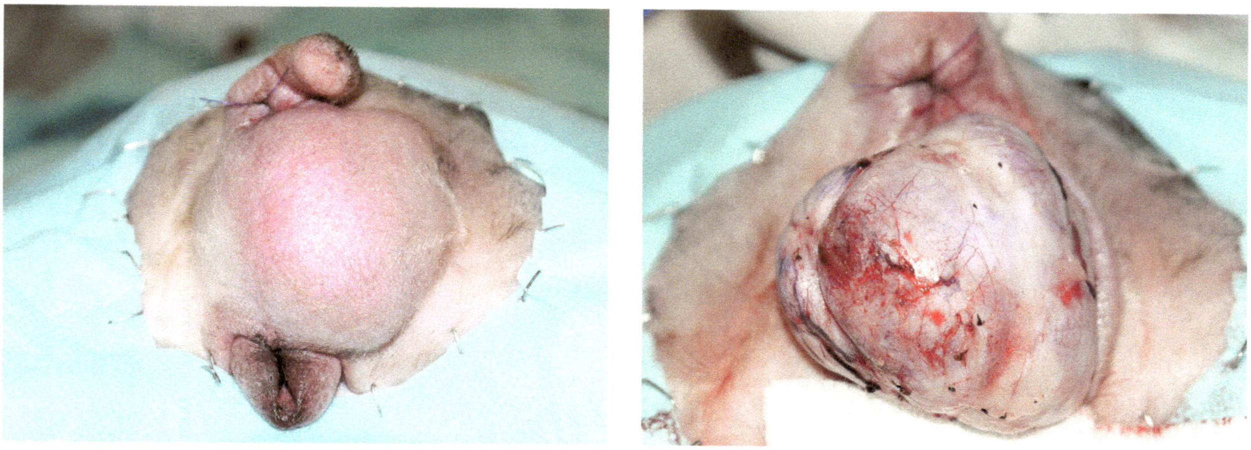

Figure 11. Images of an extraluminal vaginal tumour which can be seen as a mass in the ventral perineal region. (Images courtesy of Manuel Jiménez Peláez).

Tumours may be intraluminal or extraluminal (Figure 11).

- **Intraluminal tumours** are often associated with stranguria; owners can see the mass protruding during urination or defaecation. These are often solitary, several centimetres in diameter, and are usually pedicled. Other possible clinical signs include bleeding, secretions, dysuria, and licking the vulva.
- **Extraluminal tumours** are slow growing perineal masses.

Diagnosis

The initial diagnostic evaluation should include **vaginal and rectal palpation and a vaginoscopic examination**. Fine needle aspiration of the mass may aid in diagnosis, although **histopathological analysis is usually required for definitive diagnosis**. Thoracic radiographs and abdominal ultrasound should be considered to evaluate lymph node involvement in cases of non-pedunculated masses.

Diagnosis of pedunculated intraluminal tumours usually requires excisional biopsy by resection of the peduncle; local recurrence is very rare.

Treatment

For hormone sensitive tumours, ovariohysterectomy (OH) performed at the time of tumour removal reduces the risk of recurrence and is generally curative.

Unlike benign tumours, malignant vaginal masses usually have a broad base, which infiltrates the tissue, so they often require more extensive surgical resection. The use of simple episiotomies, a ventral laparotomy, or a combination of laparotomy, episiotomy, and osteotomy/ostectomy of the pubis have been described.

Recently, a subtotal vaginectomy technique has been described to treat invasive benign and malignant vaginal neoplasms or extensive vaginal disease with few complications and good results.

Radiation therapy and/or chemotherapy may be considered in the few cases which are malignant. According to the results obtained in a small study, the prognosis in cats with vulvar adenocarcinoma seems to be poor, since most of the patients were euthanised for progressive local disease or recurrence.

Uterus

Tumours of the uterus, including the horn, body, and cervix, are **relatively rare in dogs and cats**.

Mesenchymal tumours make up the vast majority of uterine tumours, with canine leiomyomas accounting for 85 to 90% and leiomyosarcomas accounting for 10% of all tumours, while fibroadenomas, lipomas, adenocarcinomas, lymphomas, and mast cell tumours are described less frequently. Neutered females may develop tumours that originate from the uterine stump.

Adenocarcinoma is the most common uterine tumour in cats and affects middle aged to geriatric patients, with some isolated cases described in animals younger than one year of age. German Shepherd bitches can develop a syndrome with an inherited component characterised by the presence of renal cystoadenocarcinomas, nodular and uterine dermatofibrosis associated with leiomyomas.

Most canine uterine tumours are slow growing, non-invasive and, while in the case of dogs they are not usually metastatic, in cats they are usually associated with aggressive biological behaviour and frequent metastases.

Diagnosis

In the dog, uterine tumours are rarely associated with clinical signs, although they may occur at diagnosis with signs associated with uterine enlargement with abdominal distension, vaginal discharge, and clinical urinary signs. Feline patients may also have signs related to metastatic disease.

Although abnormalities are not usually detected, chest radiographs and blood tests should be performed at initial evaluation. Abdominal radiographs may confirm the presence of a soft tissue mass in the caudal area of the abdomen, although ultrasound is more specific and precise at determining the origin of the mass (uterine body or cervical tumours). The use of CT can help plan surgeries in more complex cases.

The ultrasound appearance of uterine tumours in bitches is variable and the only way to obtain a definitive diagnosis of a uterine tumour is usually through **histopathological examination of surgically obtained samples**.

Treatment

OH, along with complete removal of the mass, is often curative for canine patients, but due to the aggressive biological behaviour in the cat it is unlikely to provide long term disease control, with a reserved prognosis if only OH is performed (Figure 12).

The effectiveness of chemotherapy in dogs and cats with these types of tumours is unknown.

Ovaries

Ovarian neoplasms are rare, probably because a large portion of the canine population in most countries is neutered at an early age. The incidence in unneutered females is 6.25% and tumours are mainly seen in bitches aged between ten and twelve years.

Ovarian tumours that do not cause clinical signs are most commonly found during routine OH in older animals. In this situation, a possible differential diagnosis which should be considered are ovarian cysts, which may have a similar macroscopic appearance. However, because some ovarian tumours are malignant, **any ovaries with an abnormal macroscopic appearance should be sent for histological examination**.

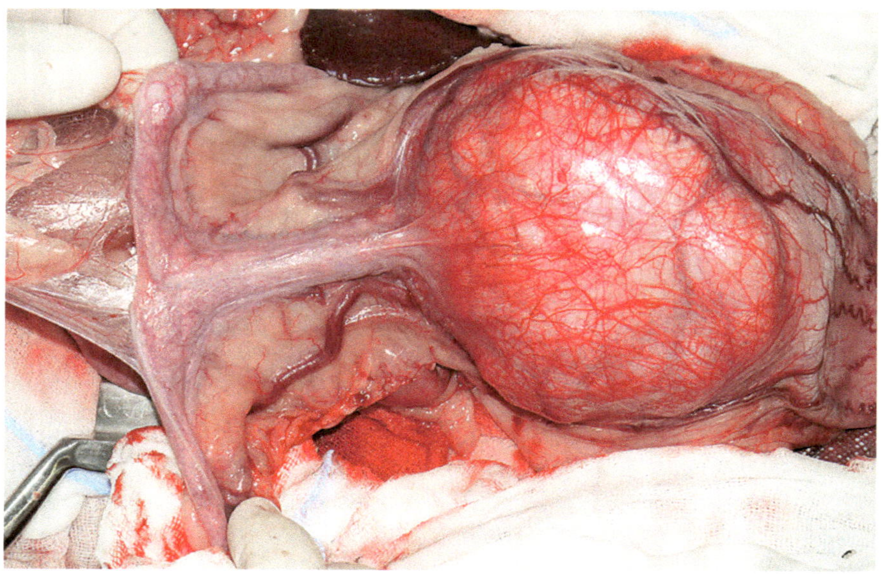

Figure 12. Image of a large sized uterine leiomyosarcoma found during a laparotomy which was removed during ovariohysterectomy.

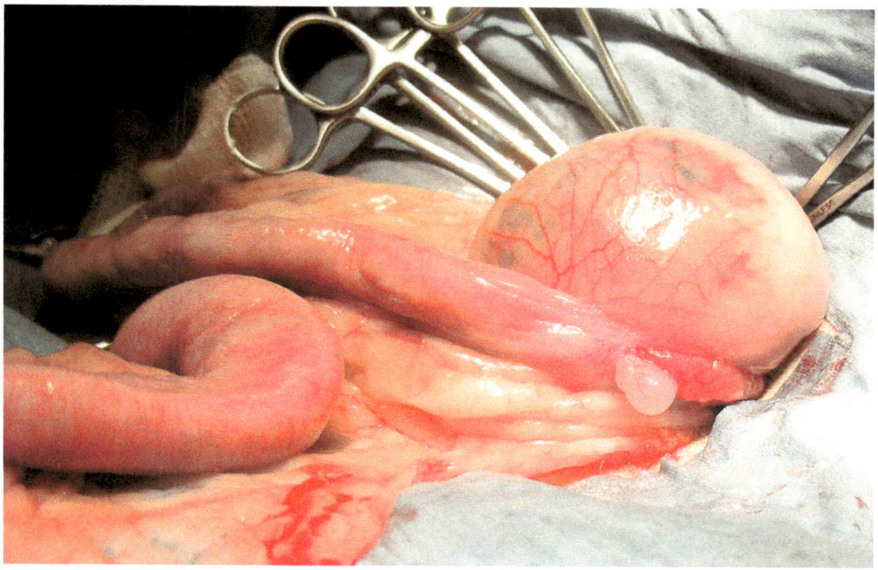

Figure 13. Image of a unilateral epithelial ovarian tumour without the presence of metastasis or local dissemination, removed via ovariohysterectomy.

Diagnosis

More specific clinical signs associated with ovarian tumours include a palpable mass, signs of ascites, or systemic effects due to hormone production. These tumours may be of considerable size before they are detected.

Ovarian tumours are classified according to the human WHO classification:

- epithelial tumours originating in the Müllerian ducts
- stromal tumours of the sex cord
- germ-cell tumours
- mesenchymal tumours.

Most are spermatic cord stroma or epithelial tumours, accounting for 80–90% of ovarian tumours. Malignant forms can metastasise to the peritoneum and can cause malignant abdominal effusion; these metastases can also be seen in the lymph nodes, liver, and lungs. Types of feline ovarian tumours are similar to canine ones, with the exception of mesenchymal types, which have not been described to date.

In the dog, 80–90% of ovarian tumours are epithelial and include histological diagnoses of papillary adenoma, cystadenoma, papillary adenocarcinoma, and undifferentiated adenocarcinoma. These tumours are typically unilateral, rarely bilateral, usually non-functional, and have a metastasis rate of approximately 50%. Epithelial tumours are rare in cats (Figure 13).

Germ-cell tumours originate from primary ovarian cells and include dysgerminomas, teratomas, and malignant teratomas (teratocarcinomas) and account for approximately 10% of ovarian tumours in dogs. Dysgerminomas (ovarian seminomas) are derived from undifferentiated germ cells, are usually unilateral and the metastasis rate described is low (10 to 30%). Teratomas consist of more than one layer of germ cells (ectoderm, mesoderm, and/or endoderm) and most are well differentiated. Teratocarcinomas have differentiated and undifferentiated components with metastases in up to 50% of cases. Approximately 15% of ovarian tumours in cats are dysgerminomas with a rate of metastasis similar to that recorded in bitches.

Granulosa cell tumour is the most common stromal tumour and the only tumour in this category that can metastasise, followed by less common histological types, such as Sertoli Leydig tumours, thecomas, and luteomas. Occasionally the presentation is bilateral, and they are functional in approximately 50% of cases, with a metastasis rate of less than 20%. These tumours can produce oestrogen and progesterone with clinical signs related to oestrogenic effects, such as enlargement of the vulva, vaginal discharge, and cystic endometrial hyperplasia. In cats, stromal tumours of the sex cords constitute approximately 50% of ovarian tumours and more than 50% of ovarian tumours are malignant. The most frequent histological type in feline patients are granulosa cell tumours, which are usually associated with hyperoestrogenism.

The incidence of neoplasms in residual ovarian tissue in bitches is higher (26.3%) than in intact ovaries, with an incidence of approximately 6%. In one study, all tumours except one cystadenoma were granulosa cell tumours.

The initial diagnostic evaluation in dogs and cats with ovarian tumours should include **thoracic radiographs and abdominal**

ultrasound. If ascites is present, cytological examination of the fluid may be very helpful in detecting whether the effusion is malignant. There is a good correlation between diagnosis by ultrasound-guided FNA and histopathology in a small number of cases, but this technique is generally not recommended due to the risk of tumour seeding and spread, especially in malignant cystic tumours if they are disturbed. Ultrasound characteristics of canine ovarian tumours have also been described, and can present with a solid to cystic appearance. Concomitant changes in the uterus, consistent with cystic endometrial hyperplasia or pyometra, are often detected.

Treatment

Treatment of ovarian tumours is mainly **based on performing an OH** and generally involves a good prognosis.

The role of conventional therapies such as chemotherapy or radiation therapy has not been sufficiently investigated. In cases of peritoneal metastases or malignant abdominal effusion, intracavitary chemotherapy with platinum derived compounds may be useful, as well as the implantation of abdominal ports that facilitate the administration of these drugs.

Mammary Gland

Mammary gland tumours are the most common **tumours in entire bitches and the third most common tumour in cats**. Their incidence varies greatly from country to country depending on neutering policies. Older females of either species are more likely to develop these tumours and the breeds most at risk include Siamese cats, Poodles, English Cocker Spaniel, Breton Spaniel, English Setter, Fox Terrier, and the Boston Terrier.

Ovarian hormone exposure during the first two years of life is a well-known risk factor for the development of these tumours, while **OH considerably decreases the risk in both species**.

- Occurrence in **dogs neutered** before their first oestrus is 0.5%. After the first oestrus the risk increases to 8% and after the second oestrus it reaches 26%. After the third oestrous cycle, OH provides only modest protection, although recent studies show a decrease in the risk of developing new tumours if performed at the same time as the removal of the tumour, suggesting a continuous effect of the hormones during the lifetime of the bitch.
- Neutering before the first oestrus in **feline patients** offers a risk reduction of up to 91%, before the second oestrus of 86% and before the third oestrus of 11%. After two years of age, there is no benefit to surgery.

Exogenous hormone exposure also increases the risk of tumour development, although they are usually benign. Oestrogen and progesterone receptors have been identified in dogs and cats with mammary tumours. Although hormonal aetiology is common, in both species male dogs and cats can develop mammary tumours that are commonly benign in canine patients, while in male cats they behave as aggressively as in females.

Diagnosis

On physical examination, animals may have **single or multiple nodules associated with the nipple or gland itself**. Benign lesions tend to be small, well defined, and firm on palpation. Caudal mammary glands are the most frequently affected in dogs and feline tumours occur with the same frequency in all glands. Mammary tumours can be mobile, attached to the skin or abdominal wall, and also become ulcerated, inflamed and oedematous, or be associated with nipple discharge. The differentials that must be considered in any mammary mass include other neoplasms (mast cell carcinoma, squamous cell carcinoma), mastitis, lobular hyperplasia and fibroepithelial hyperplasia in the case of cats.

The initial diagnostic evaluation of animals with mammary neoplasms should include a complete blood count, biochemistry profile and urinalysis. **Histopathological examination**, usually through excisional biopsy of the mass, is considered the test of choice for the diagnosis of mammary tumours. FNA and cytological evaluation of the mass may be performed which may help to distinguish benign from malignant lesions, but does not eliminate the need for histopathology because it may underestimate the malignant potential of the tumour. Cytology is more useful to rule out other differentials, for detection of locoregional nodal metastases and in cases in which spread to the skin and neoplastic emboli within the dermal lymphatic vessels are suspected (mammary tumours which have spread to the skin or inflammatory carcinomas (IC)).

Metastatic spread of malignant mammary tumours occurs through the lymph vessels to the regional lymph nodes or via the blood, and the lungs are the most frequent site of distant metastasis. Although cytology may be helpful, a histopathological evaluation of the lymph nodes is required to definitively diagnose metastases/micrometastases.

Thoracic radiographs are important for assessing the presence of metastatic lung disease or pleural effusion (common in cats). Abdominal ultrasound should be recommended in cases where a complete staging is required, in order to evaluate possible locoregional extension (superficial inguinal, axillary lymph nodes) or metastatic intra-abdominal lymphadenopathy, especially in cases where mammary tumours are located in the caudal mammary glands. **Suspicions of metastasis found on ultrasound should preferably be confirmed by FNA and cytological analysis**. Several studies have been described evaluating the usefulness of ultrasound in these masses to try to determine their biological behaviour, but the correlation with histopathological changes and the diagnosis of malignancy varies between studies.

In **bitches about 60% of mammary tumours are benign and** are most often fibroadenomas (benign mixed tumour). The most common types of malignant tumours in bitches are solid carcinomas, followed by tubular adenocarcinomas; only 3% are sarcomas and 1% are inflammatory carcinomas. Generally, 50% of malignant tumours will recur or metastasise.

Some of the prognostic factors associated with decreased survival times in female dogs with mammary tumours include histological type (poorly differentiated tumours, inflammatory sarcoma and carcinomas have a worse prognosis), tumour size greater than 3 cm, lymph node involvement, histological evidence of lymphatic or vascular invasion, previous neutering, primary tumour lymphocyte infiltration rate, ulceration, hormone receptor expression (oestrogens and progesterone), COX-2 expression, microvascular density, proliferation markers, clinical behaviour (growth pattern, fixation, ulceration), and the presence of distant metastases (Figure 14).

Most mammary tumours in cats are malignant (80–90%) **and the most frequent are adenocarcinomas** (Figure 15). ICs have also been described in feline patients: they are biologically aggressive with a high rate of metastasis, but survival times can vary significantly.

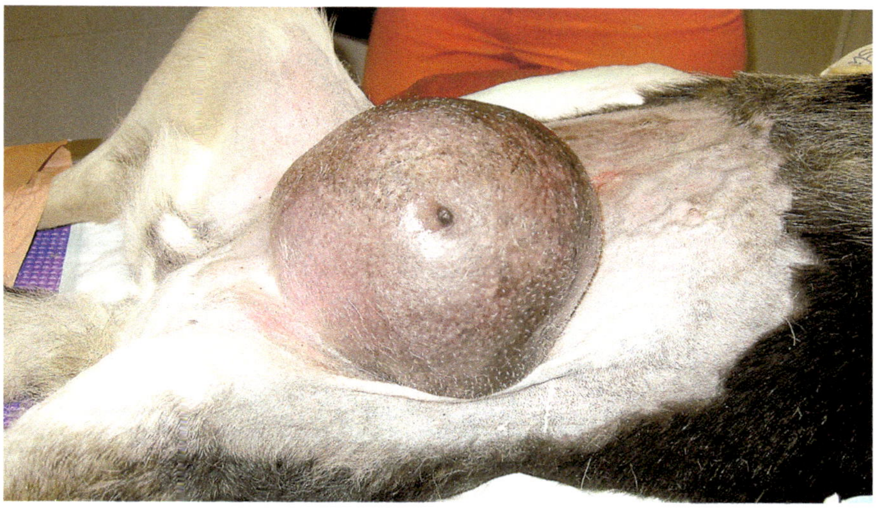

Figure 14. Image of a mammary tumour with the presence of various clinically recognised prognostic factors such as ulceration, invasion of adjacent tissues, size greater than 5 cm and locoregional lymphadenopathy, which means the biological behaviour of this tumour may potentially be more aggressive.

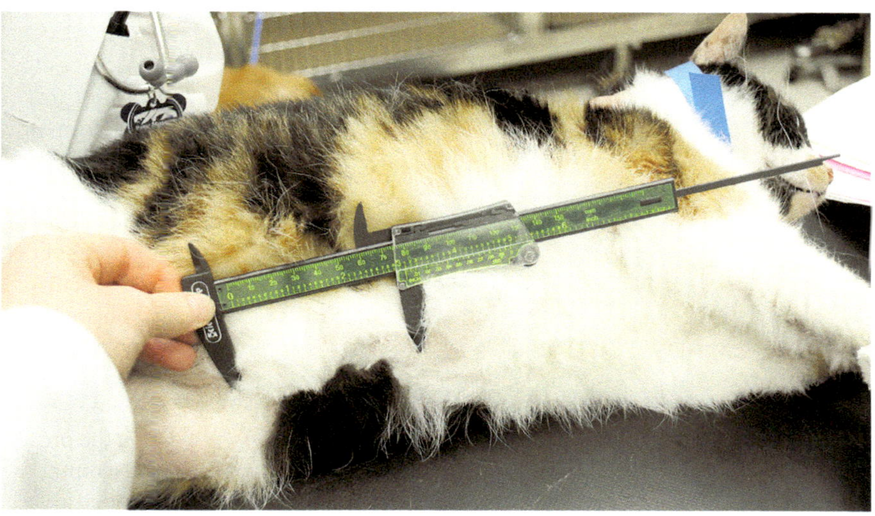

Figure 15. Presence of a mammary tumour in a feline patient measuring more than 3 cm which is a recognised negative prognostic factor in this species.

Tumour size, disease stage, histological grade, and extent of surgical intervention have been shown to influence prognosis. Large volume tumours, larger than 3 cm, have been associated with shorter survival times (4–12 months). The type of surgery performed and whether the resection is complete have been shown to be prognostic for disease-free time, but not for survival time.

Treatment

Surgery is the basis of treatment for mammary tumours in dogs and cats. One of the important contraindications when performing surgery is the diagnosis of IC since it is practically impossible to eliminate the entire tumour and recurrence can occur within a few days of surgery (Figure 16). In bitches with other types of mammary tumours, the goal of surgery is to remove the entire tumour using the simplest procedure possible. For example, a nodulectomy is acceptable for a small (<1 cm) superficial tumour, since most of them are benign, while lesions of 1 to 2 cm in diameter may require a simple mastectomy. If the masses are present in multiple glands, they can be removed individually or in a chain mastectomy, choosing the type of surgery based on the easiest way to remove all the affected tissue, when taking into account the lymphatic drainage of the affected glands. **OH should be recommended at the time of mastectomy** to prevent future pathologies in the ovary or uterus, as well as reduce the risk of developing new mammary tumours.

Prophylactic mastectomies of normal mammary glands could be considered to avoid the appearance of new mammary tumours, since bitches who undergo the removal of individual mammary tumours are likely to develop new tumours in the ipsilateral mammary chain in up to 60% of cases. **Most canine mammary tumours can be cured with surgery as the sole treatment**.

In cats, due to the possible connection between individual mammary glands and between the left and right sides, performing unilateral or bilateral complete mastectomies including the underlying fascia in a "block" surgery is recommended (Figure 17).

The extent of surgery makes a difference in disease-free and recurrence-free times, which are longer when more extensive surgery is performed. In cases where a bilateral mastectomy is performed, a minimum of two weeks between surgeries is recommended. The inguinal lymph node should always be removed in conjunction with the last caudal mammary gland, while the axillary lymph nodes should only be removed if they are enlarged. Radiation therapy is not routinely used to treat this disease in dogs or cats.

Despite how common this disease is, little information is available about the efficacy of chemotherapy in canine and feline patients with mammary tumours and most treatments are considered to be in an experimental phase, especially adjuvant treatments after surgery.

In dogs with malignant mammary tumours and with the presence of negative prognostic factors, locally advanced disease, the presence of metastases or with a histologically aggressive type, adjuvant treatments such as chemotherapy or antiangiogenic therapies are usually recommended. Several drugs have been used, as monotherapy or in combination, to combat the macroscopic presentation of the disease, with modest results and response rates of about 20–40%.

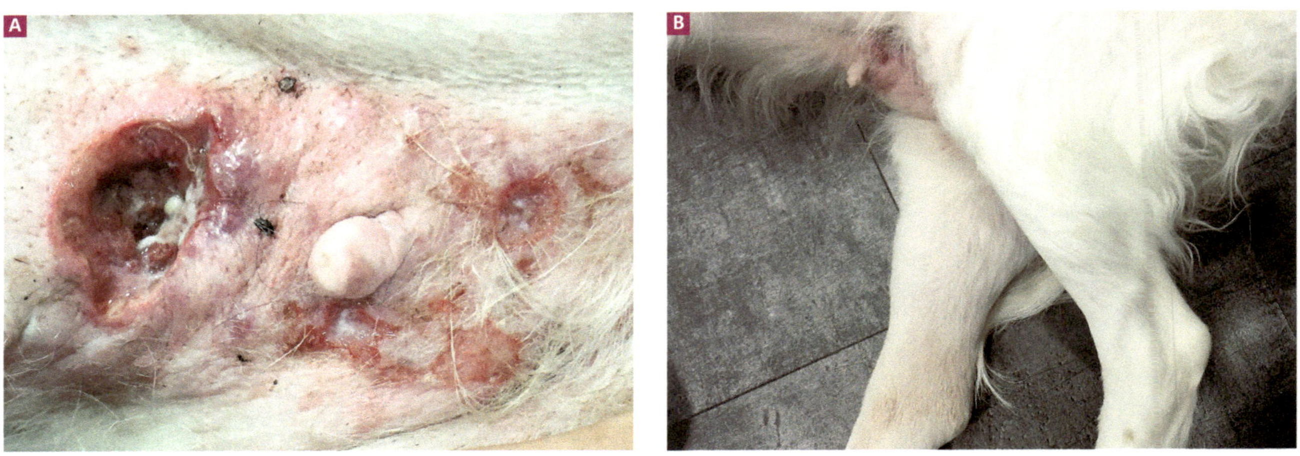

Figure 16. Images of an aggressive mammary tumour showing rapid progression (**A**) and lymphoedema of the ipsilateral limb to the affected mammary chain (**B**), corresponding with an inflammatory carcinoma.

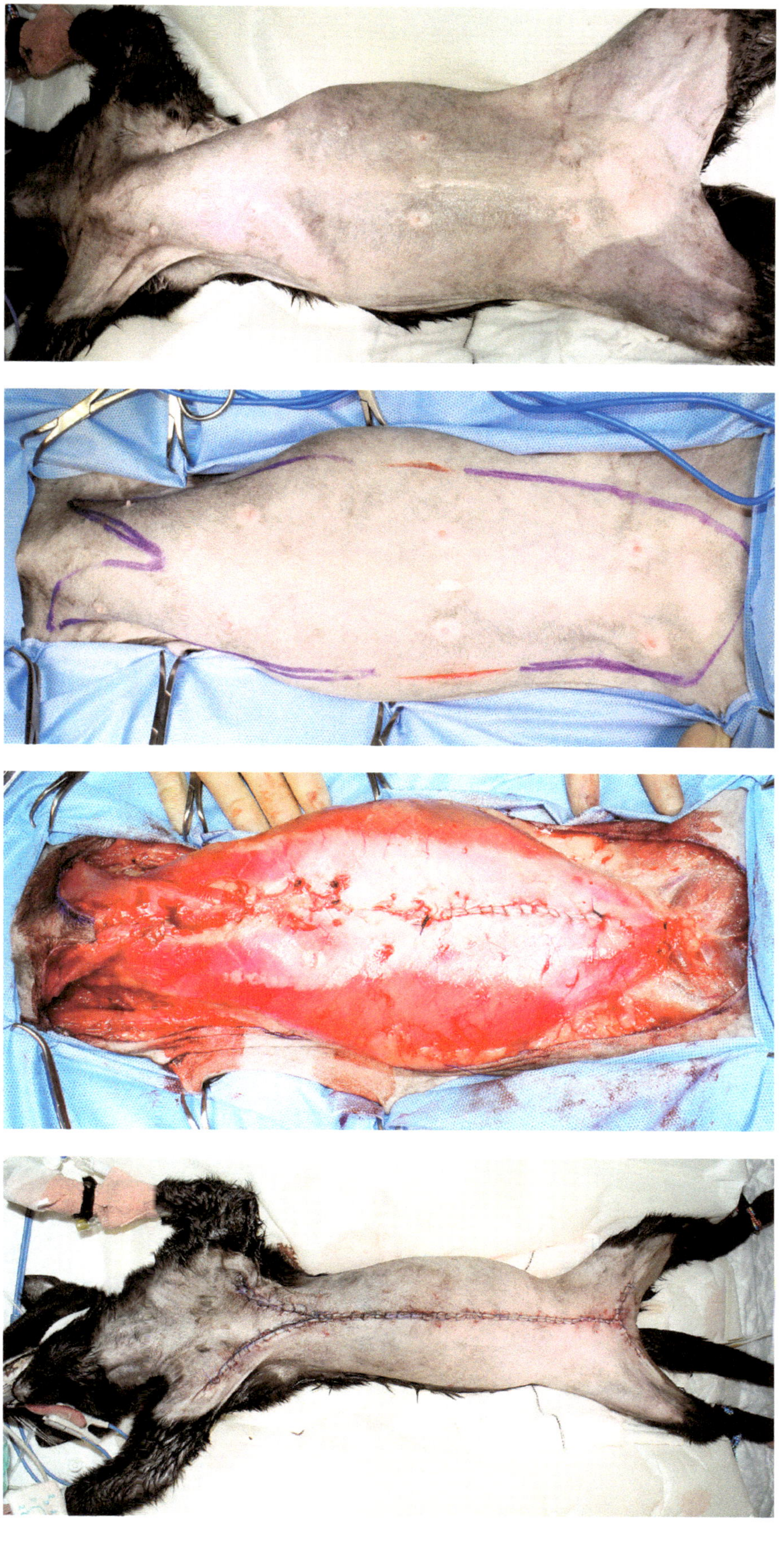

Figure 17. Complete bilateral mastectomy in a cat. In general, due to the communication between mammary glands in the same chain and even between chains, complete unilateral mastectomies are usually recommended. More recently it seems that complete bilateral mastectomies performed at once or in two procedures improve survival times in feline patients with mammary tumours. This is something which should be discussed with the owners before deciding what type of surgery to perform. (Images courtesy of Manuel Jiménez Peláez).

The most commonly used drugs are doxorubicin, carboplatin, mitoxantrone, 5-fluorouracil, or cyclophosphamide, although paclitaxel and thalidomide have also been used.

Unfortunately, there is little information available about their role in adjuvant treatment after surgery, with few published studies available, all of which look at a small number of cases. Overexpression of COX-2 has been demonstrated in malignant mammary tumours compared to benign or normal mammary tissues and is associated with a worse prognosis.

COX-2 inhibitors have only been described in the treatment of cases of IC as part of a multidrug treatment to improve quality of life that resulted in a higher survival rate over the chemotherapy only group. Additional studies in other canine mammary tumours are required before recommending the use of COX-2 inhibitors as an effective adjuvant therapy. One study showed that after administration of 1 mg/kg intravenous desmopressin 30 minutes before surgery and 24 hours after surgery, disease-free and surviva time was increased.

Antiangiogenic therapies with toceranib phosphate have shown efficacy in dogs and cats with mammary tumours in cases of macroscopic disease and their role in the treatment of mammary tumours should be evaluated. In feline patients, doxorubicin is usually used as an adjuvant treatment, although there are conflicting reports about its role in prolonging survival in these patients.

Bibliography

- Alonso-Diez Á., Ramos A., Roccabianca P. et al. (2019) Canine Spindle Cell Mammary Tumor: A Retrospective Study of 67 Cases. *Vet Pathol.* Jul;56(4):526–535.
- Anderson C.R., McNiel. E.A., Gillette E.L. et al. (2002) Late complications of pelvic irradiation in 16 dogs. *Vet Radiol Ultrasound.* 43(2):187–192.
- Armbrust L.J., Biller D.S., Hoskinson J.J. (2000) Compression radiography: an old technique revisited. *J Am Anim Hosp Assoc.* 36(6):537–541.
- Arnold E., Childress M., Fourez L. et al (2011) Clinical Trial of Vinblastine in Dogs with Transitional Cell Carcinoma of the Urinary Bladder. *J Vet Intern Med.* 25:1385–1390.
- Bacon N.J., Farese J.P., Lurie D. et al. (2010) Feasibility of stereotactic radiosurgery in the treatment of canine urethral transitional cell carcinoma. *Veterinary Cancer Society MidYear Meeting*, Las Vegas, NV, (abstr).
- Bearss J.J., Schulman F.Y., Carter D. (2012) Histologic, Immunohistochemical, and Clinical Features of 27 Mammary Tumors in 18 Male Dogs. *Vet Pathol.* 49(4):602–7.
- Bennett T.C., Matz B.M., Henderson R.A. et al. (2018) Total prostatectomy as a treatment for prostatic carcinoma in 25 dogs. *Vet Surg.* 47(3):367–377.
- Bertazzolo W., Dell'Orco M., Bonfanti U. et al. (2004) Cytological features of canine ovarian tumours: a retrospective study of 19 cases. *J Small Anim Pract.* 45(11):539–545.
- Best M.P., Frimberger A.E. (2015) Ovarian carcinomatosis in a dog managed with surgery and intraperitoneal, systemic, and intrapleural chemotherapy utilizing indwelling pleural access ports. *Can Vet J.* 58(5):493–497.
- Bigliardi E., Denti L., De Cesaris V. et al. (2019) Colour Doppler ultrasound imaging of blood flows variations in neoplastic and non-neoplastic testicular lesions in dogs. *Reprod Domest Anim.* 54(1):63–71.
- Blackburn A.L., Berent A.C., Weisse C.W. et al. (2013) Evaluation of outcome following urethral stent placement for the treatment of obstructive carcinoma of the urethra in dogs: 42 cases (2004–2008). *J Am Vet Med Assoc.* 242:59–68.
- Bommer N.X. Hayes A.M., Scase T.J. et al. (2012) Clinical features, survival times and COX-1 and COX-2 expression in cats with transitional cell carcinoma of the urinary bladder treated with meloxicam. *Journal of Feline Medicine and Surgery.* 14(8) 527–533.
- Bonsembiante F., Benali S.L., Trez D. et al. (2016) Histological and immunohistochemical characterization of feline renal cell carcinoma: a case series. *J Vet Med Sci.* 78(78):1039–1043.
- Boria P.A., Glickman N.W., Schmidt B.R. et al. (2005) Carboplatin and piroxicam therapy in 31 dogs with transitional cell carcinoma of the urinary bladder. *Vet Comp Oncol.* 3(2):73–80.
- Bradbury C.A., Westropp J.L., Pollard R.E. (2009) Relationship between prostatomegaly, prostatic mineralization, and cytologic diagnosis. *Vet Radiol Ultrasound.* 50(2):167–171. 11.
- Brown P.J., Evans H.K., Deen S. et al. (2012) Fibroepithelial Polyps of the Vagina in Bitches: a Histological and Immunohistochemical Study. *J. Comp. Path.* Vol. 147, 181e185
- Bryan J.N., Henry C.J., Turnquist S.E. et al. (2006) Primary renal neoplasia of dogs. *J Vet Intern Med.* (5):1155–1160.
- Bryan J.N., Keeler M.R., Henry C.J. et al. (2007) A population study of neutering status as a risk factor for canine prostate cancer. *Prostate.* 67(11):1174–1181.
- Burrow R.D., Gregory S.P., Giejda A.A. et al. (2011) Penile amputation and scrotal urethrostomy in 18 dogs. *Veterinary Record.* 169, 657.
- Cahalane A.K., Payne S., Barber L.G. et al. (2004) Prognostic factors for survival of dogs with inguinal and perineal mast cell tumors treated surgically with or without adjunctive treatment: 68 cases (1994–2002). *J Am Vet Med Assoc.* 225:401–408.
- Cave T.A., Hine R., Howie F. et al. (2002) Uterine carcinoma in a 10-month-old Golden Retriever. *J Small Anim Pract.* 43(3):133–135.
- Cerf D.J., Lindquist E.C. (2012) Palliative ultrasound-guided endoscopic diode laser ablation of transitional cell carcinomas of the lower urinary tract in dogs. *J Am Vet Med Assoc.* 240(1):51–60.
- Chang S.C., Chang C.C., Chang T.J. et al. (2005) Prognostic factors associated with survival two years after surgery in dogs with malignant mammary tumors: 79 cases (1998–2002). *J Am Vet Med Assoc.* 227(10):1625–1629.
- Childress M.O. et al. (2011) Results of biopsy via transurethral cystoscopy and cystotomy for diagnosis of transitional cell carcinoma of the urinary bladder and urethra in dogs: 92 cases (2003–2008). *J Am Vet Med Assoc.* 239(3):350–356.
- Chun R., Knapp D.W., Widmer W.R. et al. (1996) Cisplatin treatment of transitional cell carcinoma of the urinary bladder in dogs: 18 cases (1983–1993). *J Am Vet Med Assoc.* 209(9):1588–1591.
- Cornell K.K., Bostwick D.G., Cooley D.M. et al. (2000) Clinical and pathologic aspects of spontaneous canine prostate carcinoma: a retrospective analysis of 76 cases. *Prostate.* 45(2):173–183.
- Cunha S.C., Corgozinho K.B., Souza H.J. et al. (2015) Adjuvant chemotherapy with mitoxantrone for cats with mammary carcinomas treated with radical mastectomy. *J Feline Med Surg.* Dec;17(12):1000–4.
- Dagher E., Abadie J., Loussouarn D. et al. (2019) Feline Invasive Mammary Carcinomas: Prognostic Value of Histological Grading. *Vet Pathol.* 56(5):660–670.
- Dhaliwal R.S., Kitchell B.E., Knight B.L. et al. (1999) Treatment of aggressive testicular tumors in four dogs. *J Am Anim Hosp Assoc.* 35(4):311–318.
- DE Campos C.B., Lavalle G.E., Monteiro L.N. et al. (2018) Adjuvant Thalidomide and Metronomic Chemotherapy for the Treatment of Canine Malignant Mammary Gland Neoplasms. *In Vivo.* 32(32):1659–1666.
- De Campos C.B., Damasceno K.A., Gamba C.O. et al. (2016) Evaluation of prognostic factors and survival rates in malignant feline mammary gland neoplasms. *J Feline Med Surg.* 18(12):1003–1012.

■ Diez-Bru N., Garcia-Real I., Martinez E.M. et al. (1998) Ultrasonographic appearance of ovarian tumors in 10 dogs. *Vet Radiol Ultrasound*. 39(3):226–233.

■ Dos Anjos D.S., Vital A.F., Lainetti P.F. et al. (2019) Deregulation of VEGFR-2 and PDGFR Expression and Microvascular Density in a Triple-Negative Model of Canine Malignant Mammary Tumors with Lymph Node or Lung Metastasis. *Vet Sci*. 6(1):3.

■ Edmonson E.F., Hess A.M., Powers B.E. (2014) Prognostic Significance of Histologic Features in Canine Renal Cell Carcinomas: 70 Nephrectomies. *Vet Pathol*. 52(2), pp.260–268.

■ Feliciano M.A., Ramirez R.A., Maronezi M.C. et al. (2018) Accuracy of four ultrasonography techniques in predicting histopathological classification of canine mammary carcinomas. *Vet Radiol Ultrasound*. 59(4):444–452.

■ Feliciano M.A., Uscategui R.A., Maronezi M.C. et al. (2017) Ultrasonography methods for predicting malignancy in canine mammary tumors. *PLoS One*. 12(5):e0178143.

■ Gattino F., Maniscalco L., Iussich S. et al. (2018) PDGFR-, PDGFR-, VEGFR-2 and CD117 expression in canine mammary tumours and evaluation of the in vitro effects of toceranib phosphate in neoplastic mammary cell lines. *Vet Rec*. 18;183(7):221.

■ Gemignani F., Mayhew P.D., Giuffrida M.A. et al. (2018) Association of surgical approach with complication rate, progression-free survival time, and disease-specific survival time in cats with mammary adenocarcinoma: 107 cases (1991–2014). *J Am Vet Med Assoc*. 252(11):1393–1402.

■ Gilson S.D., Stone E.A. (1990) Surgically induced tumor seeding in eight dogs and two cats. *J Am Vet Med Assoc*. 196(11):1811–1815.

■ Glickman L.T., Schofer F.S., McKee L.J. et al. (1989) Epidemiologic study of insecticide exposures, obesity, and risk of bladder cancer in household dogs. *J Toxicol Environ Health*. 28(4):407–414.

■ Goldschmidt M., Pena L., Rasotto R. et al. (2011) Classification and grading of canine mammary tumors. *Vet Pathol*. 48:117–131.

■ Gómez A.S., Scase T.J., Foale R.D. (2014) Unilateral squamous cell carcinoma of the renal pelvis with hydronephrosis in a cat. *Journal of Feline Medicine and Surgery*. Vol 16(2) 183–188.

■ Greene S.N., Lucroy M.D., Greenberg C.B. et al. (2007) Evaluation of cisplatin administered with piroxicam in dogs with transitional cell carcinoma of the urinary bladder. *J Am Vet Med Assoc*. 231(7):1056–1060.

■ Grieco V., Riccardi E., Greppi G.F. et al. (2008) Canine testicular tumours: a study of 232 dogs. *J Comp Pathol*. 138(2–3):86–89.

■ Guil-Luna S., Sanchez-Cespedes R., Millan Y. et al. (2011) Aglepristone decreases proliferation in progesterone receptor-positive canine mammary carcinomas. *J Vet Intern Med*. 25, 518–523.

■ Gundim L.F., de Araújo C.P., Blanca W.T. et al. (2016) Clinical staging in bitches with mammary tumors: Influence of type and histological grade. *Can J Vet Res*. 80(80):318–322.

■ Hayden D.W., Barnes D.M., Johnson K.H. (1989) Morphologic changes in the mammary gland of megestrol acetate–treated and untreated cats: a retrospective study. *Vet Pathol*. 26(2):104–113.

■ Heller D.A., Clifford C.A., Goldschmidt M.H. et al. (2005) Cyclooxygenase-2 expression is associated with histologic tumor type in canine mammary carcinoma. *Vet Pathol*. 42(6):776–780.

■ Henry C.J., Flesner B.K., Bechtel S.A. et al. (2018) Clinical Evaluation of Tavocept to Decrease Diuresis Time and Volume in Dogs with Bladder Cancer Receiving Cisplatin. *J Vet Intern Med*. 32(32):370–376.

■ Henry C.J., Turnquist S.E., Smith A. et al. (1999) Primary renal tumours in cats: 19 cases (1992–1998). *J Feline Med Surg*. 1(3):165–170.

■ Henry C.J., McCaw D.L., Turnquist S.E. et al. (2003) Clinical evaluation of mitoxantrone and piroxicam in a canine model of human invasive urinary bladder carcinoma. *Clin Cancer Res*. 9(2):906–911.

■ Hermo G.A., Turic E., Angelico D. et al. (2011) Effect of adjuvant perioperative desmopressin in locally advanced canine mammary carcinoma and its relation to histologic grade. *J Am Anim Hosp Assoc* .47(1):21–27.

■ Higuchi T., Burcham G.N., Childress M.O. et al. (2013) Characterization and treatment of transitional cell carcinoma of the abdominal wall in dogs: 24 cases (1985–2010). *J Am Vet Med Assoc*. 242:499–506.

■ Itoh T., Uchida K., Ishikawa K. et al. (2005) Clinicopathological survey of 101 canine mammary gland tumors: differences between small-breed dogs and others. *J Vet Med Sci*. 67(3):345–347.

■ Iwasaki R., Shimosato Y., Yoshikawa R. et al. (2019) Survival analysis in dogs with urinary transitional cell carcinoma that underwent whole-body computed tomography at diagnosis. *Vet Comp Oncol*. 17(3):385–393.

■ Karayannopoulou M., Kaldrymidou E., Constantinidis T.C. et al. (2001) Adjuvant postoperative chemotherapy in bitches with mammary cancer. *J Vet Med A Physiol Pathol Clin Med*. 48(2):85–96.

■ Kaszak I., Ruszczak A., Kanafa S. et al. (2018) Current biomarkers of canine mammary tumors. *Acta Vet Scand*. 60(1):66.

■ Knapp D.W., Ruple-Czerniak A., Ramos-Vara J.A. et al. (2016) A Nonselective Cyclooxygenase Inhibitor Enhances the Activity of Vinblastine in a Naturally-Occurring Canine Model of Invasive Urothelial Carcinoma. *Bladder Cancer*. 2(2):241–250.

■ Knapp D.W., Richardson R.C., Bottoms G.D. et al. (1992) Phase I trial of piroxicam in 62 dogs bearing naturally occurring tumors. *Cancer Chemother Pharmacol* 29(3):214–218.

■ Knapp D.W., McMillan S.K. (2013) Tumors of the urinary system. In: Withrow SJ, Vail DM, eds. *Withrow and MacEwen's Small Animal Clinical Oncology*. 5th ed. St. Louis: Elsevier–Saunders. p 572–582.

■ Knapp D.W., Glickman N.W., DeNicola D.B. et al. (2000) Naturally occurring canine transitional cell carcinoma of the urinary bladder: a relevant model of human invasive bladder cancer. *Urol Oncol*. 5:47–59.

■ Knapp D.W., Henry C.J., Widmer W.R. et al. (2013) Randomized trial of cisplatin versus firocoxib versus cisplatin/firocoxib in dogs with transitional cell carcinoma of the urinary bladder. *J Vet Intern Med*. 27:126–133.

■ Knapp D.W., Richardson R.C., Chan T.C.K. et al. (1994) Piroxicam therapy in 34 dogs with transitional cell carcinoma of the urinary bladder. *J Vet Intern Med*. 8(4):273–278.

■ Knapp D.W., Glickman N.W., Widmer W.R. et al. (2000) Cisplatin versus cisplatin combined with piroxicam in a canine model of human invasive urinary bladder cancer. *Cancer Chemother Pharmacol*. 46(3):221–226.

■ Klein M.K., Cockerell G.L., Harris C.K. et al. (1988) Canine primary renal neoplasms: a retrospective review of 54 cases. *J Am Anim Hosp Assoc* 24:443–452.

■ Koltai Z., Szabó B., Jakus J. et al. (2018) Tyrosine kinase expression analyses in canine mammary gland tumours - A pilot study. *Acta Vet Hung* 66(2):294–308.

■ Kristiansen V.M., Nødtvedt A., Breen A.M. et al. (2013) Effect of Ovariohysterectomy at the Time of Tumor Removal in Dogs with Benign Mammary Tumors and Hyperplastic Lesions: A Randomized Controlled Clinical Trial. *J Vet Intern Med*. 27:935–942.

■ Kudo T., Kamiie J., Aihara N. et al. (2019) Malignant Leydig cell tumor in dogs: two cases and a review of the literature. *J Vet Diagn Invest*. 31(4):557–561.

■ Leffler A.J., Hostnik E.T., Warry E.E. et al. (2018) Canine urinary bladder transitional cell carcinoma tumor volume is dependent on imaging modality and measurement technique. *Vet Radiol Ultrasound*. 59(6):767–776.

■ LeRoy B.E., Nadella M.V., Toribio R.E. et al. (2004) Canine prostate carcinomas express markers of urothelial and prostatic differentiation. *Vet Pathol*. 41(2):131–140.

■ Leveille R., Biller D.S., Partington B.P. et al. Sonographic investigation of transitional cell carcinoma of the urinary bladder in small animals. *Vet Radiol Ultrasound*. 33(2):103–107.

■ Liao A.T., Chu P.Y., Yeh L.S. et al. (2009) A 12-year retrospective study of canine testicular tumors. *Theriogenology*. 71:919.

■ Liptak J.M., Brutscher S.P., Monnet E. et al. (2004) Transurethral resection in the management of urethral and prostatic neoplasia in 6 dogs. *Vet Surg*. 33(5):505–516.

■ Locke J.E., Barber L.G. (2006) Comparative aspects and clinical outcomes of canine renal hemangiosarcoma. *J Vet Intern Med*. 20(4):962–7

■ Machado M.C., da Costa-Neto J.M., Portela R.D. et al. (2018) The effect of naltrexone as a carboplatin chemotherapy-associated drug on the immune response, quality of life and survival of dogs with mammary carcinoma. *PLoS One*. 13(10).

■ Macy D.W., Withrow S.J., Hoopes J. (1983) Transitional cell carcinoma of the bladder associated with cyclophosphamide administration. *J Am Anim Hosp Assoc*. 19(6):965–969.

■ MacLachlan N.J., Kennedy P.C. (2002) *Tumors of the genital systems*. In: *Tumors in domestic animals*, ed. Meuten DJ, 4th ed., pp. 547–573. Iowa State Press, Ames, IA.

■ Marvel S.J., Séguin B., Dailey D.D. et al. (2017) Clinical outcome of partial cystectomy for transitional cell carcinoma of the canine bladder. *Vet Comp Oncol*. 15(4):1417–1427.

■ Masserdotti C., Bonfanti U., De Lorenzi D. et al. (2005) Cytologic fea- tures of testicular tumours in dog. *J Vet Med A Physiol Pathol Clin Med*. 52:339–346.

■ Matos, A.J.F., Faustino, A.M.R., Lopes, C. et al. (2006) Detection of lymph node micrometastases in malignant mammary tumours in dogs by cytokeratin immunostaining. *Veterinary Record*. 158, 626–629.

■ McAloney C.A., Sharkey L.C., Feeney D.A. et al. (2018) Evaluation of the diagnostic utility of cytologic examination of renal fine-needle aspirates from dogs and the use of ultrasonographic features to inform cytologic diagnosis. *J Am Vet Med Assoc*. 15;252(10):1247–1256.

■ McDonald R.K., Walker M., Legendre A.M. et al. (1988) Radiotherapy of metastatic seminoma in the dog: case reports. *J Vet Intern Med*. 2(2):103–107.

■ McMillan S.K., Knapp D.W., Ramos-Vara J.A. et al. (2012) Outcome of urethral stent placement for management of urethral obstruction secondary to transitional cell carcinoma in dogs: 19 cases (2007–2010). *J Am Vet Med Assoc* 15; 241(12):1627–1632.

■ McNeill C.J., Sorenmo K.U., Shofer F.S. et al. (2009) Evaluation of adjuvant doxorubicin-based chemotherapy for the treatment of feline mammary carcinoma. *J Vet Intern Med*. 23: 123–129.

■ Merlo D.F., Rossi L., Pellegrino C. et al. (2008) Cancer incidence in pet dogs: findings of the animal tumor registry of Genoa, Italy. *J Vet Intern Med*. 22(4):976–984.

■ Meuten D.J. (2002) Tumors of the urinary system. In: Meuten DJ, ed. *Tumors in Domestic Animals*. 4th ed. Ames: Iowa State Press; 509–546.

■ Miller J.M., Lambrechts N.E, Martin R.A. et al. (2008) Persistent vulvar hemorrhage secondary to vaginal hemangioma in dogs. *J Am Anim Hosp Assoc*. 44(2):86–89.

■ Miller M.A., Ramos-Vara J.A., Dickerson M.F. et al. (2003) Uterine neoplasia in 13 cats. *J Vet Diagn Invest*. 15:575–522.

■ Mills S.W., Musil K.M., Davies J.L. et al. (2014) Prognostic Value of Histologic Grading for Feline Mammary Carcinoma: A Retrospective Survival Analysis. *Vet Pathol*. 24

■ Moe L., Lium B. (1997) Computed tomography of hereditary multifocal renal cystadenocarcinomas in German Shepherd Dogs. *Vet Radiol Ultrasound*. 38(5):335–343.

■ Mooney S.C., Hayes A.A., Matus R.E. et al. (1987) Renal lymphoma in cats: 28 cases (1977–1984). *JAVMA*. 191(11):1473–1477.

■ Moore A.S., Kirk C., Cardona A. (1991) Intracavitary cisplatin chemotherapy experience with six dogs. *J Vet Intern Med*. 5:227–231.

■ Nelissen P., White R.A. (2012) Subtotal Vaginectomy for Management of Extensive Vaginal Disease in 11 Dogs. *Veterinary Surgery*. 41; 495–500.

■ Nolan M.W., Kogan L., Griffin L.R. et al. (2012) Intensity-modulated and image-guided radiation therapy for treatment of genitourinary carcinomas in dogs. *J Vet Intern Med*. 26:987–995.

■ Nodtvedt A., Gamlem H., Gunnes G. et al. (2011) Breed differences in the proportional morbidity of testicular tumours and distribution of histopathologic types in a population-based canine cancer registry. *Vet Comp Oncol*. 9:45.

■ Norris A.M., Laing E.J., Valli V.E.O. et al. (1992) Canine bladder and urethral tumors: a retrospective study of 115 cases (1980–1985). *J Vet Intern Med.* 6:145–153.

■ Novosad C.A., Bergman P.J., O'Brien M.G. et al. (2006) Retrospective evaluation of adjunctive doxorubicin for the treatment of feline mammary gland adenocarcinoma: 67 cases. *J Am Anim Hosp Assoc.* 42(2):110–120.

■ Nyland T.G., Wallack S.T., Wisner E.R. (2002) Needle-tract implantation following US-guided fine-needle aspiration biopsy of transitional cell carcinoma of the bladder, urethra, and prostate. *Vet Radiol Ultrasound.* 43(1):50–53.

■ Nyman H.T., Nielsen O.L., McEvoy F.J. et al. (2006) Comparison of B-mode and Doppler ultrasonographic findings with histologic features of benign and malignant mammary tumors in dogs. *Am J Vet Res.* 67(6):985–991.

■ Nyman H.T., Kristensen A.T., Lee M.H. et al. (2006) Characterization of canine superficial tumors using gray-scale B mode, color flow mapping, and spectral Doppler ultrasonography: a multivariate study. *Vet Radiol Ultrasound.* 47(2):192–198.

■ Overley B., Shofer F.S., Goldschmidt M.H. et al. (2005) Association between ovarihyster- ectomy and feline mammary carcinoma. *J Vet Intern Med.* 19:560–3.

■ Palmieri C., Lean F.Z., Akter S.H. et al. (2014) A retrospective analysis of 111 canine prostatic samples: Histopathological findings and classification. *Research in Veterinary Science.* 97; 568–573.

■ Parfitt S.L., et al. (2011) Radiosensitivity and capacity for radiation-induced sublethal damage repair of canine transitional cell carcinoma (CCT) cell lines. *Vet Comp Oncol.* 9(3):232–240.

■ Patnaik A.K., Greenlee P.G. (1987) Canine ovarian neoplasms: a clinicopathologic study of 71 cases, including histology of 12 granulosa cell tumors. *Vet Pathol* 24(6):509–514.

■ Patsikas M., Papazoglou L.G., Jakovljevic S. et al. (2014) Radiographic and Ultrasonographic Findings of Uterine Neoplasms in Nine Dogs. *J Am Anim Hosp Assoc.* 50:330–337.

■ Payan-Carreira R., Saraiva A.L., Santos T. et al. (2013) Feline endometrial adenocarcinoma in females <1 year old: a description of four cases. *Reprod Dom Anim.* 48, e70–e77.

■ Perez-Alenza M.D., Jimenez A., Nieto A.I. et al. (2004) First description of feline inflammatory mammary carcinoma: clinicopathological and immunohistochemical characteristics of three cases. *Breast Cancer Res.* 6: R300–307.

■ Petterino C., Luzio E., Baracchini L. et al. (2011) Paraneoplastic leukocytosis in a dog with a renal carcinoma. *Vet Clin Pathol.* 40/1; 89–94.

■ Pierini A., Millanta F., Zanforlin R. et al. (2017) Usefulness of cytologic criteria in ultrasound-guided fine-needle aspirates from subcentimeter canine mammary tumors. *J Vet Diagn Invest.* 29(6):869–873.

■ Powe J.R., Canfield P.J., Martin P.A. (2004) Evaluation of the cytologic diagnosis of canine prostatic disorders. *Vet Clin Pathol.* 33(3):150–154.

■ Queiroga F.L., Alves A., Pires I. et al. (2007) Expression of COX-1 and COX-2 in canine mammary tumours. *J Comp Pathol.* 136(2–3):177–185.

■ Radhakrishnan A. (2017) Urethral Stenting for Obstructive Uropathy Utilizing Digital Radiography for Guidance: Feasibility and Clinical Outcome in 26 Dogs. *J Vet Intern Med.* 31(31):427–433.

■ Raghavan M., Knapp D.W., Dawson M.H. et al. (2004) Topical flea and tick pesticides and the risk of transitional cell carcinoma of the urinary bladder in Scottish Terriers. *J Am Vet Med Assoc.* 225:38–394.

■ Rasotto R., Berlato D., Goldschmidt M.H. et al. (2017) Prognostic Significance of Canine Mammary Tumor Histologic Subtypes: An Observational Cohort Study of 229 Cases. *Vet Pathol.* 54(4):571–578.

■ Ravicini S., Baines S.J., Taylor A. et al. (2018) Outcome and prognostic factors in medically treated canine prostatic carcinomas: A multi-institutional study. *Vet Comp Oncol.* 16(4):450–458.

■ Reed L.T., Knapp D.W., Miller M.A. (2013) Cutaneous Metastasis of Transitional Cell Carcinoma in 12 Dogs. *Vet Pathol.* 50: 676.

■ Rippy S.B., Gardner H.L., Nguyen S.M. et al. (2016) A pilot study of toceranib/vinblastine therapy for canine transitional cell carcinoma. *BMC Vet Res.* 12(1):257.

■ Rogers K.S., Walker M.A., Dillon H.B. (1998) Transmissible venereal tumor: a retrospective study of 29 cases. *J Am Anim Hosp Assoc.* 199834:463–470.

■ Rossi F., Sabattini S., Vascellari M. et al. (2018) The impact of toceranib, piroxicam and thalidomide with or without hypofractionated radiation therapy on clinical outcome in dogs with inflammatory mammary carcinoma. *Vet Comp Oncol.* 16(4):497–504.

■ Saba C.F., Rogers K.S., Newman S.J. et al. (2007) Mammary gland tumors in male dogs. *J Vet Intern Med.* 21(5):1056–1059.

■ Saulnier Troff F.G., Busoni V., Hamaide A. (2008) A technique for resection of invasive tumors involving the trigone area of the bladder in dogs: preliminary results in two dogs. *Vet Surg.* 37:427–437.

■ Seixas F., Palmeira C., Pires M.A. et al. (2011) Grade is an independent prognostic factor for feline mammary carcinomas: a clinicopathological and survival analysis. *Vet J.* 187(1):65–71.

■ Sfiligoi G., Rassnick K.M., Scarlett, J.M. et al. (2005) Outcome of dogs with mast cell tumors in the inguinal or perineal region versus other cutaneous locations: 124 cases (1990–2001). *J Am Vet Med Assoc.* 226:1368–1374.

■ Shapiro W., Kitchell B.E., Fossum T.W. et al. (1998) Cisplatin for treatment of transitional cell and squamous cell carcinomas in dogs. *JAVMA.* 193(12):1530–1533.

■ Simon D., Schoenrock D., Baumgartner W. et al. (2006) Postoperative adjuvant treatment of invasive malignant mammary gland tumors in dogs with doxorubicin and docetaxel. *J Vet Intern Med.* 20(5):1184–1190.

■ Skorupski K.A., Overley B., Shofer F.S. et al. (2005) Clinical characteristics of mammary carcinoma in male cats. *J Vet Intern Med.* 19(1):52–55.

■ Smith J.D., Stone E.A., Gilson S.D. (1995) Placement of a permanent cystostomy catheter to relieve urine outflow obstruction in dogs with transitional cell carcinoma. *J Am Vet Med Assoc.* 206(4):496–499.

■ Smith J. (2008) Canine prostatic disease: a review of anatomy, pathology, diagnosis, and treatment. *Theriogenology.* 70:375–383.
■ Stone E.A., Withrow S.J., Page R.L. et al. (1988) Ureterocolonic anastomosis in ten dogs with transitional cell carcinoma. *Vet Surg.* 17(3):147–153
■ Sorenmo K. (2003) Immunohistochemical characterization of canine prostatic carcinoma and correlation with castration status and castration time. *Vet Comp Oncol.* 1(1):48–56.
■ Sorenmo K.U., Shofer F.S., Goldschmidt M.H. (2000) Effect of spaying and timing of spaying on survival of dogs with mammary carcinoma. *J Vet Intern Med.* 14(3):266–270.
■ Sontas B.H., Erdogan O., Enginler A.S. et al. (2013) Endometrial adenocarcinoma in two young queens. *Journal of Small Animal Practice.* 54, 156–159.
■ Stratmann N., Failing K., Richter A. et al. (2008) Mammary tumor recurrence in bitches after regional mastectomy. *Vet Surg.* 37(1):82–86.
■ Taylor A.J., lara-garcia A., Benigni L. (2014) Ultrasonographic characteristics of canine renal lymphoma. *Vet Radiol Ultrasound.* Vol. 55, No 4, pp 441–446.
■ Taylor A., Finotello R., Vilar-Saavedra P. et al. (2019) Clinical characteristics and outcome of dogs with presumed primary renal lymphoma. *J Small Anim Pract.* 31.
■ Taylor S.S., Goodfellow M.R., Browne W.J. et al. (2009) Feline extranodal lymphoma: response to chemotherapy and survival in 110 cats. *J Small Anim Pract.* 50:584–592.
■ Teske E., Naan E.C., van Dijk E.M. et al. (2002) Canine prostate carcinoma: epidemiological evidence of an increased risk in castrated dogs. *Mol Cell Endocrinol.* 197(1–2):251–255.
■ Valdes-Martinez A., Cianciolo R., Mai W. (2007) Association between renal hypoechoic subcapsular thickening and lymphosarcoma in cats. *Vet Radiol Ultrasound.* 48:357–360.
■ Verin R., Cian F., Stewart J. et al. (2018) Canine Clitoral Carcinoma: A Clinical, Cytologic, Histopathologic, Immunohistochemical, and Ultrastructural Study. *Vet Pathol.* 55(4):501–509.
■ Vlasin M., Rauser P., Fichtel T. et al. (2006) Subtotal intracapsular prostatectomy as a useful treatment for advanced stage prostatic malignancies. *J Small Anim Pract.* 47:512–516.
■ Weisse C., Berent A., Todd K. et al. (2006) Evaluation of palliative stenting for management of malignant urethral obstructions in dogs. *J Am Vet Med Assoc.* 229(2):226–234.
■ Welsh J.B., Best S.J., Yager J.A. et al. (2010) A report of 7 cases of feline vulval adenocarcinoma. *Can Vet J.* 51:764–766.
■ White R.N., Davies J.V., Gregory S.P. (1996) Vaginourethroplasty for treatment of urethral obstruction in the bitch. *Vet Surg.* 25:503–510.
■ Wilson H.M., Chun R., Larson V.S. et al. (2007) Clinical signs, treatments, and outcome in cats with transitional cell carcinoma of the urinary bladder: 20 cases (1990–2004). *J Am Vet Med Assoc.* 231(1):101–106.
■ Zambrano-Estrada X., Landaverde-Quiroz B., Dueñas-Bocanegra A.A. et al. (2018) Molecular iodine/doxorubicin neoadjuvant treatment impair invasive capacity and attenuate side effect in canine mammary cancer. *BMC Vet Res.* 14(1):87.

Test

1. **What are the most common renal tumours in dogs and cats?**
    a. Carcinoma in dogs and lymphoma in cats.
    b. Lymphoma in both dogs and cats.
    c. Carcinoma in both dogs and cats.
    d. Lymphoma in dogs and carcinoma in cats.

2. **Regarding the diagnosis of a TCC located in the cranial part of the bladder in a female, which of the following diagnostic techniques would be the best choice?**
    a. Traumatic catheterisation.
    b. Ultrasound-guided fine needle aspiration.
    c. Cystoscopy and incisional biopsy.
    d. Surgical biopsy.

3. **Regarding prostate tumours, which option is incorrect?**
    a. Prostate tumours affect neutered animals most frequently.
    b. Administration of NSAIDs appears to improve survival in these patients.
    c. The rate of metastasis is approximately 10–20%.
    d. One of the most frequent locations of metastases is the bones and, in particular, the lumbar vertebrae.

4. **What type of testicular tumour is most likely to metastasise?**
    a. Leydig cell tumour.
    b. Sertoli cell tumour.
    c. Seminoma.
    d. None metastasise.

5. **In which case should a mastectomy not be performed?**
    a. Mammary sarcoma.
    b. 5 cm ulcerated tumour.
    c. Mammary tumour with inguinal lymphadenopathy.
    d. Inflammatory carcinoma.

6. **Which chemotherapy treatment is most commonly used historically in cats with mammary tumours?**
    a. Carboplatin.
    b. Cyclophosphamide.
    c. Mitoxantrone.
    d. Doxorubicin.

7. **Which of the following chemotherapy drugs could be used to treat transitional cell carcinoma of the bladder?**
    a. Cyclophosphamide.
    b. Methotrexate.
    c. Carboplatin.
    d. Vincristine.

Answers on page 376

8. **A cat with a mammary mass which is 2 cm in size in the third left mammary gland is brought to the practice. What kind of surgery should be performed?**
    a. Regional mastectomy (third and fourth mammary gland, plus inguinal lymph node).
    b. At least one complete unilateral mastectomy.
    c. Nodulectomy due to the small size of the mass.
    d. Simple mastectomy (only the affected mammary gland).

9. **What is the most common uterine tumour in bitches?**
    a. Leiomyoma.
    b. Leiomyosarcoma.
    c. Adenocarcinoma.
    d. Haemangiosarcoma.

Clinical Case

A 6-year-old Siamese cat weighing 5 kg which has been suffering with respiratory distress over the last 2–3 days has been brought to the practice. Lethargy is also observed.

It has an ulcerated 3 cm mass in the left inguinal mammary gland that has been present for almost four months. It is an indoor cat that is up to date with vaccinations and is dewormed.

Physical examination showed inspiratory and expiratory dyspnoea at 60 bpm. The femoral pulse is strong and cardiac auscultation normal, with a heart rate of 160 beats/min and regular rhythm. Respiratory auscultation shows a decrease in respiratory sounds in both hemithoraces. Thoracic and abdominal radiographs are also performed.

Questions:

1. **Based on the clinical history and physical examination, what is the most likely cause of this cat's respiratory problem?**
    a. Congenital cardiopathy.
    b. Pulmonary neoplasia.
    c. Pleural effusion.
    d. Pulmonary neoplasm and pleural effusion.

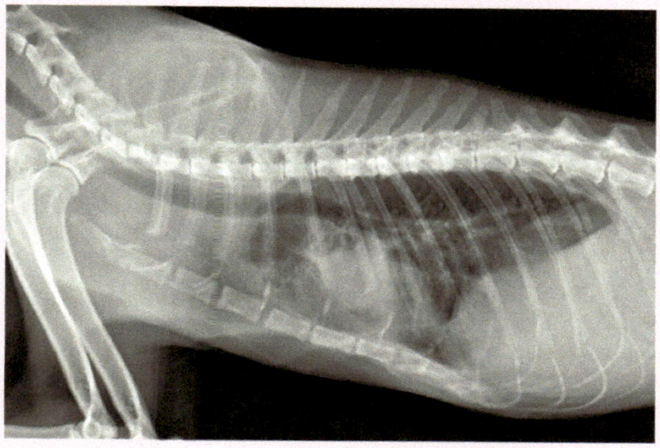

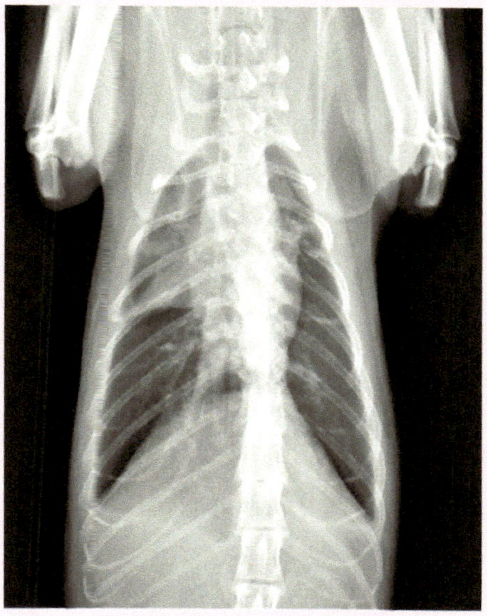

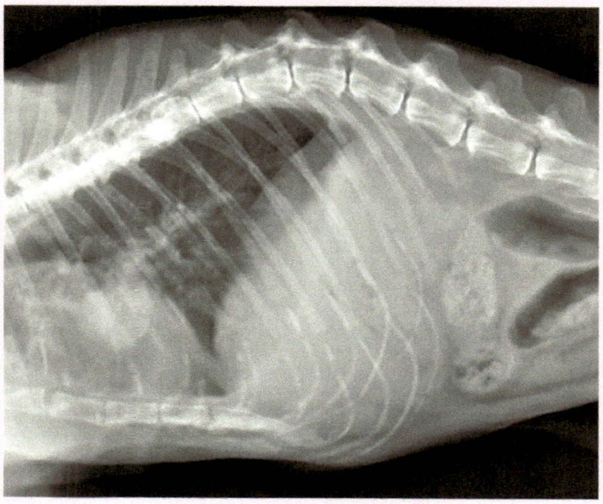

2. What action is the most appropriate and fastest way to try to reach a diagnosis?

a. Administration of a bronchodilator.
d. Sedation and subcutaneous administration of furosemide.
c. Obtain a sample of the pleural fluid and evaluate it using cytology.
d. Hospitalise with oxygen.

3. Cytology images of a sample obtained directly from the pleural fluid, such as the four images shown below are seen. What could the diagnosis be?

a. Pyogranulomatous disease.
b. Mesenchymal cell tumour.
c. Normal mesothelial cells.
d. Epithelial cells with multiple criteria of malignancy such as anisokaryosis, anisocytosis and the presence of mitosis.

4. After performing the tests, what is the most likely diagnosis?

a. Chronic inflammation.
b. Foreign body.
c. Pulmonary tumour with possible malignant pleural effusion.
d. Normal cells on thoracic puncture.

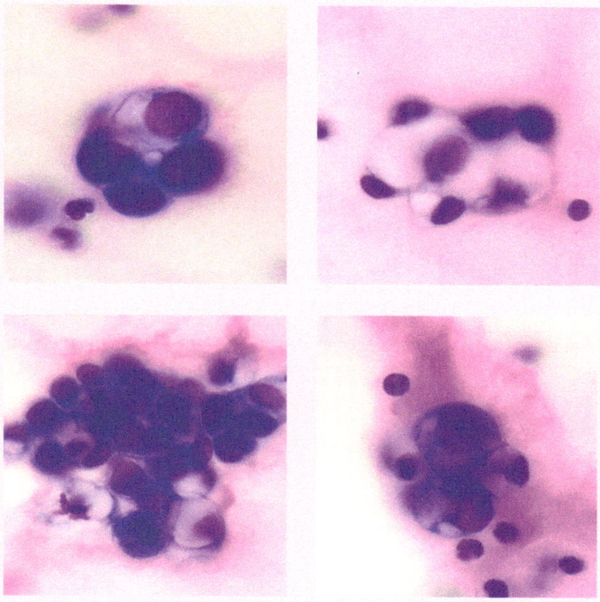

Correct Answers:

Test

1. a
2. c
3. c
4. b
5. d
6. d
7. c
8. b
9. a

Clinical Case

1. d
2. c
3. d
4. c

Notes

Tumours of the Endocrine System

Jarno Schmidt

Box 1. Classification of tumours of the endocrine system

- **Thyroid tumours:**
  - **canine thyroid tumours**
  - **feline thyroid tumours.**
- **Parathyroid tumours:**
  - **canine parathyroid tumours (primary hyperparathyroidism)**
  - **feline parathyroid tumours (primary hyperparathyroidism).**
- **Insulinoma:**
  - **canine insulinoma**
  - **feline insulinoma.**
- **Hypersomatotropism (acromegaly):**
  - **feline hypersomatotropism (acromegaly)**
  - **canine hypersomatotropism (acromegaly).**
- **Hyperadrenocorticism:**
  - **canine hyperadrenocorticism**
  - **feline hyperadrenocorticism.**
- **Canine pheochromocytoma**
- **Feline primary hyperaldosteronism (Conn syndrome).**

Oncology of the endocrine system is a very important part of veterinary oncology. Since many tumours derived from the endocrine glands have hormonal activity, they are accompanied by a wide variety of paraneoplastic syndromes. This chapter describes some of the more significant endocrine tumours of the dog and cat but given the extensive nature of veterinary endocrinology it cannot be seen as a substitute for an endocrinology textbook. Therefore, if the reader needs more information on diagnostic and treatment protocols, consulting any standard manual of internal medicine or endocrinology is recommended.

Thyroid Tumours

Canine Thyroid Tumours

Thyroid tumours **are the most common endocrine neoplasms in dogs**, accounting for 1 to 4% of all canine tumours. Typically, they appear in dogs of middle or advanced age (mean age of 9–10 years). The most affected breeds are Labrador Retrievers, Golden Retrievers, Beagles, the Siberian Husky, German Shepherd, and Boxer. There is no sex predisposition.

History and Clinical Signs

Dogs usually present because clients feel a **subcutaneous (painless) mass in the cranial region of the neck**. Less frequently, the reason for the visit is a clinical sign such as cough, dysphagia, change in voice, Horner's syndrome, swelling of the face (precaval syndrome) or due to signs related to either hyperthyroidism (such as polyphagia, weight loss, polyuria, polydipsia) or hypothyroidism (e.g. lethargy, weight gain, dermatological disorders). Very rarely, thyroid tumours can have an ectopic location, which can appear anywhere, from the base of the tongue to the heart, with clinical signs consistent with a mass in that area. For example, dogs with a mediastinal (ectopic) thyroid mass may present with dyspnoea.

Types of Tumours, Biological Behaviour, and Differential Diagnoses

Most of the apparent clinical cases (more than 80%) and of the casually detected tumours (more than 70%) are malignant (i.e. carcinomas). The rest of primary thyroid tumours are almost always adenomas. Thyroid carcinomas arise from the follicular epithelium (follicular thyroid carcinoma, 71%) or from parafollicular C cells (medullary thyroid carcinoma, 29%). Most dogs are euthyroid (more than 60%), only 10 to 30% of patients are hyperthyroid and the rest are hypothyroid or presumed hypothyroid.

The differential diagnosis of a thyroid tumour should also include other subcutaneous masses, such as an abscess, a granuloma, a lymphadenopathy, a lipoma, a soft-tissue sarcoma, a mast cell tumour, a haemangiosarcoma, tumours of the larynx and of the trachea. Thyroid carcinomas grow faster than adenomas and locally invade the tumour capsule, blood, and lymphatic vessels, and/or adjacent tissues. Initially approximately 33–50% of tumours are mobile, while the rest are adherent to the underlying tissues. A minority are bilateral tumours (15–20%). Carcinomas metastasise to regional lymph nodes (medial retropharyngeal, prescapular, sternal) and to distant sites (especially in the lungs). In approximately

15–40% of cases, there is already evidence of metastasis at initial presentation. The rate of metastasis depends mainly on the size and volume of the tumour. Also, according to some studies, bilateral tumours are more likely to metastasise at the time of presentation. In a recent study, macroscopic and microscopic vascular invasion were found to be independent negative factors for disease-free survival times.

Diagnostic Approach and Staging

Evaluation of the primary tumour is initially based on **physical examination**, to assess its mobility, size, the possibility of a bilateral tumour and detect regional metastases, if any. **Ultrasound** can also be used to better define the size and invasiveness of the primary lesion, although CT and MRI give better results for this purpose (Figure 1).

Cytology is a quick way to rule out other differential diagnoses and can sometimes even allow a presumptive diagnosis of endocrine neoplasia to be made. However, smears are often heavily contaminated with blood. The cells from thyroid carcinomas have a characteristic appearance, and are relatively monomorphic, with a round or oval naked nucleus. The cytoplasm is poorly differentiated, although it may contain a bluish black pigment. Cytology generally cannot be used to distinguish between benign and malignant endocrine neoplasia (Figure 2).

To assess the functional status of the tumour, a **panel of thyroid hormones** (for example, T4/TSH) and **calcium concentrations** (**ionised**) **should be measured. Immunohistochemistry** can be used to determine whether the tumour originates from the follicular (thyroglobulin positive) or parafollicular (calcitonin positive) epithelium, although the importance of this differentiation in establishing the prognosis is currently unclear.

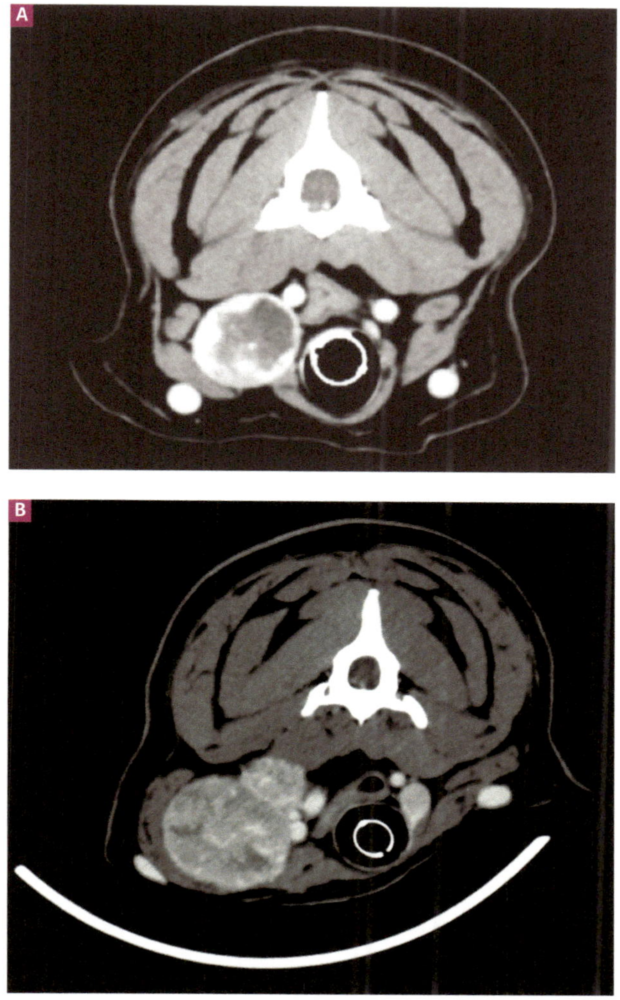

Figure 1. Dog with a unilateral thyroid carcinoma. The image (CT) shows a large 2.5 cm mass with a marked increase in peripheral contrast in the right thyroid lobe. The left thyroid gland is normal (**A**). Dog with bilateral thyroid carcinoma. The image shows an invasive, large sized mass of approximately 4 cm in the right thyroid lobe. The left thyroid gland is also enlarged (approximately 1 cm) (**B**).

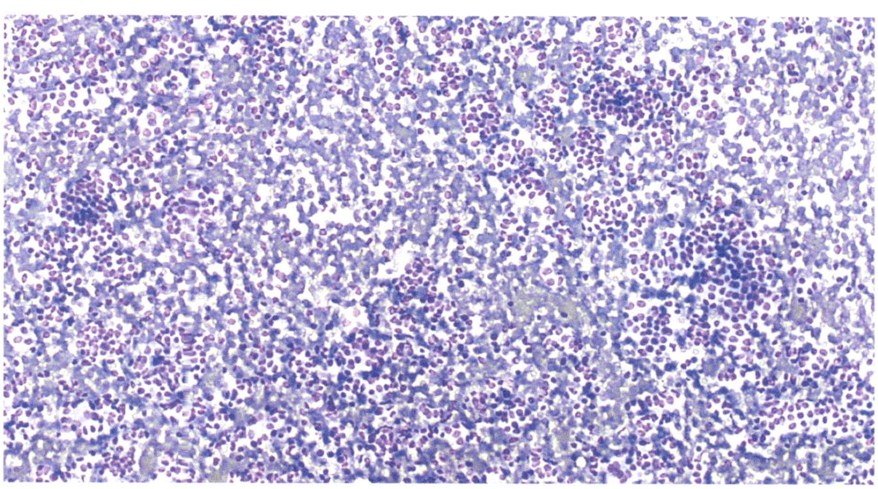

Figure 2. Cytology from a fine needle aspirate of a dog with thyroid carcinoma (200x magnification). Groups of cells which are monomorphic with naked nuclei and indistinct cytoplasmatic borders can be seen, typical of neuroendocrine tumours, and marked blood contamination.

Ideally, CT staging should include the primary tumour, regional lymph nodes, and the thorax (and occasionally the abdomen). Alternatively, a combination of ultrasound of the primary tumour and retropharyngeal lymph nodes (with or without fine needle aspiration biopsy) and three thoracic radiograph views may be helpful in some cases.

Treatment and Prognosis

Treatment options will depend on various factors, including the degree of attachment of the tumour, its staging, and the presence or absence of a bilateral condition. If there is no evidence of metastasis, treatment will depend on the mobility of the primary tumour. **Mobile masses are surgically removed**. Also, the ipsilateral retropharyngeal lymph nodes and any other enlarged regional lymph nodes should be removed for staging. If necessary, the recurrent laryngeal nerve, jugular vein, carotid artery, and both ipsilateral parathyroid glands can be removed.

Median survival time after complete surgical removal of a nonmetastatic thyroid tumour is approximately three years. Surgical removal of tumours attached to surrounding tissues is ineffective and not recommended (median survival time, 6–12 months). These tumours are best referred for radiotherapy, radioactive iodine therapy, or palliative chemotherapy (see below). Bilateral tumours can be operated on, but will require prolonged supplementation with thyroxine, vitamin D, and calcium. The median survival time in one study exceeded three years.

Tumours attached to surrounding tissues may be best treated with **radiotherapy with a linear accelerator**. Usually, the tumour response is delayed and is only seen after several months. With radiotherapy with curative intent, 80% progression free survival after twelve months and 72% progression free survival after three years of treatment can be expected. Acute adverse effects (mucositis, dermatitis, cough) appear in approximately 50% of dogs, although they usually disappear within 2–4 weeks. Late onset adverse effects (skin fibrosis, alopecia, chronic tracheitis) are rare, but up to 50% of cases may experience hypothyroidism after radiotherapy. With a palliative radiotherapy protocol, a mean survival time of 2 years has been published. **Treatment with radioactive iodine (I-131)** is an alternative if the tumour absorbs iodine (median survival time 30 months).

The role of chemotherapy in the treatment of thyroid tumours is unclear. It may be an option for nonremovable tumours if radiotherapy or iodine therapy is not available. If there are any negative prognostic factors, adjuvant therapy may also be considered. Partial remissions of macroscopic tumours treated with doxorubicin have been described, but the survival benefit is uncertain. Measurable remissions and/or stabilisations have also been described with toceranib phosphate (2.5–2.8 mg/kg every other day, PO, Palladia®, Zoetis) or metronomic chemotherapy with chlorambucil (4 mg/kg per day, PO, Leukeran®) in some cases. Some authors advocate administering oral L thyroxine indefinitely after surgery to suppress endogenous TSH secretion, which can act as a tumour promoter.

Feline Thyroid Tumours

Hyperthyroidism is the most common feline endocrinopathy. It is usually caused by unilateral or bilateral adenomatous hyperplasia of the thyroid glands. Malignant feline thyroid tumours are rare, constituting less than 5% of thyroid tumours. However, the incidence of malignancy may increase because, in treated cats, benign hyperthyroidism can progress from adenoma to carcinoma.

Thyroid carcinomas appear in older cats with a long history of benign hyperthyroidism. Non-secreting (euthyroid) tumours are very rare. Carcinomas are highly invasive, generally larger than adenomas, and moderately metastatic (metastasis rate 40–70%) (Figure 3).

Diagnosis is based on histology and/or documentation of invasion or signs of metastatis. Feline ectopic thyroid tumours can occasionally be found in the ventral area of the neck, cranial to the mediastinum (Figure 4), or in the pericardium.

Since most feline thyroid carcinomas cannot be removed, the **treatment of choice is radioactive iodine (I-131)** therapy at very high doses (e.g. 30 Ci = 1100 mBq). With this, the resolution of hyperthyroidism and remission of the primary pathology and metastases are usually achieved. Survival times range from several months to several years. Long survival times are common.

If radioactive iodine therapy is not available, palliative external radiotherapy may be beneficial in some cases. However, in these cases the general prognosis is reserved.

Parathyroid Tumours

Canine Parathyroid Tumours (Primary Hyperparathyroidism)

Primary hyperparathyroidism is an endocrine disorder characterised by autonomous secretion of parathyroid hormone

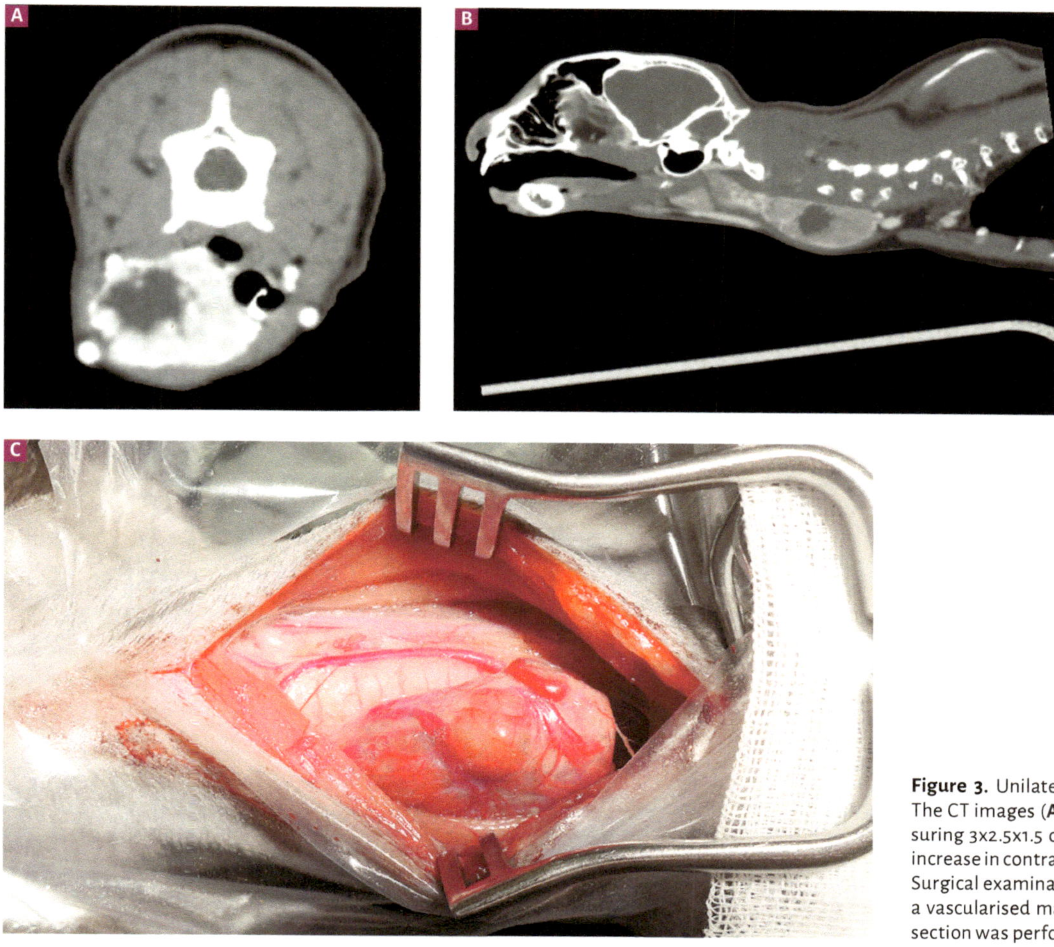

Figure 3. Unilateral thyroid carcinoma in a cat. The CT images (**A** and **B**) show a large mass measuring 3x2.5x1.5 cm with a marked heterogenous increase in contrast in the right lobe of the thyroid. Surgical examination (**C**) confirms the presence of a vascularised mass in the right thyroid lobe. Resection was performed without incident.

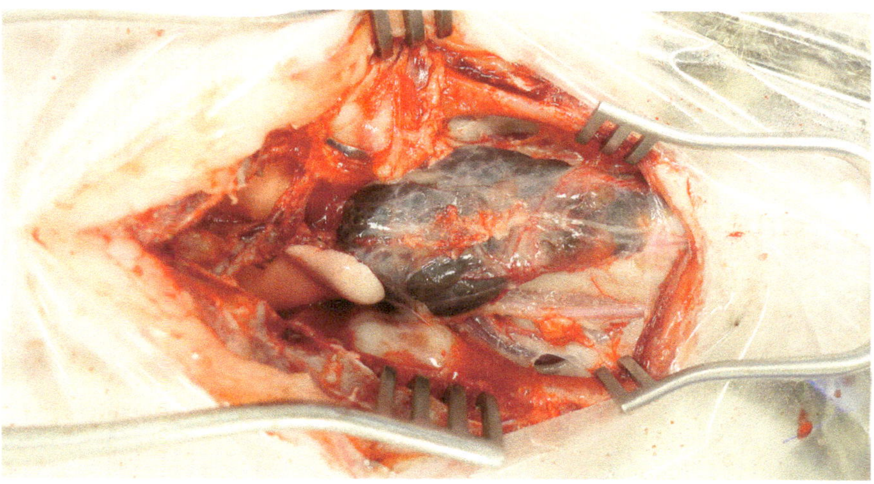

Figure 4. Intraoperative image of a cat with ectopic thyroid adenoma. Resection was performed without complications.

(PTH) by an adenoma (85%), a hyperplastic nodule (10–12%), or, more rarely, by a carcinoma (3%) of the main cells of one or two parathyroid glands. The resulting hypercalcaemia can cause clinical signs. This pathology usually affects middle aged or older dogs, and the Keeshond breed is predisposed to it.

History and Clinical Signs

Most dogs with hyperparathyroidism are clinically normal and hypercalcaemia is sometimes found incidentally on routine blood tests. In other dogs, typical signs of hypercalcaemia appear, such as polyuria and polydipsia, and lethargy. Approximately 25% of dogs with primary hyperparathyroidism present to diagnose a reason for a lack of urination control, secondary to calcium urolithiasis and/or urinary tract infection, with signs such as dysuria, pollakiuria or haematuria. In dogs the parathyroid glands commonly cannot be palpated, even when they are dilated.

Diagnostic Approach and Staging

Dogs with primary hyperparathyroidism have elevated total and ionised serum calcium levels and normal or low phosphorus levels. The diagnosis of primary hyperparathyroidism is based on ruling out other causes of hypercalcaemia and/or documenting an elevated serum PTH level. Although dogs with primary hyperparathyroidism may also have normal serum PTH levels, in these patients the level is usually in the upper half of the normal range. In patients with primary hyperparathyroidism, the serum concentration of thyroid hormone related polypeptide (PTHrp) is usually low.

An **ultrasound** performed with a high frequency linear probe allows visualisation of the parathyroid glands and helps establish the diagnosis (Figure 5). Dogs with primary hyperparathyroidism usually present with one or two dilated parathyroid nodules (≥4 mm; the mean size of a normal parathyroid gland is 3×2.2×1.7 mm). The relationship between the observation of four dilated parathyroid glands and primary hyperparathyroidism is inconsistent.

The definitive diagnosis is based on **histopathology**, after exploratory surgery of the neck and, where appropriate, the removal of the dilated parathyroid glands.

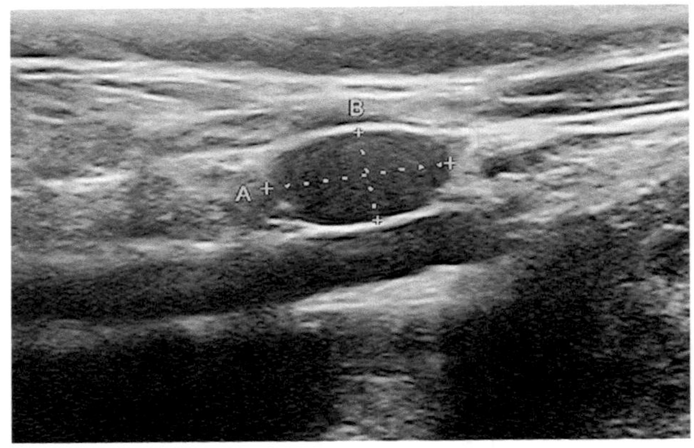

Figure 5. Ultrasound image of a caudal parathyroid nodule in the right lobe of the thyroid gland (sagittal view). The rest of the parathyroid glands were normal.

Treatment and Prognosis

The **treatment of choice for dogs with primary hyperparathyroidism depends on the clinical status of the patient**. Some incidentally detected cases of primary hyperparathyroidism can be monitored, especially if the dog is elderly and multimorbid. The definitive treatment of choice is **surgical exploration of the neck and removal** of the dilated thyroid glands.

If urolithiasis is present, the stones must be removed by cystectomy, because calcium urolithiasis cannot usually be resolved with medical treatment alone.

An alternative to surgical excision is ultrasound-guided transcutaneous radiofrequency **thermoablation** or **transcutaneous ablation** with ethanol (96%), also ultrasound-guided, of the dilated parathyroid glands. Complications of thermoablation include hypocalcaemia, Horner's syndrome (rare), and aspiration bronchopneumonia. Ethanol ablation can cause hypocalcaemia, transient changes in barks, cough, and dysphagia.

After removal or transcutaneous destruction of the autonomic parathyroid glands, patients are at **risk of hypocalcaemia (life threatening)** due to atrophy of the normal parathyroid glands. Hypocalcaemia is common within seven days after treatment. Since muscle arousal and activity can exacerbate signs of hypocalcaemia, it is imperative to keep patients quiet and resting. Serum ionised calcium concentrations should be monitored. If there are signs of hypocalcaemia, such as panting, muscle twitching, ataxia, rubbing the face with the paws, and nervousness, it should be treated.

In case of acute and severe clinical signs treatment should be administered intravenously (e.g. 10% calcium gluconate slowly IV at a dosage of 0.5–1.5 ml/kg over 20–30 minutes until observed to be effective, followed using a slow infusion of 10–15 mg/kg/hour) with ECG monitoring until the patient is stable enough to switch to oral treatment (e.g. calcium carbonate 20–50 mg/kg/day PO and calcitriol 20–30 ng/kg/day over 3–4 days, followed by 5–15 ng/kg/day as maintenance treatment). Afterwards, the supplementation should be reduced progressively over several weeks.

If the dog survives the postoperative period, the prognosis after surgery is usually excellent, even in (rare) cases of parathyroid carcinoma. Percutaneous ethanol ablation has a success rate greater than 80% while heat ablation is successful in 90–100% of cases. Occasionally, a recurrence of hypoparathyroidism can develop from one of the remaining parathyroid glands, within months to years of treatment.

Feline Parathyroid Tumours (Primary Hyperparathyroidism)

Feline primary hyperparathyroidism is **rare**. Unlike dogs, hypercalcaemic cats are unlikely to have polyuria and polydipsia. Normal parathyroid glands are not visible on ultrasound. However, in most cases enlarged parathyroid glands in cats are palpable and often present with cysts.

The **treatment of choice is surgical removal**. There are only occasional reports of ethanol or heat ablation. In some cats, palliative treatment of hypocalcaemia with alendronate bisphosphonate (1–4 mg/kg every 48–72 h PO) may be appropriate.

INSULINOMA

Canine Insulinoma

Insulinoma is the result of the neoplastic transformation of the endocrine β cells of the pancreas, which begin to secrete insulin autonomously and cause hypoglycaemia. **In dogs it is a rare disease**. It usually appears in animals of middle or advanced age and there is no apparent sex or breed predisposition.

History and Clinical Signs

Dogs usually present with **signs of hypoglycaemia**, such as polyphagia and weight gain, or **neurological deficits**, such as episodes of seizures, weakness, tremors and/or lethargy. Usually, the clinical signs are episodic and often improve with intake or are aggravated with diet or exercise.

Types of Tumours, Biological Behaviour

Insulinoma can have its origin in an adenoma, although it is most often caused by a pancreatic endocrine β-cell carcinoma. Hypersecretion of insulin causes hypoglycaemia and neuroglycopaenia, leading to weakness, ataxia, tremors, and possible seizures. Hypoglycaemia triggers the secretion of counter regulatory hormones (catecholamines, growth hormone, glucagon, cortisol, and adrenocorticotropic hormone), responsible for signs such as polyphagia and polyuria and polydipsia.

At the time of diagnosis, most dogs have **metastases**, either microscopic or macroscopic. The usual points of metastasis are the regional lymph nodes, the liver, the peritoneum, and other abdominal organs. In the more advanced stages, there may even be lung metastases.

Diagnostic Approach, Differential Diagnoses, and Staging

Often, the diagnosis of insulinoma is **based on clinical suspicion and exclusion of other causes of hypoglycaemia**. Differential diagnoses of hypoglycaemia are laboratory error, hypocortisolism (Addison's disease), liver failure, extreme leucocytosis, polycythaemia, sepsis, hypopituitarism, anorexia (puppies) and intense exercise (working dogs). Another important differential diagnosis is paraneoplastic hypoglycaemia caused by a variety of (large) extrapancreatic tumours. Such cases are usually mediated by the production of insulin like growth factor type 2 (IGF-2) in neoplastic cells and serum insulin concentrations are typically low.

The diagnosis of insulinoma can be confirmed by documenting elevated serum insulin concentrations or those in the upper half of the normal range, while the animal has moderate to severe hypoglycaemia (≤3.3 mmol/l or ≤60 mg/dl). The absence of a pancreatic nodule or mass on imaging does not rule out an insulinoma. Pancreatic nodules or masses are detected in 55% of cases using ultrasound only, while this rises to 71% of cases if a dual CT or CT angiography is performed (Figure 6). Sometimes presurgical cytology of a pancreatic nodule or mass can help with diagnosis. Unlike pancreatic adenocarcinoma, insulinoma may have a relatively monomorphic cytological appearance, with numerous bare nuclei (Figure 7).

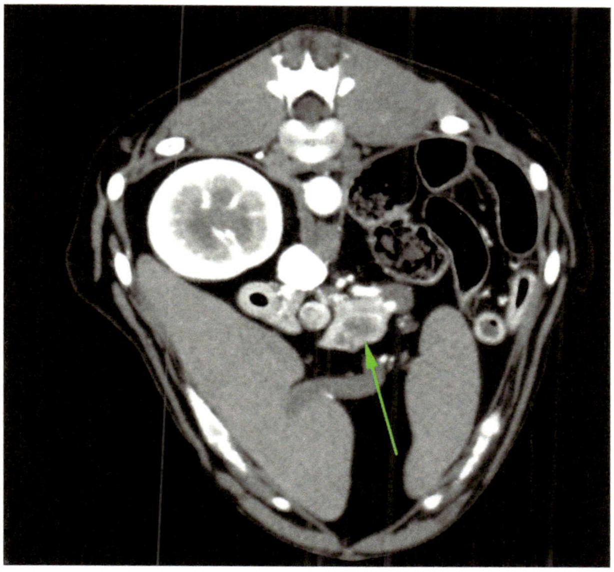

Figure 6. CT section where a pancreatic insulinoma in a dog (arrow) can be seen.

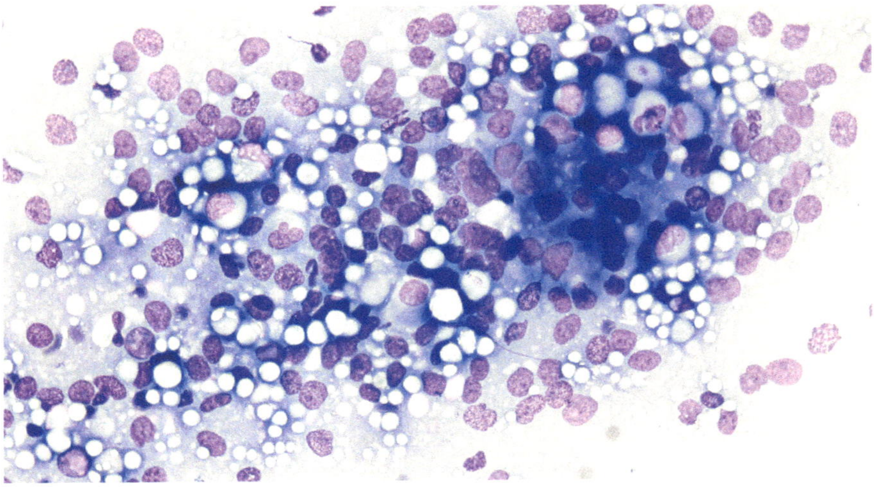

Figure 7. Cytology from a biopsy performed using fine needle aspiration of a canine insulinoma (400x magnification). Groups of cells with mild pleomorphism and cells with naked nuclei can be seen.

If serum insulin concentrations cannot be measured, surgical removal followed by histological analysis and normalisation of glucose concentrations confirm the diagnosis. Since most insulinomas are malignant, staging (Box 2) should be done before surgical removal. The usual points of metastasis are the regional lymph nodes, liver, peritoneum, and other abdominal organs and in advanced cases also the lungs. Therefore, ultrasound or CT and thoracic radiographs or CT are the staging tests of choice.

Box 2. Stages of insulinoma

- **Stage I: insulinoma limited to the pancreas.**
- **Stage II: presence of regional lymph node metastases.**
- **Stage III: presence of distal metastases.**

Treatment and Prognosis

Insulinoma therapy consists of **medical and dietary palliative treatment, surgical treatment, or both**. The benefits and risks of each option need to be carefully discussed with owners.

Medical and Dietary Treatment

Medical and dietary treatment can be given to stabilise the patient before an intervention or as an alternative to surgery. The main objective of medical and dietary treatment is to **control hypoglycaemia and associated clinical signs**. Chronic medical treatment of insulinoma patients consists of switching to a diet for diabetic patients (such as Hills m/d™ or Royal Canin Diabetic®) which is relatively rich in fat, proteins, and complex carbohydrates but low in simple sugars. Feeding frequency should be increased to 4–8 small meals a day, which can prevent episodes of hypoglycaemia between meals. Glucose intake should be limited, further avoiding excitement and strenuous exercise.

The **drugs of choice** for the treatment of insulinoma are glucocorticoids, diazoxide or both. Prednisolone is usually given as a first line drug, which acts as an insulin antagonist. It also increases glycogenolysis and gluconeogenesis. The dose can be progressively adjusted until clinical signs are controlled (typical range: 0.25–1 mg/kg every 24–48 h PO). In refractory cases diazoxide (5–10 mg/kg twice daily PO, Proglycem®) may be added, which inhibits insulin secretion from β cells.

Octeotride inhibits the synthesis of insulin and its secretion, so it may be a rescue option in some cases, although its effectiveness is unclear. Theoretically, antineoplastic chemotherapy with streptozocin, a cytotoxic agent specific to pancreatic β cells, can also be used. However, it can cause serious adverse effects and has not been shown to significantly improve survival time in small animals. Circumstantially toceranib phosphate (2.5–2.8 mg/kg every other day PO, Palladia® Zoetis) has provided partial remissions in some dogs with insulinoma.

For cases of acute hypoglycaemic seizures, 1–15 ml of 50% dextrose solution (diluted in saline at a ratio of 1:3–1:5) is administered slowly over 10–15 minutes; if the animal responds favourably, 5% dextrose is followed with a constant rate infusion. Dexamethasone sodium phosphate (e.g. 0.1–0.25 mg/kg IV) may also be administered additionally parenterally, to increase insulin resistance. In theory, a glucagon infusion can also be administered, but it is not always available in all practices. A possible home emergency treatment in case of hypoglycaemic seizures is to rub a concentrated solution of sugar (such as syrup or honey) on the dog's gums.

Surgical Treatment

Usually, the surgical intervention for a solitary insulinoma consists of a partial pancreatectomy. **The best curative option is the surgical removal of the insulinoma**. However, in most cases there are usually microscopic or macroscopic metastases. In some specific cases of macroscopic metastasis, a cytoreductive intervention aimed at the primary tumour and larger metastatic lesions may be considered to improve glycaemic control, at least temporarily. Surgery of the endocrine pancreas is associated with a number of potentially serious complications, such as the appearance of diabetes mellitus (almost always transient), pancreatitis, sepsis, thromboembolism, pneumonia, cardiac arrhythmias, and exocrine pancreatic insufficiency.

The prognosis is usually good in the short term but reserved to poor in the long term. In most cases, metastasis and/or tumour recurrence occur. The median survival time of surgically treated dogs is 13–14 months (in one study it even reached 26 months), but in cases where metastasis are present it is only 6 months. In studies the average survival with medical treatment alone is around 3–7 months. The best survival averages (more than 3 years) were published in a small series of dogs treated with medical and surgical treatment. Prognosis after surgery is better if dogs have normoglycaemia or hyperglycaemia after surgery than if they continue to have hypoglycaemia.

Feline Insulinoma

Insulinoma is **extremely rare in cats**, and fewer than 20 cases have been reported. Based on the few cases described, the diagnosis, biological behaviour, treatment, and prognosis appear to be similar to that of canine insulinoma.

Hypersomatotropism or Acromegaly

Feline Hypersomatotropism or Acromegaly

Definition and Pathophysiology

Feline hypersomatotrophism is usually **caused by a slow growing adenoma of the distal region of the anterior pituitary**, which causes excessive, chronic, and autonomous growth hormone (GH) production and secretion. Elevated GH concentration has anabolic and catabolic effects, participates in insulin resistance (and diabetes mellitus), and causes an increase in serum insulin like growth factor 1 (IGF-1). IGF-1 is produced in the liver and has indirect anabolic effects on various tissues, causing tissue growth that results in organomegaly. In the advanced stages, pituitary adenoma can also cause neurological signs due to its invasive lesion effect.

Epidemiology and Signalment

It is typical for acromegaly to be diagnosed in middle aged or older cats (mean age 11 years), especially in males (male to female ratio of 8:1).

Based on data collected in the United States and the United Kingdom, the prevalence of hypersomatotropism in diabetic cats is estimated to be around 25–33%.

History and Clinical Signs

Acromegaly is a major cause of insulin resistance and, with **very few exceptions, cats with hypersomatotropism suffer from diabetes mellitus**. Therefore, it is typical for cats to present signs related to poorly controlled diabetes mellitus, such as polyuria/polydipsia and polyphagia. It is interesting to note that most cats have a history of weight gain rather than weight loss. Mean insulin requirements in cats with acromegaly (7 IU twice daily) are typically significantly higher than those in diabetic cats without acromegaly (3 IU twice daily).

Apart from having poorly controlled diabetes mellitus, a minority of cats are only diagnosed with hypersomatotropism after the veterinarian or owner becomes aware of physical changes in the cat's size, such as large feet, wide face, protrusion of the jaw, increased interdental space and/or dilation of the abdomen. Other cats sometimes have comorbidities due to the anabolic effect of insulin like growth factor 1 in various tissues, such as arthropathies, heart, kidney, or respiratory failure. Only in very rare cases do cats present with neurological signs due to a pituitary macroadenoma (Figure 8).

Diagnostic Approach and Differential Diagnoses

Diagnosis is based on a combination of review, clinical history, clinical signs, measurement of hormone concentrations (serum IFG-1), imaging, and ruling out other differential diagnoses. Although, theoretically, the confirmation of high GH concentrations in a cat with poorly controlled diabetes mellitus is the most direct diagnostic test, it is common for GH to be secreted in waves, in addition to having only moderate sensitivity and specificity. On the other hand, no serum GH analyses are currently commercially available. This is why the **diagnosis is based on the following triad**.

1. Ruling out other causes of poor glycaemic control in cases of diabetes mellitus.
2. Identification of a mass in the pituitary gland by imaging (CT or MRI).
3. Documentation of elevated serum IGF-1 concentrations.

Rule Out Other Differential Diagnoses

Acromegaly is a major cause of insulin resistance and, apart from very few exceptions, cats with feline hypersomatotropism suffer from diabetes mellitus. Currently, more and more veterinarians are investigating possible acromegaly when they establish the diagnosis of diabetes mellitus in a cat. Until recently, however, hypersomatotropism was only suspected in cats with poorly controlled diabetes mellitus with standard doses of insulin. In cats, tests for hypersomatotropism were only performed after ruling out technical issues which were related, for example, with the administration and storage of insulin, and after ruling out other causes of insulin resistance, such as hyperthyroidism, hyperadrenocorticism, infections and inflammation, iatrogenic causes (for example, administration of corticosteroids), neoplasms and a whole series of concomitant diseases (renal, pancreatic, hepatic or cardiac insufficiencies, among other pathologies).

The differentiation of feline hyperadrenocorticism, which usually also causes diabetes mellitus, is based in part on the clinical characteristics that differentiate both conditions: clinical signs such as friable skin, changes in the coat and ecchymosis are typical of cats with hyperadrenocorticism but are not common in hypersomatotropism. In addition to the above, serum IGF-1 measurement and a low dose dexamethasone suppression test (LDDST) can help distinguish between both pathologies.

Diagnostic Imaging (CT, MRI)

Although a mass in the pituitary gland can be detected with CT or MRI, **in more than 95% of cases with hypersomatotropism these imaging modalities alone are not enough to establish a final diagnosis**, because sometimes pituitary tumours can be incidental findings or can secrete other hormones. In addition, in the initial phase of diagnosis the images obtained in some cats may be irrelevant.

Serum Concentration of Insulin Like Growth Factor

There are commercial kits available for analysis of insulin like growth factor (IGF-1) by rapid immunoassay or ELISA. Significantly high serum concentrations (greater than 1000 ng/ml) or concentrations in the upper half of the normal range are compatible with acromegaly, although occasionally false positive results are obtained. A low serum IGF-1 concentration makes acromegaly unlikely, although it does not rule it out completely.

Treatment and Prognosis

There are **medical, surgical, and radiological treatment options** for feline acromegaly, each with pros and cons. Therefore, the treatment of choice will depend on the cat's condition, owner concerns, cost, and availability of treatment options.

Although there is little information available to establish an accurate prognosis, many cats treated with insulin alone die from poorly controlled diabetes mellitus or complications or comorbidities related to acromegaly. Their life expectancy varies from a few weeks to several years.

Surgery

Transsphenoidal hypophysectomy or cryohypophysectomy techniques have been described to treat cats with acromegaly but are procedures available at only a few specialised centres worldwide.

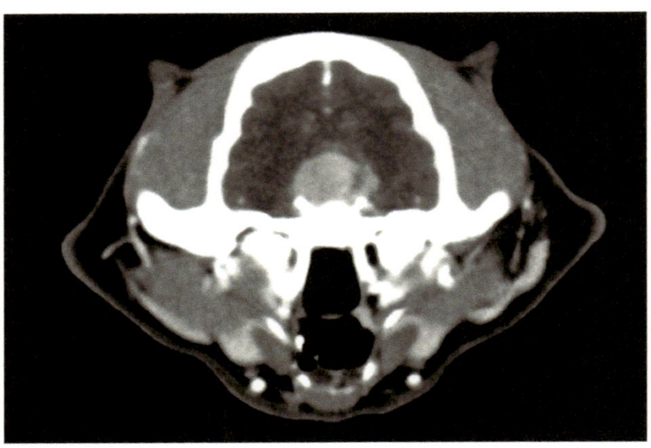

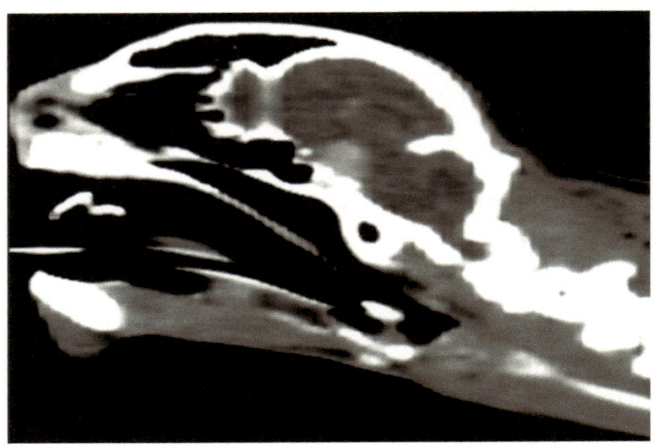

Figure 8. Two images of a CT where a macro pituitary adenoma is seen in a cat.

After the procedure, serum growth hormone concentrations drop rapidly, and insulin demand is reduced by more than 90% within seven days of the procedures and usually insulin is no longer needed three to four weeks after. Desmopressin should be administered in the ventral conjunctival sac for three weeks and the cat usually needs supplementation with cortisone acetate and L-thyroxine for the rest of its life. The intrasurgical and perisurgical mortality rate is approximately 10%.

Radiotherapy

Radiotherapeutic options are conventional fractional teletherapy or stereotactic radiotherapy, both of which are increasingly widespread.

- **Conventional fractional teletherapy** with linear accelerator (for example 10 fractions in total, 3 fractions per week) usually manages to reduce the pituitary tumour and alleviate possible neurological signs. Radiation usually leads to normalisation of high serum growth hormone concentrations, although the onset of this normalisation is unpredictable. The vast majority of cats end up with improved diabetic control or even the remission of diabetes mellitus. Despite the diabetic remission, paradoxically the IGF-1 concentrations often remain elevated and therefore cannot be used to assess response to treatment. In addition, in some cats physical changes related to acromegaly continue to progress despite improving diabetic control. Conventional radiation therapy is expensive, time consuming and requires prolonged hospitalisation, as well as repeated treatments under general anaesthesia.
- **Stereotactic radiation therapy** generates very high doses of radiation in just 1–4 fractions. To date, studies document improved diabetic control in most patients; approximately one third of cats in one study achieved complete remission of diabetes. 14% developed hypothyroidism as a result of radiation, requiring supplementation with thyroxine. In the same study, the median survival time was 1072 days.

Medical Treatment

Medical options are the **treatment of complications and comorbidities** related to acromegaly (for example, cardiac or joint pathologies), as well as the **treatment of diabetes mellitus and/or acromegaly**.

Treatment of diabetes mellitus also involves continuing high doses of parenteral insulin. While this is probably the most economical option, success is variable and involves life threatening risks, such as iatrogenic hypoglycaemia.

Medical treatment of hypersomatotropism is likely to become increasingly widespread. Recent studies have shown promising results and improved diabetic control with parenteral pasireotide (Signifor® and Signifor® LAR, Novartis), a somatostatin analogue. Currently, this drug is prohibitively expensive.

Canine Hypersomatotropism or Acromegaly

Unlike in cats, **in dogs acromegaly is usually caused by an endogenous secretion of progesterone or exogenous administration of a progestin**, which stimulate the secretion of growth hormone in the mammary gland. The cause is only rarely a growth hormone secreting adenoma in the pituitary gland. It is usually accompanied by organomegaly and/or diabetes mellitus.

Treatment is aimed at the underlying cause:

- for progesterone mediated acromegaly, appropriate treatment consists of an ovariectomy or progesterone receptor blockers; and
- in cases of acromegaly of pituitary origin, radiotherapy or hypophysectomy may be considered.

Hyperadrenocorticism

Canine Hyperadrenocorticism

Hyperadrenocorticism **is characterised by a constantly elevated concentration of cortisol in serum**. It can be caused by pituitary adenoma (or, more rarely, pituitary hyperplasia) that autonomously produces an excess of adrenocorticotropic hormone (ACTH), which causes bilateral secondary hyperplasia of the adrenal glands and cortisol secretion. This hyperadrenocorticism is the so called pituitary dependent type and constitutes more than 80% of the cases of canine hyperadrenocorticism.

Less commonly (15–20%) hyperadrenocorticism may be caused by a primary adrenal tumour, either benign or malignant (50% in each case) that autonomously secretes cortisol (adrenal dependent hyperadrenocorticism). This causes suppression of ACTH secretion in the pituitary and atrophy of normal cortical tissue of the contralateral gland. Occasionally, bilateral adrenal tumours also appear.

Older small breed dogs (over six years) are predisposed to this disease. There is no obvious sex predisposition. Signs that commonly occur are polyuria/polydipsia (greater than 90%), polyphagia, weight gain, panting, hepatomegaly, abdominal distension, muscle atrophy, dermatological disorders (such as alopecia, comedones, hyperpigmentation or thin skin). However, the severity of clinical signs varies greatly.

The diagnostic approach is based on an initial clinical suspicion based on clinical history and compatible clinical signs, as well as laboratory results suggesting disease (e.g. stress leukogram, mild thrombocytosis, elevated alkaline phosphatase, hypercholesterolaemia, or proteinuria). In other cases, the finding of unilateral or bilateral adrenal dilation on an ultrasound or abdominal CT scan (Figure 9) may lead to other diagnostic steps.

Differential diagnoses for an adrenal mass are endocrine tumours of the medulla or cortex, non-functional tumours ("incidentaloma"), myelolipoma, cyst, abscess, haematoma, and metastasis. Diagnosis is established by applying one or more screening tests (ACTH stimulation test, low dose dexamethasone suppression test, urine cortisol:creatinine ratio). **Any concomitant disease must be treated and cured before these screening tests are used**, since any concurrent pathology outside the adrenals can generate false positive results and make it difficult or even impossible to interpret the tests. Once the diagnosis of hyperadrenocorticism has been established, there are additional tests (e.g. endogenous serum ACTH analysis, high dose dexamethasone suppression test, and abdominal ultrasound) to differentiate between pituitary dependent hyperadrenocorticism or one due to an adrenal tumour. This differentiation is important because the treatment and prognosis of both forms of hyperadrenocorticism are different.

The median survival is significantly higher in treated dogs than in untreated dogs, in part due to a whole host of possible secondary complications (such as urinary tract infections, recurrent pyoderma, hypertension, thromboembolism etc.).

In the case of pituitary dependent hyperadrenocorticism there are **medical, surgical, and radiological treatment options**.

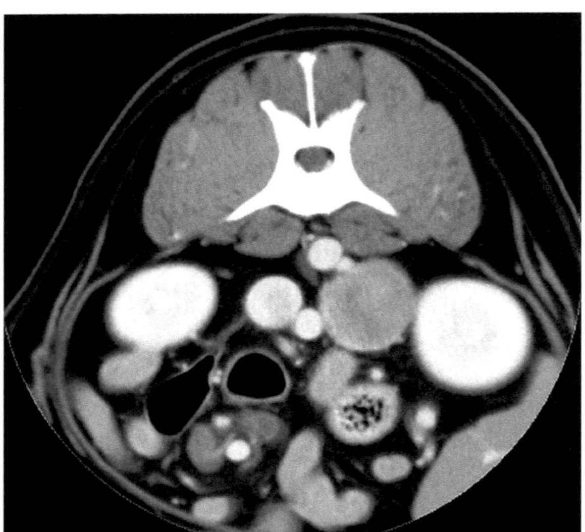

Figure 9. CT image from a dog where a 6 cm mass was observed in the left adrenal gland stained heterogeneously by the contrast.

A surgical hypophysectomy of the pituitary microadenomas may also be performed, but this treatment is only available at a very few specialised centres. Radiation therapy is usually reserved for pituitary macroadenomas that cause clinical (neurological) signs.

Currently, the treatment of choice in most dogs with pituitary dependent hyperadrenocorticism is trilostane (Vetoryl®, starting dose 1–5 mg/kg once or twice daily PO). **Trilostane** inhibits an enzyme (3 -hydroxysteroid dehydrogenase) essential for cortisol synthesis. After several months of treatment, clinical signs are fully or partially controlled in most dogs (more than 75%). The dose of trilostane is adjusted based on the clinical signs and results of the ACTH stimulation test. Generally, it is a well-tolerated drug, although it can cause gastrointestinal adverse effects and hypoadrenocorticism. Therefore, during treatment it is essential to monitor electrolyte concentrations.

Mitotane (Lysodren®) selectively destroys glucocorticoid secreting cells in the adrenal cortex. The glomerulosa area of the adrenal cortex, which secretes aldosterone, is reasonably safe. Mitotane treatment consists of an induction phase lasting one to two weeks, followed by a maintenance phase. Use of the drug is not widespread, and it is not used to treat pituitary dependent hyperadrenocorticism.

To treat hyperadrenocorticism caused by an adrenal tumour, the patient first needs to be stabilised with trilostane and then a unilateral adrenalectomy can be performed. Approximately 50% of dogs have intrasurgical or postsurgical complications (such as thromboembolism, pancreatitis, bleeding and disseminated intravascular coagulation). The average survival time after surgery is very variable (7 to 35 months).

Inoperable or metastatic tumours can be treated with mitotane at high doses if available, as it can even destroy metastatic tumour cells. Trilostane has also been used to control adrenal dependent hyperadrenocorticism. Although it does not destroy tumour cells, in one study the median survival time of dogs treated with this drug (14 months) was not significantly different from that of dogs treated with mitotane (15.6 months).

Feline Hyperadrenocorticism

Hyperadrenocorticism **is an unusual disorder in cats**. As in dogs, feline hyperadrenocorticism can also occur in two forms: pituitary dependent (80%) and adrenal origin (20%).

The clinical signs are similar to those of dogs with hyperadrenocorticism. However, the vast majority (more than 80%) of cats with hyperadrenocorticism also have diabetes mellitus, due to insulin resistance caused by excess cortisol. In addition, in cats it is frequent for fragile skin syndrome to appear. The screening test of choice is the low dose dexamethasone suppression test. There is evidence of differentiation using this test as described for canine hyperadrenocorticism. Trilostane (e.g. 10–60 mg/cat/day) has been successfully used to treat feline hyperadrenocorticism. A unilateral or bilateral adrenalectomy can also be considered.

Pheochromocytoma

Pheochromocytoma is caused by a **chromaffin cell tumour of the adrenal medulla, which produces an excess of catecholamines**. This tumour is uncommon in dogs and extraordinarily rare in cats. It most frequently affects older dogs (mean age 11 years old, range 7–16 years).

Usually, clinical signs are non-specific or absent, or episodic. When they occur, they consist of weakness, polyuria/polydipsia, nervousness, tachypnoea, tachyarrhythmias, collapses and convulsions. Initially, there is only hypertension (more than 160 mg Hg systolic blood pressure) in 50% of dogs, due to a paroxysmal secretion of hormones. Routine clinical tests are often normal or barely reveal any non-specific results (mild nonregenerative anaemia, leucocytosis, mild increase in pancreatic enzymes, moderate hyperglycaemia etc.).

Often pheochromocytoma only appears as a possible diagnosis after detection of an adrenal mass on an ultrasound scan. The definitive diagnosis is based on the histological evaluation of the adrenal mass, although a presumptive diagnosis can be made before the intervention, based on the finding of an adrenal tumour, on ultrasound, or a CT scan, ruling out other adrenal endocrinopathies and documenting a very high ratio of normetanephrine:creatinine in urine in dogs (four times normal levels).

In dogs, at least 50% of pheochromocytomas are malignant. The size of the tumours varies greatly (0.5 to more than 10 cm) and in more than 60% of cases the right adrenal is affected. Bilateral involvement is rare (5%). Typically, pheochromocytoma is locally invasive, affecting retroperitoneal tissues, including blood vessels (e.g. caudal vena cava). The points of metastasis are usually abdominal organs, regional lymph nodes and lungs.

The treatment of choice for nonmetastatic pheochromocytoma is **unilateral adrenalectomy** by laparotomy or laparoscopy. Depending on the size and invasiveness of the tumour, the technique may be difficult or even impossible. Surgical removal of a pheochromocytoma involves a number of intrasurgical and postsurgical risks, such as hypertension or hypotension, tachyarrhythmias, dyspnoea, haemorrhages, and disseminated intravascular coagulation (DIC). Therefore, starting phenoxybenzamine treatment (0.5 mg/kg twice daily; an α-antagonist), two days before surgery is recommended, which improves survival rates. One study showed that phenoxybenzamine reverses vasoconstriction and hypovolaemia and significantly reduces the mortality rate relative to untreated dogs. In another study, dogs that were still alive fourteen days after the procedure achieved 1-, 2- and 3-year survival rates of 83%, 60% and 60% respectively.

Dogs with **inoperable or metastatic pheochromocytomas have a reserved to poor prognosis**. Some dogs respond to toceranib phosphate treatment (2.5–2.8 mg/kg every other day, PO; Palladia®, Zoetis). In a recent series of cases, the clinical signs were stabilised in four out of five dogs for 11 to 36 weeks and one of them experienced a partial remission that lasted more than a year.

Feline Primary Hyperaldosteronism (Conn Syndrome)

Feline primary hyperaldosteronism (FPH) **is currently considered the most common feline adrenocortical disorder, however, in dogs it is very rare**. It is almost always caused by a functional adrenal neoplasm, capable of secreting aldosterone (adenocarcinoma) autonomously. It is rarely the result of bilateral functional adrenal hyperplasia. It almost always affects middle aged or older cats and there does not seem to be a sex or breed predisposition.

The clinical syndrome is characterised by hypokalaemia, which causes polymyopathy and/or systemic hypertension and organ damage. Hypokalaemic polymyopathy manifests itself in the form of generalised muscle weakness, plantigrade posture in the hindlimbs, inability to jump and/or respiratory failure. Systemic hypertension may exist as an incidental finding or may even cause blindness due to, for example, intraocular haemorrhage and/or retinal detachment. Hypertension can damage the kidneys, heart, or brain, which in turn leads to new clinical problems.

The diagnostic process is initiated upon detection of hypokalaemia, systemic hypertension and/or an adrenal mass (Figure 10). It is characteristic for cats with FPH to exhibit high plasma aldosterone concentrations and low plasma renin activity. Currently, the possibility of measuring plasma renin activity is not widely available. Therefore, the most practical way to substantiate the diagnosis is to document a normal or high concentration of aldosterone in plasma in the presence of hypokalaemia, while ruling out pathologies associated with secondary hyperaldosteronism (for example, renal failure).

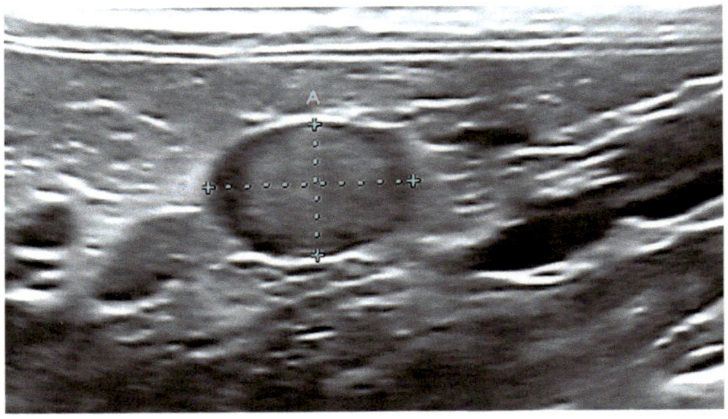

Figure 10. Ultrasound where an increase in size of the left adrenal gland can be seen in a cat with primary hyperaldosteronism.

Other diagnostic tests (aldosterone:creatinine ratio in urine, fludrocortisone suppression test) have been suggested, but their use is not widespread, and they are often not necessary to establish the diagnosis.

The **treatment of choice for FPH caused by a unilateral tumour is unilateral adrenalectomy** (Figure 11). Hypokalaemia and hypertension should be corrected before the procedure. Since the contralateral adrenal gland may be atrophied, some authors advocate perisurgical and postsurgical therapy with fludrocortisone. Usually, the prognosis for cats which are discharged is excellent. For medical treatment of a bilateral case administration of potassium gluconate orally and spironolactone (2–4 mg/kg/day PO) to treat hypokalaemia is recommended. Systemic hypertension can be treated with amlodipine besylate (0.125–0.250 mg/kg/day PO). Cases refractory to this treatment may be treated using bilateral adrenalectomy followed by medical treatment of the cat's hypocortisolism (Addison's disease) for the rest of its life.

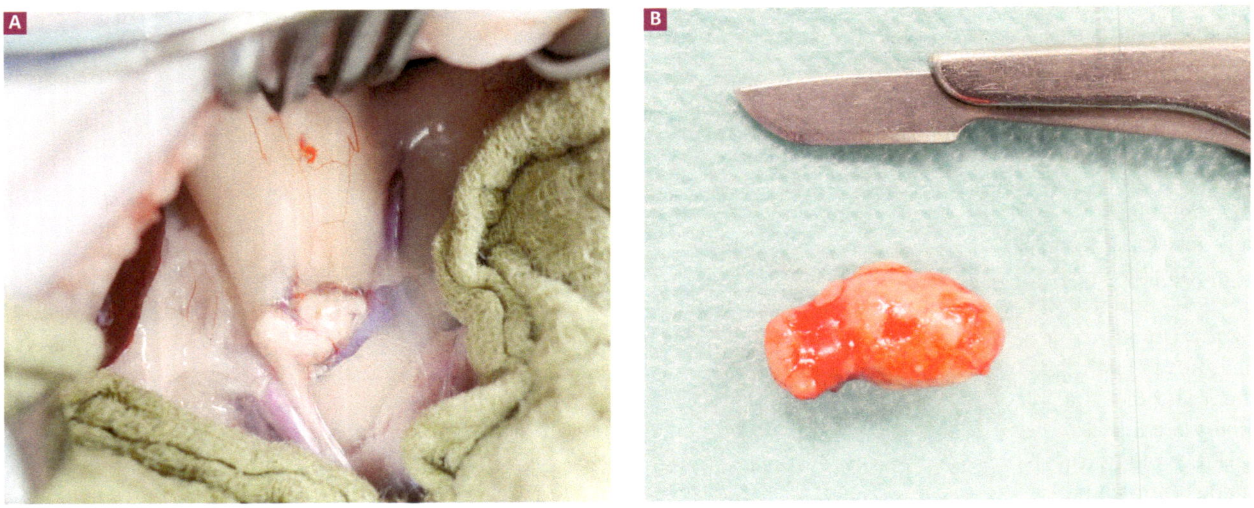

Figure 11. Intraoperative image of a unilateral adrenal mass in a cat with primary hyperaldosteronism (**A**). Resection of the adrenal gland (**B**) is performed without complications.

Bibliography

- Buishand F.O., Vilaplana Grosso F.R., Kirpensteijn J., van Nimwegen S.A. (2018) Utility of contrast-enhanced computed tomography in the evaluation of canine insulinoma location. *The veterinary quarterly*. 38(1):53–62.
- Campos M., Ducatelle R., Rutteman G., Kooistra H.S., Duchateau L., de Rooster H., et al. (2014) Clinical, pathologic, and immunohistochemical prognostic factors in dogs with thyroid carcinoma. *Journal of veterinary internal medicine*. 28(6):1805–13.
- Dear J.D., Kass P.H., Della Maggiore A.M., Feldman E.C. (2017) Association of Hypercalcemia Before Treatment With Hypocalcemia After Treatment in Dogs With Primary Hyperparathyroidism. *Journal of veterinary internal medicine*. 31(2):349–54.
- Deitz K., Gilmour L., Wilke V., Riedesel E. (2014) Computed tomographic appearance of canine thyroid tumours. *The Journal of small animal practice*. 55(6):323–9.
- Feldman E.C., Nelson R.W., Reusch C., Scott-Moncrieff J.C.R. (2015) *Canine & feline endocrinology*. Fourth edition. ed. St. Louis, Missouri: Elsevier Saunders; xi, p. 669
- Goutal C.M., Brugmann B.L., Ryan K.A. (2012) Insulinoma in dogs: a review. *Journal of the American Animal Hospital Association*. 48(3):151–63.
- Herrera M.A., Mehl M.L., Kass P.H., Pascoe P.J., Feldman E.C., Nelson R.W. (2008) Predictive factors and the effect of phenoxybenzamine on outcome in dogs undergoing adrenalectomy for pheochromocytoma. *Journal of veterinary internal medicine*. 22(6):1333–9.
- Hibbert A., Gruffydd-Jones T., Barrett E.L., Day M.J., Harvey A.M. (2009) Feline thyroid carcinoma: diagnosis and response to high-dose radioactive iodine treatment. *Journal of feline medicine and surgery*. 11(2):116–24.
- Kook P.H., Boretti F.S., Hersberger M., Glaus T.M., Reusch C.E. (2007) Urinary catecholamine and metanephrine to creatinine ratios in healthy dogs at home and in a hospital environment and in 2 dogs with pheochromocytoma. *Journal of veterinary internal medicine*. 21(3):388–93.
- Leal R.O., Frau Pascual L., Hernandez J. (2018) The Use of Percutaneous Ultrasound-Guided Radiofrequency Heat Ablation for Treatment of Primary Hyperparathyroidism in Eight Dogs: Outcome and Complications. *Veterinary sciences*. 5(4).
- Miller M.L., Peterson M.E., Randolph J.F., Broome M.R., Norsworthy G.D., Rishniw M. (2017) Thyroid Cysts in Cats: A Retrospective Study of 40 Cases. *Journal of veterinary internal medicine*. 31(3):723–9.
- Milovancev M., Schmiedt C.W. (2013) Preoperative factors associated with postoperative hypocalcemia in dogs with primary hyperparathyroidism that underwent parathyroidectomy: 62 cases (2004–2009). *Journal of the American Veterinary Medical Association*. 242(4):507–15.
- Nakamura K., Lim S.Y., Ochiai K., Yamasaki M., Ohta H., Morishita K., et al. (2015) Contrast-enhanced ultrasonographic findings in three dogs with pancreatic insulinoma. *Veterinary radiology & ultrasound: the official journal of the American College of Veterinary Radiology and the International Veterinary Radiology Association*. 56(1):55–62.
- Niessen S.J., Church D.B., Forcada Y. (2013) Hypersomatotropism, acromegaly, and hyperadrenocorticism and feline diabetes mellitus. *The Veterinary clinics of North America small animal practice*. 43(2):319–50.
- Polton G.A., White R.N., Brearley M.J., Eastwood J.M. (2007) Improved survival in a retrospective cohort of 28 dogs with insulinoma. *The Journal of small animal practice*. 48(3):151–6.
- Rasor L., Pollard R., Feldman E.C. (2007) Retrospective evaluation of three treatment methods for primary hyperparathyroidism in dogs. *Journal of the American Animal Hospital Association*. 43(2):70–7.
- Robben J.H., Pollak Y.W., Kirpensteijn J., Boroffka S.A., van den Ingh T.S., Teske E., et al. (2005) Comparison of ultrasonography, computed tomography, and single-photon emission computed tomography for the detection and localization of canine insulinoma. *Journal of veterinary internal medicine*. 19(1):15–22.
- Salesov E., Boretti F.S., Sieber-Ruckstuhl N.S., Rentsch K.M., Riond B., Hofmann-Lehmann R., et al. (2015) Urinary and plasma catecholamines and metanephrines in dogs with pheochromocytoma, hypercortisolism, nonadrenal disease and in healthy dogs. *Journal of veterinary internal medicine*. 29(2):597–602.
- Schulman R.L. (2010) Feline primary hyperaldosteronism. *The veterinary clinics of North America small animal practice*. 40(2):353–9.
- Scudder C.J., Gostelow R., Forcada Y., Schmid H.A., Church D., Niessen S.J. (2015) Pasireotide for the Medical Management of Feline Hypersomatotropism. *Journal of veterinary internal medicine*. 29(4):1074–80.
- Tuohy J.L., Worley D.R., Withrow S.J. (2012) Outcome following simultaneous bilateral thyroid lobectomy for treatment of thyroid gland carcinoma in dogs: 15 cases (1994–2010). *Journal of the American Veterinary Medical Association*. 241(1):95–103.
- Worth A.J., Zuber R.M., Hocking M. (2005) Radioiodide (131I) therapy for the treatment of canine thyroid carcinoma. *Australian veterinary journal*. 83(4):208–14.
- Zini E., Nolli S., Ferri F., Massari F., Gerardi G., Nicoli S., et al. (2019) Pheochromocytoma in Dogs Undergoing Adrenalectomy. *Veterinary pathology*. 56(3):358–68.

Test

Answers on page 394

1. **Thyroid tumours are the most frequent endocrine neoplasms in canines. What percentage of the total number of tumours in the dog do they represent?**
   a. 3–5%.
   b. 1–4%.
   c. 5–10%
   d. The statement is incorrect, they are not the most frequent.

2. **Regarding the metastatic capacity of canine thyroid tumours, which of the following answers is correct:**
   a. Up to 40% of cases already show evidence of metastasis at initial diagnosis.
   b. Tumour size hardly influences the rate of metastasis.
   c. Unilateral tumours tend to metastasise more frequently.
   d. At diagnosis the number of cases with metastases does not reach 15%.

3. **Hyperthyroidism is the most common feline endocrinopathy. Which of the following statements about this disease is false?**
   a. It is usually caused by unilateral or bilateral adenomatous hyperplasia of the thyroid glands.
   b. Malignant feline thyroid tumours are rare and constitute less than 5% of thyroid tumours.
   c. In treated cats, benign hyperthyroidism does not progress from adenoma to carcinoma.
   d. Thyroid carcinomas appear in older cats with a long history of benign hyperthyroidism.

4. **Primary hyperparathyroidism is an endocrine disorder characterised by the autonomous secretion of parathyroid hormone (PTH) by...**
   a. ...an adenoma (80%), a hyperplastic nodule (10–12%) or, more rarely, by a carcinoma (8–10%) of the main cells of one or two parathyroid glands.
   b. ...an adenoma (85%), a hyperplastic nodule (10–12%) or, more rarely, a carcinoma (3–5%) of the main cells of one or two parathyroid glands.
   c. ...an adenoma (75%), a hyperplastic nodule (15–17%) or, more rarely, a carcinoma (8–10%) of the main cells of one or two parathyroid glands.
   d. ...an adenoma (95%), a hyperplastic nodule (5–7%) or, more rarely, a carcinoma (3–5%) of the main cells of a parathyroid gland.

5. **Regarding the diagnosis of primary hyperparathyroidism in dogs, what is the correct answer?**
   a. Dogs with primary hyperparathyroidism have high concentrations of total calcium and serum ionised calcium is at normal levels.
   b. Serum phosphorus concentrations are normal or low.
   c. Dogs with this problem have normal total calcium and ionised calcium concentrations, but normal or low phosphorus concentrations.
   d. Canine patients with primary hyperparathyroidism have high concentrations of total calcium, ionised calcium, and serum phosphorus.

6. **Regarding primary hyperparathyroidism in cats, which answer is incorrect:**
   a. Primary feline hyperparathyroidism is rare.
   b. Cats with hypercalcaemia are unlikely to have polyuria and polydipsia.
   c. Normal parathyroid glands are not visible on ultrasound.
   d. The treatment of choice for this disease is conservative since surgery poses an unacceptable risk and does not improve the patient's quality of life.

7. **Canine insulinoma is a rare tumour, what is its most frequent origin?**
   a. An adenoma.
   b. A pancreatic endocrine β-cell carcinoma.
   c. Metastasis of a malignant liver tumour.
   d. In most cases, the origin is unknown.

8. **How can the presence of an insulinoma in a dog be confirmed?**
   a. This type of tumour can be detected on ultrasound in more than 70% of cases.
   b. Detecting elevated serum insulin concentrations or levels in the upper half of the normal range, while the animal has moderate to severe hypoglycaemia.
   c. Combined ultrasound and CT are diagnostic in 100% of cases.
   d. Detecting elevated serum insulin concentrations and blood glucose greater than 70 mg/dl.

9. What nonsurgical treatments can be used in a dog or cat with insulinoma?

a. Dietary treatment aimed at controlling hypoglycaemia and the clinical signs associated with it.
b. Pharmacological treatment with glucocorticoids, diazoxide or both.
c. First line treatment with prednisolone.
d. The above three options are correct.

10. What is the most common cause of feline acromegaly?

a. It is usually idiopathic.
b. An adenoma in the distal region of the anterior pituitary.
c. A liver tumour formed of IGF-1 producing cells.
d. A thyroid gland tumour.

11. What is taken into account when diagnosing a cat suffering from acromegaly?

a. All other causes of poor glycaemic control should be ruled out in cases of diabetes mellitus.
b. Whether there is identification of a mass in the pituitary gland by imaging (CT or MRI).
c. Documentation of elevated serum IGF-1 concentrations.
d. The above three signs must be present to confirm a diagnosis of feline hypersomatotropism.

12. What is the most common cause of canine hypersomatotropism?

a. An adenoma in the distal region of the anterior pituitary.
b. Endogenous progesterone secretion or endogenous administration of a progestin.
c. A liver tumour formed of IGF-1 producing cells.
d. A thyroid gland tumour.

13. Regarding canine hyperadrenocorticism, which statement is correct?

a. It is characterised by elevations in serum cortisol dependent on food ingestion.
b. Pituitary dependent canine hyperadrenocorticism accounts for up to 70% of cases of this disease.
c. Hyperadrenocorticism can be caused in 15–20% of cases in the dog by a benign or malignant primary adrenal tumour.
d. Middle aged dogs (up to six years) and small or toy breeds are predisposed to suffering from this problem.

14. Feline hyperadrenocorticism is an unusual disorder. Which of the following answers is incorrect?

a. It occurs in the same two forms as in the dog: pituitary dependent (80% of cases) or of adrenal origin (20%).
b. The clinical signs are similar to those of hyperadrenocorticism in dogs.
c. Only 20% of cats with hyperadrenocorticism have diabetes mellitus.
d. The screening test of choice is the low dose dexamethasone suppression test.

15. Which of the following is the correct answer, regarding pheochromocytoma?

a. It is a more common tumour in cats than in dogs, although it is very rare in both species.
b. Neurological clinical signs occur in all diseased animals, consistently.
c. It is not usually a malignant tumour in the dog: only 15% of canine pheochromocytomas are.
d. It is caused by a chromaffin cell tumour of the adrenal medulla, which produces an excess of catecholamines.

16. Which of the following answers is incorrect?

a. Feline primary hyperaldosteronism (FPH) is considered the most common feline adrenocortical disorder.
b. FPH is often the result of bilateral functional adrenal hyperplasia.
c. The clinical syndrome caused by FPH is characterised by hypokalaemia, which causes polymyopathy and/or systemic hypertension and organ damage.
d. The treatment of choice for FPH caused by a unilateral tumour is unilateral adrenalectomy.

Correct Answers:

1. b
2. a
3. c
4. b
5. b
6. d
7. b
8. b
9. d
10. b
11. d
12. b
13. c
14. c
15. d
16. b

Notes

Cytological Diagnosis of Neoplastic Processes

Antonio Meléndez Lazo

Cytology is a **fundamental tool for the diagnosis of neoplastic processes**. Information about lesions can be obtained quickly, noninvasively and with minimal expense.

It is important that interpretation of cytological samples is carried out by experienced personnel who are up to date with the latest knowledge in the field to ensure optimal results from this test, since in many cases there may be false negatives and positives that put the patient at risk and complicate the clinical management of the case.

It should always be considered that cytological preparations examine a very small part of lesions and that, at times, the cells that are seen under a microscope may not be representative of the lesion. Therefore, although cytology is very useful as a first approach for the management of neoplasms, confirming the diagnosis by biopsy and histopathological examination in most cases is recommended.

In this chapter the factors that influence the results of cytology, the handling of samples, the classification of neoplastic lesions and the characteristics of the most frequent neoplasms that affect the different body systems are reviewed, although it is not possible to cover them all in detail due to the extensive nature of the topic. For information on the clinical presentation and behaviour of different lesions, the reader is referred to the corresponding chapters.

Author's note. All cytologies are stained with a modified Romanowsky stain, unless otherwise noted in the figure caption. In the images in which the scale bar is not shown, the lens magnification used is indicated in the figure caption.

Sample Handling: Cytological Preparation Quality

Cytological interpretation depends to a large extent on the quality of the preparations to be examined and on the means used for the microscopic examination. Important factors include:

- obtaining a **representative sample**: when masses are detected by touch or through imaging tests in different areas, samples must be taken from all of them;
- **extension on the slide**: excessive pressure can break the cells, making evaluation impossible (Figure 1). Similarly, insufficient extension results in excessively thick samples that do not allow evaluation of cell morphology;
- **staining**: there is no universal protocol for staining cytological preparations, although poor quality stains can lead to insufficient staining of cells, making it difficult to visualise cellular details;
- **storage**: exposure to formaldehyde vapours (Figure 2), direct sunlight or keeping the preparations unfixed for

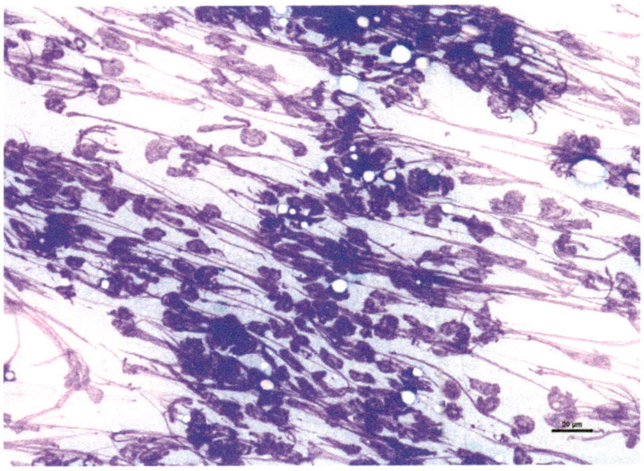

Figure 1. Lymph node sample showing damaged cells.

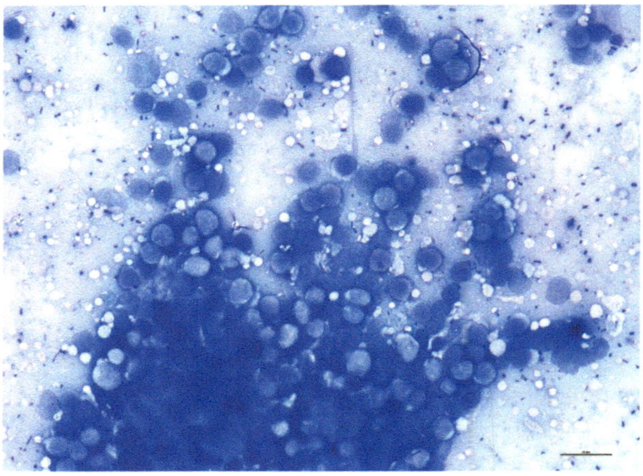

Figure 2. Incorrect staining of a lymph node cytology due to exposure to formaldehyde fumes.

long periods may hinder subsequent staining or degrade the samples; and
- **microscope**: the use of quality microscopes allows better visualisation of the cells and, therefore, a better interpretation of the cytological findings.

Sampling and Types of Preparations

Fine Needle Puncture/Biopsy

In most cases, sampling is performed using needles. The needle size should be large enough not to break the cells, but not too large, in order to minimise contamination with blood. The needle of choice is 23G for most lesions, although it is possible to successfully use 25G in small patients or lesions and 21G in large patients and/or non-exfoliating lesions.

- **Superficial (skin/subcutaneous) lesions**: it is important to immobilise the lesion and redirect the needle at least three times to take samples from different areas (Figure 3).
- **Deep lesions**: samples can be taken guided by ultrasound (Figure 4) or CT, preferably using longer needles (e.g. spinal needles) and with a stylet to prevent them from clogging with tissue between the skin surface and the lesion. "Blind sampling" is not recommended because of the risk of harm to the patient and the lower likelihood of sampling the target lesion.

Whether or not aspiration should be performed during needle sampling depends on several factors. **By default, aspiration is not recommended** to prevent haemodilution of the sample. In the case of not obtaining enough material without aspiration, the lesion should be aspirated (for example, in poorly exfoliating samples). Aspiration of internal organs or thyroid lesions is never recommended, as these locations are usually highly vascularised. Once the sample has been taken, a small amount should be deposited at the end of a clean slide and spread with another slide in a smooth manner, without sudden movements and without exerting much pressure (squash technique) (Figure 5).

Impression Smears

Impressions can be used to obtain samples of **flat and exudative lesions**, as well as to obtain rapid information from tissue samples obtained for histopathological study. It is important to remove excess blood from the tissues with a gauze or filter paper before pressing the tissue onto the slide, in order to minimise contamination with blood (Figure 6).

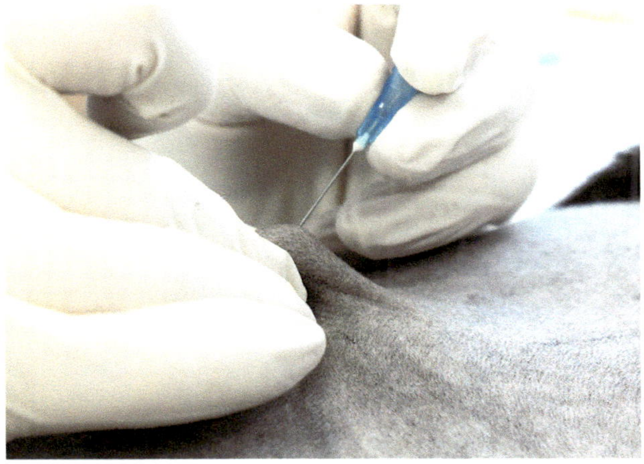

Figure 3. Firm immobilisation of a cutaneous nodule before performing a fine needle puncture.

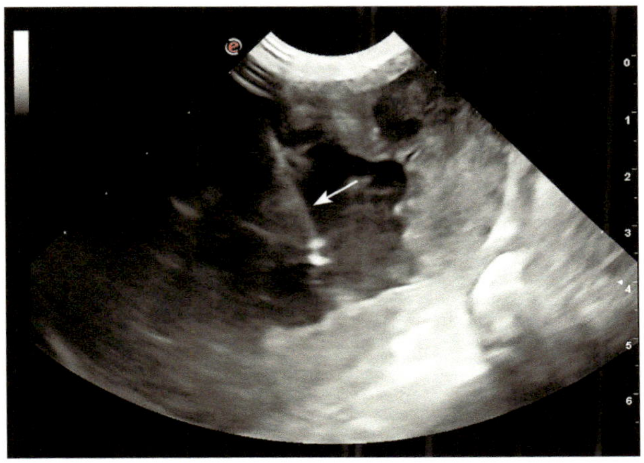

Figure 4. Ultrasound-guided puncture of a cavitated abdominal mass. The arrow indicates the location of the needle.

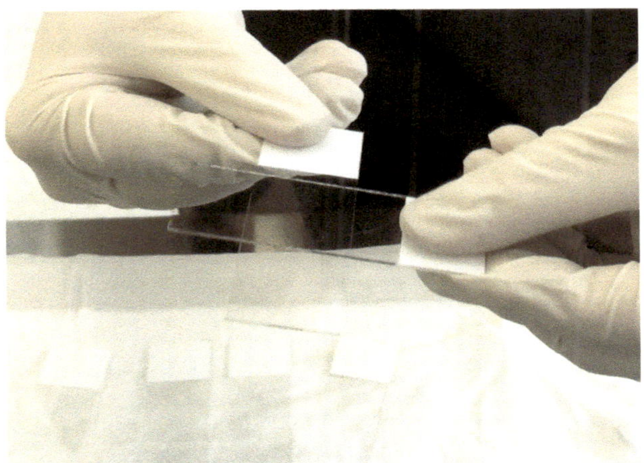

Figure 5. Squash technique for extension of cytological samples.

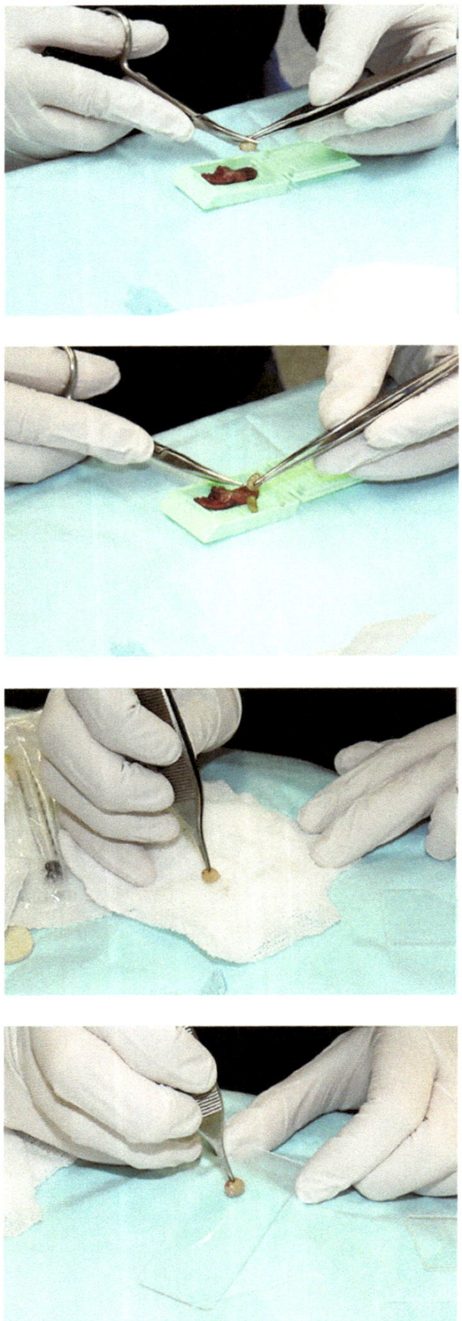

Figure 6. Steps showing how to perform an impression smear for cytology from a sample obtained using biopsy.

Fluid Handling

Although neoplasms may cause pleural, abdominal, and pericardial effusions, neoplastic cells are not always seen in the cytological examination of these fluids. Initially, the cellularity of the fluid should be measured using haematological analysers.

- If the fluid is **haemorrhagic**, it can be centrifuged in a microhaematocrit tube and the buffy coat examined, where most of the nucleated cells are located.
- If the fluid is of **low cellularity** (<15 000 cells/µl), the sample should be concentrated using cytocentrifuges or the fluid pellet should be examined.
- If the fluid is **very cellular**, examination of direct extensions should be sufficient.

Other Sample Types

- prostatic lavage
- bronchoalveolar lavage
- tracheal/bronchial brush
- traumatic urinary bladder catheterisation.

Malignancy Criteria: Neoplasm vs Non-neoplasm

Malignancy criteria are characteristics of the cell itself or of the nuclei that, when observed, suggest malignant behaviour of the lesions. The greatest challenge in interpreting these criteria is to differentiate reactive cell changes (dysplasia) from their neoplastic transformation, especially in the presence of inflammation.

The **differentiation between benign neoplasms, healthy tissue and hyperplasia is especially complicated**. It is important to know the normal appearance of cells of the different organs to be able to detect atypia in them (for example, hepatocytes normally have prominent nucleoli). In some cases, there is a tendency to count the number of malignancy criteria to make a diagnosis of malignancy. Caution should be exercised when using these criteria and they are only applicable if the studies describing the cytological findings have been compared with the histological results and a large number of patients have been included in the study.

Malignancy criteria can be classified into general or cellular and nuclear.

- General
  - **Anisocytosis**: cells of different sizes within the same cell population (Figure 7).
  - **Hypercellularity**: obtaining samples with more cells than expected for the organ from which the

sample was taken (for example, obtaining numerous lung epithelial cells).

- **Pleomorphism**: cells with very different shapes (Figure 7)
- **Cell cannibalism**: recently proposed, consists of the consumption of other neoplastic cells or inflammatory cells by the neoplasm to obtain energy that favours growth (Figure 8).

– Nuclear

- **Macronuclei and macronucleoli**: nuclei larger than whole cells from the same cell population and nucleoli larger than erythrocytes (Figure 9).
- **Increased nucleus/cytoplasm ratio**: larger nuclei and reduced cytoplasm (Figure 10).
- **Anisokaryosis**: nuclei of different sizes even within the same cell with more than one nucleus (Figure 11).
- **Multinucleated cells**: cells with more than one nucleus (Figure 12).
- **Increased numbers of mitotic figures and abnormal mitosis**: finding more mitosis than expected for the organ and presence of mitosis with abnormally distributed chromatin (Figure 13).
- **Coarse chromatin**: nuclei with a chromatin pattern with voids representing high nuclear activity (Figure 10).
- **Nuclear moulding**: nuclei deformed by the presence of other nuclei, indicating alteration of cell growth regulation mechanisms (Figure 14).
- **Irregular nucleoli and anisonucleolosis**: non-round nucleoli, with angular shapes and nucleoli of different sizes in the same nucleus (Figure 15).

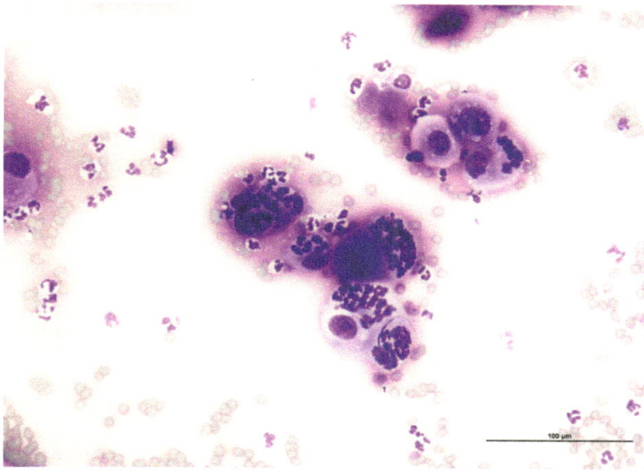

Figure 8. Metastasis of a squamous cell carcinoma where neoplastic cells accumulate neutrophils in the cytoplasm.

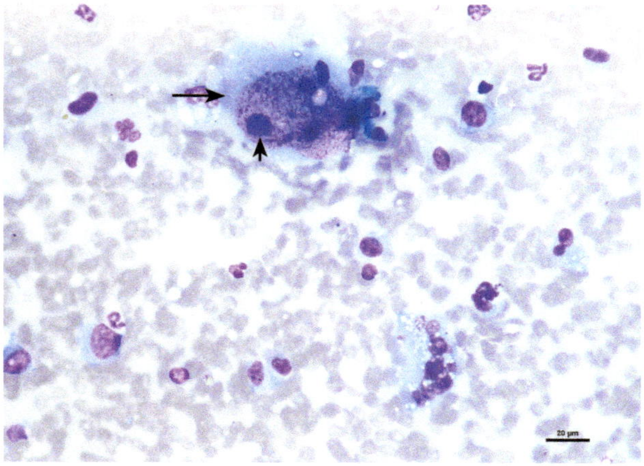

Figure 9. Macronucleus (large arrow) with macronucleolus (small arrow) from a histiocytic sarcoma.

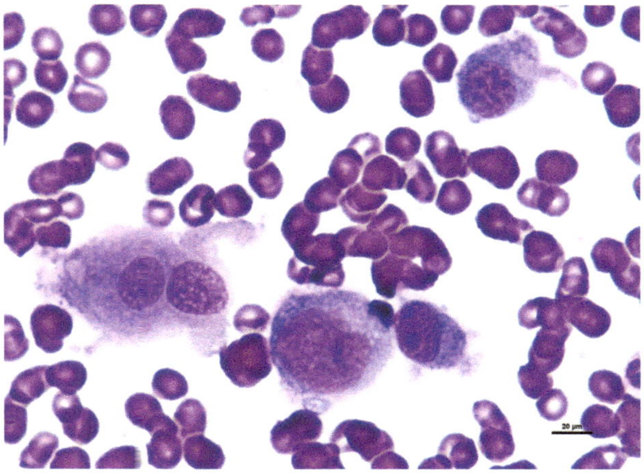

Figure 7. Cellular pleomorphism, anisocytosis and anisokaryosis in an amelanotic oral melanoma.

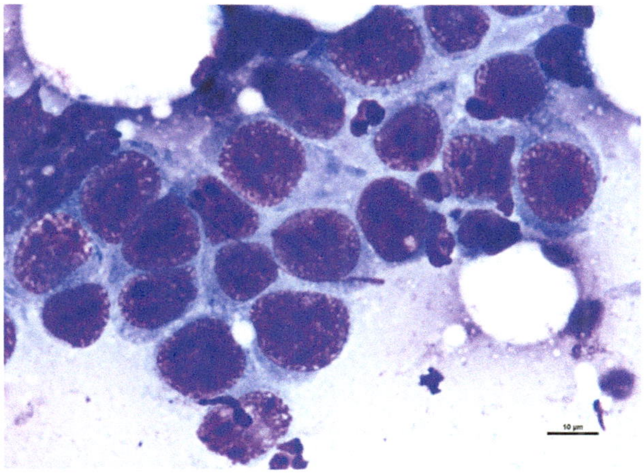

Figure 10. Malignant cutaneous neoplasia with a high nuclear/cytoplasm ratio and coarse chromatin.

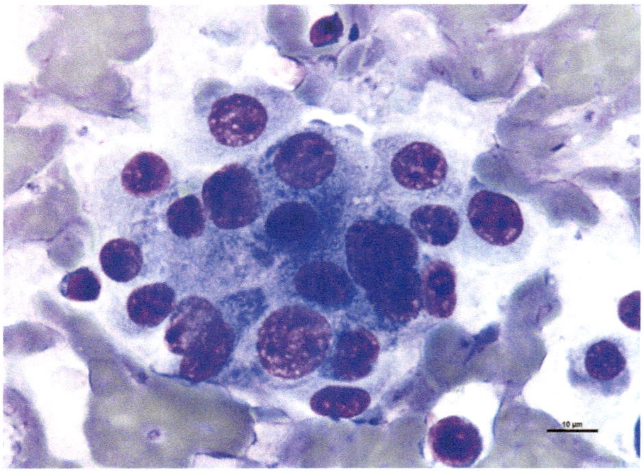

Figure 11. Anisokaryosis, prominent and multiple nucleoli in epithelial neoplasia.

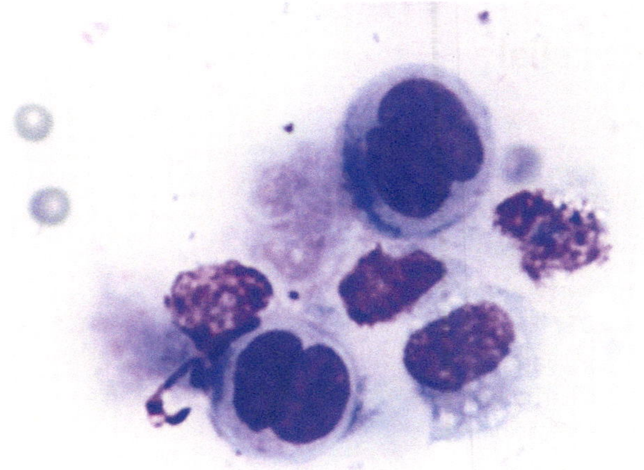

Figure 14. Two binuclear cells with nuclear moulding.

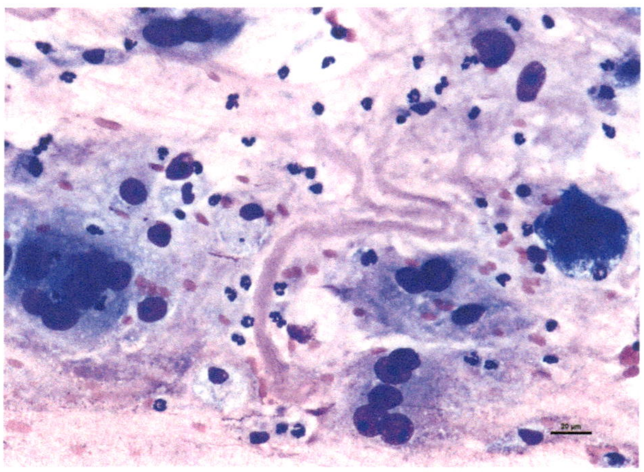

Figure 12. Multinucleated cells in malignant pulmonary neoplasia in a cat.

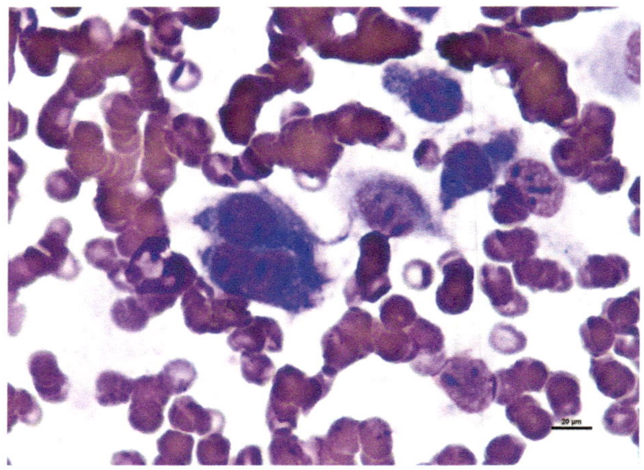

Figure 15. Prominent, multiple, and irregular nucleoli from an amelanotic melanoma.

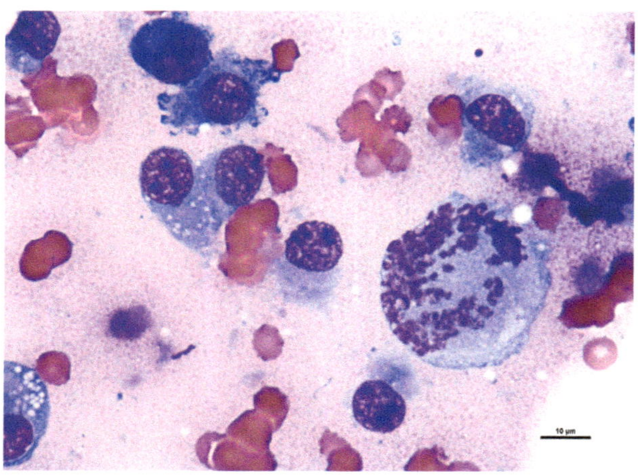

Figure 13. Atypical mitosis.

Classification of Neoplastic Lesions

Neoplasm categories are based on both the tissue of origin and, more importantly, morphological characteristics of the cells. Based on these characteristics, the clinical history and the location of the lesion, the objective is to shorten the list of possible differential diagnoses as much as possible.

Epithelial

Origin

Glandular or parenchymal tissue, lining surfaces.

Characteristics

- exfoliation in aggregates of cohesive cells or sheets
- cell arrangement pattern: pavement, honeycomb (Figure 16), acinar/pseudoacinar, palisade (Figure 17), papillary (Figure 18), trabecular
- cells attached to each other can form desmosomes (intercellular junctions)
- large, round to polygonal cells with generally well-defined cell borders
- examples: adenoma, carcinoma, mesothelioma, trichoblastoma etc.

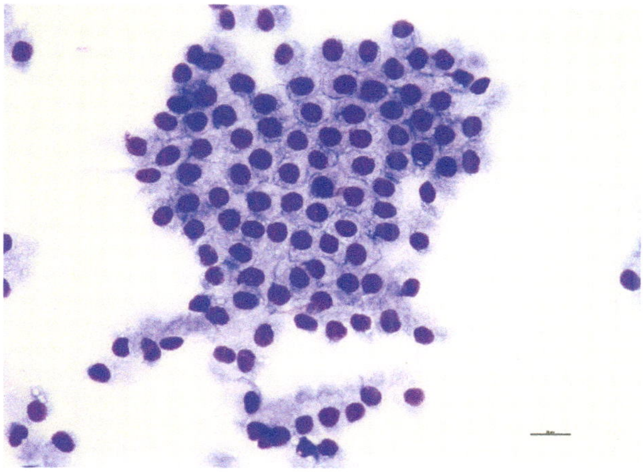

Figure 16. Honeycomb arrangement of epithelial cells from a benign prostatic hyperplasia.

Naked Nuclei

This is not a category itself but is a group of epithelial neoplasms that have peculiar cytological characteristics.

Origin

Endocrine or neuroendocrine tissue.

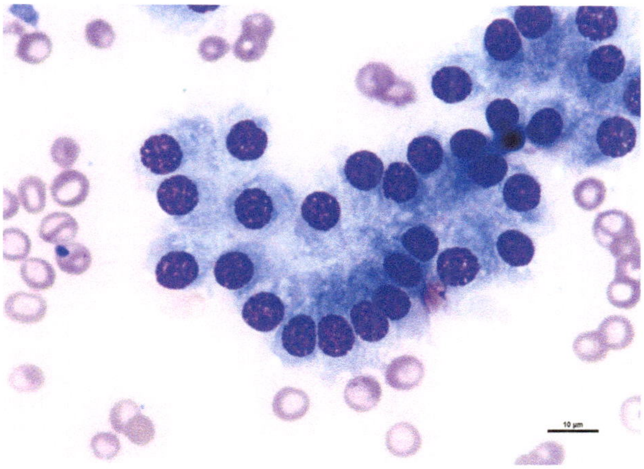

Figure 17. Palisade arrangement of epithelial cells from thyroid neoplasia.

Characteristics

- cells exfoliate into sheets of variably cohesive cells
- cell arrangement pattern: palisade, acinar/pseudoacinar or laminae
- abundant free but intact nuclei (fragile cells) (Figure 19)
- some with intact cytoplasm and variably defined borders (Figure 20)
- they usually have a vacuolated clear or bluish cytoplasm
- examples: carotid or aortic body chemodectoma, pheochromocytoma etc.

Mesenchymal

Origin

Connective tissue elements such as fibroblasts, osteoblasts, adipocytes, myocytes, vascular lining cells etc.

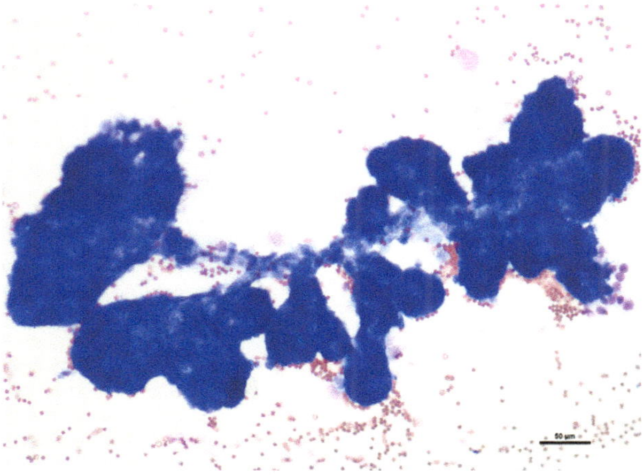

Figure 18. Papillary arrangement of epithelial cells in abdominal fluid from a bitch with carcinomatosis secondary to ovarian adenocarcinoma.

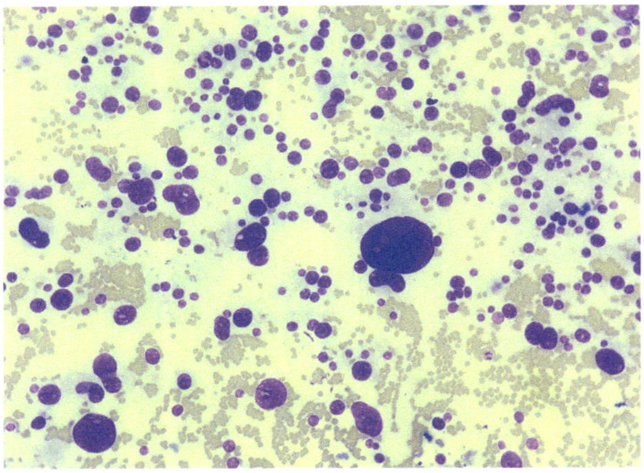

Figure 19. Numerous naked nuclei from a tumour cytology of the carotid body. 20x magnification.

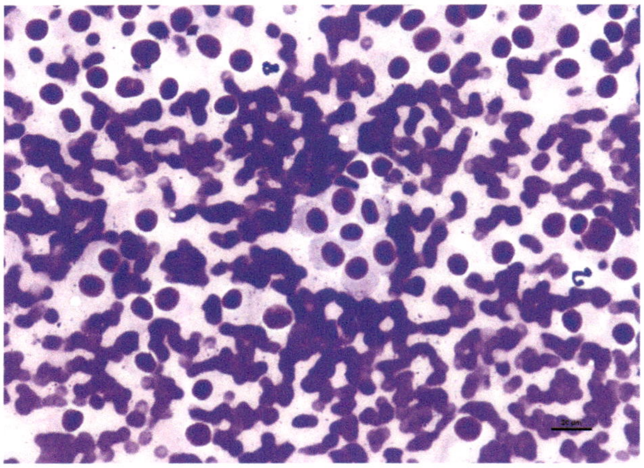

Figure 20. Endocrine neoplasm of the spleen with classic characteristics of this type of tumour.

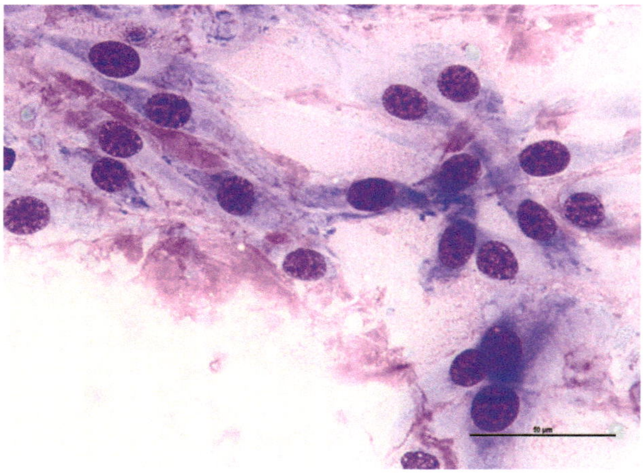

Figure 21. Malignant mesenchymal neoplasia (sarcoma) with abundant pink extracellular matrix.

Characteristics

- cells usually exfoliate individually, sometimes in non-cohesive aggregates
- low cellularity
- cell distribution pattern: storiform, perivascular
- oval cells, spindle to stellate, often with indistinguishable cell borders (Figure 21).
- smaller in size than epithelial cells
- round to oval nuclei
- usually form an extracellular matrix
- examples: haemangiosarcoma, osteosarcoma (may appear to be round cells), soft-tissue sarcoma, lipoma.

Round Cells

Origin

Round cells usually originate from haematopoietic cells.

Characteristics

- cells exfoliate individually and have well defined borders (Figure 22)
- cell distribution pattern: individual (sometimes they can appear cohesive, when overlapping)
- generally, round in shape
- moderately cellular samples
- smaller in size than epithelial cells
- round, indented or irregular nuclei
- examples: lymphoma, plasmacytoma, transmissible venereal tumour (TVT), histiocytoma, mast cell tumour.

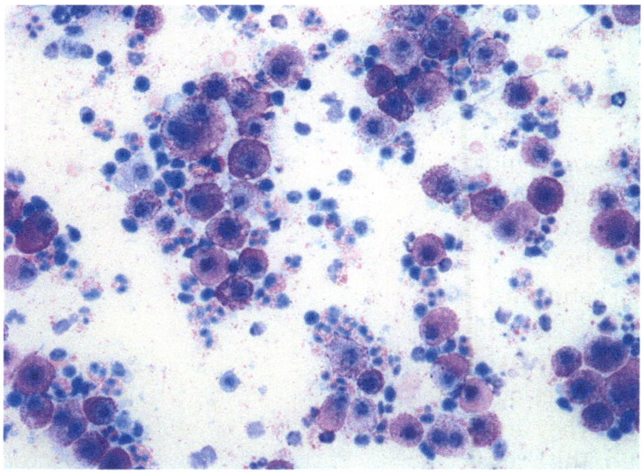

Figure 22. Mastocytic mast cell tumour with marked eosinophilic inflammation from a cat. Pappenheim stain. 20x magnification.

Cutaneous and Subcutaneous Neoplasms

Epithelial

Squamous Cell Papilloma

Origin

Squamous cell papilloma originates from the stratum spinosum layer of the epidermis.

Cytological Features

Benign looking squamous cells are often seen which commonly retain the nuclei. A type of cell called a koilocyte is seen (Figure 23), which is a squamous epithelial cell with a globoid appearance.

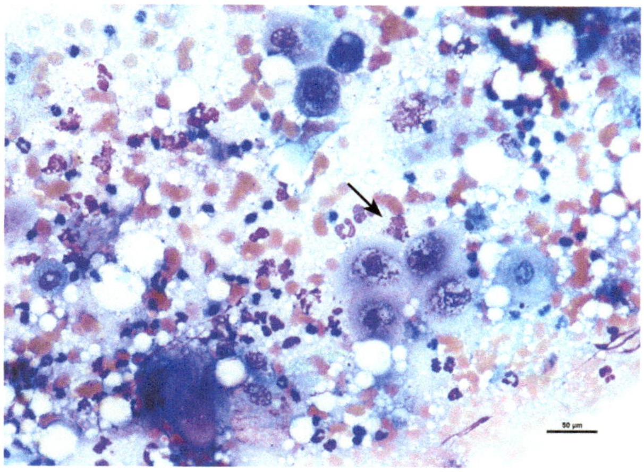

Figure 23. Squamous papilloma with koilocytes (arrow) from a dog.

Squamous Cell Carcinoma

Origin

Squamous layer of the epidermis.

Cytological Features

Samples are usually very cellular. Well-differentiated keratinocytes can be observed in variable numbers, although to make a diagnosis, cohesive cells with obvious malignancy must be located. Depending on the degree of differentiation, they may be polygonal in shape, similar to mature keratinocytes, or be rounded. Anisocytosis and anisokaryosis are moderate to marked and nucleoli are prominent. Perinuclear vacuolisation (keratohyalin granules) is common (Figure 24). In most cases they are accompanied by neutrophilic inflammation as a result of invasive growth with contact of keratin with adjacent tissues or ulceration.

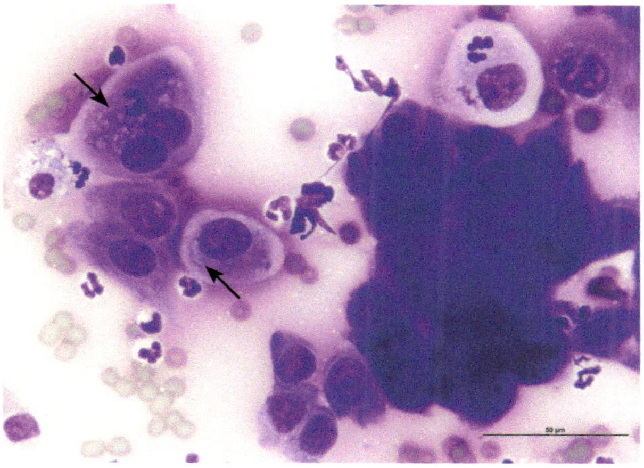

Figure 24. Oral squamous cell carcinoma. The perinuclear vacuoles are characteristic of this type of tumour (arrows). 40x magnification.

Hair Follicle Neoplasms

The most common tumour of the basal epithelium is **trichoblastoma** (Figure 25).

Origin

Hair germ cells.

Cytological Features

Aggregates of epithelial cells are observed in palisade or in rows. They are small in size, with a high nucleus/cytoplasm ratio. The scarce cytoplasm is variably blue, sometimes containing pigment. The nuclei are round and central, and the nucleoli are not usually visible.

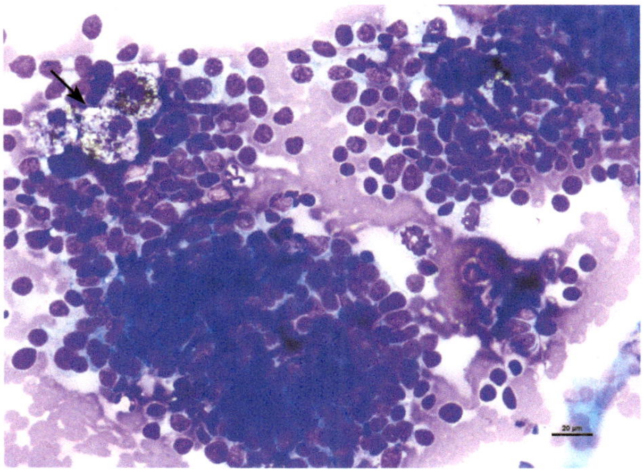

Figure 25. Trichoblastoma with associated melanophages (macrophages phagocytising melanin) (arrow).

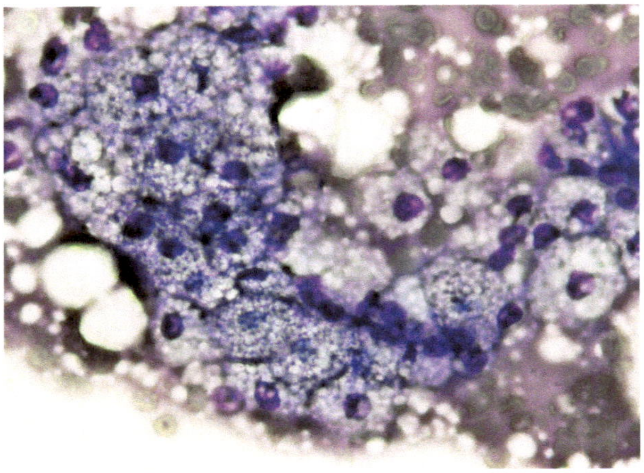

Figure 26. Sebaceous adenoma, formed by mature sebocytes. 50x magnification.

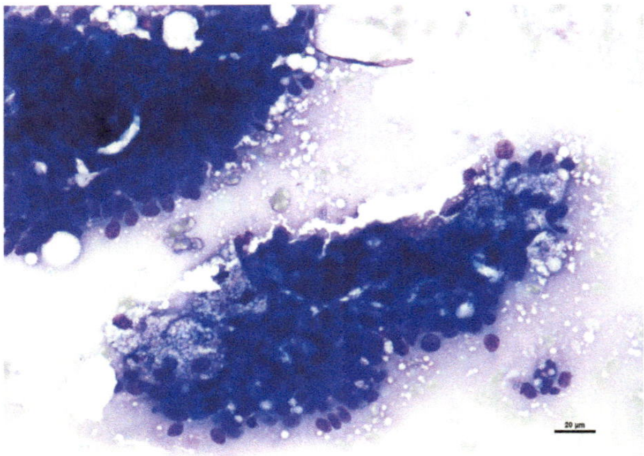

Figure 27. Sebaceous epithelioma with reserve cells and some mature sebocytes.

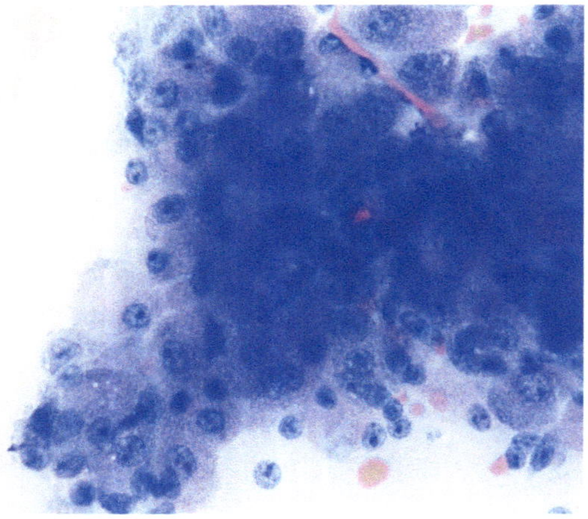

Figure 28. Perianal gland adenoma (hepatoids). Pappenheim stain. 40x magnification.

Other Hair Follicle Neoplasms

There are different benign neoplasms, such as trichoepithelioma, originating in the hair follicle. Differentiation between them cannot be reliably performed by cytology. They can be found with variable amounts in basal epithelium, squamous epithelium, and keratin aggregates, so histopathological study of lesions is recommended, although their biological behaviour is usually benign.

Sebaceous Adenoma/Carcinoma/Epithelioma

Origin

Sebocytes of the sebaceous glands of the skin.

Cytological Features

Mature sebocytes, which predominate in **adenomas**, are arranged in groups of varying size (Figure 26). They have a clear, foamy cytoplasm, and small, dense central nuclei, with no obvious nucleoli. In adenomas it is common to find cells with basal cell characteristics (such as those described in trichoblastoma). In **sebaceous epitheliomas** (Figure 27) there is a predominance of basal cells and, mature sebocytes and well-differentiated squamous epithelial cells are found in smaller numbers. If clear malignancy criteria are observed in sebocytes, **sebaceous carcinoma** (rare) should be suspected.

Adenoma/Carcinoma of Perianal (Hepatoid) Glands

Origin

Perianal glands (modified sebaceous glands).

Cytological Features

Cells have similar characteristics to hepatocytes (Figure 28). They exfoliate in aggregates and have rounded to polygonal borders.The cytoplasm is abundant, microgranular, bluish-pink (amphophilic), and the nuclei are round, central, and often have obvious nucleoli. Aggregates of cells with basal cell characteristics (reserve cells) may be found. Although uncommon, perianal gland carcinomas have similar characteristics but with malignancy criteria.

Anal Sac Adenocarcinoma

Origin

Apocrine glands of the anal gland.

Cytological Features

The cytological appearance of this type of tumour (Figure 29) is variable. In general, laminae of cells are observed that can sometimes acquire a papillary or pseudoacinar arrangement.

Cell borders are not well defined, and the cytoplasm is usually light blue with occasional vacuoles. The nuclei may be uniform in size and shape or may show malignancy criteria such as moderate anisokaryosis. Types of tumour have been described in which spindle cells predominate on cytology, which can be confused with a sarcoma.

Adenoma/Carcinoma of the Ceruminous Glands

Origin
Apocrine sweat glands of the external auditory canal.

Cytological Features
Variable amounts of cell detritus and epithelial cell aggregates are observed, which are sometimes arranged in palisades. The cytoplasm is bluish and microvacuolated and may contain a dark, granular (ceruminous) secretory material. The nuclei may be uniform in adenomas or show a varying degree of atypia in carcinomas (Figure 30).

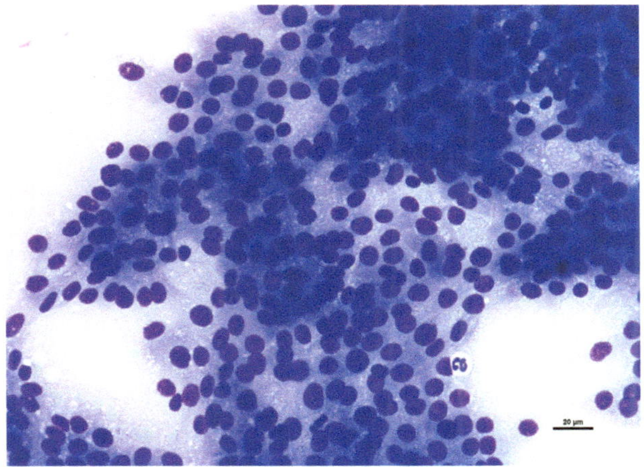

Figure 29. Anal gland carcinoma. The morphology of the cells is very different to neoplasms of the perianal glands.

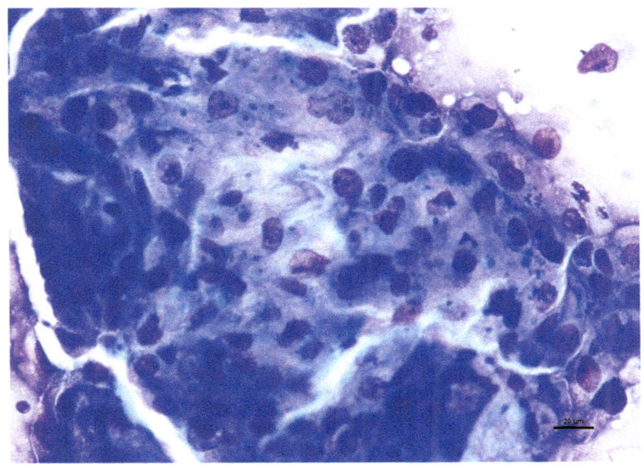

Figure 30. Ceruminous gland carcinoma with characteristic cytoplasmatic pigmentation in the external auditory canal of a cat.

Mesenchymal

Fibroma/Fibrosarcoma

Origin
Fibrous connective tissue.

Cytological Features
Usually, samples are of low cellularity.

Fibromas are rare and are characterised by the presence of well-differentiated spindle cells, with uniform, oval nuclei with dense chromatin and no obvious nucleoli. **Fibrosarcomas** (Figure 31), which are more frequent, are observed as larger mesenchymal cells, with fusiform to stellate morphology and poorly defined cell borders. Nuclear atypia is often prominent, with coarse chromatin and prominent and irregular nucleoli, and multinucleated cells can be observed. It is common to observe a collagenous amorphous or fibrillar pink material.

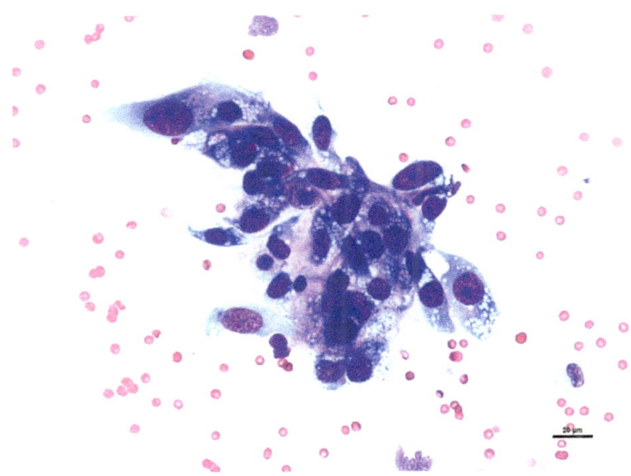

Figure 31. Injection site sarcoma on the back of a cat.

Perivascular Wall Tumours (PWTs) and Peripheral Nerve Sheath Tumours (PNSTs)

Origin
PWTs (Figure 32) originate in the walls of vessels adjacent to the endothelium and give rise to haemangiopericytomas (origin in pericytes) and myopericytomas (origin in myocytes). **PNSTs** are mainly derived from Schwann cells which surround the nerves.

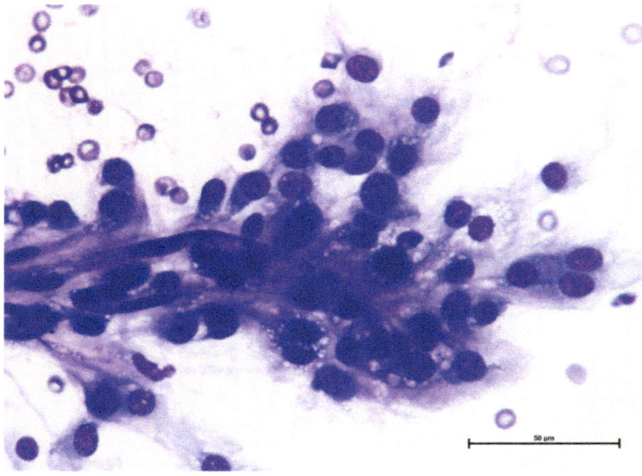

Figure 32. Perivascular wall tumour. Mesenchymal cells are arranged around capillaries.

Cytological Features

Cytologically, these tumours may show similar characteristics. Cell exfoliation is greater than in fibrosarcomas, although they also have fusiform to stellate morphology with poorly defined borders. The cytoplasm is light blue with occasional small clear vacuoles. The nuclei are round to oval, with finely stippled chromatin and prominent nucleoli. Anisocytosis and anisokaryosis are moderate.

Cells can generally be observed arranged individually, although in PWTs they may be in a perivascular pattern. In this type of tumour, crown cells can also be observed, with multiple nuclei acquiring a characteristic arrangement in a circle. The presence of binucleated cells that resemble the head of an insect are also useful for the diagnosis of this type of neoplasm, but definitive classification of soft-tissue sarcomas requires histopathological examination.

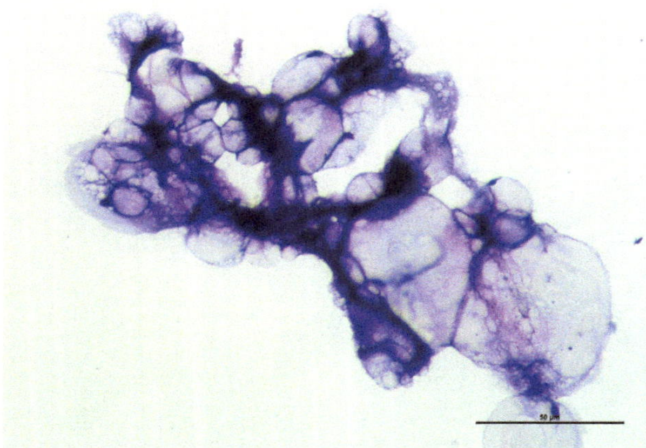

Figure 33. Lipoma formed from well-differentiated adipocytes.

Lipoma/Liposarcoma

Origin

Adipocytes from adipose tissue.

Cytological Features

While lipomas (Figure 33) are very common, liposarcomas (Figure 34) are rare. In both cases the preparations usually look greasy before staining.

Well-differentiated adipocytes are found in **lipomas**. They have a globular appearance and abundant clear cytoplasm. The nuclei appear compressed on the periphery and are small and dense in appearance. **Liposarcomas** have similar characteristics to the previously described soft-tissue sarcomas, with spindle cells with moderate atypia arranged in aggregates. The most important differential feature is the presence of lipid vacuoles of varying size in the cytoplasm.

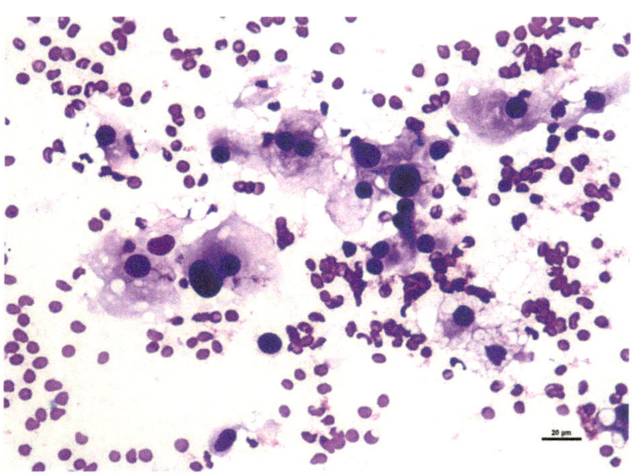

Figure 34. Liposarcoma. The malignant mesenchymal cells have large cytoplasmatic vacuoles with a lipidic appearance.

Haemangioma/Haemangiosarcoma

These tumours may appear on the skin or, in the case of haemangiosarcoma (Figure 35), may be metastatic lesions from another location, although they arise more commonly from organs such as the spleen.

Origin

Endothelial cells.

Cytological Features

Cytological preparations of these lesions often show large amounts of blood. Macrophages showing erythrophagocytosis or haemosiderin in the cytoplasm are also common. While in **haemangiomas** well-differentiated or mildly atypical mesenchymal cells can be observed, in **haemangiosarcomas**, although the samples are generally poorly cellular, there are mesenchymal cells with marked atypia. They have fusiform to stellate morphology, with a clear to bluish cytoplasm that may contain haemosiderin and small, clear vacuoles. The nuclei have finely stippled to coarse chromatin and prominent nucleoli. Anisocytosis and anisokaryosis are moderate to marked. Neoplastic cells may show erythophagocytosis and mitotic figures can be seen. Extramedullary haematopoiesis may be found.

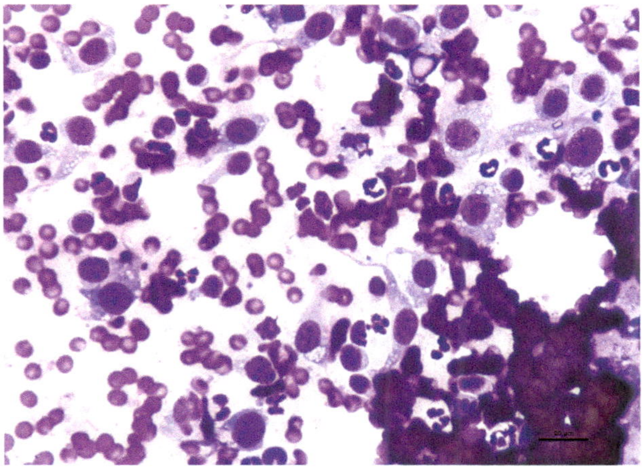

Figure 35. Haemangiosarcoma. The small clear vacuoles are seen in the cytoplasm.

Melanoma

It is important to differentiate melanomas from other types of pigmented neoplasms with a better prognosis, especially from melanocytomas and pigmented benign epithelial tumours.

Origin

Melanocytes.

Cytological Features

The **variability** in the cytological appearance of these types of tumours is enormous. Well-differentiated forms of the tumour show abundant black-greenish granular to amorphous pigmentation and uniform nuclei (Figure 36). Less differentiated forms may not exhibit melanin, or it is extremely difficult to find (Figure 37). The morphology and arrangement of cells may resemble a round, epithelial, or mesenchymal cell neoplasm.

Poorly differentiated forms show numerous malignancy criteria, including moderate to marked anisocytosis and anisokaryosis, coarse chromatin and prominent nucleoli, as well as the presence of frequent atypical mitoses. In many cases, in amelanotic forms it is not possible to make an accurate diagnosis on cytology, or even on histology, without the use of immunohistochemical techniques.

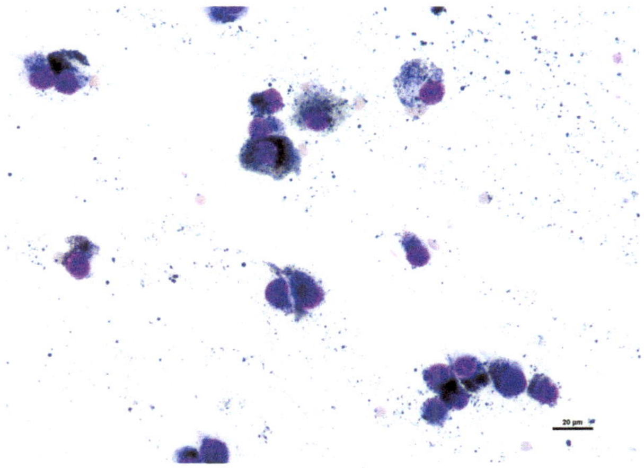

Figure 36. Well-differentiated cutaneous melanoma from the skin of a cat. The neoplastic cells show malignancy criteria and contain abundant melanin granules in the cytoplasm.

Round Cells

The cytology of round cell neoplasms makes it possible, in most cases, to reach a definitive diagnosis. However, it is not uncommon to have to provide differential diagnoses including two or more diagnoses because no clear cytological characteristics of any of the groups can be observed, which makes histological examination and the use of ancillary techniques such as immunohistochemistry necessary.

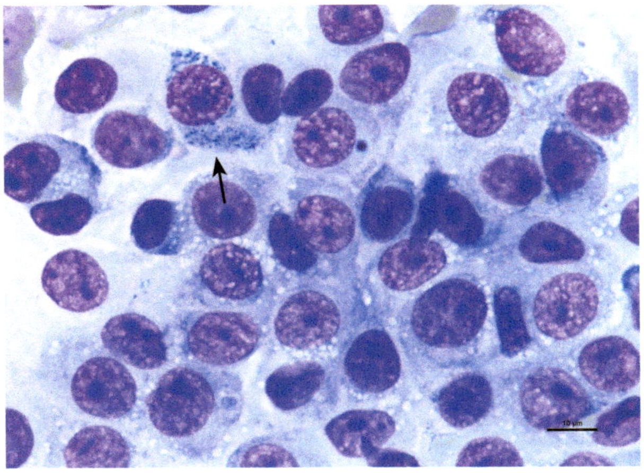

Figure 37. Amelanotic melanoma from the oral cavity of a dog. The population of neoplastic cells is highly pleomorphic. Occasionally cells containing melanin granules may be present (arrow).

Histiocytic Neoplasms

Origin

- canine cutaneous histiocytoma in Langerhans cells
- histiocytic sarcoma in interstitial dendritic cells
- haemophagocytic histiocytic sarcoma in macrophages.

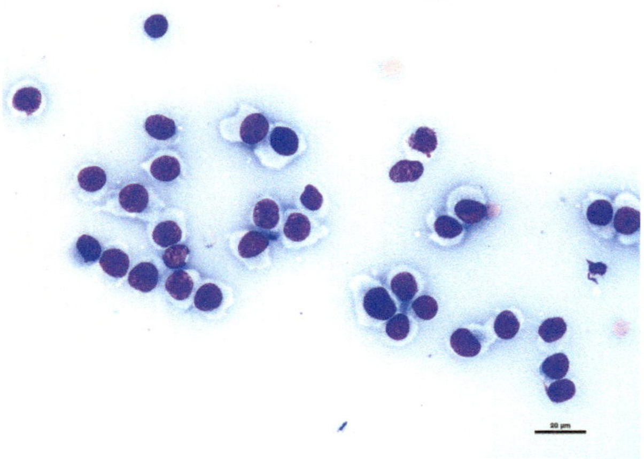

Figure 38. Cutaneous histiocytoma.

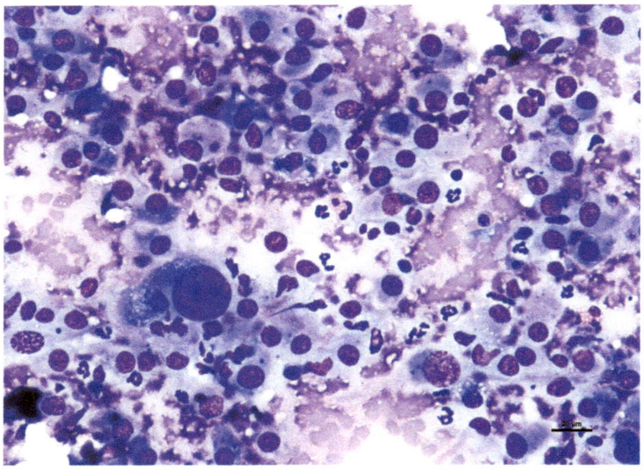

Figure 39. Histiocytic sarcoma from the spleen of a Bernese Mountain Dog.

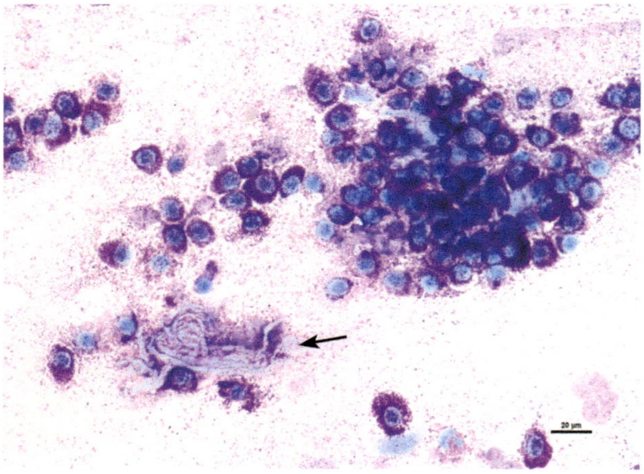

Figure 40. Low cytological grade canine cutaneous mastocytoma. Degraded fibrin can be seen (arrow). Pappenheim's stain.

Cytological Features

In histiocytomas (Figure 38) the cells have slight to moderately well-defined borders and a clear cytoplasm, with occasional vacuoles. The nuclei are round to oval, with no obvious nucleoli. Anisocytosis and anisokaryosis are mild. Mitosis can often be seen. Over time, the number of small lymphocytes in the lesion increases until it disappears (spontaneous regression) and there may be a predominance of lymphocytes in the final stages.

In histiocytic sarcoma (Figure 39) the cells may appear rounded or fusiform. They are large in size and show numerous criteria of malignancy such as marked anisocytosis and anisokaryosis and prominent nucleoli. It is common to see multinucleated cells and atypical mitosis. Sometimes phagocytosis of other cells by neoplastic cells may be observed. A characteristic of haemophagocytic histiocytic sarcomas is that their cells show prominent erythrophagocytosis.

Mast Cell Tumour

Origin

Mast cells.

Cytological Features

In well-differentiated tumours, mast cells contain numerous metachromatic cytoplasmic granules that almost completely hide the nuclei.

Generally, as tumours have fewer (more undifferentiated) granules, diagnosis is often more difficult. Criteria that may aid in the diagnosis of mast cell tumours are, for example, the presence of eosinophilic inflammation (Figure 22), reactive mesenchymal cells (fibroplasia), and degraded collagen (collagenolysis).

In **dogs**, it is possible to establish a low (Figure 40) or high (Figure 41) **cytological grade** for this tumour.

Tumours with poorly granulated mast cells are directly considered high-grade, as well as those that meet at least two of the following criteria:

- presence of mitosis
- multinucleated cells
- nuclear pleomorphism
- anisokaryosis of more than 50%.

High cytological tumour grades are associated with lower survival rates and a higher likelihood of recurrence.

In **cats**, cutaneous mast cell tumours can be classified into:

- mastocytic, when well differentiated (Figure 22)
- pleomorphic, when they have cellular and nuclear atypia
- histiocytic or atypical.

Of this last type there are no cytological imaging data, since they have only been described in two litters of Siamese cats less than 6 months of age.

Plasmacytoma

Origin
Plasma cells.

Cytological Features
In plasmacytomas (Figure 42) the cells usually have well-defined borders. Cytology often shows well-differentiated plasma cells with bluish cytoplasm and a clear perinuclear zone (Golgi zone), as well as round, eccentric nuclei with finely stippled chromatin and non-evident nucleoli.

One of the most representative features on cytology of this type of tumour is the presence of binucleated and multinucleated cells. Sometimes a pink, amorphous material may be seen between the cells (amyloid). However, plasmacytomas can be very pleomorphic, showing marked atypias which prevent their diagnosis without the use of adequate immunohistochemical techniques.

Cutaneous Lymphoma

Origin
Lymphocytes.

Cytological Features
As in all other locations, the diagnosis of cutaneous lymphoma is based on the identification of a monomorphic population of lymphocytes in the absence of significant inflammation. Lymphocytes, within the homogeneity of the cell population, may present irregular nuclei (Figure 43) with multiple indentations and, occasionally, nucleoli may be observed.

It is common to find mitosis and cytoplasmic fragments. When neoplastic lymphoid cells are seen in peripheral blood, this is called Sézary syndrome.

Confirmation of the diagnosis can be performed by a clonality test or PARR, flow cytometry (if a sufficient number of cells in suspension is obtained), histology and immunohistochemistry to differentiate between epitheliotropic and non-epitheliotropic, as well as to determine the immunophenotype (usually T cells).

Transmissible Venereal Tumour

Origin
Probably histiocytic.

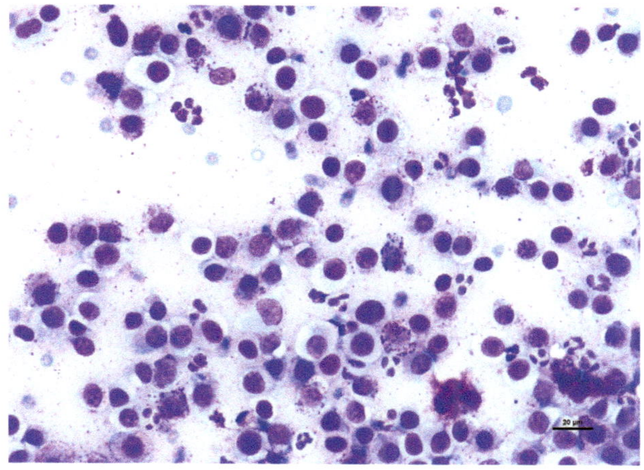

Figure 41. High cytological grade canine cutaneous mast cell tumour. Pappenheim's stain.

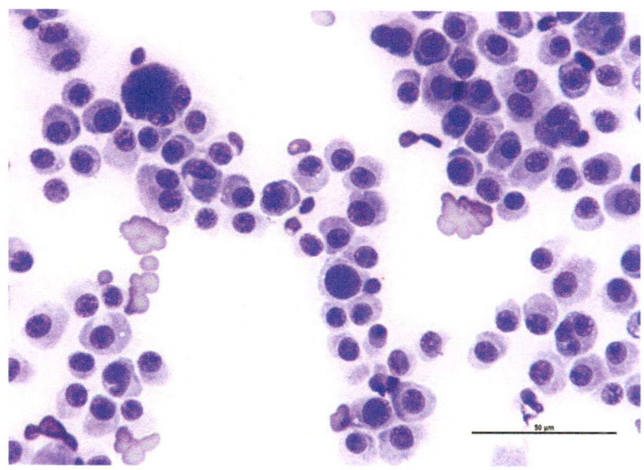

Figure 42. Plasma cell tumour (plasmacytoma). Cells with more than one nucleus and the characteristic morphology with eccentric nuclei and blue cytoplasm with a pale perinuclear area.

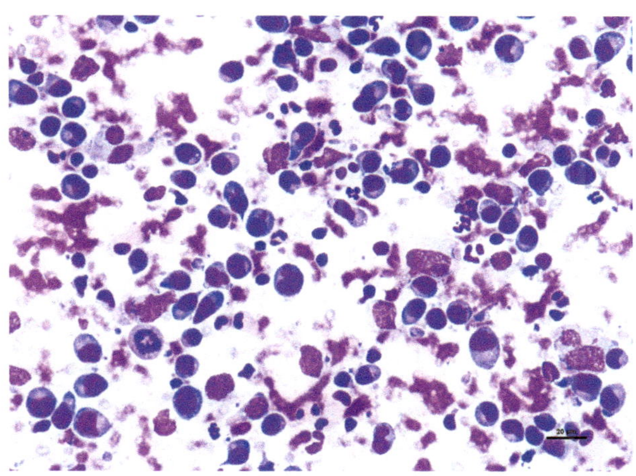

Figure 43. Cutaneous lymphoma with lymphocytes which frequently have pleomorphic nuclei.

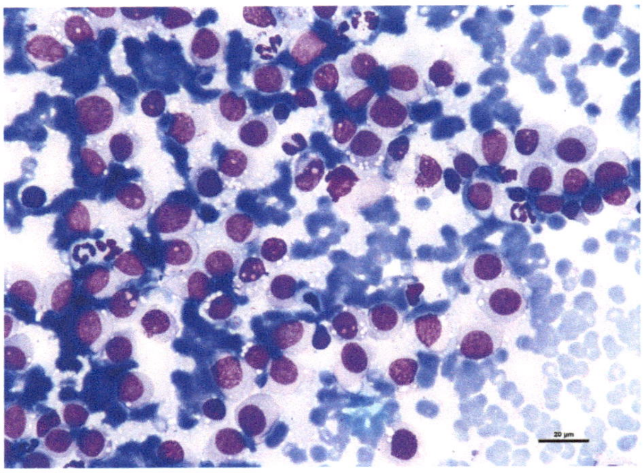

Figure 44. Transmissible venereal tumour from the penile area of a dog. The frequent mitosis and clear well-defined vacuoles are typical.

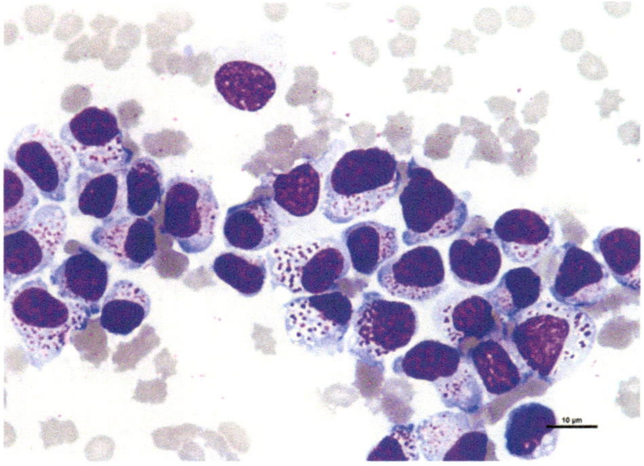

Figure 45. Granular cell lymphoma from the spleen of a cat. The lymphocytes contain magenta-coloured granules which is many cases stain in the centre.

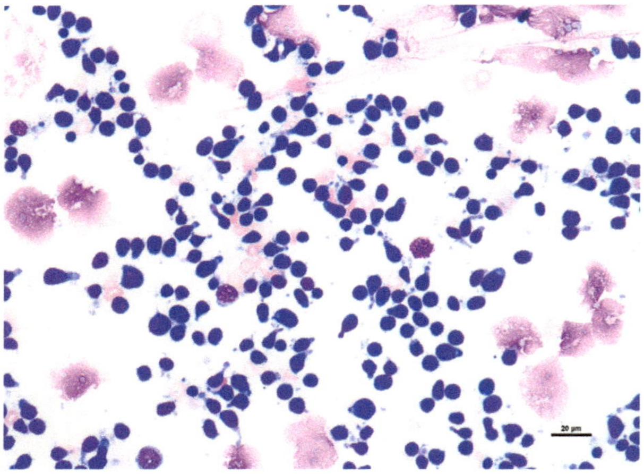

Figure 46. T-cell lymphoma from a dog, with cells with a "hand mirror" morphology.

Cytological Features

Cells from this type of tumour have well defined borders, blue cytoplasm with clear and well-defined vacuoles characteristic of this type of tumour (Figure 44). The nuclei are round to oval, generally eccentric, with finely stippled to coarse chromatin and occasionally visible nucleoli. Mitoses are common.

Neoplasms of Lymphoid Organs

Lymphoma is one of the most common neoplasms affecting lymphoid organs and has similar characteristics in all of them. The key to diagnosis is the presence of a **uniform population of lymphocytes**. When the size of the lymphocytes is intermediate to large (nucleus diameter greater than 1.5 times that of an erythrocyte), the diagnosis is relatively simple. However, in cases of lymphocytic (small cell) lymphomas, the diagnosis may be complicated (for example, in low-grade alimentary lymphomas in the cat or T zone lymphomas in the dog).

In the case of a predominance of small lymphocytes with the presence of plasma cells, complementary techniques are recommended to confirm the diagnosis if there is clinical suspicion of lymphoma (e.g. clonality test or PARR). This is especially true in the spleen, where the diagnosis of lymphoma can be particularly complex due to the heterogeneity of the cell populations that can be found.

In some cases, cytological features may be useful as a guide in establishing the prognosis and/or immunophenotype of lymphoma:

- **large granular lymphocytes** (**LGL**) **or granular lymphocytes**: azurophilic granules in the cytoplasm that, at times, may not be completely stained. These cells correspond to cytotoxic T cells or natural killer cells (Figure 45);
- **lymphocytes with "hand mirror" morphology**: lymphocytes of generally small to intermediate size (diameter of the nuclei from 1 to 2 times that of an erythrocyte) with cytoplasmic prolongations that give them the appearance of a hand mirror. They correspond to T cells (Figure 46); and
- **centroblastic and immunoblastic lymphocytes** (large in size, with several nucleoli on the periphery of the nucleus, or one which is large and central, respectively) are, in most cases, B cells (Figure 47).

Cytological differentiation between high and low-grade is also useful for establishing a prognosis, especially in cats. Cytological grade is established based on cell size (specifically nuclei) and mitotic index (Box 1).

Box 1. How is the cytological grade of a lymphoma established based on cell size and mitotic index?

- **Cell size** (comparison of the diameter of the nucleus with the diameter of an erythrocyte)
  - — Small: 1–1.5 times the diameter of an erythrocyte.
  - — Medium: 1.5–2 times the diameter of an erythrocyte.
  - — Large: >2 times the diameter of an erythrocyte.
- **Mitotic index** (estimated by examining five fields at 40x or 50x magnification)
  - — Low: 0–1 mitoses in five fields.
  - — Moderate: 2–3 mitoses in five fields.
  - — High: >3 mitoses in five fields.
- **Grade of lymphoma**
  - — Low-grade: low mitotic index and small cells.
  - — High-grade: moderate to high-mitotic index and medium to large size cells.

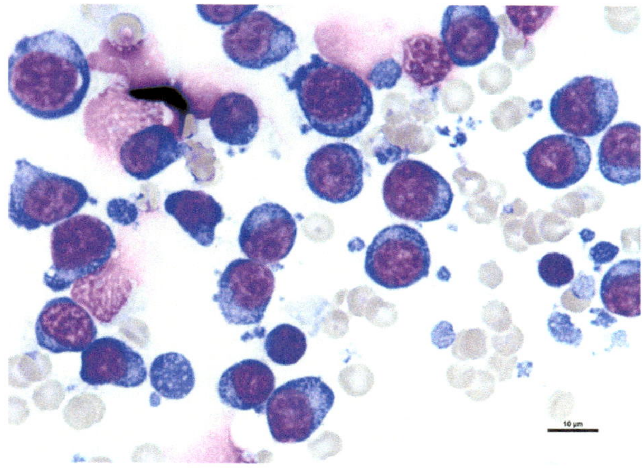

Figure 47. Lymphoma which is likely B-cell from a dog. In the image the predominance of centroblasts can be observed.

Table 1 shows other criteria that can be applied to predict the immunophenotype and grade of the tumour, although the use of complementary techniques is essential to establish both (Figure 48).

Table 1. Cytological criteria for the classification of lymphoma.

Criteria	T-cells compared to B	Low-grade (LG) compared to high-grade (HG)
Macrophages	> in B	No differences
Lymphoglandular bodies	> in B	> in HG
Mitosis	No differences	> in HG
Vacuolated cytoplasm	No differences	No differences
Plasmatic cells	> in T	> in LG

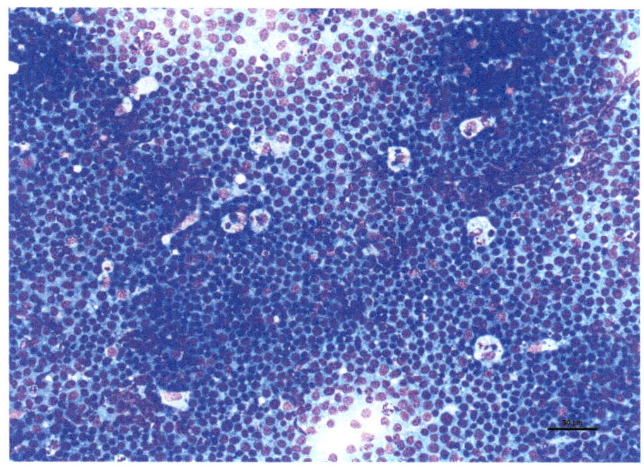

Figure 48. Low magnification image of B-cell lymphoma with a significant number of macrophages.

Lymph Nodes

Primary lymph node non-lymphoid neoplasms are rare, while metastases are relatively common. The presence of a population of cells outside the lymph node is diagnostic of metastasis (Figures 49 and 50).

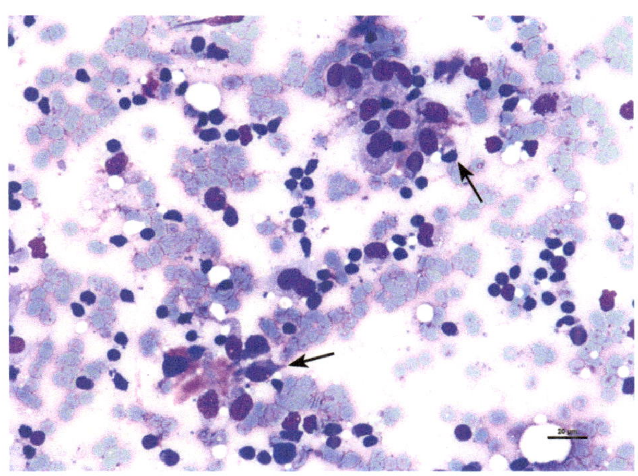

Figure 49. Mesenchymal neoplasm metastasis (arrows).

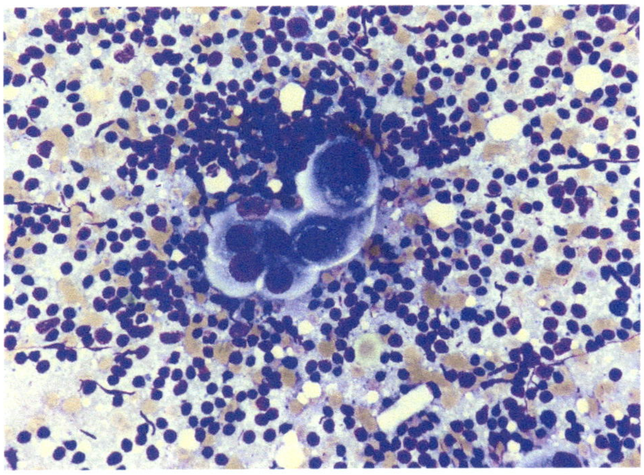

Figure 50. Epithelial neoplasm metastasis (mammary carcinoma) in an inguinal lymph node. 40x magnification.

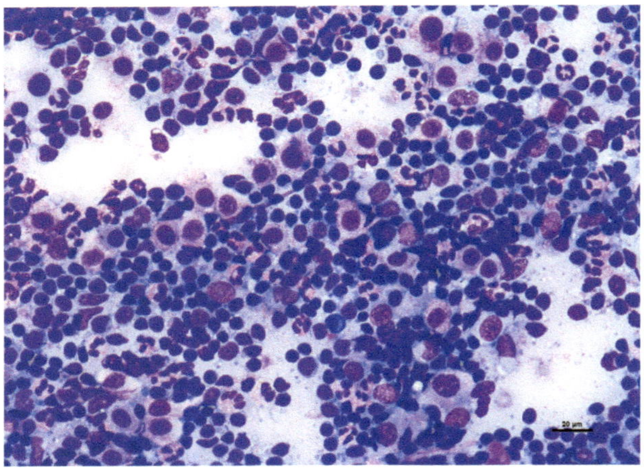

Figure 51. Poorly differentiated mastocytoma metastasis and eosinophilic lymphadenitis.

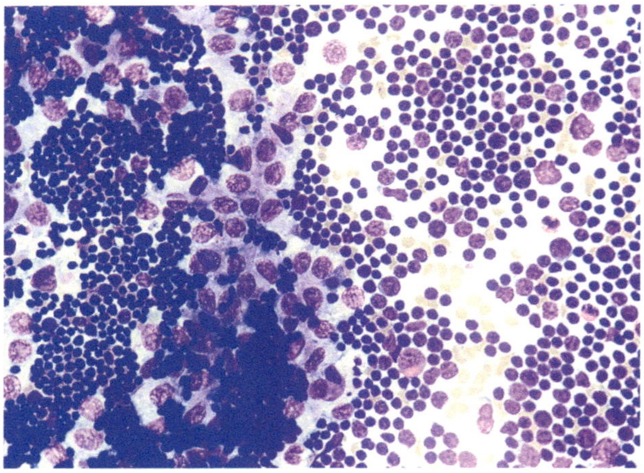

Figure 52. Lymphoepithelial thymoma. There is a similar proportion of variably sized lymphocytes with predominance of small cells and atypical epithelial cells. The presence of well-differentiated mast cells is common (not shown in this image). 20x magnification.

In some cases, such as mast cells, finding a significant number of mast cells with atypia or in groups is necessary, since mast cells can normally be found in the lymph node (Figure 51).

Spleen

Apart from lymphoma, haemangiosarcoma is the most common neoplasm that primarily affects the spleen. The cytological characteristics are similar to those described for the cutaneous form of the tumour (Figure 35).

Other relevant neoplasms are histiocytic sarcoma (primary or as part of the systemic form of the disease) (Figure 39) and mast cell tumour (especially in cats). Metastases are also relatively common.

Thymus

The most common neoplasms affecting the thymus are thymic lymphoma and thymoma. In all thymomas, the neoplastic population of origin is the reticular epithelium.

Thymomas are classified according to the predominant cells into the following categories:

- **epithelial** (epithelial predominance)
- **lymphoepithelial** (similar proportion of lymphoid and epithelial tissue)
- **lymphocytes** (predominantly lymphoid tissue).

In all cases lymphoid tissue has a predominance of small lymphocytes, with variable increases in intermediate and large cells, as well as plasma cells.

The presence of well-differentiated mast cells in this type of neoplasm is also frequent. Neoplastic epithelial cells may appear individually and with macrophage-like morphology, or in cohesive aggregates of varying size, with variably defined cell borders. Nuclear atypia may or may not be prominent (Figure 52).

Neoplasms of the Endocrine System

Endocrine and neuroendocrine neoplasms share certain cytological characteristics (see the section on classification of neoplastic lesions according to the tissue of origin).

As a rule, in the presence of cellular atypia, a diagnosis of malignancy may be established. However, malignant neoplasms may present a "benign" cytological appearance.

Thyroid Gland

Thyroid neoplasms can occur from ectopic thyroid tissue from the base of the tongue to the base of the heart, although the most common location is the ventral region of the neck. While in cats most neoplasms are benign and hormone producing, in dogs most clinically detectable neoplasms are malignant and do not produce hormones. Differentiation between follicular and medullary or C-cell neoplasms is not possible based on cytology.

Cytology of thyroid neoplasms usually shows large amounts of blood with a variable number of naked nuclei. The borders of the cells are poorly defined and exfoliate in aggregates of variable size with occasional formation of pseudoacinar structures and palisades.

Differential characteristics of thyroid neoplasms that help in their identification would be both the presence of a bluish, granular pigmentation in the cytoplasm (which would contain tyrosine) and a pink, amorphous material between the cells that corresponds to colloid (Figure 53). Generally, nuclear atypia is minimal in both benign and malignant neoplasms, although some malignancies may show moderate anisocytosis and anisokaryosis.

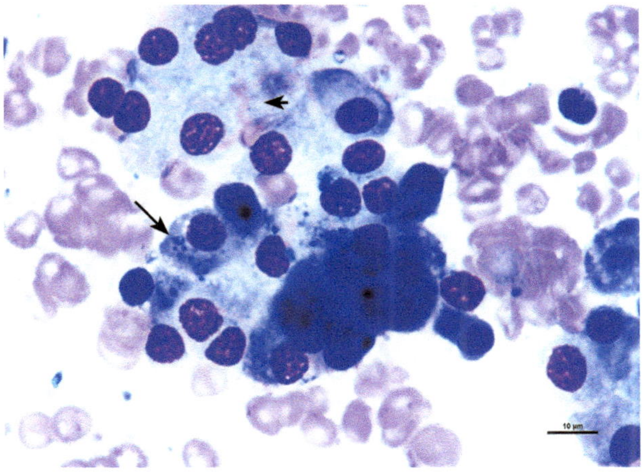

Figure 53. Thyroid neoplasia from a dog. The pink extracellular material (colloid) (small arrow) and the blue cytoplasmatic pigment (tyrosine) (large arrow) help to identify the origin of the cells.

Endocrine Pancreas

Insulinomas, tumours of pancreatic beta (β) cells, are the most frequent endocrine neoplasms of this organ (Figure 54). The cytological and histological appearance of most of these tumours is similar, so interpreting the cytological findings together with the clinical signs is necessary and, sometimes, immunohistochemical techniques to differentiate them from neoplasms such as gastrinoma or glucagonoma.

Cytologically, features similar to other endocrine neoplasms are observed, with numerous bare nuclei and light blue cytoplasm with frequent clear vacuoles. In some cases, neoplastic cells can be visualised individually and with well-defined borders. The nuclei are round and may show occasional visible nucleoli.

As in other cases of endocrine neoplasms, the absence of cellular or nuclear atypia is not useful for prediction of the biological behaviour in this type of tumour.

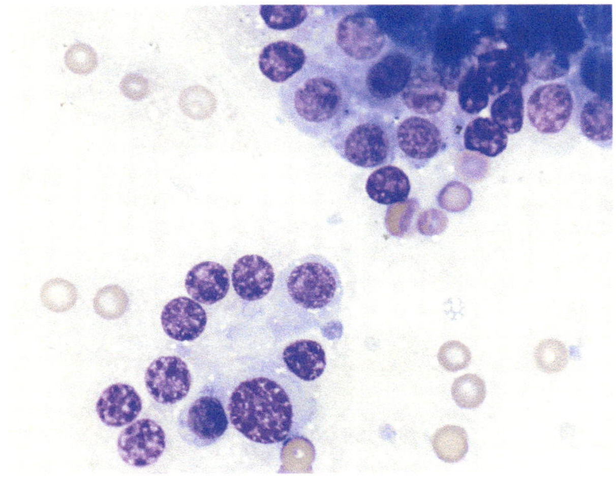

Figure 54. Pancreatic nodule from a dog with severe hypoglycaemia, compatible with insulinoma. 40x magnification.

Adrenal Glands

Neoplasms originating in the cortex and medulla of the adrenal gland have distinct clinical and cytological features.

Cortex

Adrenocortical adenomas and adenocarcinomas may show similar cytological characteristics. They exfoliate in aggregates of cells with variably defined borders and light blue cytoplasm. Clear cytoplasmic vacuoles are common. The nuclei are usually uniform, with variably visible nucleoli. The nucleus/cytoplasm ratio is low to moderate.

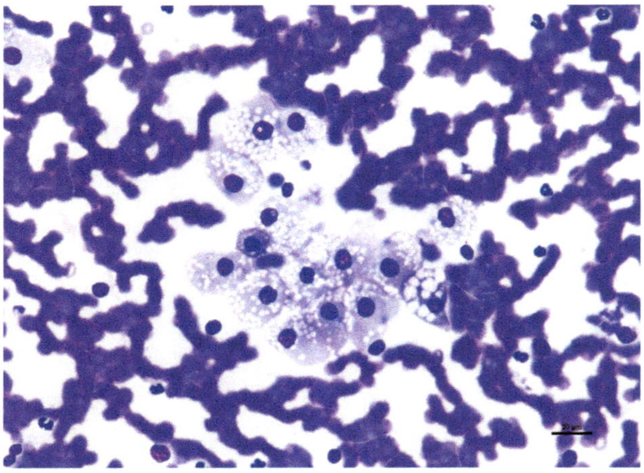

Figure 55. Adrenal mass with invasion of the caudal vena cava. Cytologically the adrenal cortex cells appear well differentiated although clinical signs were of an adrenocortical carcinoma.

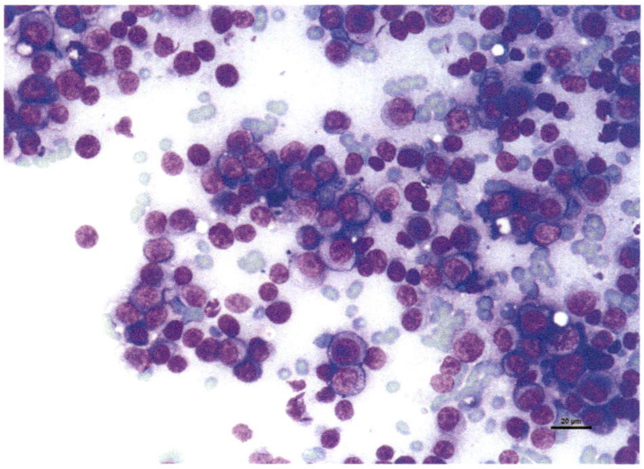

Figure 56. Pheochromocytoma. Cytology of an adrenal mass in an animal with an increase in the concentration of plasmatic catecholamines.

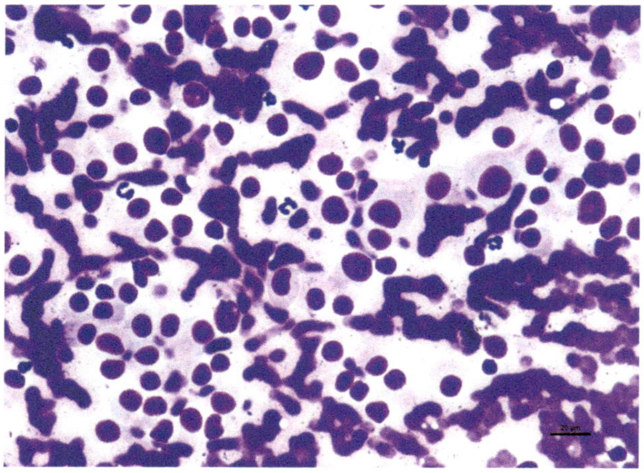

Figure 57. Splenic carcinoid. Presence of a population of cells with characteristics commonly seen in endocrine tissues.

In tumours without cytological features of malignancy, differentiation between adenoma and adenocarcinoma should be based on clinical presentation and ultrasound findings (especially invasion of the vasculature by the mass) (Figure 55).

Medulla

Pheochromocytoma is the most frequent neoplasm of the adrenal medulla and that of which the cytological characteristics are best known. The cells of this type of tumour are usually found individually or in small aggregates, with rounded and well-defined cell borders. The cytoplasm is sparse, light blue, with an occasional pinkish, granular material. The nuclei may have visible nucleoli. Anisocytosis and anisokaryosis can be mild to moderate and the nucleus/cytoplasm ratio is usually elevated (Figure 56).

Others

Carcinoid

Carcinoids (Figure 57) are neoplasms originating in the endocrine tissue of organs such as the stomach, intestine, gallbladder, liver, lung, skin etc. Despite the great variability of origins, the cytological appearance is similar regardless of location.

The carcinoid should be included in the cytological differential diagnosis of any organ in which a population of cells with endocrine tissue characteristics are found in the absence of a known endocrine neoplasia that may have metastasised.

Chemodectoma

Chemodectomas are neuroendocrine neoplasms originating in chemoreceptors present in the aortic and carotid bodies (Figure 58).

Cytology of this type of lesion is usually very cellular and with characteristics typical of other endocrine tumours, with a high number of naked nuclei. The presence of prominent nucleoli is frequent and, in this case, prominent anisokaryosis is not a reliable criterion to distinguish between benign and malignant forms of the tumour.

Differentiation between chemodectoma and an ectopic thyroid tumour can be complicated if performed using cytology alone.

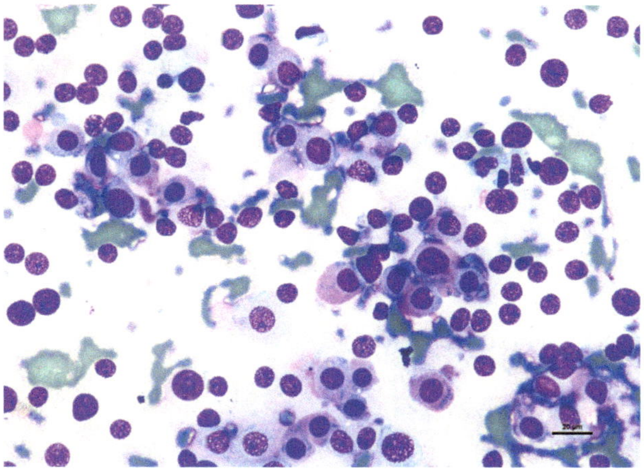

Figure 58. Chemodectoma of the carotid body.

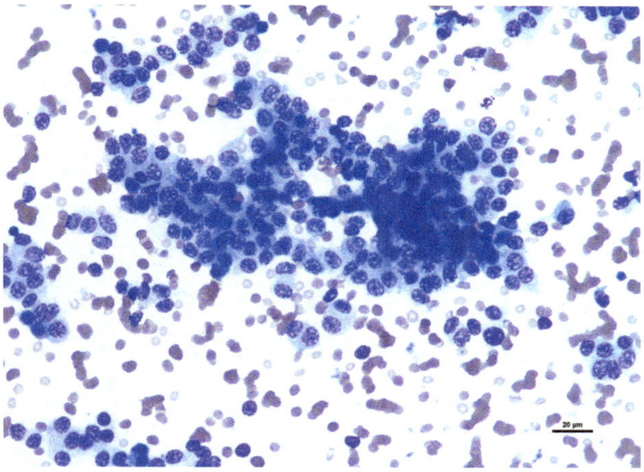

Figure 59. Neoplasm of the biliary epithelium of the liver.

Neoplasms of Internal Organs

Liver

Most primary liver neoplasms originate in the biliary epithelium or hepatocytes. Neoplasms of the biliary epithelium are characterised by being very cellular, with little bluish cytoplasm and a high nucleus/cytoplasm ratio. Anisocytosis and anisokaryosis may be mild to moderate and nucleoli may occasionally be visible.

Differentiation of biliary adenomas and cholangiocarcinomas is based on the invasion of the hepatic parenchyma by neoplastic growth, which should be determined using histology (Figure 59).

Well-differentiated hepatocellular neoplasms can be extremely difficult to differentiate from normal liver tissue (Figure 60).

Of the 33 cellular characteristics evaluated in one study, the most useful for the **diagnosis of well-differentiated hepatocellular carcinoma** were the following:

- **dissociation** of hepatocytes
- distribution of cells in **acinar structures or palisades**
- presence of **naked nuclei and capillaries**
- mild **anisocytosis and anisokaryosis**
- presence of **multinucleated cells**
- increased **nucleus/cytoplasm ratio**.

In the case of less differentiated tumours, it can be difficult to determine the origin in hepatocytes (Figure 61). The detection of greenish material among hepatocytes compatible with bile

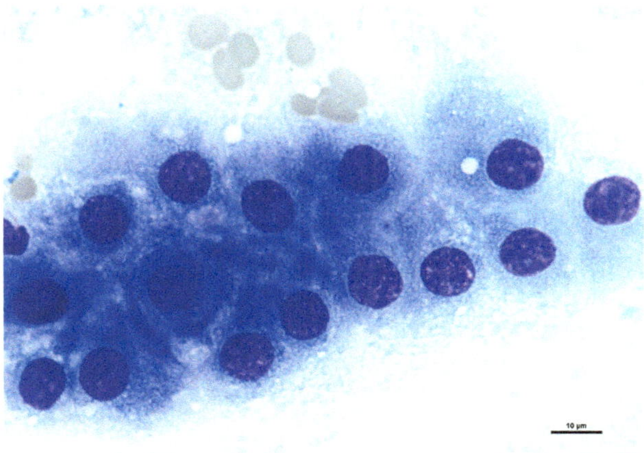

Figure 60. Palisade cells from a well-differentiated hepatocellular carcinoma in a dog.

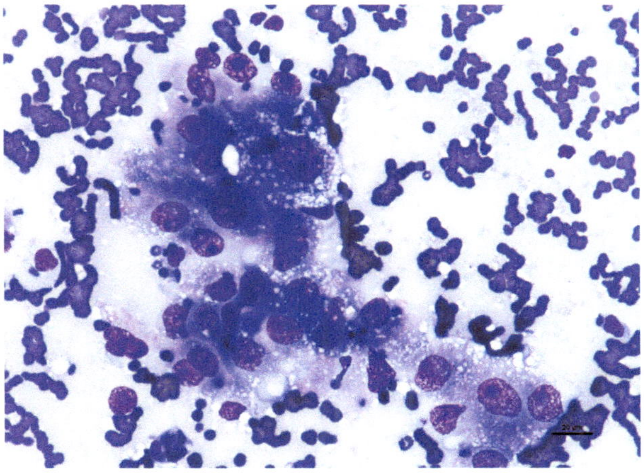

Figure 61. Hepatocellular carcinoma from a cat. The cells retain the cytomorphological characteristics of hepatocytes and show moderate anisokaryosis.

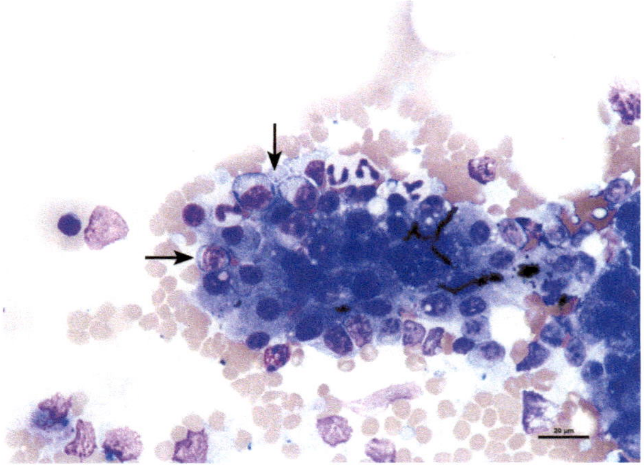

Figure 62. Hepatic involvement of a multicentric lymphoma. The large lymphocytes (arrows) appear next to the hepatocytes. Cholestasis can also be seen.

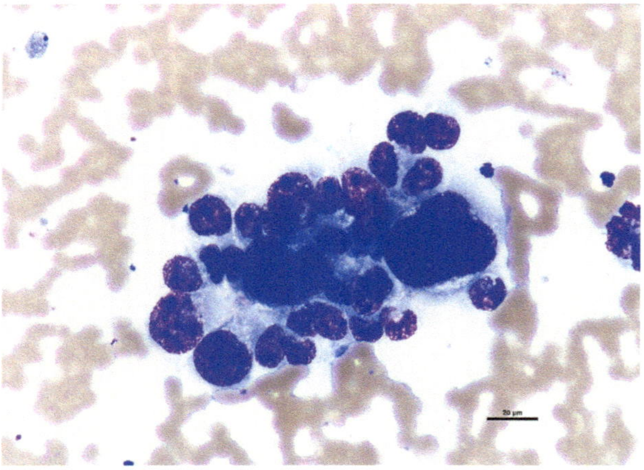

Figure 63. Pancreatic adenocarcinoma from a dog. At the time of diagnosis there were metastasis in the liver and spleen.

or a blue green and granular pigment consistent with lipofuscin inside the cells can help.

Liver metastases are also common (Figure 62).

Gastrointestinal Tract

Carcinomas of both the different regions of the gastrointestinal tract and the pancreas have similar cytological features (Figure 63). The cells are observed in cohesive aggregates of variable size, with a rounded to polygonal morphology, sometimes acquiring a papillary or pseudoacinar disposition. The cytoplasm is medium to dark blue with frequent vacuolisation. The nuclei usually show prominent nucleoli, and the nucleus/cytoplasm ratio is high.

Lymphoma can be easy to diagnose when the cells involved are large or granular lymphocytes, but it is complicated when there are small lymphocytes.

In the gastrointestinal tract, as in all organs with connective tissue, mesenchymal neoplasms may be seen (Figure 64). In the presence of proliferation of spindle to stellate cells with marked atypia, a sarcoma (e.g. leiomyosarcoma if it originates in the smooth muscle) should be suspected. In the case of gastrointestinal stromal tumours (GIST), the degree of cellular atypia can be mild to marked.

Although cytology may provide a first approximation in this type of neoplasm, the differentiation between neoplasms such as leiomyosarcoma and GIST should be made by histological examination and the application of immunohistochemistry techniques.

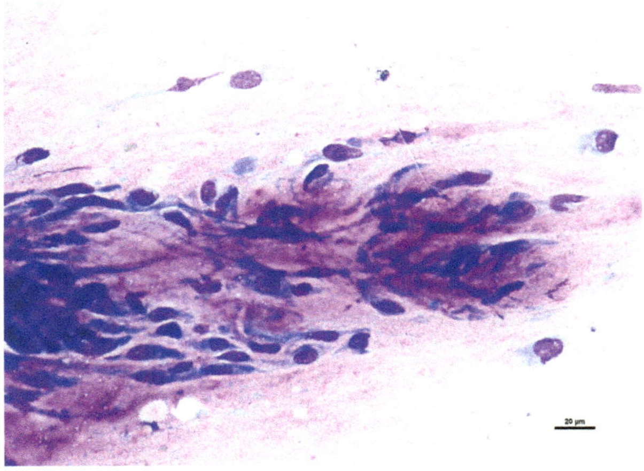

Figure 64. Gastrointestinal stromal tumour. Mesenchymal neoplasm of fusiform cells with a collagenous matrix which is pink in colour.

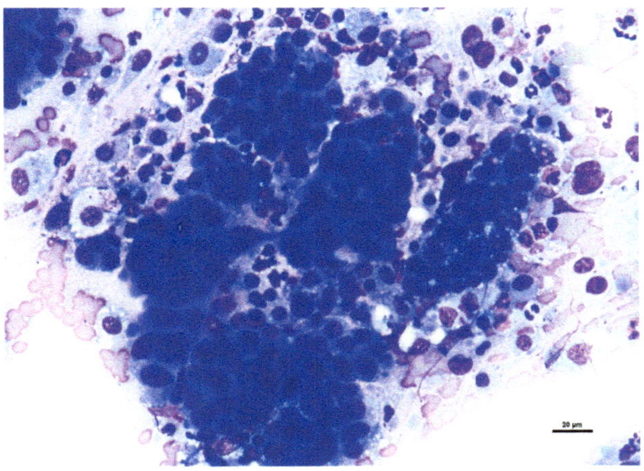

Figure 65. Pulmonary adenocarcinoma with neutrophilic and eosinophilic inflammation. The neoplastic epithelial cells form papillary structures.

Lung

Carcinomas are the most frequent neoplasms found in the lung (Figure 65). Primary tumours cannot be differentiated from metastatic tumours based on cytology, so differentiation between these must be made using clinical history.

Primary lung carcinomas may have a relatively benign cytological appearance, consisting of epithelial cells with a high nucleus/cytoplasm ratio and homogeneous nuclei (basaloid appearance) or, conversely, may exhibit classical features of a carcinoma. Associated neutrophilic inflammation and, in some cases, eosinophilic inflammation is common.

Bibliography

- Alleman, A.R., Bain, P.J. (2000) Diagnosing neoplasia: the cytologic criteria for malignancy. *Vet Med* 95:204–223.
- Bailey, D.B., Page, R.L. (2007) Tumors of the endocrine system. In: Withrow, S.J., Vail, D.M. (eds): *Withrow & MacEwen's small animal clinical oncology*, ed 4, St. Louis, Saunders, pp 583–609.
- Balkman, C. (2009) Hepatobiliary neoplasia in dogs and cats. *Vet Clin North Am Small Anim Pract*. 39(3):617–25.
- Bertazzolo, W., Didier, M., Gelain, M.E. et al. (2014) Accuracy of cytology in distinguishing adrenocortical tumors from pheochromocytoma in companion animals. *Vet Clin Pathol*, 43:453–459.
- Burkhard, M.J. (2016) Respiratory Tract. In: Raskin, R.E., Meyer, D.J. (eds): *Canine and feline cytology: a color atlas and interpretation guide*, ed 3, St Louis, Elsevier Inc, pp. 138–190.
- Camus, M.S., Priest, H.L., Koehler, J.W. et al. (2016) Cytologic criteria for mast cell tumor grading in dogs with evaluation of clinical outcome. *Vet Pathol*, 53(6):1117–1123.
- Caniatti, M., Ghisleni G., Ceruti R. et al. (2001) Cytological features of canine haemangiopericytoma in fine needle aspiration biopsy. *Vet Rec*. 149:242–244.
- Capen, C.C. (2002) Tumors of the endocrine glands. In: Meuten, D.J. (ed): *Tumors in domestic animals*, ed 4, Ames, Iowa State Press, pp. 607–696.
- Choi, U.S., Arndt, T. (2016) Endocrine/Neuroendocrine System. In: Raskin, R.E., Meyer, D.J. (eds): *Canine and feline cytology: a color atlas and interpretation guide*, ed 3, St Louis, Elsevier Inc, pp. 430–452.
- da Costa, R.C., Parent, J.M., Dobson, H. et al. (2008) Ultrasound-guided fine needle aspiration in the diagnosis of peripheral nerve sheath tumors in 4 dogs. *Can Vet J*, 49(1):77–81.
- Foster, A.P., Evans, E., Kerlin, R.L. et al. (1997) Cutaneous T-cell lymphoma with Sézary syndrome in a dog. *Vet Clin Pathol*, 26:188–192.
- Fournier, Q., Cazzini, P., Bavcar, S. et al. (2018) Investigation of the utility of lymph node fine-needle aspiration cytology for the staging of malignant solid tumors in dogs. *Vet Clin Pathol*, 47(3):489–500.
- Henry, C., Herrera, C. (2013) Mast cell tumors in cats: clinical update and possible new treatment avenues. *J Feline Med Surg*, 15(1):41–7.
- Jergens, A.E., Hostetter, S.J., Andreasen, C.B. (2016) Oral Cavity, Gastrointestinal Tract, and Associated Structures. In: Raskin, R.E., Meyer, D.J. (eds): *Canine and feline cytology: a color atlas and interpretation guide*, ed 3, St Louis, Elsevier Inc, pp. 220–246.
- La Perle, K.M.D. (2013) Endocrine system. In: Zachary, J.F., McGavin, M.D. (eds): *Pathologic basis of veterinary disease*, ed 4, St. Louis, Mosby, pp. 660–697.
- Maddux, J.M., Shull, R.M. (1989) Subcutaneous glandular tissue: mammary, salivary, thyroid, and parathyroid. In: Cowell, R.L., Tyler, R.D. (eds): *Diagnostic cytology of the dog and cat*, American Goleta, CA, Veterinary Publications, pp. 83–92.
- Masserdotti, C., Drigo, M. (2012) Retrospective study of cytologic features of well-differentiated hepatocellular carcinoma in dogs. *Vet Clin Pathol*, 41(3):382–390.
- Masserdotti, C., Ubbiali, F.A. (2002) Fine needle aspiration cytology of pilomatricoma in three dogs. *Vet Clin Pathol*, 31:22–25.
- McDonough, S.P., Moore, P.F. (2000) Clinical, hematologic, and immunophenotypic characterization of canine large granular lymphocytosis. *Vet Pathol*, 37:637–645.
- Moore, P.F. (2014) A review of histiocytic diseases of dogs and cats. *Vet Pathol*, 51(1):167–84.
- Moore, P.F., Affolter, V.K., Vernau, W. (2006) Canine hemophagocytic histiocytic sarcoma: a proliferative disorder of CD11d+ macrophages. *Vet Pathol*, 43:632–645.
- Perman, V., Alsaker, R.D., Riis, R.C. (1979) Cytology of the dog and cat. South Bend. *American Animal Hospital Association*, pp. 4–7.
- Raskin, R.E. (2016) General Categories of Cytologic Interpretation. In: Raskin, R.E., Meyer, D.J. (eds): *Canine and feline cytology: a color atlas and interpretation guide*, ed 3, St Louis, Elsevier Inc, pp. 16–33.
- Raskin, R.E. (2016) Hemolymphatic System. In: Raskin, R.E., Meyer, D.J. (eds): *Canine and feline cytology: a color atlas and interpretation guide*, ed 3, St Louis, Elsevier Inc, pp. 91–137.
- Raskin, R.E., Fox, L.E. (2003) Clinical relevance of the World Health Organization classification of lymphoid neoplasms in dogs. *Vet Clin Pathol*, 32:151 (abstract).
- Roth, L. (2001) Comparison of liver cytology and biopsy diagnoses in dogs and cats: 56 cases. *Vet Clin Pathol*. 30(1):35–38.
- Wang, K.Y., Panciera D.L., Al-Rukibat R.K. et al. (2004) Accuracy of ultrasound-guided fine-needle aspiration of the liver and cytologic findings in dogs and cats: 97 cases (1990–2000). *J Am Vet Med Assoc*, 224(1):75–8.
- Wilkerson, M.J., Chard-Bergstrom, C., Andrews G. et al. (2002) Subcutaneous mass aspirate from a dog [epithelioid hemangiosarcoma]. *Vet Clin Pathol*, 31:65–68.

Test

Answers on Page 422

1. **Regarding the collection and handling of samples for cytology:**
    a. The larger the needle gauge, the better.
    b. Aspiration is always recommended to obtain more cells.
    c. Thick preparations allow a better evaluation of the lesion as they contain more cells.
    d. There is no standard protocol for staining preparations.

2. **Among malignancy criteria on cytology, which of the following is not seen:**
    a. A low nucleus/cytoplasm ratio in cells.
    b. An increase in the number of mitoses and presence of atypical mitoses.
    c. Coarse chromatin in the nuclei.
    d. Prominent, multiple, and irregular nucleoli.

3. **Regarding the classification of neoplasms according to their morphological characteristics:**
    a. Mesenchymal neoplasms have cells with well-defined borders.
    b. Histiocytic sarcoma is considered a round cell neoplasm.
    c. The presence of bare nuclei suggests a round cell neoplasm.
    d. Epithelial tumours are usually distributed in a perivascular pattern.

4. **In squamous cell carcinomas:**
    a. Mast cells are seen frequently.
    b. Cells have poorly defined borders.
    c. Associated neutrophilic inflammation is often seen.
    d. "Koilocytes" are observed.

5. **Regarding neoplasms of the sebaceous glands:**
    a. Mature sebocytes predominate in sebaceous epitheliomas.
    b. When malignancy criteria are observed, sebaceous carcinoma should be suspected.
    c. Eosinophilic inflammation is common.
    d. Granulated cytoplasm is characteristic of sebocytes.

6. **Regarding neoplasms of the perianal glands and anal glands:**
    a. Anal gland tumours are also called hepatoids, because of the cell's resemblance to hepatocytes.
    b. The cells of anal gland carcinomas have well-defined borders.
    c. Perianal gland adenomas may show reserve cells, with basal cell characteristics.
    d. Anal gland carcinomas always show marked anisokaryosis.

7. **Regarding mesenchymal cell proliferations:**
    a. Mesenchymal cells can show numerous malignancy criteria in fibromas.
    b. Cells from haemangiosarcomas may show melanin in the cytoplasm.
    c. Adipocytes in lipomas usually show obvious nucleoli.
    d. "Crown cells" can be seen in perivascular wall tumours.

8. **In the cytological grading of canine cutaneous mast cell tumours:**
    a. If granulated mast cells predominate, they are of a low-grade.
    b. If granules are not observed in mast cells or there are very few, they are high-grade.
    c. If eosinophil numbers are high, they are high-grade.
    d. If they no do not exfoliate much, they are high-grade.

9. **In canine lymphoma:**
    a. "Hand mirror" shaped cells indicate a B-cell lymphoma.
    b. The predominance of centroblasts indicates a T-cell lymphoma.
    c. It is possible to determine the immunophenotype of lymphoma based on cell morphology with certainty.
    d. High-grade lymphoma is characterised by frequent large lymphocytes and mitosis.

10. **Thymomas:**
    a. Originate in the mediastinal lymph nodes.
    b. The neoplastic population is lymphoid.
    c. The neoplastic population is epithelial.
    d. In lymphoepithelial thymomas, lymphocytes predominate.

11. Regarding endocrine tumours:

a. In pheochromocytomas, individual round cells can be seen.
b. Pheochromocytomas originate in the adrenal cortex.
c. Insulinomas are characterised by marked cytological malignancy.
d. Carcinoids originate in the β cells of the pancreas.

12. Cytological criteria for the diagnosis of well-differentiated hepatocellular carcinoma include:

a. Marked anisocytosis and anisokaryosis.
b. Prominent nucleoli.
c. Distribution of cells forming acinar or palisade structures.
d. Decreased nucleus/cytoplasm ratio.

13. In pancreatic carcinomas:

a. Characteristics similar to those of other carcinomas are usually observed.
b. Epithelial cells usually display pink cytoplasmic granules.
c. Abundant naked nuclei are observed.
d. It is common to find mast cells.

14. Regarding tumours of the digestive system:

a. Leiomyosarcomas show cytological features very different from those of gastrointestinal stromal tumours (GIST).
b. GIST is an epithelial type.
c. In intestinal lymphoma, large numbers of plasma cells are observed.
d. It is difficult to cytologically differentiate lymphocytic inflammation from low-grade alimentary lymphomas.

15. Regarding lung carcinomas, which of the following statements is incorrect:

a. Eosinophilic inflammation can be seen.
b. Neutrophilic inflammation is common.
c. It is not possible to distinguish primary from metastatic neoplasms cytologically.
d. They always show marked malignancy criteria.

Clinical Case

An 8-year-old French Bulldog with a nodule on the metatarsus of the left forelimb is brought to the practice. The owners say that they noticed it around a month ago, but over the last few days it has grown a lot. They mention he licks it continuously and they can see it getting bigger and smaller at different t mes.

On physical examination there is a mass of 4x4 cm in diameter, which is mobile, partially alopecic, erythematous, and warm to the touch. The rest of the physical examination is normal.

A cytology sample is taken with a blue needle, without aspiration.

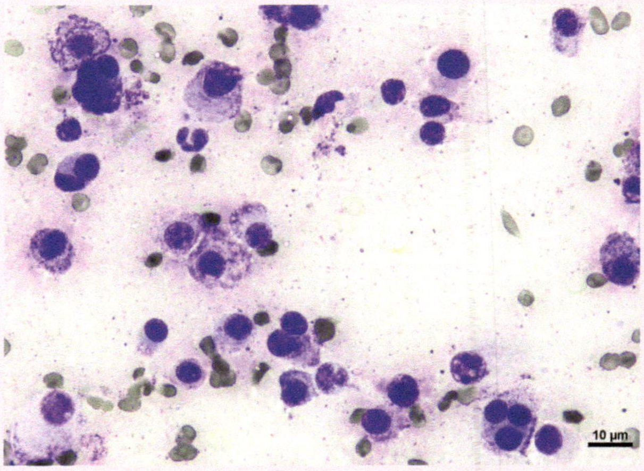

Questions:

1. What type of tumour is it?

2. What is the cytological diagnosis?

3. What is the cytological grade?

4. What criteria can be seen (or not) leading to this grade being assigned?

5. What additional tests could be performed?

Notes

Correct Answers:

Test

1. d
2. a
3. b
4. c
5. b
6. c
7. d
8. b
9. d
10. c
11. a
12. c
13. a
14. d
15. d

Clinical Case

1. **What type of tumour is it?**
   Round cell.

2. **What is the cytological diagnosis?**
   Mast cell tumour.

3. **What is the cytological grade?**
   High-grade.

4. **What criteria can be seen (or not) leading to this grade being assigned?**
   Mast cells with few granules, multinucleated cells, nuclear pleomorphism and anisokaryosis.

5. **What additional tests could be performed?**
   Biopsy and histopathological examination. Sampling of regional lymph nodes, spleen, liver, and bone marrow for staging.

NOTES

Annex 1. New Developments in Immunotherapy in Veterinary Oncology

Keita Kitagawa and Paulo Vilar Saavedra

This chapter is an overview of immunotherapy in veterinary oncology.

The Innate and the Acquired Immune Response

The immune system can be classified into two main subsystems or responses.

- The innate immune response, which occurs rapidly, but lacks specificity. It includes, but is not limited to, physicochemical barriers, the complement system, phagocytic cells (e.g. macrophages, neutrophils, dendritic cells), and cytokines (e.g. IL-2, IL-6).
- On the other hand, the acquired immune response has the ability to recognise and respond to a particular antigen amongst several different antigens (high specificity) but requires a lapse to produce an immune response. Acquired immunity differentiates self-antigens from non-self-antigens and comprises cell- and antibody-mediated responses. Cell-mediated immune responses include activation of cytotoxic T cells (CD8 positive), helper T cells (CD4 positive), and NK cells. The key to acquired immunity is memory of previous exposure, i.e. immunological memory, which allows a rapid response when the organism is exposed to the same antigen again (Bergman, 2014).

Mechanism of Immune Evasion

A concept called immunoediting illustrates how the immune system kills cancer cells. One of the important features of immunoediting is that cancer cells are immunogenic. Immunoediting consists of three phases: elimination (also called immunovigilance) (Muenst et al., 2016), equilibrium, and escape. The escape phase is also called immune evasion, which means that cancer cells evade recognition by the immune system. Cancer cells develop direct and indirect mechanisms to prevent recognition and elimination by the immune system (Drake et al., 2013; Nurieva et al., 2013). Tumour cells can directly downregulate antigen presentation by loss, decreasing MHC I expression, and antigen processing mechanisms (Drake et al., 2013; Nurieva et al., 2013).

In contrast, when indirect mechanisms are applied, tumours produce and release various immunosuppressive factors, such as TGF-β or IL-10. It is important that immunosuppressive factors stimulate or promote the differentiation or expansion of suppressor immune cells, such as T-regs and myeloid-derived suppressor cells (MDSCs) (Nurieva et al., 2013). As a result, they suppress the activity of anti-cancer T cells, allowing tumour cells to survive immune activity (Bergman, 2014; Yamaguchi et al., 2006).

Myeloid Suppressor Cells

Myeloid-derived suppressor cells (MDSCs) play a crucial role in immune evasion.

MDSCs are immature monocytes and granulocytes released from the bone marrow into the blood during pathological processes, including cancer (Murdoch et al., 2008). Not only is the percentage of MDSC in the blood significantly higher in cancer patients than in healthy individuals, but their absolute number also increases in correlation with the stage and number of metastatic tumours in cancer patients (Diaz-Montero et al., 2009). These cells suppress the local anti-tumour immune response and promote angiogenesis and tumour metastasis (Gabrilovich, 2017).

MDSCs directly suppress T cell activation and interact with tumour-associated macrophages (TAMs), to increase the IL-10 produced by the MDSCs themselves and decrease the IL-12 production of TAMs. IL-10 is a cytokine that indirectly suppresses immunity against cancer (Sinha et al., 2007). MDSCs also have the ability to suppress NK-cell activity.

T-cell Regulators (T-reg)

Regulatory T cells (T-reg) are another cell population of the immune system that play an important immunosuppressive role in cancer patients.

T-reg is defined as the cell population expressing CD4, CD25 in the cell membrane and Foxp3 intercellular transcription factor in humans and dogs (Pinheiro. et al., 2011; Pereira et al., 2017). The percentage of T-reg in cancer patients is known to be higher than in healthy dogs in both blood and locoregional lymph nodes (Biller et al., 2007).

According to these main mechanisms, the immunotherapy strategy includes recognition of tumour-specific antigens and production of tumour-specific antibodies, activation of the anti-tumour immunity itself (e.g. reduction of the T-reg population or inhibition of MDSC function).

Non-specific Immunotherapy

Non-specific immunotherapy includes:
- biological response modifiers:
  - bacillus de Calmette-Guérin
  - *Corynebacterium parvum*
  - *Salmonella typhimurium*
  - liposome encapsulated muramyl tripeptide (L-MTP-PE)
  - superantigens
  - imiquimod
- recombinant cytokine therapy:
  - interferon
  - IL-2
  - IL-12.

Bacillus Calmette-Guérin (BCG)

BCG is the live attenuated strain of *Mycobacterium bovis*. Intravesical instillation in the urinary bladder with this bacterium causes a significant local inflammatory response, resulting in anti-tumour responses in human urinary cancer.

It was used in a BCG and hGC human chorionic gonadotropin (LDI-100) study to treat canine mast cell tumours. Dogs were randomly assigned to groups and received either LDI-100 (1.35 ng BCG and 2 units hCG/24 h SC) or vinblastine (2 mg/m² IV, once weekly) for 6 weeks. The overall response rate was not significantly different between LDI-100 and vinblastine alone (28.6 and 11.7% respectively). The study did not include data on survival time, but some adverse events were recorded in the 46 dogs which received LDI-100 (zero with neutropaenia, one with lethargy, seven with gastrointestinal signs and two with increased rectal temperature). Therefore, LDI-100 provided comparable clinical responses to single-agent vinblastine chemotherapy but without myelosuppression (Henry et al., 2007).

It has been reported that treatment with intratumoural BCG may have an effect on canine transmissible venereal tumours (CTVT). BCG was administered intratumourally daily for 5 consecutive days at a dose of 2.5×10^8 CFU in 5 ml. All dogs experienced complete remission, except for the study control group (Mukaratirwa et al., 2009). Mukaratirwa *et al.* reported that CTVTs decreased by half in size within 4 weeks of initiation of treatment. In addition, combined intratumoural therapy with BCG and vincristine achieved the fastest complete remission. No side effects were observed in animals treated for CTVT with intratumoural BCG (Mukaratirwa et al., 2009).

Corynebacterium Parvum

There is limited evidence on *Corynebacterium parvum* therapy. The efficacy of surgical excision alone and surgery plus treatment with *C. parvum* was compared in dogs with malignant oral melanoma. Animals that received *C. parvum* and surgery had a longer survival time (12 months) compared to those that only underwent surgery (7.5 months) (MacEwen, 1990), for melanoma in stages II and III.

In other studies, the comparison between animals that had an incomplete surgical margin followed by a local injection of *C. parvum* and those without injection revealed that there was a similar rate of local tumour recurrence and disease-free intervals in three tumour groups (canine haemangiopericytoma, canine mast cell tumour, and feline mammary carcinomas). Recurrence rates in both *C. parvum* (9/22) and control (8/20) treated animals were similar in canine haemangiopericytoma. For mast cell tumours, the recurrence rate in the *C. parvum* group (7/26) was lower than that of the control group (6/17). In the case of feline mammary carcinomas, recurrence rates in both the *C. parvum* group (15/18) and the control group (6/8) were extremely high (Misdorp, W., 1987). These results suggest that local injection of *C. parvum* therapy may not be clinically effective in these three tumour groups.

The side effects of *C. parvum* therapy have not yet been clearly described as there are no reports to date. Side effects of treatment are supposed to include hypersensitivity, fever, vomiting, diarrhoea, etc.

Salmonella Typhimurium

Therapy with *S. typhimurium* strains has shown promising results in veterinary medicine.

In a phase 1 clinical trial, VNP20009 (modified strain of *S. typhimurium*) was administered to dogs with a variety of malignant tumours (Thamm, et al., 2005) as a weekly or fortnightly intravenous infusion over 30 minutes or 4 hours, at doses ranging from 1.5×10^5 to 1×10^8 CFU/kg. Some cases received dexamethasone (0.5 mg/kg SC) and/or paracetamol (10 mg/kg PO) before and after infusion with VNP20009 (Thamm et al., 2005). In this study, 15% of dogs achieved a general response (10% complete remission, 5% partial remission). Fever, diarrhoea, and vomiting were the most common side effects, although the frequency of occurrence was not reported in the study. These common adverse events were generally mild and self-limiting. 15% of dogs developed elevated liver enzymes, while 34% developed leucocytosis (mean white blood cell count: 25 400/µl) and peripheral blood band neutrophils appeared or increased in number in 59% of dogs. Glomerulonephritis, clinical hepatotoxicity, pancreatitis, epistaxis, and pyoderma also occurred occasionally.

Liposome-encapsulated Muramyl Tripeptide

Liposome-encapsulated muramyl tripeptide (L-MTP-PE) is a non-specific activator of monocytes and macrophages showing anti-tumour activity. For example, L-MTP-PE increases the amount of tumour necrosis factor alpha (TNF-α) and IL-6 activity.

In one study, dogs with osteosarcoma received L-MTP-PE (2 mg/m² IV twice weekly for 8 weeks, with a total of 16 doses), after amputation and followed by cisplatin therapy (70 mg/m² IV every 28 days, 4 cycles). Dogs treated with L-MTP-PE had a longer median survival (14.4 months), compared to the control group (9.8 months) (Kurzman et al., 1995). Compared to 93% in the control group, only 73% of dogs receiving L-MTP-PE developed metastatic disease (Kurzman et al., 1995).

The efficacy of L-MTP-PE in canine haemangiosarcoma (HSA) was also evaluated (Vail et al., 1995) in this study. All macroscopic abdominal HSAs were treated with surgery. After surgery, dogs were classified by clinical stage and assigned to randomised treatment groups with L-MTP-PE group or placebo. All dogs received four cycles of doxorubicin (30 mg/m² IV) plus cyclophosphamide (100 mg/m² IV) administered together once every 3 weeks. L-MTP-PE was administered twice weekly for 8 weeks slowly IV over 5–8 minutes, coinciding with the initiation of chemotherapy. The first dose of L-MTP-PE was 1 mg/m²; all subsequent doses were 2 mg/m². Dogs receiving L-MTP-PE had an overall survival time of 277 days, while dogs in the placebo group had an overall survival time of 143 days. No reports of adverse effect are included in the publication (Vail et al., 1995).

In another study, dogs with stage I oral melanoma who received L-MTP-PE had greater survival times than dogs treated with placebo. According to the study, dogs with oral malignant melanoma received an initial dose of 1 mg/m² IV over 5 to 8 minutes once a week for 8 weeks (subsequent doses were scaled according to the dog's weight: 1 mg/m² for dogs under 5 kg, 1.5 mg/m² for dogs weighing 5–10 kg and 2 mg/m² for dogs over 10 kg) (MacEwen et al., 1999). Individuals who received L-MTP-PE had longer survival times (504 days) than those treated with placebo (271 days). In dogs with oral melanoma in advanced stages, no differences in survival time were observed (258 days in dogs treated with L-MTP-PE versus 243 days in dogs treated with placebo) (MacEwen et al., 1999).

Side effects are thought to be tolerable because the only side effect associated with L-MTP-PE recorded is an elevation in body temperature (1–2 °C), which lasts for 1 to 4 hours after treatment (Kurzman et al., 1995; MacEwen, et al., 1999).

Superantigens

Superantigens (SAg) are enterotoxins produced by bacteria such as *Staphylococcus aureus*. In veterinary medicine, the efficacy and safety of SAg have been evaluated in dogs with oral melanoma and soft-tissue sarcoma (STS).

In oral malignant melanoma, there is a report indicating the efficacy of intratumoural injection of plasmid DNA encoding SAg and granulocyte-macrophage colony-stimulating factor (GM-CSF) or IL-2 every two weeks (Dow et al., 1998). The overall response rate was 46% and a longer survival time was observed in dogs with stage III disease, compared to the historical control at that time (66 weeks in the SAg group versus 22 weeks in the historical control). No serious toxicities were reported.

In another study the efficacy of a lipid DNA therapy encoding canine SAg and IL-2 in dogs with soft-tissue sarcoma is shown. Subjects received once weekly intratumoural injections at an initial dose of 240 or 480 µg of DNA in volumes of 0.8 to 1.6 ml. Treatment was administered based on tumour size and surgery was performed after the 12-week treatment (Thamm et al. ,2003). The overall response rate was 25%. Despite more than 18 months of follow-up, none of the five patients experienced disease recurrence or metastasis.

Adverse effects included diarrhoea, lethargy, lameness and vomiting and were not considered dose limiting nor did they require specific treatment.

Imiquimod

Imiquimod is an immune response modifier and cytokine inducer that enhances both innate and cell-mediated immune responses (Gill et al., 2008; Miller et al., 1999).

Imiquimod treatment has been used for feline multicentric squamous cell carcinoma in situ (MSCCIS) and cutaneous sarcoids in horses. In the case of MSCCIS, one study showed an initial response of skin lesions to imiquimod therapy, but 75% of cats developed a new recurrent lesion. In addition, 41% of animals had side effects following the application of imiquimod cream, including local erythema (25%), increased liver enzymes and neutropaenia (8%) and partial anorexia and vomiting (8%) (Gill et al., 2008). Laboratory abnormalities resolved after a brief interruption of treatment and a decrease in the frequency of application.

In the equine sarcoid study, nineteen tumours were treated in fifteen patients by topically applying imiquimod cream three times a week. There were nine complete remissions, six partial remissions, two stabilisations, and two tumour progressions (Nogueira et al., 2006).

Another study shows that imiquimod therapy can achieve long-term control: 73% of treated cases had a disease-free interval of more than 6 months (Haspeslagh et al., 2016).

The most common side effects of imiquimod are alopecia, erythema, exudation, and erosion in the application area, but recovery should be seen within 30 days of discontinuation (Nogueira et al., 2006).

Therefore, imiquimod may be effective for local control in MSCCIS and equine sarcoids (Nogueira et al., 2006; Haspeslagh et al., 2016)

Interferon

Interferons (IFNs) are proteins produced by lymphocytes that function as anticancer agents and/or immune regulators. Interferons are of two types: IFN-I (IFN-α, -β, and -ω) and IFN-II (IFN-γ).

Intratumoural administration of recombinant human α-interferon-2a (rhIFNα-2a) appears to increase the treatment effect for transmissible venereal tumours in dogs. In a recent study dogs received intratumoural injection of rhIFNα-2a (Roferon®, Roche) weekly at a dose of 1.5 million IU (5.55 μg/0.25 ml). Dogs were divided into three groups, according to the different treatment methods in the study: vincristine, rhIFNα-2a and the combination of vincristine and rhIFNα-2a. The time required to complete remission was shortened in the combined treatment group (3 to 5 weeks) compared to the vincristine-only group (5 to 11 weeks) (Kanca et al., 2018). This result indicated that treatment with intratumoural rhIFNα-2a alone is not effective in CTVT, whereas the combination of rhIFNα-2a and vincristine may achieve rapid complete regression of these tumours. Side effects were classified as described by the Veterinary Cooperative Oncology Group and grade 1 thrombocytopaenia was observed in 3/9, 1/6 and 2/6 dogs in the vincristine group, rhIFNα-2a group and combination treatment group, respectively (Veterinary Co-operative Oncology Group, 2004). Grade 1 neutropaenia was observed in one dog in each study group, as well as reduced PCV values in 2/9, 0/6 and 1/6 in the vincristine group, rhIFNα-2a group and combination treatment group, respectively. As for gastrointestinal effects, grade 1 anorexia, vomiting and diarrhoea were observed, which did not require treatment. Anorexia (2/9), vomiting (1/9) and diarrhoea (2/9) were reported in the vincristine group. Diarrhoea (1/6) was the only gastrointestinal side effect observed in the rhIFNα-2a group. One case was observed for each gastrointestinal side effect in the combination treatment group.

Interleukin-2 (IL-2)

IL-2 is a cytokine that releases activated T cells and not only activates B cells, DCs and macrophages, but also stimulates NK cells.

In a study using IL-2 gene therapy using viral vectors to treat feline fibrosarcomas and canine melanoma, treatment was shown to be safe and effective. The use of IL-2 therapy reduced the rate of tumour recurrence after surgery plus radiation therapy (Jourdier et al., 2003). Cases received an IL-2 injection after surgery and postoperative iridium brachytherapy. The treatment protocol consisted of 0.5 ml administered subcutaneously twice during the first week (day 1 and day 5), then once a week on the first day of weeks 2, 3, 4, 6 and 8. Compared to 61% in the control group, only 28% of cats receiving IL-2 therapy developed local recurrence within the following 12 months.

Another randomised, parallel clinical study revealed the efficacy and safety of a recombinant canarypox virus vaccine expressing feline IL-2, although it did not collect data on side effects. The treatment protocol mentioned that cats received one dose once a week for 4 weeks in a row and every 2 weeks for the last two doses (i.e. on days 0, 7, 14, 21, 35 and 49). IL-2 therapy was administered subcutaneously around the tumour excision site. The IL-2 vaccine resulted in a significantly longer mean recurrence time (>730 days) than in the control group (287 days) and a significant reduction in the risk of recurrence in one year of 56% and a recurrence in two years of 65% (Jas et al., 2015). No general injection site reaction or haematological changes were observed.

In another study, IL-2 therapy was found to be effective against canine transmissible venereal tumours (Den Otter et al., 2015).

Specific Immunotherapy

Tumour-specific proteins are known as tumour antigens (TAs). These proteins may be the target for a tumour vaccine and some TAs tend to be individual or tumour specific. Specific immunotherapies are treatment methods that recognise tumour antigens and produce specific immunity against tumours.

Human Tyrosinase DNA Vaccine

The human tyrosinase DNA vaccine is known as Oncept® (Merial, Duluth, GA) and is used against malignant melanoma. Oncept® uses xenogenic DNA plasmids that contain the gene encoding human tyrosinase (huTyr). Once dogs receive Oncept® intramuscularly, they produce a protein tyrosinase that is 85% homologous to canine tyrosinase to elicit an immune response (Liao et al., 2006).

The vaccination program for canine melanoma with Oncept® is recommended as follows: one treatment every two weeks for four injections, followed by booster vaccines every six months (Sarbu et al., 2017). This vaccine has been used primarily to treat dogs with stage I, II and III oral melanoma (Bergman et al., 2003; Bergman et al., 2006; Grosenbaugh et al., 2011). In one of the studies that have been conducted in the United States, the Oncept®-treated group (N = 58 dogs) had significantly greater survival than the historical control group (N = 53 dogs, previous publications) with a mean survival time of 324 days (Grosenbaugh et al., 2011). However, a more recent study reported that dogs with oral malignant melanoma treated with Oncept® showed no significant difference in survival time compared to dogs that had not received the vaccine (Ottnod et al., 2013; Verganti et al., 2017). In terms of survival, the Oncept® group with stage I-III oral malignant melanoma where locoregional disease control was achieved has been reported to have a mean survival time (MST) of 485 days, versus a MST of 585 days in the non-vaccinated group (Ottnod et al., 2013).

In terms of toxicity, adverse effects were reported in 27 of 111 dogs within fourteen days of vaccination (Grosenbaugh et al., 2011). The injection site reaction included tenderness (14 cases), heat or swelling (14), lameness or stiffness of the injected limb (14) and bruising or erythema at the injection site (13). Non-specific reactions meant that clinical symptoms occurred within 48 hours of vaccination. Clinical signs were reported to include lethargy or depression (14 cases), inappetance (4), polydipsia (5), vomiting (3), diarrhoea (2) and anxiety, increased appetite, incontinence, and mental disturbances (1 in each group). One dog had two incidents of sneezing and pruritus (Grosenbaugh et al., 2011).

This vaccine has become a popular therapy worldwide, so its effectiveness has been used or researched for species other than canines (cats, horses). Most studies emphasise the side effects of the vaccine, which is well tolerated in the species tested, but make little reference to tumour control.

Live Listeria Vector Vaccine

Canine appendicular osteosarcoma (OSA) has a high rate of metastasis: 90% of cases have microscopic metastases at diagnosis.

A phase I clinical trial has evaluated the safety and efficacy of a recombinant strain of *Listeria monocytogenes* (Lm) expressing a chimeric HER2/non-human fusion protein (ADXS31–164) to prevent metastatic disease in dogs with HER2/Neu+ appendicular OSA. In clinical trials, all dogs underwent surgery (seventeen dogs had the limb amputated and one dog had limb rescue surgery) and four doses of carboplatin before receiving ADXS31–164 (IV 30 minutes every 3 weeks) (Mason et al., 2016). The study concluded that a dose of up to 3.3×10^9 CFU ADXS31–164 is safe and provides a mean disease-free interval of 615 days, with a median survival time of 956 days (Mason et al., 2016; Gnanandarajah et al., 2014). Overall survival rates at one, two and three years for dogs treated with ADXS31–164 were 77.8%, 67% and 56% respectively (Mason et al., 2016). Adverse events were assessed according to the veterinary cooperative oncology group: Common Terminology Criteria for Adverse Events (VCOG-CTCAE) v 1.1. grade 1 hypertension (N = 19/23), grade 1 thrombocytopaenia (N = 13/23) and grade 2 (N = 8/23). ALP elevation was observed more frequently (Mason et al., 2016).

Antibody Therapy

The development of monoclonal antibody therapy (mAbs) for dogs is considerably behind, compared to the large number of mAbs available to humans, as tumour antigens have hardly been identified in canines.

Regarding nomenclature, the names of mAbs ending in -omab are murine, -ximab and -zumab are chimeric, and -umab are humanised versions of antibodies.

Anti-CD20 Antibodies

Rituximab, which targets CD20, is one of the most common monoclonal antibodies for a portion of the treatment of human non-Hodgkin lymphoma. However, rituximab does not bind to canine B cells even though they express CD20 (Impellizeri et al., 2006).

Anti-human Antigen-leucocyte Monoclonal Antibodies (HLA)-DR

In a study using the human leucocyte monoclonal antibody (HLA)-DR for canine lymphoma, the anti-HLA-DR monoclonal antibody bound to normal and malignant canine lymphocytes and produced induced apoptosis in canine lymphoma cells.

Preliminarily, stable transient disease was observed in dogs with advanced stage lymphoma after immunotherapy with anti-HLA-DR monoclonal antibodies. Immunotherapy with anti-HLA-DR monoclonal antibodies has frequently caused adverse events, which were evaluated by the veterinary cooperative oncology group according to the common terminology criteria for adverse events (VCOG-CTCAE) v1.1. 6/7 cases had grade 1 nausea or vomiting and 5/7 had grade 1 fever, although slowing infusion rate avoided adverse reactions. Two dogs received dexamethasone at 0.5–2 mg/kg IV to treat vomiting and elevated temperature. Haematological toxicity was also observed in 3/7 cases. One dog had grade 1 neutropaenia and grade 1 thrombocytopaenia two weeks after the first infusion. Grade 3 neutropaenia and grade 4 thrombocytopaenia were observed in two dogs one week after the second infusion; both received chemotherapy prior to the antibody infusion. One of the dogs was euthanased due to bleeding from multiple ulcerated cutaneous lymphoma lesions (Stein et al., 2011).

Adoptive T-Cell Transfer Therapy (ACT)

ACT is a method that harnesses autologous T cells from the tumour microenvironment, which are harvested, cultured, and activated and then transferred back to the patient. This technique has been used experimentally as a treatment for canine lymphoma.

Eight dogs were used for this preliminary study (O'Connor et al., 2012) and in seven of them a previous complete remission (CR) was achieved after receiving a CHOP protocol. The use of ACT after the CHOP protocol resulted in notable improvements in overall and tumour-free survival: animals that received ACT after CHOP had a longer overall survival time (392 days), compared to dogs that received CHOP therapy alone (167 days).

Toxicities were limited to a period of 72 hours after the second T-cell infusion. Adverse events were measured according to the VCOG-CTCAE v1.1.40: grade I or II gastrointestinal toxicity (i.e. vomiting, diarrhoea, nausea etc.). A dog with a grade III gastrointestinal adverse event required hospitalisation for dehydration.

Other Treatments

Some immune checkpoint blockers have been successful in anticancer treatment, such as programmed cell death 1 (PD-1) and cytotoxic T-cell-associated protein 4 (CTLA4). Similarly, expectations for immune checkpoint blockers are increasing even in the veterinary field. One study reported that the anti-PD-L1, monoclonal antibody, called c4G12, could be used to treat oral melanoma (Maekawa et al., 2017). As part of a study, nine dogs with oral malignant melanoma (OMM) (N = 7) or undifferentiated sarcoma (N = 2) were administered c4G12. All dogs had been treated with locoregional therapy, including surgery, radiation therapy, and a combination of radiation and chlorambucil chemotherapy prior to c4G12 treatment.

These dogs were treated with 2 or 5 mg/kg c4G12 by intravenous administration every two weeks. As a result, two out of nine dogs achieved a partial response. Among the dogs with OMM treated with c4G12, four out of seven suffering from lung metastases had disease progression. However, one dog had an unexpectedly long survival time (222 days) despite lung metastasis. Adverse events were classified according to the veterinary cooperative oncology group, common terminology criteria for adverse events (VCOG-CTCAE, v 1.1). The only adverse event was grade 1 diarrhoea.

Bibliography

- Bergman, P.J. (2014) Immunotherapy in veterinary oncology. *Vet Clin North Am Small Anim Pract*. 44:925-939.
- Bergman, P.J., Camps-Palau, M.A., McKnight, J.A. et al. (2006) Development of a xenogeneic DNA vaccine program for canine malignant melanoma at the Animal Medical Center. *Vaccine*. 24:4582–4585.
- Bergman, P.J., McKnight, J., Novosad, A. et al. (2003) Long-Term Survival of Dogs with Advanced Malignant Melanoma after DNA Vaccination with Xenogeneic Human Tyrosinase. A Phase I Trial. *Clinical Cancer Research*. 9:1284–1290.
- Biller, B.J., Elmslie, R.E., Burnett, R.C. et al. (2007) Use of FoxP3 expression to identify regulatory T cells in healthy dogs and dogs with cancer. *Veterinary Immunology and Immunopathology*. 116:69–78.
- Den Otter, W., Hack, M., Jacobs, J.J. et al. (2015) Treatment of transmissible venereal tumors in dogs with intratumoral interleukin-2 (IL-2). A pilot study. *Anticancer Res*. 35:713–717.
- Diaz-Montero, C.M., Salem, M.L., Nishimura, M.I. et al. (2009) Increased circulating myeloid-derived suppressor cells correlate with clinical cancer stage, metastatic tumor burden, and doxorubicin–cyclophosphamide chemotherapy. *Cancer immunology, immunotherapy*. 58:49–59.
- Dow, S.W., Elmslie, R.E., Willson, A.P. et al. (1998) In vivo tumor transfection with superantigen plus cytokine genes induces tumor regression and prolongs survival in dogs with malignant melanoma. *The Journal of Clinical Investigation*. 101:2406–2414.
- Drake, C.G., Jaffee, E., Pardoll, D.M. (2013) Mechanisms of immune evasion by tumors. *Adv Immunol*. 90:51-81.
- Fritz, S.E., Henson, M.S., Greengard, E. et al. (2016) A phase I clinical study to evaluate safety of orally administered, genetically engineered Salmonella enterica serovar Typhimurium for canine osteosarcoma. *Veterinary medicine and science*. 2:179–190.
- Gabrilovich, D.I. (2017) Myeloid-Derived Suppressor Cells. *Cancer immunology research*. 5:3–8.
- Gill, V.L., Bergman, P.J., Baer, K.E. et al. (2008) Use of imiquimod 5% cream (Aldara) in cats with multicentric squamous cell carcinoma in situ: 12 cases (2002–2005). *Vet Comp Oncol*. 6:55–64.
- Gnanandarajah, J.S., Ndikuyeze, G.H., Engiles, J.B. et al. (2014) A recombinant HER2/neu expressing *listeria monocytogenes* (Lm-LLO) immunotherapy delays metastatic disease and prolongs overall survival in a spontaneous canine model of osteosarcoma - a Phase I clinical trial. *Journal for ImmunoTherapy of Cancer*. 2:p55.
- Grosenbaugh, D.A., Leard, A.T., Bergman, P.J. et al. (2011) Safety and efficacy of a xenogeneic DNA vaccine encoding for human tyrosinase as adjunctive treatment for oral malignant melanoma in dogs following surgical excision of the primary tumor. *American Journal of Veterinary Research*. 72:1631–1638.
- Haspeslagh, M., Vlaminck, L.E., Martens, A.M. (2016) Treatment of sarcoids in equids: 230 cases (2008–2013). *J Am Vet Med Assoc*. 249:311–318.
- Henry, C.J., Downing, S., Rosenthal, R.C. et al. (2007) Evaluation of a novel immunomodulator composed of human chorionic gonadotropin and bacillus Calmette-Guerin for treatment of canine mast cell tumors in clinically affected dogs. *Am J Vet Res*. 68:1246–1251.
- Impellizeri, J.A., Howell, K., McKeever, K.P. et al. (2006) The role of rituximab in the treatment of canine lymphoma: An ex vivo evaluation. *The Veterinary Journal*. 171:556–558.
- Jas, D., Soyer, C., De Fornel-Thibaud, P. et al. (2015) Adjuvant immunotherapy of feline injection-site sarcomas with the recombinant canarypox virus expressing feline interleukine-2 evaluated in a controlled monocentric clinical trial when used in association with surgery and brachytherapy. *Trials in Vaccinology*. 4:1–8.
- Jourdier, T.M., Moste, C., Bonnet, M.C. et al. (2003) Local immunotherapy of spontaneous feline fibrosarcomas using recombinant poxviruses expressing interleukin 2 (IL2). *Gene Ther*. 10:2126–2132.
- Kanca, H., Tez, G., Bal, K. et al. (2018) Intratumoral recombinant human interferon alpha-2a and vincristine combination therapy in canine transmissible venereal tumour. *Veterinary Medicine and Science*. 4:364–372.
- Kurzman, I.D., MacEwen, E.G., Rosenthal, R.C. et al. (1995) Adjuvant therapy for osteosarcoma in dogs: results of randomized clinical trials using combined liposome-encapsulated muramyl tripeptide and cisplatin. *Clinical cancer research: an official journal of the American Association for Cancer Research*. 1:1595–1601.
- Liao, J.C., Gregor, P., Wolchok, J.D. et al. (2006) Vaccination with human tyrosinase DNA induces antibody responses in dogs with advanced melanoma. *Cancer Immunity*. 6:8.
- MacEwen, E.G. (1990) Spontaneous tumors in dogs and cats: Models for the study of cancer biology and treatment. *Cancer and Metastasis Reviews*. 9:125–136.
- MacEwen, E.G., Kurzman, I.D., Vail, D.M. et al. (1999) Adjuvant Therapy for Melanoma in Dogs: Results of Randomized Clinical Trials Using Surgery, Liposome-encapsulated Muramyl Tripeptide, and Granulocyte Macrophage Colony-stimulating Factor. *Clinical Cancer Research*. 5:4249–4258.
- Maekawa, N., Konnai, S., Takagi, S. et al. (2017) A canine chimeric monoclonal antibody targeting PD-L1 and its clinical efficacy in canine oral malignant melanoma or undifferentiated sarcoma. *Scientific reports*. 7:8951–8951.
- Mason, N.J., Gnanandarajah, J.S., Engiles, J.B. et al. (2016) Immunotherapy with a HER2-Targeting *Listeria* Induces HER2-Specific Immunity and Demonstrates Potential Therapeutic Effects in a Phase I Trial in Canine Osteosarcoma. *Clinical Cancer Research*. 22:4380–4390.
- Miller, R.L., Gerster, J.F., Owens, M.L. et al. (1999) Imiquimod applied topically: a novel immune response modifier and new class of drug. *Int J Immunopharmacol*. 21:1–14.
- Misdorp, W. (1987) Incomplete surgery, local immunostimulation, and recurrence of some tumour types in dogs and cats. *The Veterinary quarterly*. 9:279–286.

■ Muenst, S., Läubli, H., Soysal, S.D. et al. (2016) The immune system and cancer evasion strategies: therapeutic concepts. *Journal of Internal Medicine*. 279:541–562.
■ Mukaratirwa, S., Chitanga, S., Chimatira, T. et al. (2009) Combination therapy using intratumoral bacillus Calmette-Guerin (BCG) and vincristine in dogs with transmissible venereal tumours: therapeutic efficacy and histological changes. *J S Afr Vet Assoc*. 80:92–96.
■ Murdoch, C., Muthana, M., Coffelt, S.B. et al. (2008) The role of myeloid cells in the promotion of tumour angiogenesis. *Nat Rev Cancer*. 8:618–631.
■ Nogueira, S.A.F., Torres, S.M.F., Malone, E.D. et al. (2006) Efficacy of imiquimod 5% cream in the treatment of equine sarcoids: a pilot study. *Veterinary Dermatology*. 17:259–265.
■ Nurieva, R., Wang, J., Sahoo, A. (2013) T-cell tolerance in cancer. *Immunotherapy*. 5:513–531.
■ O'Connor, C.M., Sheppard, S., Hartline, C.A. et al. (2012) Adoptive T-cell therapy improves treatment of canine non–Hodgkin lymphoma post chemotherapy. *Scientific Reports*. 2:249.
■ Ottnod, J.M., Smedley, R.C., Walshaw, R. et al. (2013) A retrospective analysis of the efficacy of Oncept® vaccine for the adjunct treatment of canine oral malignant melanoma. *Vet Comp Oncol*. 11:219–229.
■ Pereira, L.M.S., Gomes, S.T.M. et al. (2017) Regulatory T Cell and Forkhead Box Protein 3 as Modulators of Immune Homeostasis. *Frontiers in immunology*. 8:605–605.
■ Phillips, J.C., Lembcke, L.M., Noltenius, C.E. et al. (2012) Evaluation of tyrosinase expression in canine and equine melanocytic tumors. *Am J Vet Res*. 73:272–278.
■ Pinheiro, D., Singh, Y., Grant, C.R. et al. (2011) Phenotypic and functional characterization of a CD4(+) CD25(high) FOXP3(high) regulatory T-cell population in the dog. *Immunology*. 132:111–122.
■ Sarbu, L., Kitchell, B.E., Bergman, P.J. (2017) Safety of administering the canine melanoma DNA vaccine (Oncept®) to cats with malignant melanoma – a retrospective study. *Journal of feline medicine and surgery*. 19:224-230.
■ Sinha, P., Clements, V.K., Bunt, S.K. et al. (2007) Cross-Talk between Myeloid-Derived Suppressor Cells and Macrophages Subverts Tumor Immunity toward a Type 2 Response. *The Journal of Immunology*. 179:977–983.
■ Stein. R., Balkman, C., Chen, S. et al. (2011) Evaluation of anti-human leukocyte antigen-DR monoclonal antibody therapy in spontaneous canine lymphoma. *Leuk Lymphoma*. 52:273–284.
■ Thamm, D.H., Kurzman, I.D., King, I. et al. (2005) Systemic Administration of an Attenuated, Tumor-Targeting *Salmonella typhimurium* to Dogs with Spontaneous Neoplasia: Phase I Evaluation. *Clinical cancer research*. 11:4827–4834.
■ Thamm, D.H., Kurzman, I.D., Macewen, E.G. et al. (2003) Intralesional lipid-complexed cytokine/superantigen immunogene therapy for spontaneous canine tumors. *Cancer Immunology, Immunotherapy*. 52:473–480.
■ Vail, D.M., MacEwen, E.G., Kurzman, I.D. et al. (1995) Liposome-encapsulated muramyl tripeptide phosphatidylethanolamine adjuvant immunotherapy for splenic hemangiosarcoma in the dog: a randomized multi-institutional clinical trial. *Clinical cancer research: an official journal of the American Association for Cancer Research*. 1:1165–1170.
■ Verganti, S., Berlato, D., Blackwood, L. et al. (2017) Use of Oncept® melanoma vaccine in 69 canine oral malignant melanomas in the UK. *J Small Anim Pract*. 58:10–16.
■ Veterinary Co-operative Oncology Group - Common Terminology Criteria for Adverse Events (VCOG-CTCAE) following chemotherapy or biological antineoplastic therapy in dogs and cats v1.0. (2004) *Vet Comp Oncol* 2004;2:195–213.
■ Veterinary cooperative oncology group – common terminology criteria for adverse events (VCOG-CTCAE) following chemotherapy or biological antineoplastic therapy in dogs and cats v1.1. (2016) *Veterinary and comparative oncology*. 14:417–446.
■ Yamaguchi T, Sakaguchi S. (2006) Regulatory T cells in immune surveillance and treatment of cancer. *Semin Cancer Biol*. 16:115–123.

Annex 2. Histiocytic Diseases

Keita Kitagawa and Paulo Vilar Saavedra

The term "histiocyte" is used to describe dendritic cells and macrophages. Histiocytes originate from CD34 positive stem cells in the bone marrow, express CD18 and CD1a, and play a role in phagocytosis and antigen recognition (Moore, 2014; Affolter et al., 2002). Differentiated forms of these stem cells are called Langerhans epidermal cells (epidermal dendritic cells), interstitial dendritic cells, and macrophages (Affolter et al., 2002).

Canine Histiocytic Disease

Histiocytic diseases are more common in dogs than in cats. They are classified into three groups, according to the histiocyte from which they originate:

- cutaneous histiocytoma and cutaneous Langerhans histiocytosis originate from Langerhans epidermal cells;
- reactive histiocytosis and histiocytic sarcoma arise from dendritic interstitial cells;
- histiocytic haemophagocytic sarcoma originates from macrophages (Moore, 2014; Affolter, 2002).

Cutaneous Histiocytoma and Cutaneous Langerhans Cell Histiocytosis

Cutaneous Histiocytoma (CH)

Cutaneous histiocytomas are benign tumours derived from Langerhans epidermal cells (LC) (Moore, 2014). It is one of the most common histiocytic disorders and often occurs as a single lesion in young dogs (<3 years of age) but may occur in dogs of all ages (Schmidt et al., 2010; Dobson, 2013). Purebred dogs are predisposed, especially Boxers and Dachshunds (Taylor et al., 1969).

CHs are composed of well-differentiated, round to polygonal histiocytes with abundant cytoplasm and finely dispersed chromatin (Pazdzior-Czapula, 2015). Expression of CD18, CD1a and E-cadherin can be confirmed by immunohistochemistry (Moore, 2014; Pires et al., 2013).

Cutaneous histiocytomas usually regress spontaneously (Moore, 2014), so do not require treatment except in refractory cases for which there are no therapeutic guidelines. Survival prognosis is usually excellent.

Cutaneous Langerhans Cell Histiocytosis (LCH)

The other type of histiocytic disorder originating from epidermal cells is cutaneous Langerhans cell histiocytosis (LCH), also known as multiple cutaneous histiocytoma. The prevalence of the disease is very low (<1% of all cases having histiocytic disorders originating in LC) and Shar Pei dogs are more likely to be affected.

In general, the nature of the disease is progressive, and it has the ability to affect internal and/or distant organs even if they do not present morphological criteria of histopathological malignancy.

Affected dogs suffer from moderate pruritus, redness, alopecia, and multiple skin nodules. Peripheral lymph nodes and lungs are frequently involved (Moore, 2014; Nagata et al., 2000; Faller et al., 2016).

It is often difficult to distinguish CH from LCH on histopathology. Histiocytes may show anisokaryosis and be multinucleated cells, typical characteristics of solitary histiocytomas, but these results are not consistent for LCH (Moore, 2014). LCH cells express CD18, CD1a, and E-cadherin, as well as CH (Moore, 2014; Pires et al., 2013).

Treatment recommendations include surgery, if needed, and chemotherapy. Although the efficacy of the use of lomustine (CCNU) has not been described, its use (60–70 mg/m² PO every three weeks) is suggested in refractory cases (Moore, 2014).

One study includes the clinical case of a dog with LCH successfully treated with griseofulvin (30 mg/kg BID PO), which is an immunomodulatory antibiotic. Clinical response was observed one week after initiation of treatment and complete remission occurred after 7 weeks. This dog died due to disease progression 3 months after treatment with griseofulvin was withdrawn.

In the author's experience, treatment of LCH with a combination of palliative radiation therapy (6 Gy×4 fractions once weekly) and systemic chemotherapy with CCNU (60–70 mg/m² PO every 3 weeks) results in partial skin lesion response and improved quality of life. In addition, radiotherapy for LCH in human patients has been shown to stabilise or ameliorate injury-related symptoms (Kotecha et al., 2014) in 90.4% of treated individuals. Therefore, radiation therapy could be a local LCH control option.

The prognosis for LCH is not well defined. A recent study found that three out of eight dogs were still alive and without severe disease, based on palpation diagnosis and physical examination, at 1682 days, 570 days, and 318 days after diagnosis, respectively. One case had a progressive clinical course and was euthanised 2 weeks after diagnosis. The others were removed from the study or died of unknown causes (Faller et al., 2016) However, another study noted that dogs had a survival time of 3 months after discontinuation of therapy (Nagata et al. 2000).

Reactive Histiocytosis

Reactive histiocytosis includes cutaneous histiocytosis (CH) and systemic histiocytosis (SH). Both types originate from activated interstitial dendritic cells (Affolter et al., 2000). The defective interaction of dendritic cells and T cells is considered to cause the development of canine reactive histiocytosis (Moore, 2014).

Cutaneous Histiocytosis

Cutaneous histiocytosis (CH) is an early stage of reactive histiocytosis that presents as limited skin lesions (Affolter, et al., 2000). Canine CH tends to occur in younger individuals but has been seen in animals from 2 to 11 years of age. No breed predisposition has been reported, although a study in thirty-two dogs noted that the Golden Retriever, Great Dane, and Bouvier des Flandes are the breeds that suffer from CH most frequently (Palmeiro et al., 2007).

Lesions consist of multiple skin nodules, plaques, and papules on the head, neck, trunk, and extremities, which present with swelling, erythema, depigmentation, and, occasionally, spontaneous regression of lesions may occur (Moore, 2014; Affolter et al., 2000; Palmeiro et al., 2007).

Histologically, activated interstitial dendritic cells predominate in the mid/deep dermis and subcutis. Cells have large nuclei and abundant pale cytoplasm with occasional cytoplasmic vacuoles (Affolter et al., 2000; Palmeiro et al., 2007). Activated interstitial dendritic cells express CD1, CD11c, CD4, CD18, MHC II and CD90. CD8+ T cells can account for up to 50% of the cell infiltrate in the lesion (Affolter et al., 2000).

Treatment is primarily with immunosuppressants or immune system modulation. One study recorded an initial excellent response to therapy, with complete resolution of lesions in all patients (N = 32). Initial treatment included prednisone (1–2 mg/kg/day PO) or in combination with antibiotics (azathioprine and/or tetracycline/niacinamide) (Palmeiro et al., 2007).

Approximately 30% of cases experience disease recurrence. CHs affecting the nares/nasal plane have a higher recurrence rate (67%) (Palmeiro et al., 2007). To prevent recurrence, Palmeiro et al. (2007) proposed the use of tetracycline/niacinamide at a dose of 250 mg/animal TID <10 kg or 500 mg/animal TID >10 kg as maintenance therapy for cutaneous histiocytosis (Palmeiro et al., 2007). However, it is doubtful whether this maintenance therapy is effective, as the recurrence rate in dogs with tetracycline/niacinamide maintenance therapy (36.4%) was higher than in those who did not receive it (23.8%) (Palmeiro et al., 2007). About 81% of dogs were alive at the end of the study, with a median follow-up time of 25 months (Palmeiro et al., 2007).

Systemic Histiocytosis

Systemic histiocytosis (SH) is an advanced stage of reactive histiocytosis that affects other organs (Affolter et al., 2000) in addition to the skin. Systemic histiocytosis (SH) has a familial predisposition in the Bernese Mountain Dog (Moore, 1984), a breed also predisposed to suffering from histiocytic sarcoma. Interestingly, progression from SH to histiocytic sarcoma has not been observed (Affolter et al., 2000).

The age of onset of SH ranges from 1 to 9 years. It is most often seen in the skin, subcutaneous tissues, nasal cavity, eyes, and peripheral lymph nodes, although it can sometimes affect the spleen, testicular tissue, bone marrow, lung, and gingiva (Affolter et al., 2000; Paterson et al., 1995). Skin lesions due to SH are similar to those seen in cases of CH (e.g. well circumscribed nodules, alopecia, and erythema), but in SH (Affolter, et al., 2000) they are often more widespread and follow the vessels in the skin. The difference with CH is that SH does not spontaneously regress. Clinical signs depend on the organs involved: for example, bilateral episcleritis, scleritis and conjunctivitis with marked chemosis in the eyes, anorexia, weight loss, rattlesnake respiration (Moore, 1984; Paterson et al., 1995). The histological characteristics of SH are the same as those of CH and express CD1, CD11c, CD4, CD18, MHC II and CD90 (Affolter et al., 2000).

Therapy based on immunosuppressants such as azathioprine (2.2 mg/kg/day), cyclosporine A, leflunomide or a 0.1% dexamethasone topical ointment achieves long-term control in some cases (Affolter et al., 2000; Paterson et al., 1995). The treatment protocols for cyclosporine A and leflunomide have not been adequately described, although it is reasonable for cyclosporine A to be used at an initial dose of 5 mg/kg PO once daily and leflunomide at 3–4 mg/kg PO once daily (Plumb, 2015).

In the most refractory cases, the use of chemotherapeutic agents such as CCNU (Palmeiro et al., 2007) is suggested.

Histiocytic Sarcoma

Histiocytic sarcoma (HS) is derived from dendritic interstitial cells and has aggressive and rapid biological behaviour (Moore et al., 2017; Klahn et al., 2011). Currently, HS is considered a systemic disease, although there are localised and disseminated forms (Affolter et al., 2002). Localised HS and disseminated HS are considered as distinct clinical stages: localised HS is an early stage which affects a single organ, without metastasis, while disseminated HS is an advanced stage, in which multiple organs are affected.

Localised HS is classified into periarticular, pulmonary, and other locations (Affolter et al., 2002; Skorupski et al., 2009; Klahn et al., 2011; Kagawa et al., 2016; Marlowe et al., 2018).

Periarticular Histiocytic Sarcoma (PAHS)

PAHS is a localised sarcoma that occurs in the joint/periarticular region of the extremities (Moore, 2014; Klahn et al., 2011). It often affects older dogs (8.8 years on average) and large breeds, such as Labrador and Golden Retrievers, with more likely involvement of Smooth Hair Retrievers. There is no sex predisposition for PAHS.

The elbow joint is often affected, and it is less likely to occur in the tarsal, hip, and carpal joints. Lameness (79%) or soft tissue inflammation (68%) are common clinical signs at initial presentation.

Diagnosis should include basic tests (complete blood tests, serum chemistry profile and urinalysis), regional and thoracic radiography, abdominal ultrasound, and surgical biopsy. Approximately 60% of dogs have radiographic osteolysis. Distant metastatic sites include regional lymph nodes, lung, liver, kidney, and spleen. Cytological analysis describes typical HS cells, with a large, pleomorphic cytoplasm, eccentric nucleus, marked atypia and numerous nuclei and nucleoli or mitotic figures. PAHS are definitively diagnosed by histopathology-immunohistochemistry (IHC), since they are positive for CD1a, CD11c and CD18. The lack of CD3, CD79a and CD11d allows the possibility of lymphoma and haemophagocytic HS to be excluded (Moore, 2014; Klahn et al., 2011; Pazdzior-Czapula et al., 2015).

For treatment, both amputation for local pain control and systemic chemotherapy for microscopic disease control should be considered: treating PAHS with amputation followed by chemotherapy is recommended, which allows an increased survival time (Moore, 2014; Faller et al., 2016).

A chemotherapeutic adjuvant protocol including lomustine (60–80 mg/m^2 PO every 3 weeks) or doxorubicin (30 mg/m^2 IV every 3 weeks) is recommended. The use of lomustine is suggested because a 46% response rate has been recorded in dogs with gross HS lesions (Skorupski et al., 2007; Skorupski et al, 2009).

Survival time is relatively long, averaging 391 days (48–980 days). The presence of metastases at the time of diagnosis is a negative prognostic factor for survival. One study found that dogs that did not have metastases and received chemotherapy had a median survival time of 980 days, compared to 253 days in dogs with evidence of metastases. Another negative prognostic factor is concurrent administration of prednisone, according to one publication (Dervisis et al., 2017).

Pulmonary Histiocytic Sarcoma (PHS)

PHS is defined as a localised HS affecting the lung, without abdominal lesions (Kagawa et al., 2016; Marlowe et al., 2018). Old dogs (9–10 years) are more likely to be affected.

Regarding the prevalence, it is more frequent in Bernese Mountain Dogs, Rottweilers, Flat-Coated Retrievers, Miniature Schnauzers, and the Pembroke Welsh Corgi (Kagawa et al., 2016; Lenz et al., 2017). Clinical signs include coughing (37.8%), lethargy (24.3%), lack of appetite (27%) and dyspnoea (9.3%).

Minimum tests (complete blood counts, serum chemistry profile, and urinalysis), complete staging, computed tomography (CT), and biopsy are required to reach a diagnosis. Most dogs with PHS are likely to be affected in the right or accessory lung lobes, as seen by thoracic radiography and/or computed tomography in several studies (Kagawa et al., 2016; Marlowe et al., 2018).

Histologically, poorly differentiated histiocytes are observed in PHS, which means cells are densely arranged, pleomorphic, round, with prominent anisokaryosis, and many mitotic figures (Kagawa et al., 2016). In PHS the cells show the same IHC findings as in PHS (Moore, 2014; Affolter et al., 2002; Pazdzior-Czapula, 2015).

In a study in which surgery and chemotherapy (CCNU-based protocol) were combined, cases with PHS had significantly greater increases in injury-free time (276 days) and survival time (374 days). When chemotherapy alone was used, the overall response rate was 44.5%, injury-free time was 91 days, and mean survival time was 131 days. The presence of clinical signs in the diagnosis negatively affected progression-free survival (Marlowe et al., 2018).

Other Localised Histiocytic Sarcomas

Visceral and cerebral histiocytic sarcomas have been reported as a rare form of localised histiocytic sarcoma.

Although the clinical signs are different depending on the anatomical sites involved, the clinical pathological findings, diagnostic imaging and histopathological findings are similar to those for PAHS and PHS. In particular, the IHC findings are the same because they originate from the same type of histiocyte (Moore, 2014; Affolter et al., 2002; Pazdzior-Czapula, 2015).

Regarding treatment, chemotherapy is required, and surgery may be suggested. The combination of surgery and chemotherapy allows for longer survival time than surgery alone (Moore et al., 2017; Skorupski et al., 2009).

Disseminated Histiocytic Sarcomas

Disseminated histiocytic sarcoma (DHS) is an advanced stage HS in which cells spread beyond the regional lymph node to distant sites (Moore, 2014; Affolter et al., 2002; Dervisis et al., 2017). The average age of appearance is 7 years (Moore et al., 1986) and breeds which appear to be predisposed are the Bernese Mountain Dog, Rottweiler, Golden and Labrador Retriever (Affolter et al., 2002; Moore et al., 2006). Regarding clinical signs, they are non-specific and include anorexia, weight loss and lethargy (Moore et al., 1986). Depending on the anatomical location affected, dyspnoea, lameness, and ataxia may also be seen (Affolter et al., 2002). DHS is most often found in the spleen, liver, lung, bone marrow, and lymph nodes. Both DHS and the localised form originate from interstitial dendritic cells, so histopathology reveals round, pleomorphic cells, with various sizes of eccentric nuclei, many mitotic figures, and prominent anisokaryosis. Immunohistochemistry provides evidence of expression of CD1a, CD11c and CD18 and shows absence of CD3, CD79a and CD11d (Moore, 2014; Moore et al., 2017; Klahn et al., 2011; Skorupski et al., 2007).

Chemotherapy is the recommended treatment modality to prevent cancer progression in DHS. Lomustine (CCNU) is the most common chemotherapeutic agent reported to treat it. The overall response rate to CCNU varies between published studies from 46 to 58% and, in patients which respond (Skorupski et al., 2007; Cannon et al., 2015; Mason et al., 2018), the median survival time is 172–195 days. Gastrointestinal toxicity, hepatotoxicity and mild to moderate haematotoxicity (Cannon et al., 2015) are the most common adverse effects.

Haemophagocytic Histiocytic Sarcoma

Haemophagocytic histiocytic sarcoma (HHS) is a special form of sarcoma that arises from the red pulp of the spleen and originates in macrophages from the bone marrow (Moore et al., 2006). The mean age of onset is 7 years old (with a range of 2.5 to 13 years old). The Bernese Mountain Dog, Golden Retriever, Rottweiler, and the Flat-Coated Retriever are the breeds that are most frequently affected. This extremely aggressive form of sarcoma can cause several clinical signs, but symptoms associated with severe anaemia are more likely to be observed, including lethargy, exercise intolerance, shallow and rapid breathing, respiratory exertion, etc. HHS usually involves the spleen and can also affect the liver, bone marrow, lymph nodes, and/or lungs (Moore et al., 2006). Common haematological findings in dogs with HHS are Coombs-negative anaemia (94%), thrombocytopaenia (88%), hypoalbuminaemia (94%), and prolonged partial thromboplastin time (PTT) (Moore et al., 2006). Patients with HHS are more likely to have disseminated intravascular coagulation (DIC).

Cytology of HHS shows atypical histiocytes, which means that these cells are erythrophagocytic and often contain haemosiderin. HHS cells express CD18 and CD11d but have low or inconsistent CD1a expression on immunohistochemistry. The absence of CD3 and CD79a can help distinguish HHS from lymphoma (Moore et al., 2006).

No optimal treatment for HHS has been described, although there is a recent study in which dogs with HHS treated with lomustine (CCNU) (70 mg/m² PO every 3–4 weeks) (Elliott, 2018) showed a median survival time of 24 days from diagnosis (range from 4 to 67 days) (Moore et al., 2006; Elliott, 2018). Blood transfusion may be used as a supportive treatment, but it should only be used temporarily if it works.

Feline Histiocytic Disease

Histiocytic diseases are much less common in cats than in dogs. However, there are three major histiocytic diseases in domestic cats: progressive feline histiocytosis, pulmonary Langerhans cell histiocytosis, and feline histiocytic sarcoma (Moore, 2014).

Feline Progressive Histiocytosis

Feline progressive histiocytosis (FPH) is the most common histiocytic disease in cats. Immunohistochemically, it expresses CD1a and CD18, as well as CD5 in 50% of cases. Most FPHs also have a lack of E-cadherin expression. It is characterised clinically by multiple nodules and plaques primarily on the face or extremities (Affolter et al., 2006; Day et al., 2000). Affolter et al. summarised the clinical, morphological, and immunohistochemical characteristics of FPH.

Old cats are more likely to be affected by the disease, especially short-haired cats. The mean age at which it is reported is 8 years old (ranging from 2 to 17 years). Around 60–70% of cases have solitary or multiple nodules and/or plaques on the extremities and face. Nodules are not usually painful, have a firm consistency and are up to 1.5 cm in diameter. Sometimes they may be ulcerated.

Histologically, nodules are composed of a dense population of large round to polygonal cells with discrete edges. Tumour cells can infiltrate from the superficial dermis to the deep dermis (Affolter et al., 2006). Lesions can be found in lymph nodes, lungs, kidneys, pancreas, spleen, liver, heart, adrenal glands, and the mediastinum.

Immunosuppressive treatment such as corticosteroids may be used as part of therapy, but in these cases, it should be ruled out that the patient is not suffering from an infectious disease before treatment begins. Attempts to treat FPH with interferon gamma (γ), cyclosporine, leflunomide, retinoid, vincristine, L-asparaginase and vinblastine have been made, although in all cases skin lesions progressed over time (Affolter et al., 2006).

Another study showed that cats with FPH have a longer survival time. Patients were treated with lomustine, tyrosine kinase inhibitors and/or prednisone and in four out of five cats follow-up was performed over 350 days (Treggiari et al., 2017).

Langerhans Cell Pulmonary Histiocytosis

Langerhans cell pulmonary histiocytosis (LCPH) in cats is derived from epidermal Langerhans cells, which express not only CD18 but also E-cadherin (Moore, 2014) and Birbeck granules. There are a number of cases of this disease which have been published (Busch et al., 2008): older cats (10–15 years old) and short-haired ones tend to be affected by LCPH. Cats with this disease show chronic clinical signs, including respiratory difficulty, which consists of tachypnoea, increased respiratory effort and open mouth breathing.

For diagnosis, blood testing and abdominal ultrasound should be used to detect the condition. Thoracic radiography is needed to reveal pulmonary lesions with severe diffuse bronchointerstitial patterns. To reach a definitive diagnosis, a biopsy is necessary. Lungs affected with LCPH show consistent extensive infiltration with diffuse lesions in the pulmonary lobes. The lesions consist of numerous coalescing nodular masses which are pink in colour and poorly defined. Nodules range from 2 to 5 mm. Histologically, obstruction of the terminal airways and adjacent alveoli by adhesive layers of histocytes with immunochemical characteristics and microscopic Langerhans cells can be observed in cases of LCPH.

The study published reported no response to treatment, including corticosteroids and/or theophylline (Busch et al., 2008). The prognosis for animals with LCPH is poor, it is considered a serious disease.

Feline Histiocytic Sarcoma

Feline histiocytic sarcoma can originate from both dendritic cells and macrophages (Firedrichs et al., 2008; Ide, 2009). The average age of affected cats is 10 years old. Clinical signs are non-specific or tumour dependent and neurological signs such as drowsiness, tripping, blindness, and cluster seizures may be observed if histiocytic sarcoma affects the brain (Ide et al., 2010; Santifort, 2018). Anorexia, weight loss and respiratory distress are also observed when it is disseminated (Ide et al., 2009; Bell et al., 2006). In some cases, there may be no clinical signs or only ipsilateral uveitis and hyphaema. Most commonly, the spleen, liver, and bone marrow are affected, although the condition has also been reported to affect the nasal cavity, trachea, kidney, eyes, and CNS (Friedrichs, 2008; Ide et al., 2009; Ide et al., 2010; Santifort et al., 2018; Bell et al., 2006; Scurrell et al., 2013).

Diagnosis includes blood tests (CBC, chemistry profile), thoracic radiographs and abdominal ultrasound. Magnetic resonance imaging may be performed if cats have neurological signs. Severe anaemia and thrombocytopaenia may be observed in cases of disseminated feline histiocytic sarcoma. Usually, multiple masses are seen in abdominal organs by abdominal ultrasound. Magnetic resonance imaging allows intranasal and intracranial lesions to be visualised well, which are characterised as T1-hypotensive and T2-hyperintensive heterogeneous lesions/masses with strong contrast enhancement (Ide et al., 2010; Santifort et al., 2018). Definitive diagnosis requires cytology or histopathology. The tumour is composed of round, spindle-shaped polygonal cells, with moderate amounts of vacuolated eosinophilic cytoplasm and finely dotted chromatin. Anisokaryosis is also seen frequently. Immunohistochemistry can provide a definitive diagnosis and show cells positive for CD18 and negative for CD3 and CD79a (Friedrichs, 2008; Ide et al., 2009; Ide et al., 2010; Scurrell et al., 2013).

Standard treatment options include surgery, radiation therapy, and chemotherapy. Chemotherapy to treat feline histiocytic sarcoma includes a combination of lomustine (50–60 mg/m^2 PO every 3 weeks) and prednisone (1.5 mg/kg/day PO) (Ide et al., 2009), cytosine arabinoside, doxorubicin, and toceranib (Treggiari et al., 2017; Ide et al., 2009; Ide et al., 2010).

However, it is difficult to control as there is no standard treatment protocol in place and there is little detailed information on treatment protocols.

In several studies, some animals were euthanised at diagnosis due to malignancy, the progressive nature of histiocytic sarcoma or for concurrent disease (Friedrichs et al., 2008; Santifort et al., 2018; Bell et al., 2006) and, in any case, the prognosis is poor if it affects the brain, extends throughout the body or occurs in its haemophagocytic variant. One study recorded a survival time of 43 days (feline histiocytic sarcoma in the brain) and 107 days (disseminated feline histiocytic sarcoma), although it did not describe the response to treatment (Ide et al., 2009; Ide et al., 2010). Haemophagocytic feline histiocytic sarcoma has the worst prognosis (survival time <10 days).

Only one cat treated with radiation therapy and lomustine had a survival time of 1704 days free of progression and this case was still alive at the end of the study (Treggiari et al., 2017).

Histiocytic sarcoma located in the nasal bridge may have a better prognosis (Treggiari et al., 2017): in a study that included two cats with histiocytic sarcoma in the nasal bridge, who received radiation therapy (6 Gy×6 fractions every 2 weeks and 3.75 Gy×12 fractions daily), the follow-up period was 247 and 253 days, respectively, and they were still alive at the end of the study. Another cat with histiocytic sarcoma on the carpus who received surgery and NSAIDs (Treggiari et al., 2017) alone survived 226 days from the time of presentation. In another recorded case, a cat with a histiocytic sarcoma located in the stomach received prednisone as the only treatment and survived 402 days (Treggiari et al., 2017).

Bibliography

- Affolter, V.K., Moore, P.F. (2000) Canine Cutaneous and Systemic Histiocytosis: Reactive Histiocytosis of Dermal Dendritic Cells. *Am J Derm*, 22:40–48.
- Affolter, V.K., Moore, P.F. (2006) Feline progressive histiocytosis. *Vet Pathol*, 43:646–655.
- Affolter, V.K., Moore, P.F. (2002) Localized and disseminated histiocytic sarcoma of dendritic cell origin in dogs. *Vet Pathol*, 39:74–83.
- Bell, R., Philbey, A.W., Martineau, H. et al. (2006) Dynamic tracheal collapse associated with disseminated histiocytic sarcoma in a cat. *J Small Anim Pract*, 47:461–464.
- Busch, M.D, Reilly, C.M., Luff, J.A. et al. (2008) Feline pulmonary Langerhans cell histiocytosis with multiorgan involvement. *Vet Pathol*, 45:816–824.
- Cannon, C., Borgatti, A., Henson, M. et al. (2015) Evaluation of a combination chemotherapy protocol including lomustine and doxorubicin in canine histiocytic sarcoma. *J Small Anim Pract*, 56:425–429.
- Day, M.J., Lopatkin, I., Lucke, V.M. et al. (2000) Multiple cutaneous histiocytomas in a cat. *Veterinary Dermatology*, 11:305–310.
- Dervisis, N.G., Kiupel, M., Qin, Q. et al. (2017) Clinical prognostic factors in canine histiocytic sarcoma. *Vet Comp Oncol*, 15:1171–1180.
- Dobson, J.M. (2013) Breed-predispositions to cancer in pedigree dogs. ISRN *Vet Sci*, 941275.
- Elliott, J. (2018) Lomustine chemotherapy for the treatment of presumptive haemophagocytic histiocytic sarcoma in Flat coated Retrievers. *Australian Veterinary Journal*, 96:502–507.
- Faller, M., Lamm, C., Affolter, V.K. et al. (2016) Retrospective characterisation of solitary cutaneous histiocytoma with lymph node metastasis in eight dogs. *Journal of Small Animal Practice*, 57:548–552.
- Friedrichs, K.R., Young, K.M. (2008) Histiocytic sarcoma of macrophage origin in a cat: case report with a literature review of feline histiocytic malignancies and comparison with canine hemophagocytic histiocytic sarcoma. *Vet Clin Pathol*, 37:121–128.
- Ide, K., Setoguchi-Mukai, A., Nakagawa, T. et al. (2009) Disseminated histiocytic sarcoma with excessive hemophagocytosis in a cat. *J Vet Med Sci*, 71:817–820.
- Ide, T., Uchida, K., Tamura, S. et al. (2010) Histiocytic sarcoma in the brain of a cat. *J Vet Med Sci*, 72:99–102.
- Kagawa, Y., Nakano, Y., Kobayashi, T. et al. (2016) Localized pulmonary histiocytic sarcomas in Pembroke Welsh Corgi. *J Vet Med Sci*, 77:1659–1661.
- Klahn, S.L., Kitchell, B.E., Dervisis, N.G. (2011) Evaluation and comparison of outcomes in dogs with periarticular and nonperiarticular histiocytic sarcoma. *J Am Vet Med Assoc*, 239:90–96.
- Kotecha, R., Venkatramani, R., Jubran, R.F. et al. (2014) Clinical outcomes of radiation therapy in the management of Langerhans cell histiocytosis. *Am J Clin Oncol*, 37:592–596.
- Lenz, J.A., Furrow, E., Craig, L.E. et al. (2017) Histiocytic sarcoma in 14 miniature schnauzers - a new breed predisposition? *J Small Anim Pract*, 58:461–467.
- Marlowe, K.W., Robat, C.S., Clarke, D.M. et al. (2018) Primary pulmonary histiocytic sarcoma in dogs: A retrospective analysis of 37 cases (2000–2015). *Vet Comp Oncol*, 16:658–663.
- Mason, S.L., Finotello, R., Blackwood, L. (2018) Epirubicin in the treatment of canine histiocytic sarcoma: sequential, alternating and rescue chemotherapy. *Vet Comp Oncol*, 16:E30–E37.
- Moore, A.S., Taylor, D.P., Reppas, G. et al. (2017) Chemotherapy for dogs with lymph node metastasis from histiocytic sarcomas. *Aust Vet J*, 95:37–40.
- Moore, P.F., Affolter, V.K., Vernau, W. (2006) Canine hemophagocytic histiocytic sarcoma: a proliferative disorder of CD11d+ macrophages. *Vet Pathol*, 43:632–645.
- Moore, P.F., Rosin, A. (1986) Malignant histiocytosis of Bernese Mountain dogs. *Vet Pathol*, 23:1–10.
- Moore, P.F. (2014) A review of histiocytic diseases of dogs and cats. *Vet Pathol*, 51:167–184.
- Moore, P.F. (1984) Systemic histiocytosis of Bernese Mountain dogs. *Vet Pathol*, 21:554–563.
- Nagata, M., Hirata, M., Ishida, T. et al. (2000) Progressive Langerhans' cell histiocytosis in a puppy. *Veterinary Dermatology*, 11:241–246.
- Palmeiro, B.S., Morris, D.O., Goldschmidt, M.H. et al. (2007) Cutaneous reactive histiocytosis in dogs: a retrospective evaluation of 32 cases. *Vet Dermatol*, 18:332–340.
- Paterson, S., Boydell, P., Pike, R. (1995) Systemic histiocytosis in the Bernese Mountain dog. *J Small Anim Pract*, 36:233–236.
- Pazdzior-Czapula, K., Rotkiewicz, T., Otrocka-Domagala, I. et al. (2015) Morphology and immunophenotype of canine cutaneous histiocytic tumours with particular emphasis on diagnostic application. *Vet Res Commun*, 39:7–17.
- Pires, I., Rodrigues, P., Alves, A. et al. (2013) Immunohistochemical and immunoelectron study of major histocompatibility complex class-II antigen in canine cutaneous histiocytoma: its relation to tumor regression. *In Vivo*, 27:257–262.
- Plumb, D.C. (2015) *Plumb's veterinary drug handbook*. Wiley Blackwell: Chichester, West Sussex.
- Santifort, K.M., Jurgens, B., Grinwis, G.C. et al. (2018) Invasive nasal histiocytic sarcoma as a cause of temporal lobe epilepsy in a cat. *JFMS Open Rep*, 4:2055116918811 79.
- Schmidt, J.M., North, S.M., Freeman, K.P. et al. (2010) Canine paediatric oncology: retrospective assessment of 9522 tumours in dogs up to 12 months (1993–2008). *Vet Comp Oncol*, 8:283–292.
- Scurrell, E., Trott, A., Rozmanec, M. et al. (2013) Ocular histiocytic sarcoma in a cat. *Vet Ophthalmol*, 16 Suppl 1:173–176.
- Skorupski, K.A., Clifford, C.A., Paoloni, M.C. et al. (2007) CCNU for the treatment of dogs with histiocytic sarcoma. *J Vet Intern Med*, 21:121–126.
- Skorupski, K.A., Rodriguez, C.O., Krick, E.L. et al. (2009) Long-term survival in dogs with localized histiocytic sarcoma treated with CCNU as an adjuvant to local therapy. *Vet Comp Oncol*, 7:139–144.
- Taylor, D.O., Dorn, C.R., Luis, O.H. (1969) Morphologic and biologic characteristics of the canine cutaneous histiocytoma. *Cancer Res*, 29:83–92.
- Treggiari, E., Ressel, L., Polton, G.A. et al. (2017) Clinical outcome, PDGFRbeta and KIT expression in feline histiocytic disorders: a multicentre study. *Vet Comp Oncol*, 15:65–77.

Notes

Annex 3. Biopsy

Sofia Carvalho

Treatment options for the cancer patient may be influenced by various factors, such as the histopathological characteristics of the tumour. There are also several factors that can affect the quality and histological interpretation of tissue samples, so it is important that the clinician in charge of the patient has extensive knowledge of the different techniques for obtaining tissues by biopsy through to the interpretation of the histopathological diagnosis. The objective of the biopsy is to acquire a tissue fragment to obtain a histopathological diagnosis. It is important to obtain a good quality biopsy sample, as this greatly impacts the histopathological interpretation and obtaining a final diagnosis for the patient. There are also several factors that can influence histopathological interpretation such as the presence of inflammation, necrosis, and haemorrhage.

Types of Biopsy

There are different types of biopsies that can be performed and, depending on the location, type of lesion and clinical status of the patient, the most appropriate technique should be chosen. Biopsies can be performed as a method of diagnosis (pre-treatment biopsy) and/or as a form of treatment (post-treatment biopsy) and it is essential to know when to opt for one or the other, as performing the biopsy at an incorrect time and manner can have a negative effect on the prognosis of the cancer patient.

Pre-treatment Biopsy

It is well known that in the cancer patient it is important to be as well informed as possible regarding the type of tumour that is being dealt with before considering different treatment options. Pre-treatment biopsy is indicated to better understand the patient's neoplasm and to help make the most appropriate treatment recommendations.

If the results of fine needle aspiration have been questionable and more information is needed about the type and stage of the tumour to plan treatments such as surgery, radiation therapy, and/or chemotherapy, a pre-treatment biopsy should be performed. The type and grade of the tumour also greatly influence decisions about the type of surgery to be performed, especially if the tumour is in an area where surgical reconstruction is difficult.

However, pre-treatment biopsy may be contraindicated in some cases, such as when the risk of complications, morbidity and mortality associated with biopsying is high. In this situation, other diagnostic methods, such as fine needle aspiration or excisional biopsy should be considered, as long as this does not have any negative impact (Figure 1). There are also cases in which the histopathological results of a pre-treatment biopsy will not affect the final treatment options recommended for the patient. In these cases, the most appropriate method may be an excisional biopsy. An example of this would be a dog with a single lung tumour with no evidence of regional or systemic metastatic disease.

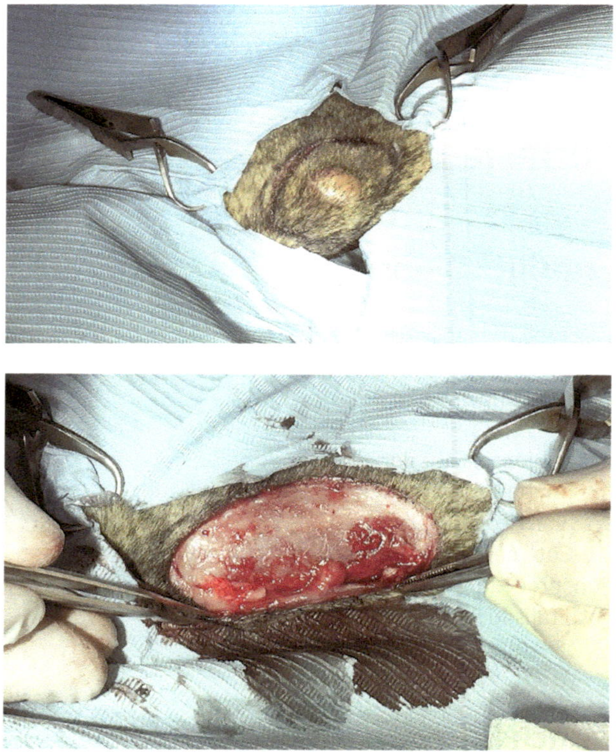

Figure 1. Excisional biopsy of a canine mast cell tumour with margins. The lesion had previously been evaluated using cytology, which was very suggestive of a well-differentiated mast cell tumour. Histopathological diagnosis confirmed the cytology diagnosis. (Image courtesy of David Díaz DVM, GPCert Oncology).

Post-treatment Biopsy

Post-treatment or excisional biopsy refers to the process of obtaining histopathological information after surgical tumour resection. The histopathological interpretation of excisional biopsy is more comprehensive and detailed and includes information on specimen margins.

Although excisional biopsy can be a form of definitive treatment, there are cases in which performing excisional biopsy as a form of initial treatment can result in incomplete histopathological margins that will seriously affect the patient if not carefully planned. An example is the resection of a high-grade feline soft-tissue sarcoma without aggressive surgical margins, resulting in incomplete histopathological margins. This example may subsequently require a second, more aggressive surgery, with a higher rate of complications and a negative impact on the patient's prognosis (Davidson et al., 1997; Hershey et al., 2000).

This reiterates that it is essential to study the type of tumour under consideration and what type of biopsy should be performed before proceeding with any surgery, especially if the excision may be incomplete, and compromise the clinical case negatively in any way.

Methods for Performing Biopsies

Tru-Cut® Biopsy

This type of biopsy uses several types of needles that can be manual or automatic. The needles are usually 14 G in diameter and the samples 1 mm thick by 10–15 mm in length.

These biopsies are **very useful for some external lesions or for image-guided internal biopsies** (ultrasound, CT, and/or fluoroscopy), for example, lung masses or liver lesions. Tru-Cut® needles are usually cheap and easy to use. In addition, procedures are usually performed without the need for hospitalisation (Figure 2).

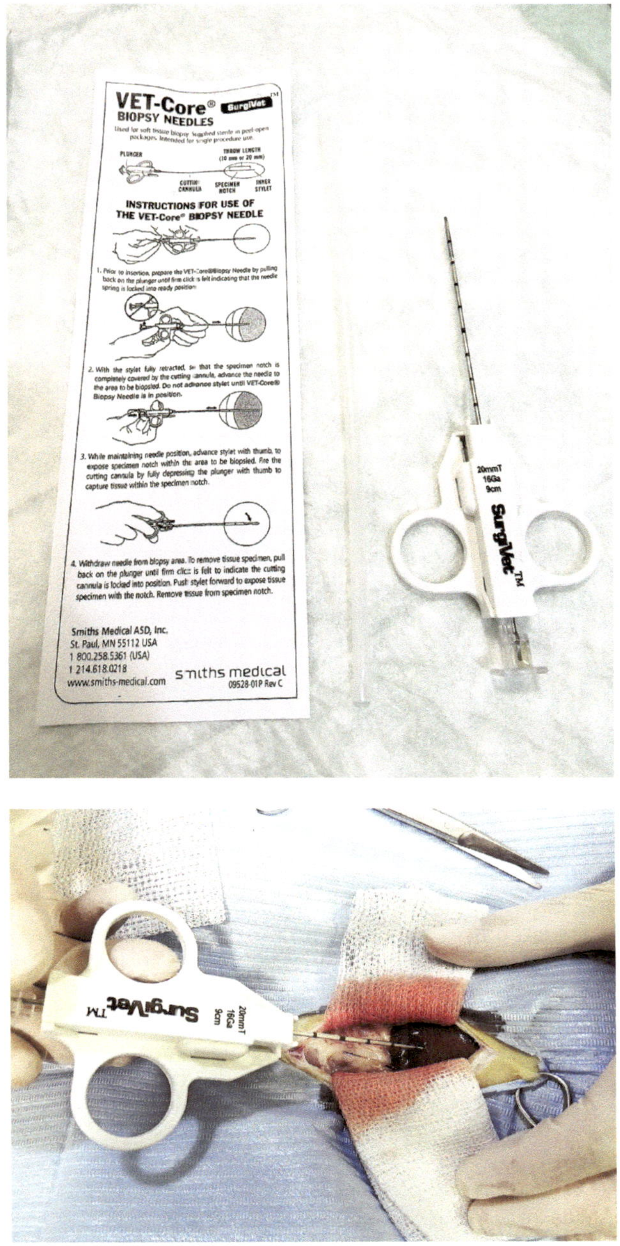

Figure 2. Collection of a sample obtained using Tru-Cut® in a feline patient with the presence of a hepatic nodule measuring 2.6 cm in the right lobule, with a heterogenous appearance which caused deformation of the capsule. (Image courtesy of David Díaz DVM, GPCert Oncology).

Punch Biopsy

This type of biopsy is **used on external tissues** (such as skin and the oral cavity) **or where full visual access of the organ is possible** (for example, during an exploratory abdominal laparotomy to perform liver biopsy).

Punch biopsy allows a fragment of tissue approximately 2–8 mm in length to be taken. If the lesion is external and covered with intact skin, a skin incision should be made with a scalpel before proceeding with the punch biopsy (Figure 3).

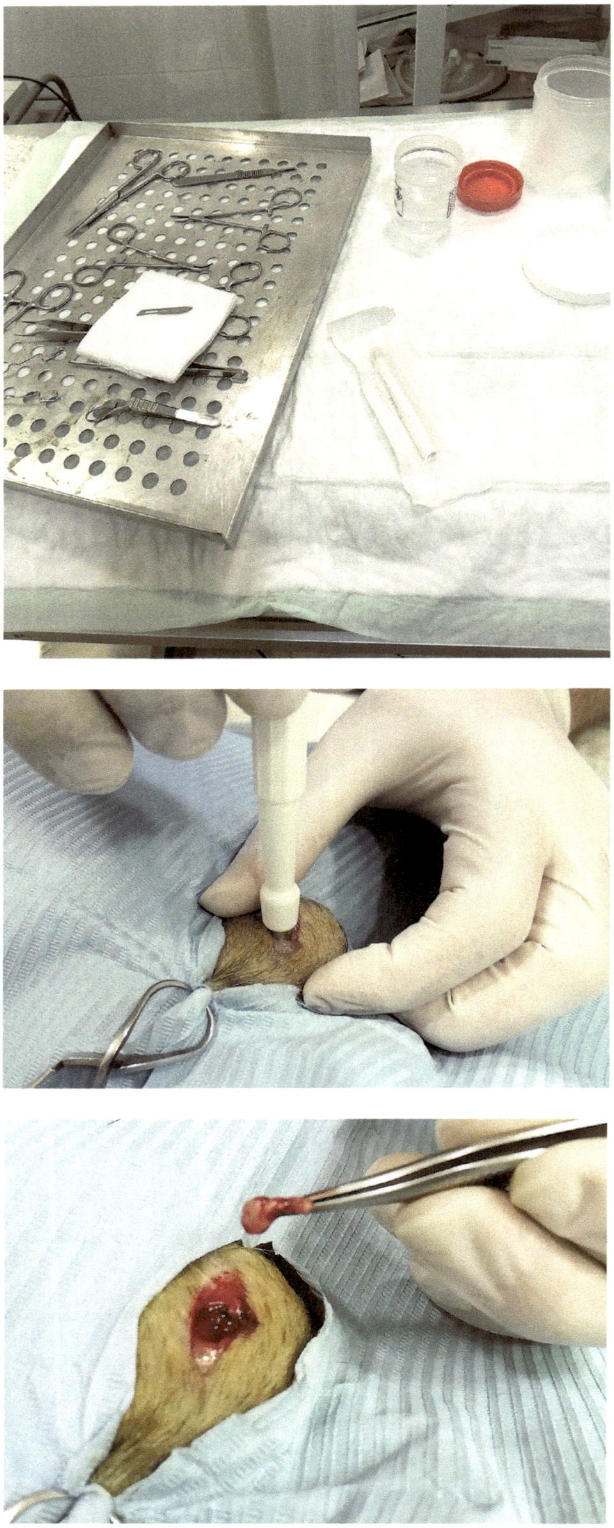

Figure 3. Punch biopsy sample collection from a prescapular lymph node in a dog diagnosed with multicentric lymphoma for histology and immunophenotyping. (Image courtesy of David Díaz, DVM, GP-Cert Oncology).

Incisional Biopsy

This type of biopsy is performed, for example, **when the results of the Tru-Cut® biopsy are inconclusive**. Incisional biopsy is **also useful in cases where the tumour lesion is ulcerated and necrotic**, as a more representative tissue fragment can be obtained.

If the lesion is external and covered with intact skin, a skin incision should be made with a scalpel, as in the case of punch biopsy, and then a wedge of tissue representative of the tumour lesion should be removed. It is not necessary to remove the skin if it is intact.

If possible, several tissue samples should be removed through the same incision, so that the sample is as representative as possible of the lesion. The surgeon must be very careful not to contaminate healthy tissues around the tumour, which may compromise future surgical procedures and hinder reconstruction procedures and/or radiation therapy protocols. The biopsy tracts should always be removed during definitive surgical treatment (Figure 4).

Endoscopic Biopsy

This type of biopsy is very useful and is **often used to obtain samples from lesions in the gastrointestinal, respiratory, and urogenital tracts**. It should be noted that sometimes the samples obtained by endoscopy are not representative of the tumour process due to the small size of the sample, the difficulty visualising the lesion and/or in cases of lesions with severe inflammation and ulceration.

Thoracoscopy and Laparoscopy Biopsy

This type of biopsy consists of a **minimally invasive surgical** method that allows for smaller incisions and faster recovery of the patient while obtaining tissue for biopsy or aiding in lesion removal.

The visualisation of the thoracic and abdominal cavities means this technique also helps in staging the tumour disease.

Imaging Guided Biopsies

The use of **ultrasound, CT scan, radiography, MRI and/or fluoroscopy** are very useful in helping to obtain a diagnostic sample. This is particularly important in cases of very

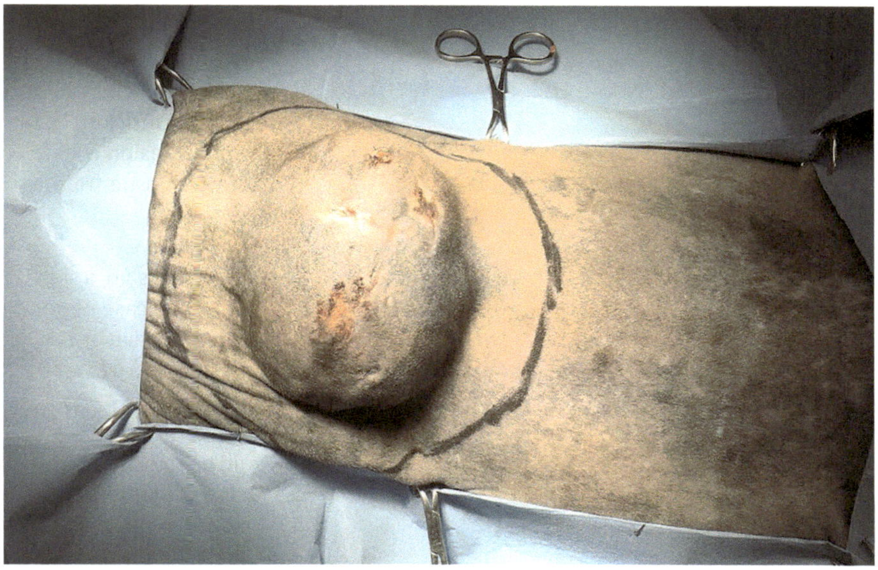

Figure 4. High-grade feline injection site sarcoma. In the image, the margins for the surgical planning can be observed and also evidence of previous incisional biopsies used to reach a diagnosis before proceeding with an aggressive excisional surgery. (Image courtesy of Ignasi Rodríguez, PhD, MVetMed, Dip. ACVIM Oncology).

heterogeneous masses, with extensive areas of necrosis/inflammation and cysts.

Recommendations for Sample Collection, Presentation, Cutting and Histopathological Margin Evaluation

The performance of **a pre-treatment biopsy should not cause any negative impact on the patient** and therefore taking some precautions when performing it is essential, including careful haemostasis, obliterating the dead space and avoiding the development of seromas or haematomas. Definitive surgery should include all previous biopsy tracts and, if possible, drains should not be put in place.

When the biopsy is performed on the tail or extremities, the incision should be made on the long axis and not the transverse one, since the latter is more difficult to remove at a later date. **Removing the junction between diseased and healthy tissue should be avoided in pre-treatment biopsies**.

Tumours are usually heterogeneous and may have various areas of necrosis, inflammation, and/or reactive tissue. Therefore, to increase the possibility of obtaining a final diagnosis for the patient, several tissue samples should be obtained from different areas of the lesion.

After performing the biopsy, the sample obtained must be inspected to confirm that it appears appropriate. If it is a pre-treatment biopsy or the biopsy has been performed with a Tru-Cut® needle, **the sample must be of sufficient size and consistency to remain intact in the formalin solution**. Samples smaller than 1 mm^3 are not usually suitable, although Tru-Cut® samples of 1 mm thickness and 5 mm in length may be sufficient.

The electric scalpel or laser should not be used to obtain biopsy samples, as both can damage cell architecture. Care must also be taken with the handling of samples before fixation, especially with tweezers.

Stainless steel vascular clips or staples should be removed from samples, because they can damage microtomes in the laboratory.

Correct fixation of samples is essential. A 10% solution of neutral formalin buffered in water should be used. Each sample should be placed in a separate, well-identified container. Samples must not be more than 1 cm thick, or fixation will not be sufficient. The thickest lesions should be cut like a loaf of bread, leaving the deep margin with the ink that delineates the margins intact. Large lesions can be cut incompletely, left in a large formalin container for 2 to 3 days, and then sent to the laboratory in a container with 50% formalin. Another option for large lesions is to choose some representative areas of the lesion to send to the laboratory, but this is not ideal because important information can be lost. In this case, the rest of the tissue should be stored at the practice until a reliable histopathological diagnosis has been reached with the samples sent to the laboratory.

In cases of post-treatment biopsies or after surgery with curative intent the **surgical margins should be evaluated**. This is why samples should be stained with ink at the surgical margins using a cotton swab, after drying the sample with a tissue (so that the ink adheres more easily). The ink is allowed to dry for about twenty minutes before putting the stained sample in the formalin solution.

Interpretation of Histopathology Results and Some Examples

Whenever a biopsy is performed, it **should be sent to the laboratory for histopathological evaluation, even in cases of suspected benign tumours**, such as lipomas.

Histopathological diagnosis should provide information on whether a tumour process is being dealt with, if the tumour is benign or malignant, what the type and grade of the tumour is, in addition to information about the surgical margins in the case of excisional biopsies. However, **there are some cases in which the histopathological diagnosis does not correlate with the clinical presentation of the patient**, and it is very important that the veterinarian in charge seeks the final and most correct histopathological diagnosis for their patient, so that treatment is most effective. This can be done in a variety of ways, including discussing the case with the pathologist, requesting new sections and/or immunohistochemical tests, and/or asking for a second histopathology opinion. The clinician should provide the pathologist with detailed information about the patient, including a complete clinical history, a description of gross lesions and lesions seen using imaging techniques, as well as suspected clinical diagnosis.

A second opinion should be requested whenever there is any doubt around the histopathological diagnosis or if the diagnosis needs confirmation. In medicine this is a very common practice that can lead to a big change in the treatment options and prognosis of cancer patients. A veterinary study (Regan et al., 2010) that evaluated the interpretation of first and second opinion histopathology found that in 30% of cases there was a discrepancy between the results of the first and second opinion. The discrepancy was partial in 20% of cases, which meant a change in the degree or presence of lymphatic or vascular infiltration. In the remaining 10% of cases the discrepancy was total, which meant that there was a disagreement between a malignant versus a benign process (7%) or a disagreement regarding the cellular origin of the tumour (3%). This study proved that, as long as the histopathological diagnosis does not correlate with the biological behaviour of the tumour, measures to confirm the diagnosis must be implemented. However, if after other diagnostic methods or a second opinion in histopathology the diagnosis remains questionable, a second biopsy should be carried out if possible.

The **interpretation of the histopathological report is fundamental**. For most tumours, histopathological grade has a great impact on their biological behaviour. The histopathological grade together with the presentation and clinical stage of the patient (for example, presence of regional or systemic metastases) help the clinician in charge to decide on the type of treatment and, at the same time, provides more information about the prognosis of the patient.

Histomorphological features commonly used to classify tumour grade include cell differentiation, number of mitotic figures, degree of invasiveness, necrosis, cell pleomorphism, size, number of nuclei, stromal reaction, and cellularity level, etc. There are grading systems published in the veterinary literature for many of the canine and feline tumours and it is important that clinicians are aware of these for a correct interpretation of the histopathological report. Some examples of these include canine mastocytomas, soft-tissue sarcomas, and mammary gland neoplasms.

Whenever a grading system is not available for a certain neoplasia the histopathology report should still be throughly studied for all the histopathological caractheristics and cell morphology including factors such as mitotic index, presence of lymphactic invasion, etc., which may help predict the most likely biological behaviour in the given patient and decisions regarding possible therapies.

Canine Mast Cell Tumours

In canine mastocytomas, **histopathological grade is considered the most important prognostic factor**. There are two main types of grading systems for these tumours, Patnaik and Kiupel, based on histological grade mast cells. They are usually referred to as low, intermediate and high-grade when assessed by the Patnaik grading system and low versus high-grade when assessed by the Kiupel grading system. Both grading system classifications are often provided on the histopathology reports.

Most dogs with well or moderately well-differentiated tumours enjoy a long survival time and a good prognosis after complete surgical excision. In contrast, dogs with undifferentiated mast cell tumours typically suffer from high metastatic rates (55–96%) (Mullins et al., 2006; Murphy et al., 2004; Michels et al., 2002; Seguin et al., 2001; Weisse et al., 2002; Schultheiss et al., 2011; Bostock, 1973; Hume et al., 2001).

Soft-tissue Sarcomas

In soft-tissue sarcomas, **tumour grade also greatly influences recommended treatments and the patient's prognosis**.

The metastatic rate of canine soft-tissue sarcoma is influenced by histopathological grade: 0–13% for grade I tumours, 7–17% for grade II tumours and 22–44% for grade III tumours (Kuntz et al., 1997).

A study in cats (Porcellato et al., 2001) showed that patients with tumours with more than 20 mitoses per 10 HPF (high power field) had median survival times of 994 days, while in patients with tumours with less than 20 mitoses per 10 HPF the survival rate exceeded the study period. The same has been confirmed in dogs with soft-tissue sarcomas, in which the likelihood of tumour related death was three times more likely in dogs with tumours with more than 10% necrosis and with more than 20 mitoses per 10 HPF (Kuntz et al., 1997).

Neoplasms of the Mammary Gland

The grade of canine and feline epithelial tumours of the mammary gland is also prognostic.

These tumours are classified according to the most recent Elston and Ellis system, which incorporates information on tubule formation, nuclear pleomorphism, and number of mitoses per 10 HPF. Other histopathological factors also have an impact on the prognosis of these tumours, such as the presence of vascular and lymphatic invasion.

Bibliography

- Bostock, D.E. (1973) The prognosis following surgical removal of mastocytomas in dogs. *J Small Anim Pract.* 14:27-41.
- Davidson, E.B., Gregory, C.R., Kass, P.H. (1997) Surgical excision of soft tissue fibrosarcomas in cats. *Vet Sur.* 26: 265-269.
- Hershey, A.E., Sorenmo, K.U., Hendrick, M.J. et al. (2000) Prognosis for presumed feline injection-site sarcoma after excision: 61 cases (1986-1996). *J Am Vet Med Assoc.* 261:58-61.
- Hume, C.T., Kiupel, M., Rigatti, L. et al. (2001) Outcomes of dogs with grade 3 mast cell tumours: 43 cases (1997-2007). *J am Anim Hosp Assoc.* 47:37-44.
- Kuntz, C.A., Dernell, W.S., Powers, B.E., et al. (1997) Prognostic factors for surgical treatment of soft-tissue sarcomas in dogs: 75 cases (1986-1996). *J Am Vet Med Assoc.* 21: 1147-1151.
- Michels, G.M., Knapp, D.W., DeNicola, D.B. et al. (2002) Prognosis fol owing surgical excision of canine cutaneous mast cell tumours with histopathologically tumour-free versus nontumour-free margins: a retrospective study of 31 cases. *J Am Anim Hosp Assoc.* 38:458-466.
- Mullins, M.N., Dernell, W.S., Withrow, S.J., et al. (2006) Evaluation of prognostic factors associated with outcome in dogs with multiple cutaneous mast cell tumours treated with surgery and without adjuvant treatment: 54 cases (1998-2004). *J Am Vet Med Assoc.* 228: 91-95.
- Murphy, S., Sparkes, A.H., Smith, KC. et al. (2004) Relationships between the histological grade of cutaneous mast cell tumours in dogs, their survival and the efficacy of surgical ressection. *Vet Rec.* 154:743-746.
- Porcellato, I., Menchetti, L., Brachelente, C. et al. (2017) Feline injection-site sarcoma: matrix remodeling and prognosis. *Vet Pathol.* 54: 204-211.
- Regan, R.C., Rassnick, K.M., Balkman, C.E. et al. (2010) Comparison of first opinion and second opinion histopathology from dogs and cats with cancer: 430 cases (2001-2008). *Vet Comp Oncol.* 8:1-10.
- Schultheiss, P.C., Gardiner, D.W., Rao, S. et al. (2011) Association of histologic tumour characteristics and size of surgical maguns with clinical outcome after surgical removal of cutaneous mast cell tumours in dogs. *J Am Vet Med Assoc.* 238:1464-1469.
- Seguin, B., Leibman, N.F., Bregazzi, V.S. et al. (2001) Clinical outcome of dogs with grade-II mast cell tumours treated with surgery alone: 55 cases (1996-1999). *J Am Anim Hosp Assoc.* 218:1120-1123.
- Weisse, C., Shofer, F.S., Soremo, K. (2002). Recurrence rates and sites for grade II canine cutaneous mast cell tumours following complete surgical excision. *J Am Hosp Assoc.* 38:71-73.
- Withrow, S.J., Vail, D.M. (2007). *Withrow & MacEwen's Small Animal Clinical Oncology*. Saunders Elsevier, St. Louis, Mo.